Global Handbook on Noncommunicable Diseases and Health Promotion

David V. McQueen

Editor

Global Handbook on Noncommunicable Diseases and Health Promotion

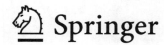 Springer

Editor
David V. McQueen
Emory University
Atlanta, GA, USA

ISBN 978-1-4614-7593-4   ISBN 978-1-4614-7594-1 (eBook)
DOI 10.1007/978-1-4614-7594-1
Springer New York Heidelberg Dordrecht London

Library of Congress Control Number: 2013941727

Printed on acid-free paper

Springer is part of Springer Science+Business Media (www.springer.com)

Introduction to the Book

It is a daunting task to prepare, edit, and contribute to a global handbook on such broad topics as noncommunicable diseases and health promotion. First and foremost one recognizes the enormity of the subject areas and realizes that it could easily be an encyclopedia. Each of the critical words in the title (global, handbook, noncommunicable diseases, health promotion) is subject to discussion and elaboration.

The word "global" itself has many possible meanings beyond simple geography. Often the word "international" is used; however that usage implies a nation-based perspective. Such a perspective drives one to think in terms of countries. The word "global" implies a broader, less narrow political, view. The subtle distinction between international and global will become apparent throughout the book and specifically in the chapters where authors take a country-based perspective while others think more about borderless issues in public health. Authors were not instructed to take one view or another with regard to the meaning of global and it remains for the reader to sort out the individual author's perspective. As the editor I chose the word "global" because of its broader meaning and because I believe it is more relevant for today's public health.

Defining a "handbook" is equally challenging. In reviewing numerous "handbooks" on a number of topics both related and unrelated to public health it became clear that the term is loosely applied to any number of monographs. In general one thinks of a handbook as a type of reference document where a student or a researcher in the field can go for a definitive understanding or documentation of the key components, issues, and challenges in the field. That is part of the underlying conceptualization of this work. Nonetheless, it will be clear to any expert in the field of public health that not all issues and challenges can be represented in a single monograph that is produced even by a representative sample of the experts in the field. At best it can only be a well-chosen representative sample.

The term "noncommunicable diseases" is a conscious choice. It is a clumsy and in many ways an unfortunate term. Many of those working in public health have struggled over and debated this terminology. It is unfortunate that we are left with a procrustean situation. It is not the point to debate the merits of the term here; it will be taken up in other venues and in some chapters. There is not even agreement globally about whether the appropriate term is noncommunicable diseases or the hyphenated non-communicable diseases and quite often simply NCDs. The spelling of the term is not even the fundamental problem with the term. The real problem is that the term has the concept of disease etiology built into it. It implies that diseases that have an infectious origin are not within the term's domain. Unfortunately many diseases commonly placed in the NCD category, e.g., cancer, heart disease, and many others, often have an infection-related etiology. In many places, e.g., the CDC (Atlanta), the term "chronic diseases" is used to represent many of the NCDs. My workplace for 20 years was the CDC National Center for Chronic Disease Prevention and Health Promotion (NCCDPHP). But the "chronic disease" term is not without its handicaps in defining the field of work. Institutions and researchers across the globe freely use the various forms of the term. In short, no NCD terminology seems to totally capture the dimensions that are the topics of this handbook. Furthermore, no terminological wizardry will really make it clear to the lay public.

The term "health promotion" also rests uncomfortably in its procrustean bed. Since its origins in the latter part of the twentieth century those in the field of health promotion have struggled over its definition and, in particular, over its content area. Lacking a core discipline has meant a proliferation of topics and roles that are salient for the field. Nevertheless, there are two chief characteristics about health promotion that define it. The first is that its primary focus is on health rather than disease. The second is that it is an area of action in contrast to description. As with the other terms, the components and subtleties of this area of work will be discussed in considerable detail in chapters throughout this handbook.

Why assemble a global handbook on noncommunicable diseases and health promotion? The salient answer is because both of these hard-to-define areas have particular problems that can be solved, in part, by the necessary unification of the two fields of work. The CDC in its wisdom saw the virtue a quarter century ago of combining chronic disease prevention and health promotion into one large and effective center of work (the NCCDPHP). Still, many topical areas in NCDs were not included. One problem that haunts NCDs and health promotion is, despite the efforts to point out with alarm the enormous global burden of NCDs and the need for health-promoting actions, there has been a marked inability to create a sense of urgency about the need to address this burden and take up the needed actions. In short, the "burden" argument does not have a certain *je ne sais quoi* that translates to people. This is unfortunate because unlike many areas of global public health concern such as AIDS, malaria, and tuberculosis, NCDs have not generated the same level of concern. That lack of concern is manifested in a lack of global resources dedicated to NCDs and the global lack of capacity to deal with NCDs and the lack of sustainable programs to create an appropriate public health infrastructure. These problems are most critical in lower and middle-income countries (LMICs).

Health promotion as a field has its own burdens. Similar to the NCD area it lacks resources globally; it has a decidedly undeveloped global capacity and infrastructure. If, as one can argue, the NCD area is marginally represented in the public health infrastructure of most LMICs, then one should recognize, by comparison, that the field of health promotion is even less part of such infrastructure. In many places health promotion is marginalized as an area in public health. Yet, it is the area of public health that is most concerned with addressing the broad health issues and focusing public health away from a concern with treating rather than preventing disease, particularly in the area of NCDs where, as we shall see argued in many of the chapters, many of the causes and solutions lie outside the area of clinical medicine. Health promotion with its emphasis on social action would seem to be the logical partner to the disease-oriented specialists. One reason for this handbook is to show how, synergistically, these two areas are in need of both perspectives. In the long run both those working in NCDs and in health promotion recognize a common concern with some key underlying values that relate to health and disease globally, principally issues of poverty, equity, and social justice.

The saying, "all models are wrong, some are useful," can characterize some of the dilemmas found in NCDs and health promotion work. The NCD world operates essentially out of a biomedical model of public health. Through recent elaborations of this model by epidemiologist and in particular social epidemiologists, this model has been extended to cover areas that seem to go well beyond a biomedical model. However these extensions are fraught with difficulties both methodological and theoretical. Much of this discussion will be found in this monograph. In a similar fashion health promotion suffers from a proliferation of models, many of which not well supported by traditional empirical findings. The problem with modeling in both fields of work is that there are too many variables, often ill defined, and in search for empirically defined relationships. Nonetheless, the literature and in particular the policy and strategic areas for work in NCDs and health promotion, whether in the academic or the institutional literature, are profligate with models. The models that are lacking and could be useful are those that link the empirical base of the NCD burden to the action areas of health promotion at the population level. To the extent that models are related to the relevant academic disciplines that underpin the NCDs and health promotion, they represent a continuum from biology through biomedicine, public health, and epidemiology on to the social sciences of psychology, social psychology, sociology, anthropology, and political science. Each of these areas and disciplines has its own theoretical and methodological paradigm. The challenge for the area of NCDs and health promotion is that these multiple paradigms provide multiple approaches to understanding the complexity of the real world, but they remain at best as useful approaches to guide the researcher and practitioner. Many chapters in this monograph address these issues and provide, in many cases, new and unique insights into these conceptual problems.

There are many ways to design the organization and content of a global handbook on NCDs and health promotion. Several obvious choices presented themselves. It could take a straightforward disease orientation with chapters focused on each of the noncommunicable diseases. Alternatively, it could take an international approach, looking at NCDs and health promotion in country after country. It could approach the area from the causes perspective, from behavioral and social factors to the so-called causes of the causes. It could consider only those action areas where there are biomedical health promotion interventions taking place. Or, it could describe how international,

national, and local agencies are addressing NCDs and health promotion. In the end the decision was made to define four sections that would try to encompass the critical aspects of the research and practice related to NCDs and health promotion that need to be known and examined by present-day researchers and practitioners. Section I is on theoretical and methodological issues arising with both NCDs and health promotion. This section is seen as critical because these fields still struggle to define their theoretical bases and therefore also struggle with what are the appropriate methodologies. Section II is called "lenses for understanding NCDs." This section addresses mainly the descriptive work of epidemiologists, social scientists, and health promoters to try and understand noncommunicable diseases. Section III focuses on approaches to try and change the burden of NCDs using perspectives ranging from treatment to policy. Finally Section IV looks at institutions and organizations that have NCDs and health promotion in their remit. These are the agencies and organizations whose work deals with NCDs and health promotion on a daily basis. These four sections provide a distinctive, if not totally comprehensive, insight into present-day research and practice in NCDs and health promotion.

Tucker, GA, USA   David V. McQueen

Contents

Contributors

Thomas Abel Division of Social and Behavioural Health Research, Institute of Social and Preventive Medicine, University of Berne, Bern, Switzerland

Karim Abu-Omar Institute of Sport Science and Sport, Friedrich-Alexander-University Erlangen-Nürnberg, Erlangen, Germany

Laurie Anderson Department of Epidemiology, School of Public Health, University of Washington, Olympia, Washington, DC, USA

Rebecca Armstrong Melbourne School of Population and Global Health, The University of Melbourne, Carlton, Victoria, Australia

Margaret M. Barry Health Promotion Research Centre, National University of Ireland Galway, Galway, Ireland

Barbara Battel-Kirk BBK Consultancy, Rabat, Malta

Adrian Bauman Prevention Research Collaboration, School of Public Health, Sydney University, Sydney, NSW, Australia

Fiona Bull Centre for Built Environment and Health, The University of Western Australia, Perth, WA, Australia

Belinda Burford Melbourne School of Population and Global Health, The University of Melbourne, Carlton, Victoria, Australia

Bronwyn Carter School of Public Health, La Trobe University, Melbourne, VIC, Australia

Stefano Campostrini University Ca' Foscari Venice, Venice, Italy

Evelyne de Leeuw Faculty of Health, Deakin University, Geelong, VIC, Australia

Ligia de Salazar FUNDESALUD, Cali, Colombia

Colette Dempsey Health Promotion Research Centre, National University of Ireland, Galway, Galway, Ireland

Christina Dietscher Ludwig Boltzmann Institute Health Promotion Research, Health Promoting Hospitals, Vienna, Austria

Jodie Doyle Melbourne School of Population and Global Health, The University of Melbourne, Carlton, Victoria, Australia

Michael Eriksen Institute of Public Health, Georgia State University, Atlanta, GA, USA

Annika Frahsa Institute of Sport Science and Sport, Friedrich-Alexander-University Erlangen-Nürnberg, Erlangen, Germany

John Frank Scottish Collaboration for Public Health Research and Policy (SCPHRP), Centre for Population Health Sciences, University of Edinburgh, Edinburgh, UK

Katherine L. Frohlich Département de médicine sociale et préventive, Université de Montréal, Montréal, QC, Canada

Peter Gelius Institute of Sport Science and Sport, Friedrich-Alexander-University Erlangen-Nürnberg, Erlangen, Germany

Ruth Jepson Scottish Collaboration for Public Health Research and Policy (SCPHRP), Centre for Population Health Sciences, University of Edinburgh, Edinburgh, UK

Darwin R. Labarthe Department of Preventive Medicine, Northwestern University Feinberg School of Medicine, Chicago, IL, USA

Ronald Labonté Institute of Population Health, University of Ottawa, Ottawa, Canada

Marie-Claude Lamarre International Union for Health Promotion and Education, Saint-Denis, France

Becky H. Lankenau Centers for Disease Control and Prevention (CDC), Atlanta, GA, USA

Raphael Lencucha Faculty of Health Sciences, University of Lethbridge, Lethbridge, AL, Canada

Vivian Lin School of Public Health, International Union for Health Promotion and Education, Melbourne, VIC, Australia

La Trobe University, Melbourne, VIC, Australia

Erma Manoncourt International Union of Health Promotion and Education, Paris, France

David V. McQueen Rollins School of Public Health, Emory University, Atlanta, GA, USA

K.S. Mohindra Institute of Population Health, University of Ottawa, Ottawa, Canada

Sania Nishtar Heartfile, Islamabad, Pakistan

Jürgen M. Pelikan Ludwig Boltzmann Institute Health Promotion Research, Health Promoting Hospitals, Vienna, Austria

Tahna Pettman Melbourne School of Population and Global Health, The University of Melbourne, Carlton, Victoria, Australia

Louise Potvin Department of Social & Preventive Medicine and Institut de recherche en santé publique, University of Montreal, Montreal, QC, Canada

Johanna Ralston World Heart Federation, Geneva, Switzerland

Dennis Raphael York University, Toronto, ON, Canada

Irving Rootman School of Public Health and School Policy, University of Victoria, Vancouver, BC, Canada

Alfred Rütten Institute of Sport Science and Sport, Friedrich-Alexander-University Erlangen-Nürnberg, Erlangen, Germany

Hermann Schmied Ludwig Boltzmann Institute Health Promotion Research, Health Promoting Hospitals, Vienna, Austria

Trevor Shilton Cardiovascular Health Programs, National Heart Foundation, Western Australia Division, Subiaco, Australia

Michael Sparks Faculty of Health, University of Canberra, Australia

Sylvie Stachenko Centre for Health Promotion Studies, School of Public Health, University of Alberta, Edmonton, AL, Canada

Maria D. Stefan CHASEAMERICA GROUP, Philadelphia, PA, USA

Sandra Vamos Innovative Health Inc., Vancouver, BC, Canada

Elizabeth Waters Melbourne School of Population and Global Health, The University of Melbourne, Carlton, Victoria, Australia

Lauren Weinberg Ecole des Hautes Etudes en Santé Publique, Rennes, France

Carrie Whitney Institute of Public Health, Georgia State University, Atlanta, GA, USA

Section I

Theoretical and Methodological Issues

High-Risk Versus Population Prevention Strategies for NCDs: Geoffrey Rose Revisited in the Twenty-First Century

John Frank and Ruth Jepson

Background

Working as an epidemiologist in the 1960s through the 1980s, Geoffrey Rose brilliantly grasped and compellingly articulated that there are two contrasting, but complementary, prevention strategies for any chronic disease with well-validated and modifiable risk factors (Rose 1985, 1992). (The term "validated" here is intended to mean prospectively validated, ideally through large, well-designed cohort studies, of which he was a master.) Taking the example of coronary heart disease—still a major premature killer in most Western countries—he showed that one could use either of the following:

1. *The High-Risk Approach*: Identify and then treat individuals at high risk of coronary heart disease, long before disease symptoms develop. Identification is undertaken through systematic screening, often in the primary care setting, to detect measurable and medically remediable cardiovascular risk factors. Such factors include serum cholesterol levels,

high blood pressure, smoking, excess weight, sedentary lifestyle, and many more less powerful or common risk factors, validated over the last half-century by cardiovascular epidemiologists, including Rose himself.

2. *The Population-Based Approach*: Alter the price, availability, and desirability of products and services that impact on cardiovascular risk factors before they even develop in individuals. Such an approach can shift entire populations' distributions of risk factors, by actually preventing—ideally in early life—their development in the first place through the adoption of harmful eating and physical activity patterns, smoking and excess alcohol consumption, etc.

Notably, the latter approach, when successful, also leads to the effective prevention of many other important chronic diseases, such as obesity, hypertension and its complications, type 2 diabetes (T2DM) and its complications, and several common types of cancer (Lee et al. 2011; McCormack and Boffetta 2011; Parkin et al. 2011; Psaltopoulou et al. 2010). Ergo this approach has inherent public health advantages, in terms of its overall population impact on much more than the common cardiovascular diseases (myocardial infarction and stroke). For this reason, such an approach is sometimes termed "primordial" prevention (Starfield 2001). In fact, the quarter-century since Rose first published this thinking has seen the advent of a new pandemic of chronic diseases for which the validity of these

J. Frank (✉) • R. Jepson
Scottish Collaboration for Public Health Research and Policy (SCPHRP), Centre for Population Health Sciences, University of Edinburgh,
20 West Richmond Street, Edinburgh EH8 9DX, UK
e-mail: john.frank@scphrp.ac.uk;
ruth.jepson@scphrp.ac.uk

D.V. McQueen (ed.), *Global Handbook on Noncommunicable Diseases and Health Promotion*,
DOI 10.1007/978-1-4614-7594-1_1, © Springer Science+Business Media, LLC 2013

same risk factors, apart from smoking, was in Rose's time much less apparent than is the case now, and/or the diseases themselves were less important burdens of illness at the global level (obesity, metabolic syndrome, and T2DM).

Despite widespread acknowledgment in the public health, clinical prevention, and epidemiological communities that Rose's views have never been proven wrong, a subtle controversy persists in the preventive health policy world about those views, and indeed in larger "lay" society. That controversy has to do with the apparently strong and persistent preference for the implementation of large-scale, expensive, risk factor screening and management programs in community-based primary care and public health settings, in contrast to the implementation of population-level legislative and regulatory interventions designed to reduce the dietary, activity-related, and tobacco-driven pandemic of chronic disease in later life. That pandemic has affected wealthy nations since at least WW II, and is now looming in developing nations, especially in its urbanized and more westernized subpopulations (Mendez et al. 2005; Murray and Lopez 1997; WHO 2011; Yusef et al. 2004).

Of special concern now is the perpetuation in poor- and middle-income countries of the rich world's prevailing, high-risk approach to chronic disease prevention. The current levels of funding, coverage, quality, and continuity of primary care in these countries are far below what is required to effectively and efficiently deliver the expensive, multiyear clinical preventive regimens, which have repeatedly been pursued in wealthy countries over the last few decades to control chronic disease. In addition, risk factor detection and management programs at the heart of the *high-risk approach* must virtually always be *perennial*—i.e., they must be offered and paid for at regular intervals, indefinitely into the future, in order to target successive new birth cohorts in every society, as their aging process brings them into susceptibility to these risk factors. As others have written (Ebrahim et al. 2011) there is thus now a considerable risk that the individualized, costly, and logistically demanding approach to chronic

disease risk factor detection and management, delivered through long-term, intensive, one-on-one clinical services, will be exported holus-bolus to poorer societies. This exportation is proceeding apace, despite the fact that those societies' primary care services are profoundly unsuited, and underfunded, to providing long-term preventive care, in the face of often overwhelming need for urgent curative care for symptomatic conditions. That approach, as we will show, can be predicted to be rolled out regardless of such legitimate concerns, driven by both new cultural expectations among these societies' elites of "Western preventive medicine" and also global commercial and local medical and pharmaceutical business interests, who stand to gain much more from this approach than from legislative or regulatory approaches aimed at primordial prevention.

Rose's Key Arguments, Revisited

In his initial, masterful paper on the subject (Rose 1985), Geoffrey Rose dispassionately laid out the pros and the cons of each of these two complementary approaches to chronic disease prevention. In the spirit of faithfulness to his original phrasing, the four tables summarizing those pros and cons are presented here.

Table 1.1 summarizes the advantages of the high-risk strategy, which centers on the relatively favorable risk–benefit balance for individuals already screened and found to have risk factors for chronic disease. This approach is especially apt when the corrective intervention to reduce risk is medically intensive—i.e., lifelong drug daily treatment, as is usual in primary care for

Table 1.1 Prevention by the "high-risk strategy": Advantages

(a) Intervention appropriate to individual
(b) Subject motivation
(c) Physician motivation
(d) Cost-effective use of resources
(e) Benefit:risk ratio favorable

Table 1.2 Prevention by the "high-risk strategy": Disadvantages

(a) Difficulties and costs of screening
(b) Palliative and temporary—not radical
(c) Limited potential for (1) individual and (2) population
(d) Behaviorally inappropriate

clinically significant hypertension, T2DM, and—increasingly (see below)—hypercholesterolemia. In other words, when the intervention target population for preventive measures is composed only of persons at very high risk of future disease, they still can obtain net health benefits, at reasonable cost, from relatively intensive and expensive medical treatments that are not without some risks (Chen et al. 2009; Grosso et al. 2011; Herman et al. 2005; Li et al. 2010; Tucker and Palmer 2011). This favorable benefit/risk/cost balance for such targeted preventive interventions in turn helps motivate patients and their physicians, and indeed high-level policymakers—there is no "cognitive dissonance."

Table 1.2 explains, however, that this strategy for prevention has a number of distinct disadvantages, some of which are so counterintuitive that very few writers on this subject had identified them clearly prior to Rose's seminal 1985 paper. First, the screening process itself, to accurately detect validated chronic disease risk factors, is rarely straightforward, or without error or costs. For example, even widely accepted "traditional" risk factors such as elevated LDL cholesterol levels have inherent "false-positive" and "false-negative" error rates, in that some persons with high LDL levels never experience clinically manifest (i.e., symptomatic) cardiovascular disease (and vice versa), at least during the first eight decades of life when it causes "premature" death and disability. This anomaly occurs simply because atherosclerotic vascular disease is inherently multifactorial, in that many aspects of both one's genetics and one's environment combine their complex influences over the life-course so as to make precise prediction of who will succumb nearly impossible. The extent of this "misclassification of risk" by serum cholesterol testing is not

appreciated by many primary care physicians, despite the fact that the first author and many other epidemiologists were publishing detailed accounts of this problem more than 20 years ago (Naylor et al. 1990). As well, the act of clinical screening only detects risk factors that have already manifested in a patient, usually due to his/her having passed through a life-course stage in which particular dietary and exercise and/or smoking/drinking habits have interacted with his/her genetic inheritance, to cause high blood pressure, blood sugar, or cholesterol levels to develop. But the age at which this occurs is not fixed, and some persons start smoking or gain a great deal of body weight much later in life than others—so that repeated risk factor screening efforts are often required throughout life, greatly increasing the logistic burden on, and costs to, the care system. Furthermore, since this approach does nothing to change the societal cultural and commercial forces that perpetuate unhealthy eating, physical activity, and smoking/drinking patterns, each generation develops anew the risk factors as it ages, requiring (as noted above) "perennial prevention efforts" decade after decade. It is for this reason that Rose calls such high-risk strategies "palliative and temporary—not radical."

Secondly, and strikingly, there are many more persons in the entire population at risk, who have only slightly elevated levels of (usually) normally distributed risk factors such as LDL cholesterol level, or blood pressure, than there are persons with very high levels. Rose elegantly showed that the inevitable algebraic consequence of this fact is that more cases of full-blown chronic disease arise from the much larger number of persons with only borderline or slightly elevated risk factor levels than from those with severely elevated levels, purely because the latter are so few in number in any population. This implies of course that a strictly high-risk approach cannot achieve effective prevention of the majority of future disease cases, especially if the optimal benefit/risk/cost balance cutoffs for treating high-risk cases are such as to only allow the identification of the small number of persons at exceptionally high risk.

Table 1.3 Prevention by the "population strategy": Advantages

(a)	Radical
(b)	Large potential for a population
(c)	Behaviorally appropriate

Table 1.4 Prevention by the "population strategy": Disadvantages

(a)	Small benefit to individual ("prevention paradox")
(b)	Poor motivation of subject
(c)	Poor motivation of physician
(d)	Benefit:risk ratio worrisome

Finally, Rose notes that the high-risk strategy is "behaviorally inappropriate" for the individual whose high levels of detected risk factors lead to being prescribed a strict diet, active exercise program, and/or smoking cessation or moderation in alcohol consumption. This is because that the person, sometimes purely because he/she has "unlucky susceptibility genes" for obesity, T2DM or its precursors, hypertension, or hypercholesterolemia, is being asked to forgo what are usually considered key pleasures by many persons in his/her society. Such lifestyle-change prescriptions are often therefore covertly resented, and sometimes actively resisted, so that long-term compliance is usually far below optimal. Yet such noncompliance is quite understandable, given that these subjects are asked, after their positive risk factor screening results, to give up fundamental aspects of life that others around them continue to enjoy.

Tables 1.3 and 1.4 summarize the converse of the above arguments: the advantages and disadvantages of the population-based strategy of prevention for chronic disease. Since these largely follow logically from what has been written above, we need not belabor them here. However, it is worth noting that the first-listed disadvantage, in Table 1.4, is not obvious to most lay persons: it is that the population strategy's inclusion, in its target audience for lifestyle behavior-change, of the entire population of a society that has developed unhealthy cultural norms for eating, exercise,

smoking, and drinking is inherently problematic from the point of view of those individuals who do *not* have elevated chronic disease risk (Rose's "prevention paradox"). That is because, of course, those low-risk individuals are being asked to forgo these "societally normed pleasures," largely for the benefit of others who do have elevated risks. They themselves stand to benefit very little, in terms of reduced chronic disease risk in the future, since their own personal baseline disease risks are so low. This inherent "injustice"—or mal-distributional aspect for risks, costs, and benefits of lifestyle modification, as economists would label it—cannot readily be overcome by any epidemiological sleight of hand. And, as Rose's Table 1.4 points out in the last three line-items, it often leads to low compliance with public health messages urging an entire society to shift its lifestyles, and—to an even greater extent—frank opposition in some quarters to economic or regulatory disincentives directed at shifting those lifestyles, by those in the general population who are aware that they personally do not have high-risk profiles, and resentful of having to change their behaviors to help others achieve health benefits. Indeed, this argument, posed by many media pundits, has proved one of the most difficult to counter in the recent Scottish public discourse about the merits, or otherwise, of putting a minimum price on alcohol. The intent of such legislation is to deliberately shift the entire population distribution of alcohol consumption downwards, in hopes that that will help de-normalize its widespread use and abuse, and also shift downwards the consumption of problem-drinkers (Black et al. 2011; Purshouse et al. 2010). But, at least in Scotland, those who feel they "drink responsibly" resent having to pay more for their drink, just to help "the family down the street" where someone has a drinking problem.

More technically, the unpromising benefit/risk ratio (Table 1.4, last line-item) for those included in the population strategy's broad intervention target-group, who are at low risk, means that public health officials can only recommend under this strategy relatively "hygienic" measures—such as the reversal of historically global-outlier patterns of eating, exercise, smoking, and drinking, not "natural" to healthy human populations in the past—as opposed to strongly medicalized interventions, such as lifelong daily prescription-drug use, for reducing chronic disease risk. What is remarkable, however, is that a body of expert opinion, further discussed below, has developed in the last decade, which argues that it is essential, given the shortcomings of the high risk strategy described above, to actually administer such daily drugs (e.g., statins, aspirin, and/or antihypertensive drugs (Lazar et al. 2011; Powlson 2003; Wald and Law 2003))—albeit at a lower dose than is normally used in clinical preventive practice—to every adult person in whole societies, in order to achieve major reductions in future chronic disease burden. Of course, from the point of view of those in the population who know they have relatively low risks, and appreciate the as yet poorly characterized risks of this radical recommendation, this is hardly an acceptable solution!

Two Examples of Current "Rose-ian" Controversies in Chronic Disease Prevention

Rose clearly understood that health policymakers and practitioners would generally need to use a judicious mix of *both* of these two approaches to chronic disease prevention, in that each approach carries associated advantages and disadvantages (Rose 1992). The precise optimal mix of the two would sometimes, he foresaw, arise purely from the state of scientific knowledge about the amenability of risk factors to both accurate detection and cost-effective clinical management. For example, if a powerful and common risk factor for a major chronic disease does not have an affordable, cost-effective, and socially acceptable screening test and medical treatment that can successfully manage it, over the remaining lifetime of persons discovered by screening to have that risk factor, the high-risk approach is immediately compromised. In that situation, the population approach clearly needs to be thoroughly explored for the cost-effectiveness and risks—if any—of

higher level policy interventions to change diet, promote physical activity, reduce smoking onset and spur successful quitting, reduce alcohol consumption, etc. in the entire population.

Conversely, as has been repeatedly shown for tobacco control (McNeill et al. 2011; Paynter and Edwards 2009) there are major health benefits, and net societal economic benefits, from systematically increasing the price of that unequivocally hazardous substance, and simultaneously reducing its availability and marketing. In the face of this evidence, individually targeted therapies directed at clinical diagnosis and management of those who already have a clear dependency problem (with all its associated treatment challenges difficulties, in terms of achieving long-term medical or psychological quit-success) should be seen as an ethically mandated but rather second-rate option for tobacco control. "The horse is well out of the barn door" by the stage of clinical nicotine dependency, and usually that "horse" is not much motivated to change the addictive behavior, until pressing health, income, or social threats present themselves, usually after decades of daily tobacco use (McBride et al. 2003). In addition, health inequalities may be unintentionally widened with individually targeted programs, as smokers from lower socioeconomic groups are less likely to be successful in a quitting than more educated and affluent smokers, even when they access smoking cessation services (Hiscock et al. 2011).

Case Study #1: Elevated LDL Cholesterol and Statin Drug Treatment

Sometimes, as has happened with serum cholesterol control by medical treatment over the last two decades, the debate on major screening programs has substantially shifted due to the advent of very effective, relatively safe risk factor treatments. Statins, and particularly the much less expensive generically manufactured statin drugs, are a case in point (however see below for a recent and worrisome caveat on the assertion that they are completely safe). In the 1980s, many experts favored population-based approaches, involving dietary and physical activity habit-changes, in preference to lifelong, daily, individualized drug treatment to lower harmful serum lipids. This preference was in large part based on the fact that no really effective, safe, and palatable drugs for that purpose were available, prior to the advent of routinely prescribed statins, just over 20 years ago. In addition, the early statins (produced under patent) were very expensive, considering that they usually need to be taken daily for the rest of a relatively well person's lifetime. However, extensive clinical experience in those two decades and now quite long and careful follow-up of statin-treated patients inside randomized control trials (Ford et al. 2007) have demonstrated (again, until very recently—see below) virtually no clinically serious and common side effects, as well as a bewildering and previously unanticipated set of putative health benefits, beyond cardiovascular risk reduction, from chronic statin use—including reductions in cancer rates (Cauley et al. 2006; Demierre et al. 2005), hospital mortality from influenza (Vandermeer et al. 2012), and improvements in markers of widespread tissue inflammation that are independently associated with cardiovascular and other chronic disease risks (Kones 2010).

These studies have left many physicians and health policymakers, and even some researchers, with the view that statins are so safe and now, in the wake of their off-patent, generic manufacture, relatively inexpensive (at less than $5.00–$10.00 per person per month)—that they can ethically be recommended to *virtually every adult past midlife in all developed countries* (Lazar et al. 2011; Powlson 2003; Wald and Law 2003). Although other experts would question the universal administration of statins to all developed country citizens past their mid-forties, in the last decade an almost ubiquitous clinician acceptance of the view has developed that this lifelong daily drug treatment should be routinely offered in primary care in wealthy countries to asymptomatic persons with (as this thinking has progressed over time) lower and lower levels of baseline LDL serum cholesterol. In short, "indication creep"

has led to a situation where "evidence-based" primary care treatment guidelines have moved steadily since the 1980s in the direction of recommending indefinite, daily statin treatment of a very large fraction (up to 25 % of the entire elderly population under some recent US guidelines, tellingly always the most aggressive in the world) (Manuel et al. 2006; National Cholesterol Education Program 2002).

To provide a historical perspective on this long-term trend, the first author was a contributor to a widely cited clinical policy review of the cholesterol screening and treatment controversy in 1990 (Naylor et al. 1990). That monograph recommended—in retrospect rather conservatively—quite cautious use of the rather unpleasant and ineffective cholesterol-lowering drugs available in primary care up to that time (this was prior to widespread statin use in primary care). That recommendation was based largely on clinical efficiency calculations ("number needed to screen and treat"). These recommendations have stood the test of time remarkably well. While some might say "How much things have changed!" in this field since that time, the first author's 22 years of personal experience give a different impression. As argued quantitatively in our 1990 analysis, it is still very unclear whether lifelong daily statin treatment of a healthy young adult (even a man, who has a much higher risk of premature cardiovascular disease than a woman), who has only a moderately elevated LDL cholesterol level and no other cardiovascular risk factors, actually represents a competitively cost-effective use of resources (Greving et al. 2011). And that cost-effectiveness assessment is before the recent (2011–2012) findings of a potential unexpected, serious, and common chronic side effect of statin use (see next paragraph) have yet been taken into consideration, in revised practice guidelines.

Notably, and predictably from the point of view of the history of adoption and diffusion of new health technologies in the past (Packer et al. 2006), a new and very careful cohort study (Culver et al. 2012) has shown what many observers of previous waves of widespread, overly enthusiastic, preventive drug prescribing have feared might eventually come to light. Specifically, just in the last year or so, strong epidemiological evidence has emerged that the risk of acquiring a relatively serious and already very common chronic disease in this same population, type II diabetes (T2DM), is substantially increased in those prescribed virtually any type of statin for a long period, by 9 % (odds ratio [OR] 1.09; 95 % CI 1.02–1.17) of the baseline incidence (Sattar et al. 2010) (also consider the findings re muscular pain and other side effects now found with statins). While some experts have called for calm and "no change in the clinical indications for statin use" (Mason 2012), many in the primary care and public health community are pointing out that this new finding means that there is a very high resultant attributable (arithmetically additional) risk—with perhaps 5–10 % of statin-prescribed patients consequently developing a profoundly life-altering disease, even just over the limited periods of follow-up studied thus far. Even lay persons are well aware that T2DM greatly reduces life span, and brings with it after some years' duration, the risk of many serious and disabling complications. If T2DM is found to be convincingly causally linked to statin use per se, by further studies (including, ideally, some basic science evidence of a biological mechanism by which this side effect occurs), one could therefore safely estimate that perhaps one in twenty persons prescribed statins (depending on their age and other baseline risk factors for diabetes) will suffer T2DM as a result. This "number needed to harm" statistic (Laupacis et al. 1988) implies in turn that it would not be prudent to administer statins to the entire middle-aged and older population of developed countries (for example, in the poly-pill, and certainly not via "the water supply," as is done with fluoride for dental caries prevention, as some have suggested!). As well, this new finding means that the clinical cardiovascular risk-threshold for prescribing lifelong statin treatment—based on the cumulative risk of heart attack or stroke, over each primary care patient's next 10 years of life, now often computed by physicians, using widely available online risk-calculators (Nandish et al. 2011)—must necessarily be substantially raised (Mason 2012).

What then is the moral of this story? Surely it is that our *initial* scientific knowledge of the long-term consequences of powerful chemical agents, especially those taken regularly for decades for preventive purposes, is necessarily quite limited—especially in the first decade or two after such use begins to be widespread. As all pharmaco-epidemiologists know, we "see through a glass darkly" in relation to subtle and long-term drug side effects, especially if they effect rather rare health outcomes. Ironically, this is also true if such agents lead to modest (but important at the population level) increases in the occurrence of very common diseases. For example, most clinicians would not be surprised to see any older patient, who is already on statins for cardiovascular risk, develop T2DM. Indeed, this was precisely the reason it took so long to suspect Vioxx of heart disease side effects—the anti-inflammatory drug taken by millions. Only very large case–control and cohort studies conducted after the drug was brought to the market and widely used showed that it led to clinically important, and often fatal, cardiovascular problems. The problem was that the disease-complex which happened to be increased in incidence in Vioxx users—coronary heart disease and heart failure—was already by far the most likely cause of hospitalization and death in the age-group and class of patients put on Vioxx, even before they were prescribed the drug. Thus no clinician could readily twig to the modestly but importantly elevated risk in patients taking the drug, until sensitive epidemiological studies revealed that something like an additional 88,000–140,000 excess cases of serious coronary heart disease, in the USA alone, had probably been caused by Vioxx (Graham et al. 2005). That finding, of course, led to Vioxx's prompt withdrawal by the manufacturer, who is still dealing with class-action suits and individual tort cases in some jurisdictions (Krumholz et al. 2007). In the modern world of pharmaco-vigilance, especially for preventive medications prescribed to relatively well people for decades, only prolonged and assiduous follow-up of hundreds of thousands of persons taking the drug, as part of post-marketing surveillance, reveals such side effects.

This is achieved best by large cohorts (the US Women's Health Study reporting diabetes in statin users, after following 153,000 subjects for many years) OR sensitive, population-level record-linkage studies—ideally between pharmaceutical prescription/purchase and subsequent, routinely collected hospitalization and mortality records. Only such massive, long-term pharmaco-epidemiological studies are likely to show us subtle (or substantially delayed) harms not previously suspected in premarketing studies, which are always of much shorter duration, smaller sample size, and limited outcome ascertainment (in terms of the range of health outcomes sought). *Caveat emptor* …

Case Study # 2: Smoking Cessation Treatment Versus Population Measures to Reduce Smoking Initiation and Continuation

It is informative to examine a clinical preventive intervention of proven worth, which does not necessarily entail chronic daily drug treatment, with its inevitable and uncertain risks. Let us explore the case of individualized smoking cessation treatment, with or without initial short-term use of nicotine replacement therapy, or other prescription drugs to reduce craving and dependency. This preventive maneuver for widespread primary care use has also come a long way in the last two decades, the same period in which statins have revolutionized serum lipid management (Aveyard et al. 2012; Villanti et al. 2010). Indeed, many experts cite smoking cessation treatment as the single most *effective* preventive intervention (in terms of the magnitude of the population-burden of disease prevented) and also the most *cost-effective* one (in terms of QALYs per unit of intervention cost) available to primary care clinicians, throughout the life-course—for it is never too late in life to reap some benefits, and also reduce your household expenditures, by stopping smoking (NICE 2009).

Much less frequently discussed is the fact that clinically delivered smoking cessation treatment has been quite impotent at reducing—and indeed,

it may under normal primary care conditions, increase (Honjo et al. 2006)—the already steep social class gradient in smoking in developed countries. Furthermore, as Rose himself would be quick to point out, treating established smokers tends to be most successful only after some decades of smoking, when daily symptoms of resultant disease start to frighten the patient into actively fighting their tobacco addiction. Such a strategy does absolutely nothing to reduce the societal rate of new smoker formation in early life (90 % of smokers in rich countries start before the end of their teens (Mitka 2009)).[1]

Thus, confirming Rose's edict that both high-risk and population-based prevention strategies are usually required for effective and efficient chronic disease prevention, many experts now advocate, in addition to accessible, high-quality and well-managed smoking cessation services, the implementation of a combination of high tobacco taxes, restricted supply and marketing, as well as tough laws on public smoking (by legislation or regulation) and active promotion of sophisticated antismoking messages, especially to the young (Brinn et al. 2010; Lantz et al. 2000). These experts know that these two Rose-ian approaches are complementary, and critical to achieving any long-term, real reduction in the steep "social gradient" in smoking, as well as to reducing the continued high rates of uptake of this very addictive habit by the young, and especially by girls—who seem, in many settings, to continue to be enthralled by Big Tobacco's shrewd marketing of smoking, as a sign of self-determination and autonomy in women (Tobacco Free Kids 2009). Indeed, a recent review concluded that population-level tobacco control interventions have the potential to benefit more disadvantaged groups and thereby contribute substantially to reducing health inequalities (Thomas et al. 2008).

---

[1] A recent paper by one of the authors, and Canadian colleagues who work full time on tobacco control (Chaiton et al. 2008) points out the extraordinary relevance of Rose's thinking to tobacco control, despite the slight epidemiological complication that smoking is not usually thought of as a continuously distributed risk factor, in statistical terminology.

Alternative Ways of Looking at the Controversy

The above examples illustrate the "shifting balance of evidence over time," for and against the use of each Rose's two approaches to controlling the common risk factors for chronic diseases. Overall, however, there is increasing concern among public health experts that the individual high-risk approach keeps preferentially "getting the nod" from health policymakers, in country after country, era after era, even when there are clear arguments for the population approach. We hypothesize here some possible reasons for this widely observed phenomenon. In particular, we cite patterns of culturally embedded thoughts, beliefs, and attitudes—and vested interests' influence—neither of which are generally made explicit in public discourse.

The Subtle Importance of Moral Views About Fault and Responsibility

It has been asserted that public health and health promotion have introduced a new moral meaning around risk (Lupton 1995; 90) and the dominant theme of lifestyle risk discourse in health promotion focuses on the individual's responsibility to avoid health risks, for the sake of their own health as well as for the greater good of society as a whole. On this view, there is a moral obligation to be "healthy citizens" (Petersen and Lupton 1996; 65), the dimensions of which are apparent in health campaigns around cigarette smoking and passive smoking, diet and physical activity patterns, and—especially—the excessive consumption of alcohol or any illegal drug. Indeed, recurrent debates in countries with publicly funded health care systems (The Guardian 2011; The Telegraph 2012) surround the legitimacy of the rights of smokers, alcoholics, drug-abusers, and now obese persons to be treated at the public's expense for complications of their "self-imposed" unhealthy habits.

Perhaps unsurprisingly, in some of these same societies there is a widespread legacy of "quasi-Calvinist" beliefs about where the principal fault lies—typically, entirely within persons engaging in such unhealthy behaviors. Often, these beliefs derive from historical religious and moral views about what constitutes "good" and "bad" behavior (and harken back to a long tradition in social welfare policy, of discourse about the "worthy and unworthy poor"). Medical historian Roy Porter describes the attitudes common in the post-industrialized period:

> Government should uphold the law, the individual should be provident, and charity should rectify hardships. Even if the trade you worked was deadly, wasn't that a personal choice, freely taken? When workers fell sick, blame was often laid upon their faulty constitution, regarded or rationalised as the cause of disease. (Porter 2002).

There has long been a commonly held perception that poverty was due to "idleness and fecklessness." Such moralistic views have often become subtly conflated with interpretations of the actual evidence, in the modern discourse about what needs to be done by "public health authorities," in order to change self-harming behaviors that lead, over decades, to major preventable diseases. This is, rather remarkably, true even though social scientists have shown that many of these behaviors are largely driven by cultural and societal norms, the control of which is arguably well beyond the individual in many cases, and heavily influenced by commercial advertising and marketing practices. This is particularly evident for those "lifestyle" habits that are strongly formed before we become adults, which include many of our food preferences and eating habits, and most of our drinking and drug-taking habits (cf. the usual age for starting smoking in the preteens or teenage years, above). Certainly, our fundamental personal approach to keeping physically active, and taking care with what we eat and drink, is largely formed at this age. This is of course not to say that these habits cannot be altered after the end of teenage life. Rather, most such habits are rather fully formed in the first two decades of life, and require considerable motivation and effort to change subsequently, especially in the sustained way required to confer major health benefits.

A good example of the complexity of such broader cultural influences is the wide international diversity in legislation aimed at restricting the marketing of unhealthy foods to children, and indeed regulating all advertising aimed at young children, which is currently in place in only in a very few societies. Sweden and the Canadian province of Quebec are frequently cited (Mooney et al. 2011) as positive exemplars of Rose's "population-based prevention" model for combating the current obesity pandemic, especially in children, where international statistics reveal a very worrisome trend. Sweden has for some time banned all marketing of "energy-dense" foods without other nutritional benefit. Quebec, on the other hand, has taken the more general view that children cannot discern when media messages come from marketers, and are purely designed to sell them something. They are unable, for example, to distinguish such advertising messages from those of public health authorities intended to give them advice from a neutral, scientifically reliable perspective. Quebec has therefore for 32 years banned the advertising of *any* products or services, aimed at children. (Unfortunately, the massive importation into Canada, via the airwaves and Internet, of US-based advertising on radio, satellite TV, the Web, and social media, and now through cell-phone broadcasting, makes this Quebec provincial policy rather ineffective. Indeed, more than ever in modern Quebec, because of such global marketization of childhood, the vast majority of francophone children understand English sufficiently to grasp those foreign, anglophone marketing messages only too well.)

On the other hand, most Western jurisdictions have either never contemplated such legislation or it has been explicitly defeated at some point (usually by vested interests) in the policy-development process (Rayner and Lang 2009). So what is going on here?

One possible interpretation has to do with how any given society tends to view childhood and children, as a whole. Recent UNICEF comparisons of child health and well-being outcomes, across more than twenty developed countries, reveal a striking tendency for English-speaking countries, especially the UK and the USA, to rank at the bottom of these league tables (Adamson et al. 2007). A subsequent qualitative analysis of cultural and social factors influencing these rankings (Nairn 2011) reveals an interesting underlying phenomenon—the profound rise in materialistic criteria for children's own assessment of their self-worth, in English-speaking cultures. Notably, it is these same cultures, within Europe, which historically persisted longest in the view that childhood is merely an earlier stage of adulthood, with no special claim to being treated as worthy of particular protections, or being spared major responsibilities. The elimination of child labor in the UK was in fact not completed until close to the end of the nineteenth century (Ostry and Frank 2010). A lingering consequence of those historical views is perhaps reflected in the current international league-table rankings of child health and well-being, in that there appears to be a special penalty associated with being born into those cultures, one marked by the poor quality of children's relationships, in particular with their significant others (Nairn 2011). The policy analogue for this regrettable cultural tradition seems to be a persistent reluctance in these jurisdictions to intervene with legislation, to protect children from commercial influences, whether they arise from the food, drink, tobacco, or alcohol marketing sectors. It is as if the "age of legal consent"—while ironically enshrined clearly in medical research consent guidelines—does not apply to healthy children, even though they can hardly be expected to be able to discern the predictably misleading elements of most advertising.

Whatever the case, it is striking that legislation to protect children and youth, from the adverse health influences of unhealthy food, beverage, and tobacco marketing practices, seems to last implemented in English-speaking societies. This suggests that deeper cultural values, rather than current scientific evidence, are the critical factors in determining how any given society responds to threats such as the current, persistent epidemic of smoking in young persons (especially those from disadvantaged groups—see above), and the relatively recent pandemic of overweight and obesity.

The Importance of Commercial and Professional Forces as Interest Groups

Strong economic and political forces, exemplified by both medical diagnostic and treatment commercial interests, as well as many health professional lobby groups, stand to benefit economically from the implementation of massive programs of individualized risk factor screening. This is especially the case when one remembers that successful risk factor detection, by such screening, is generally followed by lifelong clinical management (including much drug treatment) of the commonest chronic disease risk factors such as hyperlipidemia, hypertension, overweight, and smoking. Indeed, many clinicians appear to think of individualized, clinically situated, high-risk prevention as the only sort that they can legitimately implement or take a role in. This is particularly true where they see themselves as "small businessmen" engaged in self-employed practice, rather than potential social activists in the local community. This view of themselves, on the part of many health professionals and especially physicians, is still reinforced by their *self-employment status* within the dominant primary care delivery systems of both the UK and Canada, despite legislation in both countries now 65 and 45 years old, respectively, that transferred all insuring responsibilities to the state, for first-dollar, comprehensive medical care insurance.

Screening is also an area where major technological advances have been made. Industry is aware of the public's interest in risk reduction and screening and therefore creates new technologies to meet that demand. It has been argued that, in the USA, preventive services such as screening are marketed to healthy women using a language and a style that mimics that of the women's movement. They emphasize the right of all women to have access to health services and to be actively involved (Lupton 1995; 94). Thus, this is perhaps a cynical marketing device to attract women to services such as mammographic screening. In addition, new screening technology can potentially expose every part of our body to medical scrutiny and make us feel that we are at danger from a range of diseases.

Obviously, the ever-enlarging set of indications for lifelong, individualized risk factor screening and preventive treatment present an attractively bottomless pit of potential new clinical activity that can happily contribute substantially to the incomes of physicians—especially under the fee-for-service payment schedules still routine in North America, but ironically now also true in the UK NHS, under the Quality Outcomes Framework contract, which pays GPs extra for each recommended preventive intervention delivered. Screening has been described as "the institutionalization of risk" (Thornton et al. 2003) and for many people, it is viewed as a way of eliminating risk and uncertainty. The physician-income windfall is being created by the advent of evermore preventive practice guidelines, exemplified by the most aggressive on the planet which typically come—not surprisingly—from the US medical professional bodies (Bellizzi et al. 2011) as well as naive cancer-survivor charities. Such guidelines perennially create large number of new "patients," out of persons who previously thought of themselves as completely well, in that they had no symptoms of disease. This magical transformation is achieved simply by shifting the threshold values of laboratory and radiological screening tests to include less and less severe perturbations of body function and structure as "at risk" and "requiring management." The list of proposed screening tests for all middle-aged to elderly adults, especially in the USA, has now moved far beyond simple serum lipid levels and blood pressure (which have been validated to be worthy of detection and treatment, at least at some level of abnormality, for some decades now) to include such novel—but un-validated as net-beneficial—screening measures as a blood test for nonspecific "inflammation" (C-reactive protein—Kones 2010); routine bone-mineral-density scanning for osteoporosis; and aggressively marketed whole-body scans for "whatever they find is wrong." This transformation has been referred to by screening commentators for more than two decades as "the medicalization of normal life and aging" (Skrabenek 1994; Raffle and Muir Gray 2007), through the promulgation of progressively more aggressive screening policies. Such policies are also driven by litigation-sensitive medical practice that lives—at least in the USA—in constant fear of civil action by patients who may develop a disease alleged to be preventable, by a screening test which *was not offered* by the physician some years earlier, predictably always leading to the same regrettable pattern of preventive care. Such testing detects a burgeoning array of poorly understood subclinical risk factors in patients without symptoms, who then are duly offered cancer treatments, or put on lifetime preventive medications, diets, and other strict regimens, but who were previously living much less medicalized lives. If these patients clearly benefit, of course, there is no problem—but such is often not the case with newer, poorly researched tests, the use of which is quite unregulated in most countries.

Our point here is not that all such "secondary prevention" programs are worthless, but rather the extraordinary international variation in locally recommended thresholds for treatment (Rosser et al. 1990), and in the ways in which they are rolled out and paid for, strongly suggests that much more than epidemiological evidence, of effectiveness or cost-effectiveness, is at play in determining what citizens of various countries, localities, and social classes are routinely offered as "recommended preventive care." A case in point is routine mammography screening to detect breast cancer in healthy, low-risk women aged 40–70, where there is literally a war going on between scientists with equally impressive credentials but completely opposing views on who should be mammogrammed, and how often, with widely varying national and professional body guidance as a result (Board of Faculty of Clinical Radiology 2003; Canadian Taskforce on Preventive Health Care 2011; Hendrick and Helvie 2011; US Preventive Services Task Force 2009). A potentially more distressing example is presented in the text-box, of a particularly pernicious (i.e., scientifically proven harmful) but very widespread screening implemented in the entire USA, decades before the first robust study of its effectiveness was published in 2009, showing that such screening of low-risk, healthy, older men is almost certain to do more harm than good.

Case Study of PSA Screening for Prostate Cancer: "More Harm than Good, at High Price?"

Since the publication in 2009 (Schroder et al. 2009) of a definitive, adequately powered and assiduously followed-up trial of PSA testing in 182,160 healthy European men aged 50–69 (the age-group thought most likely to benefit), virtually all public health experts now agree that such screening—at least for men at usual risk, as opposed to high risk—should be avoided. The reason is simple: after painstaking completion of 9 years of follow-up, for each 10,000 men who were screened in the study with this blood test, which had been thought capable of detecting early prostate cancer, 340 extra cases of prostate cancer were actually detected, and in 117 cases managed by "watchful waiting," or in 223 cases by chemo/radiotherapy and/or aggressive surgery. However, only *7 men per 10,000 screened had their deaths by prostate cancer delayed at all*, leaving the balance of some 216 screened men, per 10,000 screened, effectively worse off after screening than before, since they were told that they had cancer when they felt well, in many cases aggressively managed for it, but in the end died at the same age as they would have anyway. In short, they were "victims of unvalidated screening" by a particularly inaccurate test now known to detect many prostate cancers growing so slowly that most of these men would continue to have no symptoms at all until they died of another condition. Clearly the considerable costs of the screening and subsequent confirmatory needle biopsies, as well as the complex treatments for those offered to them, were associated to an extremely unfavorable benefit-to-risk ratio—the money could have been much better spent elsewhere.

While the NHS in the UK has never officially sanctioned PSA screening in healthy

(continued)

(continued)

men, recent time-trends in prostate cancer incidence, which show a rapidly increasing rate, particularly in wealthier and more educated men (just the sort to inquire about or openly ask to be screened), are unlikely to be explained in any other way, and have been seen in every developed nation where the use of PSA screening has grown. This is especially true in the USA—where an enthusiastic lobby of scientifically ill-informed cancer survivors and urological specialists has trumpeted the test's benefits for years. In fact, a recent editorial (Vickers A. Medscape 2011: posted December 15) points out that over half % of men over 65 in the USA had been PSA-screened at least once by the mid-1990s, and a more recent commentary suggests that the screening rate is currently over 25 %, even among men over 85 years of age in whom no one would ever expect any mortality benefits from PSA screening due to both the long lag-time before benefit appears (more than 8 years) and the limited life span of such patients.

This then is an example of a current health care expenditure which cannot be justified, and which requires more effective regulation of the test's use—for example by restricting its use to specialists in charge of diagnosing symptomatic prostate cancer cases, or following up cases already diagnosed. Although the test itself may appear to have a modest cost, it sets in motion a very expensive—and potentially upsetting (for the patient and his family)—"cascade" of further investigations and treatments in about 3.4 % (1 in 29) of those screened, even though only 7 per 10,000 appear to benefit.

Despite this new evidence that PSA screening for prostate cancer probably does more harm than good, and at quite a price, a recent national newspaper supplement on cancer, paid for by the Graham Fulford Charitable Trust, took an unabashedly positive stance on the issue, urging all older men to go for screening (REF). This pattern fits perfectly, of course with the insightful point made by Raffle and Muir Gray in their superb textbook on screening: the worse the screening test's accuracy—and especially the more likely it is to generate many false positives requiring confirmatory diagnostic testing of those screened as positive, to determine that there is no cancer present after all—the more "cancer survivors" result from the screening program, who will always believe that they would now be dead without having undergone the test (Raffle and Muir Gray 2007).

Current analyses of "who benefits" from such medicalization, of clinically normal older persons' lives, must include the vested interests, relatively newly arrived-on-the-scene, of the growers/manufacturers, and marketers of very profitable "alternative health products" that modern society purchases, although there is very little unbiased science available to guide the consumer, on precisely how to use them to lead a longer and healthier life. A recent visit to the authors' local health food store in the UK reveals *hundreds—nay, thousands*—of superbly selling supplements, nutraceuticals, and herbal concoctions that are claimed—although not always directly, on the label, due to strong legislation about claims—to prolong life and improve health, despite usually much weaker legislation about marketing! Even for a trained physician-epidemiologist, finding robust, published scientific evidence, on the risks and benefits of many of these products, is virtually impossible. Yet those with the resources to buy them are doing so in great numbers—although it appears that they rarely tell their general practitioner what they are taking and also that they chop and change these medicaments with great frequency. They thereby expose themselves to the hazards of a new kind of "lay/self-prescribed poly-pharmacy"—while ironically also depriving themselves of potential health benefits of certain truly effective preparations (Farmer et al. 2007;

Marik and Varon 2009; Turner et al. 2007; Woods et al. 2002) which need to be taken daily, for some years to decades, for maximum benefit.

Finally, it almost goes without saying that most preventive health guidelines for avoiding premature chronic disease, and thereby living longer and healthier lives, entail the consumption of much *less* of very widely sold—but profoundly unhealthy—foods and beverages. Given their sales figures, these products must confer (no doubt on the basis of skillful product engineering to achieve precisely this goal) much immediate pleasure, but surely not nutritional "value for money." Examples include all sugar-sweetened beverages; virtually all candy and commercial baked goods (which have evolved, presumably on the grounds of optimal shelf-life, to be replete with entirely artificial, and proven harmful, trans fats); most salty and unhealthy fat-laden, but essentially nonnutritious, snack food; heavily salted prepared foods, including most soups and many ready-to-eat dinners; and all animal products containing large amounts of saturated fat. The corollary of these unhealthy but apparently pleasurable products' seeming stranglehold, on Westernized societies' total food budgets, is that any move to reduce their consumption, whether by "social marketing" or the potentially more potent device of selective taxation, is immediately opposed by powerful commercial and sometimes agricultural interests. Furthermore, these interests control an amazingly large part of many countries' productive economies. It comes therefore as little surprise that the current UK Government's ideological predilections have recently resulted in both the appointment under the Government's "Responsibility Deal" of multiple food and drink industry representatives to the major public health advisory bodies in England, concerned with healthier food and drink consumption (UK Faculty of Public Health 2011) and the subsequent recent complaints by independent public health professional and scientific experts that the alcohol industry pledges towards reduced marketing and selling to those at risk of overconsumption are "disappointing." It is hard to guard the hen house when someone has given the foxes keys.

Conclusion

The authors, based on some decades of experience in this field between them, offer the following concluding advice to those working in public health and health promotion, who seek to improve the fit of preventive health policies to the empirical evidence, and rein in the less salutogenic influences mentioned above:

> Evidence is good … but much of the time it is up against, first, potent underlying values and beliefs (sometimes quite covert or subconscious) held by both the electorate and policymakers, as well as, secondly, powerful economic and social forces, that render rational debate—as a sole or primary method of setting controversial prevention policy—almost useless. Professionals in public health and health promotion would do well to spend more time studying the arts of persuasion mastered by both politicians and the media, as well as the darker arts of the advertising and marketing field, if they are to be more successful in shifting chronic disease preventive policies towards an appropriate balance between the two approaches, as laid out by Rose so presciently, a quarter century ago.

References

Adamson, P., Bradshaw, J., Hoelscher, P., & Richardson. (2007). *Child poverty in perspective: An overview of child well-being in rich countries*. Unicef Innocenti Research Centre, Florence, Italy, Innocenti Report Card, vol. 7

Aveyard, P., Begh, R., Parsons, A., & West, R. (2012). Brief opportunistic smoking cessation interventions: A systematic review and meta-analysis to compare advice to quit and offer of assistance. Addiction no available from: http://dx.doi.org/10.1111/j.1360-0443.2011.03770.x

Bellizzi, K., Breslau, E., Burness, A., & Waldron, W. (2011). Prevalence of cancer screening in older, racially diverse adults. Still screening after all these years. *Archives of Internal Medicine, 171*(22), 2031–2037. doi:10.1001/archinternmed.2011.570.

Black, H., Gill, J., & Chick, J. (2011). The price of a drink: Levels of consumption and price paid per unit of alcohol by Edinburgh's ill drinkers with a comparison to wider alcohol sales in Scotland. *Addiction, 106*(4), 729–736.

Board of Faculty of Clinical Radiology. (2003). *Guidance on screening and symptomatic breast imaging*. (2nd ed.). Retrieved January 8, 2012 from: http://www.rcr.ac.uk/publications.aspx?PageID=310&PublicationID=184

Brinn, M., Carson, K., Esterman, A., Chang, A., & Smith, B. (2010). Mass media interventions for preventing smoking in young people. *Cochrane Database of Systematic Reviews Issue 11*. Art. No., CD001006. doi: 10.1002/14651858.CD001006.pub2.

Canadian Taskforce on Preventive Health Care. (2011). Screening for breast cancer. Summary of recommendations for clinicians and policy-makers. Retrieved January 8, 2012 from: http://www.canadiantaskforce. ca/recommendations/2011_01_eng.html

Cauley, J. A., McTiernan, A., Rodabough, R. J., LaCroix, A., Bauer, D. C., Margolis, K. L., Paskett, E. D., Vitolins, M. Z., Furberg, C. D., Chlebowski, R. T., & For the Women's Health Initiative Research Group. (2006). Statin use and breast cancer: Prospective results from the women's health initiative. *Journal of the National Cancer Institute, 98*(10), 700–707. http:// jnci.oxfordjournals.org/content/98/10/700.abstract.

Chaiton, M., Cohen, J., & Frank, J. (2008). Population health and the hardcore smoker: Geoffrey Rose revisited. *Journal of Public Health Policy, 29*, 307–318.

Chen, Y. F., Jowett, S., Barton, P., Malottki, K., Hyde, C., Gibbs, J. S., Pepke-Zaba, J., Fry-Smith, A., Roberts, J., & Moore, D. (2009). Clinical and cost-effectiveness of epoprostenol, iloprost, bosentan, sitaxentan and sildenafil for pulmonary arterial hypertension within their licensed indications: A systematic review and economic evaluation. *Health Technology Assessment (Winchester, England), 13*(49), 1–320.

Culver, A. L., Ockene, I. S., Balasubramanian, R., Olendzki, B. C., Sepavich, D. M., Wactawski-Wende, J., Manson, J. E., Qiao, Y., Liu, S., Merriam, P. A., Rahilly-Tierny, C., Thomas, F., Berger, J. S., Ockene, J. K., Curb, J. D., & Ma, Y. (2012). Statin use and risk of diabetes mellitus in postmenopausal women in the women's health initiative. *Archives of Internal Medicine, 172*(2), 144–152. http://archinte.ama-assn. org/cgi/content/abstract/172/2/144.

Demierre, M. F., Higgins, P. D. R., Gruber, S. B., Hawk, E., & Lippman, S. M. (2005). Statins and cancer prevention. *National Review Cancer, 5*(12), 930–942. doi:10.1038/nrc1751.

Ebrahim, S., Taylor, F., Ward, K., Beswick, A., Burke, M., & Davey Smith, G. (2011). Multiple risk factor interventions for primary prevention of coronary heart disease. *Cochrane Database of Systematic Reviews*, (1) Art. No., CD001561. doi: 10.1002/14651858. CD001561.pub3.

Farmer, A., Montori, V., Dinneen, S., & Clar, C. (2007). Fish oil in people with type 2 diabetes mellitus. *Cochrane Database of Systematic Reviews*, (3), CD003205, doi: 10.1002/14651858.CD003205

Ford, I., Murray, H., Packard, C., et al. (2007). Long-term follow-up of the west of scotland coronary prevention study. *New England Journal of Medicine, 357*, 1477–1486.

Graham, D., Campen, D., Hui, R., Spence, M., Cheetham, C., & Levy, G. (2005). Risk of acute myocardial infarction and sudden cardiac death in patients treated with cyclo-oxygenase 2 selective and non-selective non-steroidal anti-inflammatory drugs: Nested case-control study. *Lancet, 365*(9458), 457–481.

Greving, J. P., Visseren, F., de Wit G. A., & Algra, A. (2011). Statin treatment for primary prevention of vascular disease: Whom to treat? Cost-effectiveness analysis. *British Medical Journal, 342* doi: 10.1136/bmj. d1672

Grosso, A. M., Bodalia, P. N., Macallister, R. J., Hingorani, A. D., Moon, J. C., & Scott, M. A. (2011). Comparative clinical- and cost-effectiveness of candesartan and losartan in the management of hypertension and heart failure: A systematic review, meta- and cost-utility analysis. *International Journal of Clinical Practice, 65*(3), 253–263.

Hendrick, R. E., & Helvie, M. A. (2011). United States preventive services task force screening mammography recommendations: Science ignored. *American Journal of Roentgenology, 196*(2), W112–W116. Retrieved from http://www.ajronline.org/content/196/2/W112.abstract

Herman, W. H., Hoerger, T. J., Brandle, M., Hicks, K., Sorensen, S., Zhang, P., Hamman, R. F., Ackermann, R. T., Engelgau, M. M., Ratner, R. E., & Diabetes Prevention Program Research Group. (2005). The cost-effectiveness of lifestyle modification or metformin in preventing type 2 diabetes in adults with impaired glucose tolerance. *Annals of Internal Medicine, 142*(5), 323–332.

Hiscock, R., Judge, K., & Bauld, L. (2011). Social inequalities in quitting smoking: What factors mediate the relationship between socioeconomic position and smoking cessation? *Journal of Public Health, 33*(1), 39–47. http://jpubhealth.oxfordjournals.org/content/33/1/39.abstract.

Honjo, K., Tsutsumi, A., Kawachi, I., & Kawakami, N. (2006). What accounts for the relationship between social class and smoking cessation? Results of a path analysis. *Social Science & Medicine, 62*(2), 317–328. http://www.sciencedirect.com/science/article/pii/ S0277953605002935.

Kones, R. (2010). Rosuvastatin, inflammation, C-reactive protein, JUPITER, and primary prevention of cardiovascular disease—a perspective. *Drug Design Development and Therapy, 4*, 383–413.

Krumholz, H., Ross, J., & Egilman, D. (2007). What have we learnt from Vioxx? *BMJ, 334*, 120.

Lantz, P. M., Jacobson, P. D., Warner, K. E., Wasserman, J., Pollack, H. A., Berson, J., & Ahlstrom, A. (2000). Investing in youth tobacco control: A review of smoking prevention and control strategies. *Tobacco Control, 9*(1), 47–63. http://tobaccocontrol.bmj.com/ content/9/1/47.abstract.

Laupacis, A., Sackett, D. L., & Roberts, R. S. (1988). An assessment of clinically useful measures of the consequences of treatment. *New England Journal of Medicine, 318*(26), 1728–1733. Retrieved March 26, 2012, from: http://dx.doi.org/10.1056/NEJM198806303182605

Lazar, L. D., Pletcher, M. J., Coxson, P. G., Bibbins-Domingo, K., & Goldman, L. (2011). Cost-effectiveness of statin therapy for primary prevention in a low-cost statin era. *Circulation, 124*(2), 146–153.

Lee, C. D., Sui, X., Hooker, S. P., Hebert, J. R., & Blair, S. N. (2011). Combined impact of lifestyle factors on cancer mortality in men. *Annals of Epidemiology, 21*(10), 749–754.

Li, R., Zhang, P., Barker, L. E., Chowdhury, F. M., & Zhang, X. (2010). Cost-effectiveness of interventions to prevent and control diabetes mellitus: A systematic review. *Diabetes Care, 33*(8), 1872–1894.

Lupton, D. (1995). *The imperative of health. Public health and the regulated body.* London: Sage.

Manuel, D. G., Kwong, K., Tanuseputro, P., Lim, J., Mustard, C. A., Anderson, G. M., Ardal, S., Alter, D. A., & Laupacis, A. (2006). Effectiveness and efficiency of different guidelines on statin treatment for preventing deaths from coronary heart disease: Modelling study. *BMJ, 332*, 1419. http://www.ncbi.nlm.nih.gov/pmc/articles/PMC1479685/.

Marik, P. E., & Varon, J. (2009). Omega-3 dietary supplements and the risk of cardiovascular events: A systematic review. *Clinical Cardiology, 32*(7), 365–372.

Mason, J. (2012). Statin medications and increased risk for diabetes mellitus. What clinicians and patients need to know. Retrieved from http://www.medscape.com/viewarticle/756688

McBride, C. M., Emmons, K. M., & Lipkus, I. M. (2003). Understanding the potential of teachable moments: The case of smoking cessation. *Health Education Research, 18*(2), 156–170. http://her.oxfordjournals.org/content/18/2/156.abstract.

McCormack, V. A., & Boffetta, P. (2011). Today's lifestyles, tomorrow's cancers: Trends in lifestyle risk factors for cancer in low- and middle-income countries. *Annals of Oncology, 22*(11), 2349–2357.

McNeill, A., Lewis, S., Quinn, C., Mulcahy, M., Clancy, L., Hastings, G., & Edwards, R. (2011). Evaluation of the removal of point-of-sale tobacco displays in Ireland. *Tobacco Control, 20*(2), 137–143.

Mendez, M., Monteiro, C., & Popkin, B. (2005). Overweight exceeds underweight among women in most developing countries. *American Journal of Clinical Nutrition, 81*(3), 714–721.

Mitka, M. (2009). FDA exercises new authority to regulate tobacco products, but some limits remain. *The Journal of the American Medical Association, 302*(19), 2078–2081. http://jama.ama-assn.org/content/302/19/2078.short.

Mooney, J., Haw, S., & Frank, J. (2011). Interventions to tackle the obesogenic environment—focusing on adults of working age in Scotland. *Scottish Collaboration for Public Health Research & Policy: Edinburgh.* Retrieved from www.scphrp.ac.uk

Murray, C., & Lopez, A. (1997). Alternative projections of mortality and disability by cause 1990–2020: Global Burden of Disease Study. *Lancet, 349*(9064), 1498–1504.

Nairn, A. (2011). Children's well-being in UK, Sweden and Spain: The role of inequality and materialism. A qualitative study, IPSOS Mori. Retrieved January 8, 2012, from: http://www.unicef.org.uk/Documents/Publications/IPSOS_UNICEF_ChildWellBeingreport.pdf

Nandish, S., Wyatt, J., Bailon, O., Smith, M., Oliveros, R., & Chilton, R. (2011). Implementing cardiovascular risk reduction in patients with cardiovascular disease and diabetes mellitus. *The American Journal of Cardiology, 108*(Suppl 3), 42B–51B. http://www.sciencedirect.com/science/article/pii/S0002914911012161.

National Cholesterol Education Program. (2002). Detection, evaluation, and treatment of high blood cholesterol in adults (adult treatment panel III). Retrieved January 8, 2012, from: http://www.nhlbi.nih.gov/guidelines/cholesterol/atp3full.pdf

National Institute of Clinical Effectiveness (NICE). (2009). Guidance on smoking cessation in people at risk of dying prematurely. Retrieved January 8, 2012, from: http://guidance.nice.org.uk/PH15/QuickRefGuide/pdf/English

Naylor, C., Basinski, A., Frank, J., & Rachliss, M. (1990). Asymptomatic hypercholesterolaemia: A clinical policy review. *Journal Clinical Epidemiology, 43*, 1029–1121.

Ostry, A., & Frank, J. W. (2010). Was Thomas McKeown right for the wrong reasons? *Critical Public Health, 20*(2), 233–243.

Packer, C., Simpson, S., & Stevens, A. (2006). International diffusion of new health technologies: A ten-country analysis of six health technologies. *International Journal of Technology Assessment in Health Care, 22*(4), 419–428.

Parkin, D. M., Boyd, L., & Walker, L. C. (2011). The fraction of cancer attributable to lifestyle and environmental factors in the UK in 2010. *British Journal of Cancer, 105*(81), S77–S81.

Paynter, J., & Edwards, R. (2009). The impact of tobacco promotion at the point of sale: A systematic review. *Nicotine and Tobacco Research, 11*(1), 25–35.

Petersen, A., & Lupton, D. (1996). *The new public health. Health and self in the age of risk.* London: Sage.

Porter, R. (2002). A history of public health. King's fund lecture. Retrieved January 8, 2012, from: http://www.phn-bradford.nhs.uk/NR/rdonlyres/117ADE1F-4D4B-449C-BA2E-B56ABCF3F6F6/0/Ahistoryofpublichealth.pdf

Powlson, M. (2003). "Polypill" to fight cardiovascular disease: Universal polypharmacy goes against recent beliefs in prescribing practice. *British Medical Journal, 327*(807), 3.

Psaltopoulou, T., Ilias, I., & Alevizaki, M. (2010). The role of diet and lifestyle in primary, secondary, and tertiary diabetes prevention: A review of meta-analyses. *The Review of Diabetic Studies, 7*(1), 26–35.

Purshouse, R. C., Meier, P. S., Brennan, A., Taylor, K. B., & Rafia, R. (2010). Estimated effect of alcohol pricing policies on health and health economic outcomes in England: An epidemiological model. *Lancet, 375*(9723), 1355–1364.

Raffle, A., & Muir Gray, J. A. (2007). *Screening: Evidence and practice.* Oxford: Oxford University Press.

Rayner, G., & Lang, T. (2009). Obesity: Using the ecologic public health approach to overcome policy cacophony. In P. G. Kopelman, I. D. Caterson, & W. H. Dietz (Eds.), *Clinical obesity in adults and children* (3rd ed., pp. 452–470). Oxford: Wiley.

Rose, G. (1985). Sick individuals and sick populations. *International Journal of Epidemiology., 14*, 32–38.

Rose, G. (1992). *The strategy of preventive medicine.* Oxford: Oxford University Press.

Rosser, W., David, C., & Slawson, A. (1990). *Information mastery: Evidence-based family medicine* (Vol. 1). New York: BC Decker Inc.

Sattar, N., Preiss, D., Murray, H. M., Welsh, P., Buckley, BM., de Craen, AJ., et al. (2010). Statins and risk of incident diabetes: A collaborative meta-analysis of randomised statin trials. *Lancet.* Retrieved from http://dx.doi.org/10.1016/S0140-6736(09)61965-6

Schroder, F., et al. (2009). Screening and prostate-cancer mortality in a randomized European study. *New England Journal Medicine, 360*, 1320–1328.

Skrabenek, P. (1994). *Follies and fallacies in medicine.* UK: Prometheus Books.

Starfield, B. (2001). Basic concepts in population health and health care. *Journal of Epidemiology and Community Health, 55*(7), 452–454. http://jech.bmj.com/content/55/7/452.short.

The Guardian. (2011). Obesity and the NHS: People here are in big trouble. Retrieved January 8, 2012, from: http://www.guardian.co.uk/society/2011/jul/11/obesity-nhs-people-big-trouble

The Telegraph. (2012). Obese and smokers denied treatment "to save money." Retrieved January 8, 2012, from: http://www.telegraph.co.uk/health/healthnews/9127486/Obese-and-smokers-denied-treatment-to-save-money.html

Thomas, S., Fayter, D., Misso, K., Ogilvie, D., Petticrew, M., Sowden, A., Whitehead, M., & Worthy, G. (2008). Population tobacco control interventions and their effects on social inequalities in smoking: Systematic review. *Tobacco Control, 17*, 230–237. doi:10.1136/tc.2007.023911.

Thornton, H., Edwards, A., & Baum, M. (2003). Women need better information about routine mammography. *BMJ, 327*(7406), 101–103.

Tobacco Free Kids. (2009). Deadly in pink: Big tobacco steps up its targeting of women and girls. Retrieved January 8, 2012, from: http://www.rwjf.org/files/research/20090218deadlyinpink.pdf

Tucker, D. M., & Palmer, A. J. (2011). The cost-effectiveness of interventions in diabetes: A review of published economic evaluations in the UK setting, with an eye on the future. *Primary Care Diabetes, 5*(1), 9–17.

Turner, D., Steinhart, A. H., & Griffiths, A. M. (2007). Omega 3 fatty acids (fish oil) for maintenance of remission in ulcerative colitis. *Cochrane Database of Systematic Reviews,* (3), CD006443.

UK Faculty of Public Health. (2011). Press release March 15, 2011. Available from http://www.fph.org.uk/uk_faculty_of_public_health_rejects_alcohol_pledges

US Preventive Services Task Force. (2009). Screening for breast cancer: U.S. preventive services task force recommendation statement. *Annals of Internal Medicine., 151*(10), 716–726. http://www.annals.org/content/151/10/716.abstract.

Vandermeer, M. L., Thomas, A. R., Kamimoto, L., Reingold, A., Gershman, K., Meek, J., Farley, M. M., Ryan, P., Lynfield, R., Baumbach, J., Schaffner, W., Bennett, N., & Zansky, S. (2012). Association between use of statins and mortality among patients hospitalized with laboratory-confirmed influenza virus infections: A multistate study. *Journal of Infectious Diseases., 205*(1), 13–19.

Villanti, A. C., McKay, H. S., Abrams, D. B., Holtgrave, D. R., & Bowie, J. V. (2010). Smoking-cessation interventions for US young adults: A systematic review. *American Journal of Preventive Medicine, 39*(6), 564–574. http://www.sciencedirect.com/science/article/pii/S0749379710004757.

Wald, N., & Law, M. (2003). A strategy to reduce cardiovascular disease by more than 80 %. *British Medical Journal, 326*, 1419–1424.

WHO. (2011). Global status report on non communicable diseases 2010. Description of the global burden of NCDs, their risk factors and determinants. Retrieved January 8, 2012, from: http://www.who.int/nmh/publications/ncd_report2010/en/

Woods, R. K., Thien, F. C., & Abramson, M. J. (2002). Dietary marine fatty acids (fish oil) for asthma in adults and children. *Cochrane Database of Systematic Reviews,* (3), CD001283.

Yusef, S., Hawkens, S., Ôunpuu, S., Dans, T., & Avezum, A. (2004). Effect of potentially modifiable risk factors associated with myocardial infarction in 52 countries (the INTERHEART study): Case-control study. *Lancet, 364*(9438), 937–952.

Current and Future Theoretical Foundations for NCDs and Health Promotion

Thomas Abel and David V. McQueen

Introduction: The Burden of Noncommunicable Diseases

The UN General Assembly in September 2011 recognized at the highest levels the global challenge of noncommunicable diseases (NCDs) for the globe. This recognition, long in coming, was in part the result of considerable efforts over the past two decades to make the global public health community and the public aware to the huge global disease burden of NCDs and the lack of sustainable capacity to address these burdens in most countries. Loss of quality of life in individuals and reduced capacities of social development in whole populations are related to the burden of NCDs. Globally, the economic impact of NCDs has been estimated to be staggering over the next 20 years, according to a recent Harvard/World Economic Forum study (Bloom et al. 2011). "The evidence gathered is compelling. Over the next 20 years, NCDs will cost more than US$30 trillion, representing 48 % of global GDP in 2010, and pushing millions of people below the poverty line. Mental health conditions alone will account for the loss of an additional US$16.1 trillion over this time span, with dramatic impact on productivity and quality of life."

The Need for Health-Promoting Interventions

Despite this dire prediction there are also compelling arguments of proven interventions at the population level that could alleviate this burden impact and set a course for all nations to better address NCDs. Many public health practitioners have long recognized the need to change health-related behaviors and health systems. In particular there are those calling for addressing some primary disease-related risk factors such as tobacco use, unhealthy diet, physical inactivity, and harmful use of alcohol. Increasingly there are those calling for system-level changes and attention to the underlying social and political factors that are related to NCDs. Both within the biomedical world as well as in civil society there are those who argue for a health promotion approach to those causal aspects that are deeply embedded in the fabric of society, and related to causes that lie largely outside the health sector, such as the way we live and work, public policies, private sector forces, and environmental factors. Finally, increasing attention across all sectors is being aimed at issues of equity and social justice and how they relate to health and illness of populations.

T. Abel (✉)
Division of Social and Behavioural Health Research, Institute of Social and Preventive Medicine, University of Berne, Niesenweg 6, 3012 Bern, Switzerland
e-mail: abel@ispm.unibe.ch

D.V. McQueen
2418 Midvale Court, Tucker, GA 30084, USA

The Need for Theory

In recent years there has been recognition of the need for a theory that considers NCDs and health promotion in the context of modernity (McQueen and Kickbusch 2007). While the burden of NCDs is now recognized as well as the need to have active health promotion efforts to reduce it, what is lacking is a sound theoretical base that addresses how the causes of NCDs and the ways to change these causes relate to each other in terms of their complex relationship. It is not that we lack any number of theoretical insights to inform many components of this complexity; it is that we lack a sound theoretical base for linking the etiological arguments to the theories to change the causes. We need a theoretical base to deal with highly dynamic processes that link the social to the biological. We need to incorporate theories that line structure and agency, risks and resources, and description to intervention. As the conditions of NCDs are largely social, an appropriate theoretical perspective is societal and starts with the social, and brings in the nonsocial in order to arrive at a basis for interventions in the contexts in which health is produced. The problem is that we do not have many extant social theories to explain or illuminate NCDs and as we show later in this chapter, there is no theory of NCDs that adequately explains the social. Even more challenging, there is to date very little theoretical guidance available which helps to move from explanation to intervention.

Definition(s) of Health

There are many definitions of NCDs or noncommunicable disease and these are covered well in several chapters of this book; however "health" is trickier to define and is challenging theoretically. Of course there is the well-cited WHO definition from the Preamble to the Constitution of the World Health Organization as adopted by the International Health Conference, New York, 19–22 June 1946, signed on 22 July 1946 by the representatives of 61 States and entered into force on 7 April 1948, that states "Health is a state of complete physical, mental and social well-being and not merely the absence of disease or infirmity." This definition has not been amended since 1948 and despite its widespread use the controversy on a definition of health continues (Huber et al. 2011; Shilton et al. 2011).

A significant problem conceptually is that health is often defined by what it apparently is not. Thus there are statements that mix disease occurrence, disability, death, and health (Krieger 2011). In fact there is a mixture in the literature of terms such as "well-being," "positive health," as well as negative health terms such as ill health and premature morbidity. Our approach applies a broad conceptualization of health reaching beyond a particular physical or mental status and addressing the bodily, social, and mental means and conditions which human beings need to enjoy a good quality of life, to achieve their full capacity and allowing them to positively contribute to and benefit from their social contexts they live in. Furthermore, from a public health perspective health as a concept does not just belong to the individual, but exists and is addressed at the population level (cf. Chap. 1).

From a health promotion point of view the International Union of Health Promotion and Education defines health more broadly:

> Health is a basic human need. It is fundamental to the successful functioning of individuals and of societies. Health promotion aims to empower people to control their own health by gaining control over the underlying factors that influence health. The main determinants of health are people's cultural, social, economic and environmental living conditions, and the social and personal behaviors that are strongly influenced by those conditions. (IUHPE 2007).

Epidemiology as a Basis of NCD Research

In general NCD research has depended on epidemiological methodologies rather than explicit theories. But even without an explicit theory all approaches resting on epidemiology have implicit ideas about disease and causation that help define the variables used to describe causal factors. Thus, if only implicit, a fundamental theory of causation operates as a guiding perspective. Related to this is a discussion of theory and causation found in Chap. 3 of this monograph and in the excellent summation of epidemiological theory by Nancy Krieger (2011). In any case, it can be asserted that much of epidemiological theory is based on a methodological approach that rests on the underlying philosophical logic of experimental science. Further it can be noted that the search for a more profound theory of epidemiology has been enhanced in recent years by the concern with the so-called social determinants of disease and the role of social factors in health and illness. However, it is also safe to assert that few epidemiologists have looked to the writings of social scientists and health promoters as sources for a theoretical underpinning. It remains for historians of public health in the future to tease out how theory has developed in the field of epidemiology over the past few decades.

With regard to NCDs, the work and report by the WHO Commission on the Social Determinants of Health have spurred attention on NCDs, their causal origins, and most notably the so-called causes of the causes (WHOCSDOH 2008). In reality it has regenerated an interest in the causal role of social factors in disease etiology that was at the center of public health at the time of Virchow: a time when many conceptualized public health as a political science, a concept that was, with the emergence of infectious disease theory and the rise of the hygiene movement, eclipsed for much of the twentieth century. The more recent biomedical and clinical perspectives greatly affected global public health in both the academy and in governmental institutions. As a result, studies by social scientists, epidemiologists, and other public health professionals into the social aspects of health and disease have been marginalized institutionally and in terms of resources. It also meant that any theoretical discussion regarding possible social aspects would also be marginalized. It does not mean, however, that there was not some developmental work on social factors and theory.

The Limitations of Established Theories in NCD

Most of today's NCD research data are based on epidemiological studies, i.e., grounded in "theories of disease distribution" (Krieger 2011, p. 30). They are primarily produced to determine NCDs' incidence and prevalence rates and as such they are helpful for targeting public health interventions focused on risk and harm reduction. At the same time, most approaches to NCD research to date also show particular features in their theoretical foundations that significantly limit the usefulness of their data. This holds true especially for those approaches that strive to assess and eventually intervene on the role of social conditions determining to large degrees the unequal distribution of NCDs on the population level. There are three major limitations of this approach.

The first major limitation is the *focus on the individual*. The concept of NCDs derives fundamentally from biomedicine and the assumptions of biomedical practice; at the heart of that medicine is the patient and the disease. A central focus of Western medicine are fundamental assumptions of causality, environment, and the individual as a patient; thus it is not surprising that most of today's NCD approaches focus on risk "expositions of individuals." We would note here that risk is itself a notion, and within the biomedical approach, every individual has the risk of obtaining every disease—this is especially the case for NCDs where almost every human alive will sooner or later be classified bio-medically as having one of the NCDs. Those approaches operate on a guiding perspective that includes some specific underlying assumptions: The focus in this perspective is on individuals and ultimately on what is happening to and inside the human body. Trying to understand the complex disease processes inside the human body requires application of bioscience models and methods. Those are based on distinct assumptions, e.g., about strict causalities and dose–response relationships. Many of those assumptions are limiting (even incompatible) with the state of the art in social science understanding of the complexities and dynamics prevailing in the social world. Given its logical matters of interest and with the ultimate criterion (i.e., diseases) being biological in nature established theories of NCDs provide a particular focus on where and how we search for answers. The risk concept considers the risk of exposure to a causal factor that arises because of actions and conditions on the individual level. And even if some of the answers are thought to be found in the social only those parts of the social will be studied which show causal relationships to the medical biological matter of interest, leaving the researcher blind for central aspects in NCDs such as noncausal factors in the context or multidimensional consequences of chronic diseases. Much of this underlying perspective confers to the established concept of humans as "hosts," a concept in which the biological "agent" is studied as playing the only (or at least the ultimately decisive) active part. A logical consequence stemming from this focus is that public health interventions should either control (or at least manage) the activity of that agent in a given environment or protect the human host against that biological agent.

To study individuals as "being risk exposed" pays attention to humans primarily in their definition of (more or less) passive recipients of something negative that happens to them beyond their control. Thus the part on the side of the individual is often reduced to being a "carrier of risks." The fact that people actively manage their lives, including health issues, does not receive particular attention, nor do questions on how people do that. And, with little interest in the individual as a social being and social actor, this perspective promotes a further neglect of social context factors in many current public health approaches to NCDs.

Historically this means a shift from classical public health, which especially in the ninetieth century placed much attention on the social. This tradition lasted long in the efforts of "social medicine" throughout the early twentieth century. Over the last century however, a particular epidemiological focus has led to more and more precise measures of risk assessment relevant for

the biological-pathological processes inside the individual body (Susser and Susser 1996). Unfortunately, much less attention was allocated to the analysis of the social factors and processes involved (cf. Chap. 6).

Indeed, late-twentieth-century and present-day public health approaches to NCDs pay less attention to the contextual factors relevant for the incidence and prevalence of NCDs and concentrate on describing the behavioral risks found in the population. Often contextual conditions are either completely ignored or merely understood as confounding factors that should be statistically "controlled." Both approaches lead to an underutilization of the potential explanatory power of NCD models and to limited applicability in public health interventions.

A similar "under-attention" can be observed when it comes to mediating and moderating effects of contextual factors such as community characteristics, infrastructures, and social support. These types of factors are often assumed to be important background variables but their effects on the occurrence of a certain risk factor and on the relative strength of its effect on a health outcome are not included in the models. Instead they are seen as not directly measurable in the individual and thus treated as negligible. However, those are important factors in the explanatory models needed for a more comprehensive understanding to guide public health and health promotion interventions.

The second major limitation is the *focus on disease and risk of disease*—not on health and health resources. With this focus, there are at least two additional conceptual limitations reducing the explanatory and intervention-guiding power of many current bio-medically based NCD approaches.

1. Their guiding interest in (ultimately) understanding the occurrence and distribution of diseases has led most of today's NCD research to focus on risk factors and negative health outcomes (mortality, morbidity) and at the same time neglect positive health (see our definition of health above). This can be seen as too limited in two respects: First, NCDs are

often chronic diseases with an increasing number of people living longer periods in their life with both illness and health. This health part needs attention as well in public health approaches to NCDs, because positive health is interrelated to chronic conditions through health practices and resources needed for more health and better human development. A second aspect relates to the fact that many NCD-relevant behaviors (e.g., drinking, smoking) are practiced for other than risk reasons and often linked to an emphasis on their positive outcomes such as well-being, social engagement, enjoyment, and personal development. In point of fact many of these so-called individual risk factors are practiced in a social context and could be considered in that form a social factor—such as eating as a family, drinking in a sport club, and smoking as a rite-of-passage phenomena. Current approaches to NCDs have not dealt with those aspects.

2. Their guiding focus on illness not only applies to their outcome measures but also directs and limits the explanatory side of their models to pathogenic factors. As a consequence NCD risk exposure models are quite limited when it comes to observing the resources for health and health practices (e.g., income, social support). And even if they include resources at all (e.g., "education"), risk exposure approaches often run on the implicit assumption that resource factors are sufficiently considered and measured by defining and observing the "lack of a particular resource" as a risk factor. This approach is based on the implicit assumption that it makes little or no difference if one thinks of, e.g., poor education as a risk factor or higher education as a resource. Void of any explicit theoretical consideration it "technically" transforms resources into risk factors. Being primarily interested in negative health outcomes (mortality, morbidity) those studies have then consequently included (low) education as a risk factor, which certainly does not cover the full meaning of education for health status and

health practices. Being focused on illness and disease, obviously, the risk factor approach leaves little room for conceptualizing resources and to subsequently develop a better understanding of the mechanisms through which resources (education, money, social support, etc.) become effective in human action, i.e., for people to improve their health.

The third major limitation is a *focus on linear causal thinking*. Most models that have been developed to understand the causalities involved in disease and health outcomes are linear. That is, health and disease are conceptualized as outcomes and as the end point of a process that begins with variables that are attained or inherited by the individual during his/her life course. The one-way linearity is explicit in that having one of the NCDs does not cause the risk behavior or the social factor that precedes the attainment of the bio-medically defined disease condition. This is a very limited view of causality that will be discussed in detail in the following chapter.

While more can be said on the individual-oriented approaches to NCDs, this brief discussion can help to understand the roots of some of its important limitations: current public health approaches to NCDs tend to be built on a paradigm of the "risk-exposed individual." A model of individuals as hosts of medically relevant processes shapes their prevailing focus. Individuals are studied as carriers of risk while their role as social actors and coproducers of health is mostly ignored. With a disease (as a bio-medically defined condition) as the starting point for the search for explanations and with disease reduction as the ultimate evaluation criteria for successful public health interventions, (positive) health and its resources receive only minor attention. With their subsequently poorly developed concepts and measurement of contextual factors, those approaches are not likely to provide appropriate data for an approach to NCDs that could fully account for the social context factors and human social action that are, however, crucial in both explanations of and interventions in NCDs at a population level.

Social Epidemiology and the Social Determinants of Health: More Recent Developments

Social epidemiology introduces social factors into epidemiological models; to this end it aims to integrate social thinking into a perspective ultimately concerned with biomedical outcomes (i.e., occurrence of disease). Such outcomes are postulated to be unequally distributed across (sub)populations and when such populations can be meaningfully defined and characterized by some social properties the link to the social is established. The more recent social determinants of health (SDOH) approach is a good example of attempts to advance in a direction by giving increasing attention to the social causes of diseases including NCDs. It uses empirical evidence to argue convincingly that the "causes of the causes" need to be addressed and that those causes are basically social in nature. In terms of health outcome measures the SDOH approach looks mostly at mortality and morbidity to make the case that these are unequally distributed within and across societies. It also argues that the inequalities in the causes and consequences are to be considered unfair and generally avoidable, i.e., inequitable.

Another approach to questions on the unequal distribution of health more recently developed is Nancy Krieger's eco-social theory of disease distribution (Krieger 2011). Based on 6 core propositions it presents an advanced social epidemiological approach towards understanding the complex conditions and processes that determine population health levels. It aims to overcome the earlier somewhat limited understanding of embodiment processes (how social conditions "get under the skin" … or become "biologically embedded" and argues instead that embodiment "is far more active and reciprocal … our bodily engagement (soma and psyche combined), individually and collectively, with the biophysical world and each other" (p. 222). The eco-social theory also stresses the importance of contextual conditions of this embodiment by recognizing that "socially-structured causal links between exposures and outcomes can vary over time and place …" (p. 216). Without going into any elaborate account of the eco-social theory we observe here that it brings in more social factors than ever, aims at integrating different societal levels, and refers to the importance of the social and historical context for understanding the production and distribution of population health. Yet, it does not provide a systematic account on the key role of context not only for embodiment of social factors but also for any processes relevant for health including those that lead to the societal conditions directly or indirectly affecting health, its production, and distribution. And unfortunately not much has followed yet, from the eco-social theory's suggestion to include more comprehensive measures of context, social factors, and agency in the current epidemiological models.

Both the SDOH and the eco-social theory have opened up NCD-relevant research to the inclusion of more social factors by adding these to the epidemiological paradigm in an attempt to explain the distribution of diseases across time and space. Both approaches have pushed this perspective further and argue for social causes; as a consequence this perspective calls for political action. However, from a theoretical perspective the social epidemiological perspective presents a blessing and a curse at the same time: while stressing the social it remains heavy reliant on bio-medically based epidemiological principles with the typical consequence that only those factors and processes which can be causally linked to a bio-medically defined condition are admitted in explanatory models. With restrictions like these the social epidemiological perspective does not and cannot account for the complex social processes involved in risk and resource distribution. Even for the SDOH and the eco-social approaches the pathology perspective still functions as an anchor, allowing and in fact requiring the approach to keep its focus on medically relevant outcomes. The price is of course that all (social) extensions of the epidemiological model are bound back to its basic paradigm and particular methods (such as excluding those dynamics not causally related to a medical condition). The fact that the scientific basis (empirical data in particular) of both approaches is mainly provided by the knowledge about risk factor distributions with the meaning of social context in a secondary role and only vaguely understood makes them a good representation of the limits of those approaches which rely strongly on epidemiology and lack a broader theoretical foundation.

Because the "fundamental causes" (Link and Phelan 1995) of the unequal distribution of diseases refer to not medical but to social problems a comprehensive solution is unlikely to be found in the knowledge about medically defined outcomes linked to a corporeal body, but instead in the social processes that precede them and that may follow from them. Thus social-based answers to the above question on the bodily consequences of social conditions will be more likely to provide sufficient answers for public health action and provide some important contributions to research needed on the more comprehensive public health questions such as the following: How do societies create the social, economic, and cultural conditions that make up for large parts of the unequal distribution of health in populations? If it is social change that we think is needed to improve the health of populations, then we need better social theories and better ways to integrate social epidemiological knowledge into social theories about the production and distribution of health.

The approach of this chapter in the context of this book is to provide starting points for this integration by offering a perspective in which epidemiologically based knowledge on NCDs becomes part of a social science framework and is linked to health promotion theory and action to connect this body of knowledge more directly to action for social change (cf. our own definition of health below).

Those theoretical observations also have potential consequences for NCD-monitoring systems aiming at the collection of meaningful and public health-relevant data. In light of the critical appraisal above on the limitations of individual focused models, we argue that in fact, approaches which focus on the social patterning of health resources would appear more appropriate for the monitoring of health inequalities and the social

determinants of health as was earlier called for by the WHO *Commission* in 2008 (WHOCSDOH 2008). While the Commission's call has produced more requests and further action towards producing individual longitudinal data (e.g., cohort studies) we have also described above that individual-focused data have their severe limitations with respect to their relevance for timely interventions into the social conditions of health. Consequently, here we argue for new approaches to the social determinants of health with a clear focus on contextual information and social resources for health.

A Life Course Theoretical Perspective

Recent reports by the US National Academy of Sciences imply the need for a different theoretical approach, one that takes a lifelong view of social context (NRC/IOM 2013). Although the life course perspective owes its origins largely to demography, the social sciences, and biology it is not entirely new to epidemiology (Kuh et al. 2003). Today there are increasing calls for individual longitudinal data that focuses on measures of illness and contextual risks. Moreover, many of those interested in NCD inequalities today have a keen interest to include measures of social determinants of health in life course studies. But while longitudinal individual data are helpful to identify potentially harmful social conditions and give insight into causal pathways, when it comes to the social patterns (and "patterning") of health we cannot rely on data that rest only on individual life histories. Instead, data are needed that can show how the social conditions for NCDs, health, and health practices develop over time at the population, not individual, level. For obvious reasons, data that measure changes in the same individuals over time can—at best—provide only limited answers to questions on the structural contextual conditions and how they change over time.

Moreover, some of the questions we want to answer in the field of NCDs cannot be answered at all with individual longitudinal data. Many of their shortcomings are related to the fact that these studies have to wait for the health consequences to become observable in the human body and must rely on a retrospective confirmation to determine the relevance of the social conditions. That is because of the causal linear model that underlies the field—if this model is applied one has to wait—there is no way to look back. Here we list three problems most relevant for our search for better NCD approaches: (1) data from individual longitudinal observations are too time-lagged to be useful for NCD monitoring. Of course the NCDs themselves can be observed longitudinally without any problem because they are physical entities and the vessel, the individual, which carries them is irrelevant. If in public health however, we want to intervene (a) early and (b) on the social conditions of health than we need data that detects early onset of the changes in the conditions relevant for health (e.g., on changes in urban environment relevant for mental health through increasing social exclusion). The typical individual longitudinal data on the over-time consequences of risk exposure in human bodies would be of no use for monitoring social conditions of NCD and health, because by the time the associations are scientifically estab-lished the damage to the health of the population has already been done; (2) those data rarely tell us about the contextual conditions of health, e.g., if the social determinants of health themselves have changed over time, e.g., have become more frequent or may have disappeared (e.g., the num-ber of playgrounds for kids in a city); (3) they do not tell us if the factors which are (retrospectively) found to be causally related to a certain outcome (a risk factor, a health practice, or health status) would have the same or similar effect in another context, in another culture, etc.; a question, how-ever, that is key when acknowledging that chang-ing contexts may lead to significant alterations of mediating factors in causal relationships between a risk factor (or a resource) and a particular health outcome. Consequently, any attempts to use longi-tudinal individual data for public health monitor-ing are likely to lose sight of the overtime social changes at the structural level which (by defini-tion) ought to be targeted in structurally oriented public health interventions.

Interim Summary

In sum there remain some serious theoretical limitations in the life course perspectives and in any primarily epidemiology-based approaches when they are applied to the social aspects related to health and in particular to those related to strat-egies for changing the social causes and conse-quences of health. Moreover, it is not just that this perspective is poorly equipped on the side of the social explanations; the problem goes deeper: the epidemiological perspective rests on and starts out with a biomedical definition of the initial problem, and as such narrows down, limits, and potentially even misdirects the search for social explanations. The same focus often applies to the evaluation criteria for public health interventions, e.g., when the definition of success is ultimately limited to changes in the prevalence and incidence rates. With this dominance of the biomedical one might even say that in this approach the social is "theoretically subordinated." Even social epidemi-ology that takes a rather broad approach to factors impacting on disease distribution (e.g., Krieger 2011) and its social "causes" still looks for social causes for medical problems and this focus nar-rows any consecutive theoretical reasoning and empirical investigation. In brief the approach taken is looking back, from the diseases to see what is the purported origin of them and at assumptions carried back about these particular illnesses (outcome). Fundamentally these assumptions are drawn from their basic a priori base in biology, chemistry, and physics.

In a social science-based theory of NCD causa-tion we do not make assumptions from the so-called disease outcomes; instead theory is driven from the social not from the biomedical. The sec-ond major difference is that we do not make the assumption that the biomedical outcome is any more important than many other outcomes. As a consequence we argue that there is a need for a theoretical perspective that is not rooted in the "risk exposure" paradigm. Further it cannot be a theory that simply adds on the social. The social must be an inherent fundamental concept within the theory. Further, the natural sciences are no more primary in the design than the social sciences. This of course will allow for the development of both a different understanding of causality necessary for work in NCDs and health promotion and the ability to broaden the narrow evidence base used to date. Only if we can open up and allow the social to be the matter of primary interest, incorporating biomedical knowledge where needed, can we adequately address the challenges of NCDs in public health. This social science-based approach allows new questions, questions addressing issues of (a) health (not reduced to disease reduction) in its social contexts (rather than controlled for contextual effects) as the determining perspective, (b) social resources and conditions (not just illness risk factors) as the issue we need to understand for our public health/health promotion interventions, (c) nonlinear reciprocal relationships (not "consecutive" causality) among the factors involved in the reproduction of the social patterns of health practices, and (d) complexity in structure–agency dynamics (instead of explanations dividing structure and behaviors).

Established Theories in Health Promotion

While there have been many publications in the field of health promotion since the adoption of the 1986 Ottawa Charter for Health Promotion, there has been little systematic attempt to examine the theoretical knowledge that the post-Ottawa field of health promotion builds on. It is not simply that health promotion as a field of practice tends to regard theory as less important than taking action; it is also partly due to the fact that health promotion sees itself as multidisciplinary and draws from a wide range of disciplines, in particular the social sciences. Very few health promotion practitioners have the time or the opportunity to study the whole scope of theoretical insight that has led to the development of health promotion. In addition, as we have noted, there is a tendency in public health to underestimate (and frequently ignore) fields of knowledge that do not concur with the ruling paradigm and the methods of scientific exploration accepted

by the biomedical community. The often seen conflict between the natural and the social sciences is particularly common with regard to health promotion practice.

Nonetheless, the list of major theoretical thinkers whose work has helped shape the health promotion approach is impressive indeed. It encompasses classics like Emile Durkheim and Max Weber, Hannah Arendt and Marie Jahoda, Niklas Luhmann and Anthony Giddens, Pierre Bourdieux and Paolo Freire, and Gregory Bateson and Thomas Luckmann to name but some of them. Their theoretical contributions lie in the understanding of the construction and organization of everyday life, the interaction between individuals and their environments, the understanding of policy making and the role of social movements, the social construction of risk, the meaning of culture, and finally the meaning of health itself as a social and cultural construct.

It would be difficult to list all the major theoretical currents that have impacted the development of health promotion in the past half century. There are, however, certain key theoretical threads that have been developed and used during this time. A detailed discussion of some of these theoretical threads is given in Chap. 22 of this book. The following summary is illustrative of some of the key theoretical notions that have influenced the field.

One influential theory source for health promotion stemmed from the notion of health in everyday life, or what is sometimes termed the sociology of everyday life. This is a wide area of social science application with many prominent contributors. Among the components of this line of theoretical thinking are theories of symbolic interactionism, dramaturgy, phenomenology, and ethnomethodology. Representative of this work is that of Goffman (1959). A second important theoretical foundation for health promotion comes from much of the developmental work in health education. Much of this concerns the shaping of individual health behaviors, behavioral theory, and individual–environment interaction. This is a large area of work, but perhaps best represented by the work of Prochaska and DiClemente (1984) and others in the development of the transtheoretical model and in the work of Green et al. (1980)

in the precede–proceed model. These approaches remain widely used in health education and health promotion research and practice. A third source of theory came from the development of the theory of salutogenesis by Antonovsky (1979). This is an approach that focuses on human health and well-being, rather than on disease. More specifically, the "salutogenic model" looks at the relationship between health, stress, and coping. It remains an active field of research in contemporary health promotion, notably in northern Europe. Work on well-being and happiness is a continuation of this theoretical trend (cf. http://www.ophi.org. uk/wp-content/uploads/OPHI-RP-37a.pdf). A fourth theoretical source for health promotion relates to health promotion research on settings. Stimulated greatly by research and interest in school health, this area draws from a broad array of theories related to institutions as well as child development. In addition it moves theoretically to broader aspects of settings that relate to the workplace, the community, and some general concepts of institutions as a place to link health promotion theory and practice (Poland et al. 2001; Dooris 2006). A fifth theoretically rich area concerns issues of empowerment and learning. Stemming in part from theoretical writings of Brazilian educational philosopher Paulo Freire as well as many others, this area presents a perspective that is particularly well developed in health promotion in Latin America (Potvin and McQueen 2008; Wallerstein 1988). A sixth theoretically influential area has been that of social action theory. Although many Americans may resonate with Talcott Parsons, The *Structure of Social Action* (1937), as a key source for this theoretical perspective, it has deeper roots in the works of Max Weber and in the twentieth-century writings on systems theory by Niklas Luhmann (1964). Although many contemporary health promoters may not explicitly state this perspective, the underlying notion that social action theory stresses the ability of individuals to shape social meaning and social behavior is a powerful component in health promotion thinking. Nonetheless, within this perspective there is always a challenging interplay between structure, systems, and individual behavior and how these relate to each other

(cf. Abel and Frohlich 2012). The increasing complexity of the theoretical underpinnings revealed in this thinking introduces a seventh emerging theoretical concept underpinning modern health promotion, and that is complexity. This notion is discussed in more detail in Chap. 22 and in the book *Health and Modernity* (McQueen and Kickbusch 2007). Finally, an eighth critical theoretical source, arising notably after the 1986 Ottawa Charter (WHO 1986), comes from theoretical thinking within the field of political science. This is, namely, the whole area of policy theory, institutional theory, and the role of governance. These theoretical notions are discussed in more detail in Chap. 26 on policy and governance. It is arguable that many other sources of theory for health promotion could be listed, but the point here is that while health promotion has relatively little direct discussion of theory, primarily because it is an area of action and practice above all, there is a wealth of underlying theoretical assumptions that guide the work of the field.

Unifying NCDs and Health Promotion: A Social Science Approach in Public Health

NCDs pose major challenges to the functioning of modern societies. Public health is called upon to suggest appropriate responses to this challenge. Any promising interventions should be based on comprehensive knowledge about the problem to be solved. But understanding NCDs, their causes, and consequences is a horrendous task. Until today, the knowledge base in the NCD area is considerably limited with most of it based on descriptive data on the distribution of NCDs over time and space, across and within populations. This knowledge, mostly generated through the application of biomedical thinking and epidemiological methodologies, allows fairly accurate estimates of the prevalence and incidence rates and is as such useful to suggest when and where to intervene. The limitations of those contributions, however, arise from their fare reaching neglect of social context factors crucial for any health promotion intervention beyond the individual level.

As a consequence current NCD approaches seem to lag behind from what has been called the "third revolution" in health promotion (Breslow 2004), i.e., the "shift from individual behavioural change to a focus on the social context of health and on the levers of societal change" (cf. Carroll 2012, p. 37). In fact, the major societal forces that are at the roots of the conditions of NCD and which determine the range of option and define the ways in which NCDs are to be dealt with (i.e., public health) cannot be explained with knowledge generated within the paradigm of biomedicine or derived from approaches that rely on biomedical definitions of the core matter. What is needed therefore in NCD public health research and practice are approaches that can appropriately account for the social context factors and the role of the active individual.

As there is no medical solution in sight to stop the rise of NCDs, public health measures on NCD ought to focus on the social conditions and intervene basically in the social realm. In order to do this successfully and to best marshal the collective field of present-day public health we need to (1) understand the social context in which the distributions occur, a task requiring the application of sound social science theory; (2) describe the distributions of NCDs in and across different contexts, a task requiring sophisticated epidemiological modeling; and (3) apply the combined knowledge on the social conditions and distributions of NCDs in systematic public health interventions into the contextual conditions relevant for NCDs, a task requiring a comprehensive health promotion framework.

To achieve progress in this direction, obviously new theories and methodologies spanning across disciplines are needed. Those theories need to better account for the dialectic between theoretical and methodological concerns and should aid NCD studies with respect to key challenges in their epistemology (how can we know) and methodology (e.g., the selection of appropriate, meaningful methods for acquiring this knowledge) (Carroll 2012, p. 34).

Respective future work can draw on three existing bodies of knowledge: (ad 1) knowledge on social action and the social functioning of a

society and its institutions including the social conditions relevant for NCDs. Applying a social science paradigm (theories from sociology, political sciences) should allow one to study and understand better the societal contexts in which NCDs and health emerge. Social epidemiology and demography are well equipped for mapping NCDs in and across societies, taking into account its most basic structural conditions.

Knowledge and Methodologies on the Practice of Social Change for Health

Much of this can be drawn from definitions, concepts, principles, and practical experience in health promotion. Health promotion (as framed in the Ottawa Charter) is focused on actions towards improving the conditions, social and behavioral, for health including those most relevant for NCDs. Therefore health promotion appears appropriately equipped to define the starting points for interventions on the social conditions and to evaluate respective NCD public health interventions.

Unfortunately until today, neither the social sciences nor epidemiology nor health promotion provide a theory base apt to a straightforward coalesce of the three approaches. The need is to suggest some starting points for a new and more comprehensive approach. This new approach should allow us first (a) to define the challenge of NCDs and health as basically a social problem, then (b) bring in epidemiology as well as other empirical approaches to observe and monitor the distribution of the medically defined outcomes as well as to provide more of the NCD-relevant social data, and, finally, (c) draw on health promotion's expertise on how to change the social conditions for health.

There are key substantive and methodological issues a social science-based approach to NCDs and health should and can address. Perhaps the most fundamental among them is the definition of health. On that we claim that population health is a social issue which, in a health promotion perspective, cannot be reduced to an individual-oriented perspective nor sufficiently dealt with on the basis of definitions which originate from the question on what pathology applies inside the human body, even if next to biological also psychological and social risk factors are included. Instead what is in health promotion defined as health and illness is ultimately dependent on the value systems of a society. The conditions and distribution patterns, the perception of the problem, and actions taken by a society all indicate that population health issues including those on NCDs are inherently social in nature.

Accepting the proposition of health as inherently social two major theoretical challenges arise, the question of the role of "context" and the "active human being" as part of the NCD challenge. A social science approach can, so we claim, deal with both substantive challenges in a fruitful way. In terms of methodology we suggest here to focus on issues around complexity, causality, and dynamic associations (cf. Chap. 3) and offer some clues as to what the contributions of social science could be.

Context as a Frame of Reference

Contextual conditions can and need to be part of any models of NCDs and health. Advanced epidemiological approaches acknowledge the importance of context emphasizing that "understanding disease distribution requires analyzing it in dynamic context" (Krieger 2011; p. 216). In most NCD approaches however, if considered at all, context is included as a descriptive variable (e.g., "nation") or studied as an ensemble or a pattern of risk exposures (e.g., "poor neighborhood"). Yet, given its paramount importance ranging from the definition of the problem to its description and understanding to the models on where and how to intervene, there is an obvious need to develop a new approach to the meaning of context in NCD research and practice (cf. Chap. 6).

In social science "context" is an analytical concept of primary importance, basically referring to the circumstances and dynamics of social actions incl. those relevant for health. Applied to NCDs context can comprise a set of conditional factors that can, e.g., moderate or mediate the

effects of certain risk factors and resources on a health outcome. For example, the effects of education on health seem to be stronger under conditions of financial deprivation (Mirowsky and Ross 2003; Lahelma et al. 2004) and the effects found between income and health inequality may be different for people with high or low educational achievements (Schnittker 2004). And also, context can be decisive for certain health practices while the health practices themselves make up parts of that social context. In other words contextual factors on health and disease cannot easily be reduced to one-directional (linear) associations.

1. Contexts are multifaceted; they include material and nonmaterial conditions, risk factors, as well as economic, cultural, and social resources relevant for the unequal distribution of NCDs.

2. Context is a multilevel concept; on the level of individual and collective behaviors (health practices) it refers to the material and nonmaterial conditions as perceived by the individuals; on the structural level it refers to the material and nonmaterial conditions of social differentiation and stratification as identified by the researcher. As such the concept of context helps us to systematically explore the individual and structural conditions of social stratification of NCDs and health.

3. Contexts allow, promote, or discourage health practices relevant for NCDs. Human beings are social actors that function with and through their bodies. Their health-relevant behaviors and agency depend on the contexts in which they act and those contexts are most often coined by their socioeconomic and social-cultural class or status, linking health, its production, and distribution to social inequality.

4. Contexts provide the conditions for human agency relevant in the production and distribution of health. We refer here to the term agency to mean those forms of (collective) human action which are linked to social structures in a reciprocal way: behaviors that are systematically linked to structural conditions as their determinants and/or their consequences. Human agency can have structurally reproductive or structurally transformative effects (Hays 1994; Abel and Frohlich 2012). What follows from

that is that whole population groups are not just passive targets or recipients of the external forces which determine their health but are coproducers of health at the population level (for more on health-relevant agency see, e.g., Freese and Lutfey 2011; Chap. 5).

From a health promotion perspective those factors suggest to conceive of context as the primary explanatory perspective for understanding health and disease. In particular, without a better understanding of the context in which health and illness emerge our explanation of the interplay between NCD-relevant structural conditions and individual and collective health practices will remain rudimentary at best. The new approach would suggest, in contrast, developing context as the basic "frame of reference" for NCDs and health. In doing so health promotion research and interventions might be better prepared to accept and positively respond to key challenges such a complexity, structural determination, and human agency.

Defining health promotion as a field of practice focused on "social change for better health," context emerges as the "natural" choice for health promotion interventions: Since its framing in the Ottawa Charter health promotion is geared towards understanding and acting on contextual conditions for health-relevant human action with individuals as agents and coproducers of health.

Arising Needs: Changing the Paradigm, Broadening the Database

The discussion above suggests that new approaches to NCDs and health promotion should first develop an adequate "theory of the problem": For health promotion the problem is that the social conditions which affect the health chances of whole populations are not as good as they could be. Consequently, health promotion is about addressing the social conditions and social processes of health: How health is socially produced in the first place, how the social structures and conditions distribute the chances to maintain good health, etc. On that background a theory of the problem that starts with bio-medically defined risk factors would

appear inadequate in fact, potentially misleading. Instead social and political theories of resource and risk distribution (e.g., Hall and Lamont 2009), theories of structure–agency processes in the reproduction of social and health inequalities (e.g., Abel and Frohlich 2012), and alike are needed. Such theories can guide NCD research and also more appropriate health promotion interventions by providing a perspective which keeps the focus on where it needs to be: on the social contexts in which health is produced and put on risk. Health promotion when drawing on its original concepts and principles appears open as a field of practice to move in this direction. Here we proffer a context-oriented definition of health promotion as the *collective endeavor to systematically shape social systems in a way that they facilitate the production and maintenance of health in whole populations.*

Conclusions: The Way Forward

Given the recognized burden that NCDs pose in societies today, public health faces the need to develop appropriate responses that help to reduce its occurrence and alleviate its consequences. While it appears obvious that theoretical guidance is needed in particular to support new research directions, one can observe that the current theory base is rather poor in NCD research and public health practice including health promotion. Moreover, as developing a social perspective on NCDs requires the acceptance and accounting for considerable complexity in any explanatory and intervention models, the task of developing such new approaches appears ambitious. The aim of this chapter was not to resolve the issues around theory development for NCDs and health promotion but to open up new ways of thinking about them.

The need to find new ways is described earlier in this chapter, with an assessment which shows fundamental theoretical and methodological limitations of established epidemiology-based approaches and showing that current health promotion approaches are often theoretically insufficiently developed.

On the one hand, mostly data-driven NCD epidemiology with its "relentless focus on risk factors" (Freese and Lutfey 2011, p. 70), a far-reaching neglect of resources and context dynamics, cannot provide a research or an intervention perspective that would have the social in its center. On the other hand, we note that there are major deficits in health promotion theory, especially when it comes to defining an appropriate empirical base, with requisite data, necessary for social approaches to NCDs. And clearly, both epidemiology and health promotion lack a sufficient examination of their theoretical underpinnings as guidance in their research and practice. The most fundamental deficit is, however, that we currently lack an adequate definition of the problems around NCDs and health. From a disease- and risk-oriented public health perspective NCDs are first and foremost a biomedical phenomenon; from a health- and resource-oriented health promotion perspective these same NCDs are seen as a social phenomenon; consequently a problem definition which is focused on the social conditions and processes linked to the fundamental causes could provide a new starting point for future research and a way which will help identifying promising intervention points. For that we suggest developing a new theory-based approach that starts with a social definition and theoretical account of the problem and integrates epidemiologically based knowledge and other empirical data on NCDs in a social science framework. To connect this body of knowledge to action for social change for better health at the population level the framework should include a link to health promotion action. Starting from a social science definition of health, establishing context as the frame of reference for NCD research and action, including all relevant resources and risk factors is one way of opening up for new approaches in NCDs and health promotion.

References

Abel, T., & Frohlich, K. L. (2012). Capitals and capabilities: Linking structure and agency to reduce health inequalities. *Social Science & Medicine, 74*(2), 236–244.

Antonovsky, A. (1979). *Health, stress and coping*. San Francisco: Jossey-Bass.

Bloom, D. E., Cafiero, E. T., Jané-Llopis, E., Abrahams-Gessel, S., Bloom, L. R., Fathima, S., Feigl, A. B., Gaziano, T., Mowafi, M., Pandya, A., Prettner, K., Rosenberg, L., Seligman, B., Stein, A. Z., & Weinstein, C. (2011). *The global economic burden of noncommunicable diseases*. Geneva: World Economic Forum.

Breslow, L. (2004). Perspectives: The third revolution in health. *Preface to Annual Review of Public Health, 25,* 13–18.

Carroll, S. (2012). Social theory and health promotion. In I. Rootman et al. (Eds.), *Health promotion in Canada* (pp. 33–52). Toronto: Canadian Scholars Press. Chapter 3.

Dooris, M. (2006). Healthy settings: Challenges to generating evidence of effectiveness. *Health Promotion International, 21*(1), 55–65.

Freese, J., & Lutfey, K. (2011). Fundamental causality: Challenges of an animating concept for medical sociology. In B. A. Pescosolido, J. K. Martin, J. McLeod, & A. Rogers (Eds.), *Handbook of the sociology of health, illness, and healing*. New York, NY: Springer.

Goffman, E. (1959). *The presentation of self in everyday life*. New York, NY: Doubleday-Anchor.

Green, L. W., Kreuter, M. W., Deeds, S. G., & Partridge, K. B. (1980). *Health education planning: A diagnostic approach* (1st ed.). Mountain View, CA: Mayfield.

Hall, P. A., & Lamont, M. (Eds.). (2009). *Successful societies: How institutions and culture affect health*. New York, NY: Cambridge University Press.

Hays, S. (1994). Structure and agency and the sticky problem of culture. *Sociological Theory, 12*(1), 57–72.

Huber, M., Knottnerus, J. A., Green, L., van der Horst, H., Jadad, A. R., Kromhout, D., et al. (2011). How should we define health? *BMJ, 343*, d4163.

IUHPE. (2007). *Shaping the future of health promotion: Priorities for action*. Paris: International Union for Health Promotion and Education & Canadian Consortium for Health Promotion Research.

Krieger, N. (2011). *Epidemiology and the peoples health*. New York, NY: Oxford University Press.

Kuh, D., Ben-Shlomo, Y., Lynch, J., Hallqvist, J., & Power, C. (2003). Life course epidemiology. *Journal of Epidemiology & Community Health., 57,* 778–783.

Lahelma, E., Martikainen, P., Laaksonen, M., & Aittomaki, A. (2004). Pathways between socioeconomic determinants of health. *Journal of Epidemiology & Community Health, 58,* 327–332.

Link, B. G., & Phelan, J. (1995). Social conditions as fundamental causes of disease. *Journal of Health and Social Behavior, 35,* 80–94.

Luhmann, N. (1964). *Funktionen und Folgen formaler Organization*. Berlin: Duncker & Humblot.

McQueen, D., & Kickbusch, I. (Eds.). (2007). *Health and modernity: The role of theory in health promotion*. New York, NY: Springer.

Mirowsky, J., & Ross, C. (2003). *Education, social status, and health*. Hawthorne, NY: Aldine de Gruyter.

NRC/IOM, National Research Council and Institute of Medicine. (2012). In S. H. Woolf & L. Aron (Eds.), *US health in international perspective: Shorter lives, poorer health. Panel on understanding cross-national health differences among high-income countries.* Washington, DC: The National Academies Press.

Parsons, T. (1937). *The structure of social action.* New York, NY: McGraw-Hill.

Poland, B., Green, L., & Rootman, I. (Eds.). (2001). *Settings for health promotion: Linking theory and practice.* London: Sage.

Potvin, L., & McQueen, D. (Eds.). (2008). *Health promotion evaluation practices in the Americas: Values and research.* New York, NY: Springer.

Prochaska, J. O., & DiClemente, C. C. (1984). *The transtheoretical approach: Crossing the traditional boundaries of therapy.* Melbourne, FL: Krieger Publishing Company.

Schnittker, J. (2004). Education and the changing nature of the income gradient in health. *Journal of Heath & Social Behavior, 45*(3), 286–305.

Shilton, T., Sparks, M., McQueen, D., Lamarre, M.-C., & Jackson, S. (2011). Proposal for new definition of health. *BMJ, 343,* 5359. letter to the editor.

Susser, M., & Susser, E. (1996). Choosing a future for epidemiology. I. Eras and paradigms. *American Journal of Public Health, 86,* 668–673.

Wallerstein, N. (1988). Empowerment education: Freire's ideas adapted to health education. *Health Education & Behavior, 15,* 379–394.

WHO (World Health Organization). (1986). *The Ottawa charter for health promotion.* Retrieved November 21, 1986, from http://www.who.int/healthpromotion/conferences/previous/ottawa/en/

WHOCSDOH. (2008). *Closing the gap in a generation. Health equity through action on the social determinants of health.* Geneva: WHO.

The Nature of Causality: Beyond Traditional Evidence

David V. McQueen

Introduction

Regarding NCDs and health promotion there have been some significant conceptual changes in the past quarter century. Two such changes are in the realm of causality and evidence. The basic notion of causality has been infused with the complexity of the real world. The very simple idea that factor "x" causes outcome "y" has come to be regarded as far too simplistic and within the world of chronic disease etiology this is particularly true. Similarly in health promotion the ideology of such fundamental documents as the Ottawa Charter and others argued for a multi-causal world (WHO 1986, 2009; WHO EURO 1984, 1998). At the same time that there was growing recognition of the complexity of causality in the medical world there was a powerful movement towards what was termed evidence-based medicine (Sackett et al. 1996). As a result the field of public health, including the NCDs and health promotion, was faced with showing evidence in the face of increasingly complex models of causality. This, in turn, has resulted in an ongoing "evidence debate" (McQueen 2001, 2002, 2003; McQueen and Anderson 2001) that to date remains largely unresolved.

Often the debate is confusing because of discussions that treat causality and evidence as if they are independent. Undoubtedly this results from the widely accepted notion that causation is seen as an event that determines a second event that is termed the effect, and it follows that evidence is the knowledge that that these are related in a linear fashion. This notion, referred to often as temporality, was clearly outlined in the epidemiologist Bradford Hill's criteria for causation that is the hallmark of much of the beginning of the debate on causality in the NCD area (Hill 1965). However the discussion of causality is an old philosophical discussion, whereas the evidence debate, particularly in the public health sciences, is relatively recent and links more to earlier philosophical discussions on proof. The elaborated discussion of causality in terms of the effectiveness of interventions in NCDs and the relationship to epidemiological perspectives is taken up in more detail in Chap. 6.

As mentioned, causality and causal thinking have a long and distinguished history in philosophy. The origins of causal thinking date back to the ancient Greek philosophers. Even among the pre-Socratics there was an intense concern with causation and theories related to the fundamental forces in nature were well developed (Kirk et al. 1983). Moving towards modern times, many of the philosophical origins of present-day thinking find their origins in the eighteenth-century works of David Hume (Hume 2007) and Immanuel Kant (Harper and Meerbote 1984; Kant 1781). Much of the underlying epistemological basis for

D.V. McQueen (✉)
2418 Midvale Court, Tucker, GA 30084, USA
e-mail: davidmcqueen07@gmail.com

D.V. McQueen (ed.), *Global Handbook on Noncommunicable Diseases and Health Promotion*,
DOI 10.1007/978-1-4614-7594-1_3, © Springer Science+Business Media, LLC 2013

modern-day evidence-based medicine rests on a number of assumptions about theory and observation discussed by these philosophers. A careful explication of this background in relation to evidence-based medicine and the more recent efforts following the work of Archie Cochrane (1972) are found in the excellent analysis by Kelly and Moore (2012); they argue in their conclusion: "thinking about EBM in a framework of some of the ideas of Hume and Kant casts it into a different light. Therefore, intriguingly, the evidence-based approach as applied in EBM … offers an illustration of Kant's fundamental epistemological concepts in action." There is no doubt that the RCT and its relationship to EBM have a profound dependence on the work of these two earlier philosophers and their work. It was updated by the sociologist Cochrane and his incorporation of logical positivism. Much of the detailed discussion of these dimensions of scientific empiricism, logical positivism, and their relationship to causality is taken up in detail in the masterful book edited by Frederick Suppe decades before EBM became popular in the public health world (Suppe 1977).

Of course, one of the widely held beliefs in the EBM argumentation is the superiority of evidential proof that is based on the randomized controlled trial, the RCT. Despite the inherent strength of the RCT for clinical medicine applications and drug testing in particular, its limitations are clear in much work associated with NCDs, their causes, and their possible interventions. It is to that discussion that we now turn, leaving the world of the RCT's strengths and entering into the world of multi-causality and complexity.

Complexity and Causality

Complexity has many implications for NCDs and health promotion as it relates to the notion of causality. As mentioned, causality has often been treated in a simplistic manner. In part this is because in the early twentieth century the initial parameters of causality were set by logical positivism to fit an emergent view of science based on linear cause and effect. Although the modern notion of causality can be traced to David Hume, the modern world transformed causality into a notion that demanded axiomatic structure, notions such as precedence of actors and a linear relationship to effect. Even as science, both social and physical, developed models of causation with many variables arranged in reciprocal and curvilinear structures, causality essentially was based on an underlying philosophical basis in logical positivism.

The current effort to reexamine causality in many fields of public health and particularly in health promotion has arisen in parallel to thinking about complexity. In part this is due to challenging findings and theories in many areas of the physical sciences, notably in cosmology where the notion arises that causality may not be totally knowable or perhaps even describable. This does not imply that causality cannot be understood, but that the understanding lies more with the interpreter of causality and with extrapolations of theory rather than with the events being described. Thus much of causality may be more dependent upon theory than observation.

Complexity challenges some common notions of causality. For example, in trying to understand a phenomenon, scientists have often argued that complex systems might be broken down, or "reduced" to an understanding of the smaller causal units. That is, after one has understood all the single-factor causal units, the smaller units can be linked or "summed" in order to see the whole causal picture. On this basis it is seen as legitimate to understand pieces of the whole causal picture in order to understand the whole. However, the alternative notion that the "whole is the whole" and that the whole is complex challenges this fundamental reductionist procedure in the practice of modern science. Nonetheless, the notion that the whole can be "reduced" to its components is fundamental to the idea of reductionism as developed by logical positivists. Much of the work on NCDs utilizes this reductionist approach to causality but, in contrast, much of the practice of health promotion uses more of a non-reductionist approach.

The idea of complexity and its role in an approach to NCDs and health promotion is seen in other forms. In the mid-twentieth century Ludwig von Bertalanffy (1969), taking what we now recognize as systems theory, argued for a new analytical, methodological approach to dealing with the component elements of systems and in particularly with the limitations of linear causality. Systems approaches introduced critical new concepts of interaction, transaction, and understanding of relationships in multivariate systems. It certainly has been argued that general systems theory is a general science of wholeness. Because of this the fit of a systems theory approach to NCDs and health promotion has much to offer. However, the key epistemological question concerns the extent to which systems theories, however fashioned, represent another form of reductionism and/or deconstructionism.

Determinism

Another feature that relates to causality is the distinction between that which is probabilistic and that which is deterministic. In the language of positivistic causality, most causal relationships, whatever their character, may be seen as deterministic that is essentially that all causal relationships between variables are essentially knowable and could be determined if we had the appropriate measurements and had appropriately assessed all of the relationships. Just because determinism is difficult does not mean it is nonexistent. For example, the many-body problem in astrophysics may not currently be solvable, but arguably it could be solved. The idea that relations among variables are only knowable statistically is at the heart of most modern science, and public health in particular as it is practiced. In a sense probability explanations are often the best approximation of a complexity, given that we neither know nor have the skills or mathematical procedures to completely determine relationships in a complex, multicausal relationship. As will be discussed often in this book, whether one takes a probabilistic or a deterministic approach assumes a perspective about knowledge and causality. Given the current state of public health science and epidemiological knowledge in particular it should

be noted that most of that knowledge is based upon a probabilistic understanding of relationships among variables. It is a weaker form of causality than that which is deterministic. Nonetheless, as will be seen in discussions throughout Section II of this book, many use a deterministic terminology. This is notably the case with the notion of social "determinants" of health. However the use of the stronger word does not change the underlying epistemology that is deterministic and the reality of most of the observations, which are probabilistic.

Causality and Evidence in Current Context of Interventions

Given what has been said about the multi-causality above, public health interventions provide another puzzle for complexity and causality. The puzzle is what constitutes the whole context of an intervention, that is, what are the boundaries of an intervention and, in particular, what is the context prior to the intervention and what does the intervention do to the context. (In physical science this is analogous to measuring the temperature of a liquid in a container; the liquid's temperature is not independent of the thermometer inserted in the liquid to measure the temperature.) When something is perceived as a complexity it has a certain wholeness. When a new parameter is introduced into that complexity, the whole changes. This is logical because something has been added to the whole. This added "part" may be seen as an "intervention." The epistemological question then becomes to what extent the whole has changed. Framed in this way, the reductionist, or approach to understanding what has happened, is most appealing, primarily because one can then "examine" pre- and post-intervention how the whole or in turn its subcomponents have changed over time. Indeed, time and the dynamic of change appear to be the only relevant considerations. The belief is that one has observed an effect, but from a wholeness perspective you now observe a different whole entity.

From a causality perspective health-promoting interventions as well as preventive interventions on NCDs have been difficult to define. The types and varieties of such practices are taken up extensively in Section III of this book. At best the practices may be characterized as eclectic, encompassing a wide range of research types and approaches that imply various epistemologies of causation. Most interventions and notably the intervention settings may be characterized as complex. Areas such as policy research, evaluation research, survey research, action research, and social epidemiology all work within complex causal settings. Causality issues arise in several areas, notably theories and concepts implied or articulated; the methodological style of research or intervention; and the translation of research and practice into something useful to improve population health.

Consider the critical issue of methodology, particularly when applied to carrying out or assessing interventions in public health. There is unease as to what constitutes acceptable methods. In addition, there is a tendency to think that methodological design itself is coterminous with a methodological approach. Despite its often inappropriateness as a methodological approach suitable to NCD and health promotion public health interventions, the RCT remains for many as an ideal to which intervention research should aspire. When control of the setting of a population receiving an intervention can be achieved for the duration of the intervention, and where there is a focus on a simple intervention with an expected dichotomous (or an interval level that is very linear), outcome of success or failure, the RCT is a powerful design for intervention research in health promotion (Rosen et al. 2006). Clearly, the rejection of the RCT by many health promotion researchers has not convinced everyone. Nevertheless, the strength of the RCT is directly related to rigidly meeting the restrictive assumptions of experimental design. When the severe restrictions of experimental design are not met, the utility, validity, and power of the RCT diminish rapidly. Given the types of interventions in health promotion the potential misapplication of the RCT remains a problem (Bhaskar 1997; McQueen and Jones 2007; McQueen 2007). In health promotion interventions applied to NCDs,

control and experimental populations are unlikely if not impossible. It is part of the very nature of health promotion interventions that they operate in everyday life situations, involving changing aspects of the intervention as it is occurring; outcomes are often decidedly different from expectations; unanticipated consequences of the intervention are common and predictability is often low. Even if one rejects the strictest classical RCT model, the notions of experimental and control groups remain in studies and projects that use quasi-experimental designs, controls, and all the subliminal trappings of the RCT. Unfortunately, for many at the so-called hard end of the hard to soft science spectrum, a softer health promotion methodology may be viewed as a limitation of the field. The discussion and debate regarding conflicting ideas about how more "rigid" methods, such as the RCT, should be applied to health promotion and NCD interventions in the population continue. At the base of this debate lies a fundamental conflict in background orientation of the researchers and practitioners working in these fields.

Conflicting Orientations

Over the years different orientations towards public health have developed in the research community. Roughly speaking, a separation exists between two views which could be termed "biomedical public health" and "social public health." These two orientations are not necessarily conflicting, but they frequently give rise to differing interpretations of the underlying mission of public health. Essentially, a public health steeped in the biomedical tradition tends to view epidemiology as the basic science of public health. It tends to view causation as linear and relies heavily on "evidence" gathered by a set of limited methodological approaches that use mainly experimental designs and rely on a numerate tradition. Often the stress is on the individual as the focus of public health programs with the intent of influencing behavioral change. In contrast, a public health in the social tradition considers that there are many sciences that are "basic" to public health and particularly relevant disciplines are the social sciences such as sociology, politics, and economics. In these disciplines direct causation is less relevant than patterns of change and complexity is expected; linearity in causality is not expected. Although this different orientation has been discussed in many sources (Hofrichter 2003; Kelly and Moore 2012; Tones 1997; Venkatapuram 2011) there is yet to be a satisfactory resolution of the separation of views. In most of the literature regarding the causes of NCDs and the approaches to ameliorating their effects there remain quite separate literatures with regard to background disciplines and training of the researchers and practitioners involved. What follows is an effort to tackle some of the causal and evidence problems that override these differences and that hold for either orientation.

In considering causality and evidence in NCDs and health promotion there are two major challenges. The first is to discover the causes of the problem. Historically, epidemiology has excelled in this from a biomedical perspective. It has successfully shown many of the strong links between certain variables and disease outcomes. In the area of chronic disease few would doubt the clearly delineated relationship between the behavior of cigarette smoking and the disease outcome of lung cancer. Beyond lung cancer the relationship of this behavior has been well demonstrated for other cancers as well as cardiovascular diseases (USDHHS 2010). Clearly the success of the epidemiological methodologies to illuminate causality between some individual behaviors and disease outcomes is clear. Even in those cases where the behavioral causation and disease are far from a strong causal prediction, as for example in the relationship between diet and cancers to physical activity and CVD, the level of influence of these variables on disease outcomes is quite well articulated such that few would deny that there is some kind of correlational relationship occurring that is significant. The growth of the subfield of social epidemiology has pushed the epidemiological causal chain to greater length and identified that behaviors such as smoking may also be highly linked, i.e., correlated, to social factors such as socioeconomic class.

Much of this effort was well established already by the mid-twentieth century in the work of many epidemiologists (Berkman and Breslow 1983; Hollingshead and Redlich 1958; Syme et al. 1964). In recent years we have witnessed the work of many social epidemiologists (e.g., Braveman et al. 2010; Diez Roux 2007; Krieger 2011) in the Americas and the combined efforts of many in the UK (cf. Black et al. 1988; Kuh et al. 2003). With the publication of the WHO Commission on the social determinants of health (WHOCSDOH 2008) and the accompanying work of the nine knowledge networks on early childhood development, globalization, health systems, measurement and evidence, urbanization, employment conditions, social exclusion, priority public health conditions, and women and gender equity the field of challenges for social epidemiology was greatly enhanced. Of these networks the most relevant for the discussion of causation and evidence was the network on measurement and evidence. This group published three critical documents regarding this area that are available as Internet files at www.who.int/social_determinants/resources/mekn_final_report_102007.pdf; www.who.int/social_determinants/knowledge_networks/add_documents/mekn_final_guide_112007.pdf; and www.who.int/social_determinants/resources/mekn_paper.pdf. This documentation gives elaborate and detailed information on the underlying principles and perspectives used to carry out the Commission's work on causality. Suffice it to say, there is now a broad base of information that illustrates the implied causal relations between multiple social and behavioral variables and disease outcomes. Still, complexity and multivariate patterns enter into the picture and ultimately we are left with many inferences of causality, some strong, some weak, but few, if any, that would rise to the level of deterministic causal relationships. This should not be seen as a criticism or an indictment of this evidentiary work, but rather that absolute specification of causality has not been obtained. As an example, there is a strong judgment, based on much empirical data massed over years of research, that low social class may result in a poor and/or inadequate diet in a population and that poor diet, in turn, may result in multiple health-related problems. The basic premise that poor diet leads to health problems is rather forceful; the statement that poor diet causes health problems is a much weaker statement and can be partially supported probabilistically, but certainly cannot be reduced to a deterministic formulation. That there is an inequitable distribution of healthy food in a population is easier to prove than that the distribution *causes* poor health in that population. This is not just a pedantic argument; such argumentation results in serious issues regarding decisions made concerning interventions in public health. It is this type of outcome that separates the problems of causal description from the problems of intervention design. Thus enters the second major challenge with regard to evidence evaluations, namely, evidence concerning the effectiveness of interventions.

It is one thing to know the causes. It is another to believe you have a very good idea of the causes. It is something else to know what to do about the causes. It is still something else to produce evidence that your attempt to intervene in the causation process is effective. As mentioned, social epidemiology has been quite successful in delineating the causes when, all things being equal, little is changing, nor are any efforts being made to change anything. In short, it is a quite effective methodology to ascertain a static picture of the situation. It is a point in time view of implied and found causal relationships. Unfortunately, the real world is highly dynamic, as is causality. Two fundamental problems are faced. The first is that the causation structure changes through time and second, any intervention introduced into the whole context changes the causation structure through its action. This is neither an uncommon nor a trivial problem. It has haunted philosophers since the beginning; witness the fragment from Heraclitus (Kirk et al. 1983, pp. 181–202), the pre-Socratic (535–c. 475 BCE), that "you can't step into the same river twice." The second point, which may be seen as instrument attributable error is also a well-known problem; however when the instrument is something as untidy as a community-based intervention, the problems are exacerbated. Nonetheless, these are easily recognizable sources

of error in interpreting causality. There are many other sources of error that need to be detailed in any attempt to understand causality and evidence when applied to the area of seeking evidence for the effectiveness of interventions (cf. Groves and Lyberg 2010).

This discourse implies that there are some chief differences in emphasis between an epidemiological approach to the world of NCDs and that of health promotion. Epidemiology's strength is its concern with methodology. It has through the years built a sophisticated approach to understanding the causes of diseases. Health promotion, in contrast, is primarily concerned with interventions and efforts to change the causes. Of course both fields are concerned with cause and with change, but it is the leading emphasis on practice that is the primary characteristic of health promotion. It is worthwhile to recapitulate and review this difference in terms of the sources of causal errors.

Sources of Causal Errors

In any purported causal relationship, whether it is a rather simple two-variable linear causal relationship or, as is the case in most NCDs and health promotion causal relationships, complex multivariate relationships, there are many sources of errors that will impinge on ascertaining the *true* causation pattern that exists. The point of this discussion is not to enumerate all the possible sources of error, but to introduce the important concept of total error and to mention a few of the numerous sources of error in assessing causality. The most fundamental source of error in estimating causality stems from the fact that the causal relationship between variables, no matter how apparently strong, is always perturbed by all the other variables that could be influencing the variables of interest. This relates to what in classical physics is called the "n body problem" and in quantum mechanics the "many-body problem." In the social sciences this is the problem of exogenous variables, that is, those potentially causal variables that lie outside the causal model being studied, but may be still operating on the causal model under study. With large multicausal systems or models there is always potential for exogenous variables to be important. In approaches using large models, in which complex causal explanations are postulated (cf. WHOCSDOH 2008), the problem of the many components is particularly salient. A solution often tried is to add more potential causal variables to the model, that is, to make the purported exogenous causal factors endogenous to the model. This usually results in overdetermined models that are exceedingly complex to analyze and understand. There is an even more fundamental problem with exogenous variables: many important ones may not be known to be important or may be outside of the theoretical background of those building the model. This source of error stems from the underlying epistemological orientation and training of those building the model. No amount of jiggery-pokery can rescue a model of causality from this source of error and it remains the primary cause why no model to explain causes can fully delineate all the causal relationships. It is wise to honor the Box maxim that "essentially, all models are wrong, but some are useful" (Box and Draper 1987, p. 422).

Another fundamental issue in assessing causality is the relationship of time to causal relationships. There is little reason to expect causal relationships, no matter how strong or well explained, to remain constant over time. In science, constant values are unusual, variability is more common, and over time the variability often expresses itself in various temporal patterns. There is a distinction made over whether this variability is predictable, probabilistic, or, in the toughest case, chaotic. Without observations of variables over an extensive period of time one cannot know. Furthermore, outside of astrophysics where observation of systems in different points of time is possible, there are few examples of observations that have been systematically made for any great length of time. Simply put, one may observe and infer a relationship between variables, for example social class and poor diet, but that observed causality is usually made at a point in time and with weak measurements of both key variables (in fact, neither social class nor diet would be construed by any researcher as a simple

variable; rather they are both complex variables). Further, these variables have been measured differently over time and for a rather short period of time, that is, primarily only during the last century to the present.

Another issue is the type of variable and how it is assessed. Type of variable in most models varies from those that are at the individual level, e.g., traditional biomarkers as for example blood pressure as well as self-reported or observed behaviors such as smoking and self-reported social type variables such as socioeconomic status (SES) to those that are at the population level ranging from neighborhood status to health policy. Each of these types of variables comes complete with its own theoretical underpinnings and measurement issues. SES is a classic variable that is often measured by asking an individual questions regarding residence, occupation, education, and income. As a result of this it is actually a very complex variable that has many dimensions. Each of these dimensions has its own complexity; for example occupation varies throughout the lifetime of any individual, is affected by events related to his/her cohort, and it is often difficult to classify and the meaning difficult to ascertain. Furthermore many individuals live within a household of varying size and other occupants with varying degrees of education and income. So attributing a household's SES is not a simple matter. It parallels the many-body problem discussed above. In addition there is a huge and rich sociological literature on SES that needs to be taken into account in assessing the meaning of SES, a literature that is unfamiliar to most who work in the public health sector.

The Organizational Search for Evidence

Given the complexity of assessing causality and what constitutes evidence in NCDs and health promotion there have arisen many approaches beyond individual researchers attempting to assess evidence and understand complexity. In recent decades an organizationally based evidence industry has developed to try and apply a systematic basis to showing evidence and effectiveness in public health and medicine. This chapter cannot provide a guide or review all of these efforts. There is a huge literature accumulating from this collective work and it continues to grow. Much of the work has been accumulating through the Cochrane efforts and this is elaborated in detail in Chaps. 20 and 21. Similarly there is considerable work that has been carried out by governmental institutions. The reader who wants in-depth insight into these efforts should consult the numerous Web sites, documents, and the considerable literature that has accumulated (e.g., www.cochrane. org/, www.thecommunityguide.org/, www.nice. org.uk/). In some cases organizational subsets of public health specialties have developed as seen in the development of the Canadian National Collaborating Centres for Public Health that were established specifically to carry out knowledge synthesis and translate it into programmatic use for practitioners (www.nccph.ca/en/home. aspx). One center in particular, the National Centre for Methods and Tools (www.nccmt.ca/), conducts work that is highly relevant to the discussion found in this chapter. In other cases, nongovernmental type organizations (NGOs) such as the IUHPE have developed global programs on evidence and health promotion effectiveness (GPHPE, www.iuhpe.org/?page=510&lang=en). These efforts and others have been accumulating knowledge on causality and evidence for years. Some are discussed below in more detail as they pertain to NCDs.

Notwithstanding the greatly increased knowledge-synthesis base provided by all these organizational efforts, there is still much to be done and it would be wrong to assume that there is any completeness to this effort to assess evidence and effectiveness. The relevant topic areas for examination in the fields of NCDs and health promotion are almost boundless; everything from single diseases to issues of policy and climate change are potential subjects. Further, with specific regard to NCDs and the assessment of causality of intervention effectiveness there remains much to be done. It is notable that when we look to see the efforts on building evidence in interventions outside the biomedical context, for example interventions

where the focus is on changing social determinants or communities or interventions that are complex and multivariate, the situation is less satisfactory.

In the United States, initially using a somewhat restrictive methodology, the ongoing efforts of the independent Task Force on Community Preventive Services continue. After several years of diligent and time-consuming work the task force produced a comprehensive guide to Community Preventive Services: What Works to Promote Health (Zaza et al. 2005) that summarizes and rates the quality of evidence on the effectiveness of population-based interventions and in many different public health settings. The guide summarizes the literature on the effectiveness and cost-effectiveness of population-based interventions for prevention and control, provides recommendations on these interventions and methods for their delivery based on their analysis of evidence, and identifies a research agenda. Current work of this task force is easily accessible at http://www.thecommunityguide.org/index.html. This effort is an example of an approach that took a strong biomedical/epidemiological definition of evidence (Briss et al. 2000) at first, but in later years broadened its methodological approach. Much of the guide's work has gone into relating evidence to the design of interventions. What this effort has revealed is that finding evidence of intervention effectiveness is not an easy task and that methodological decisions steer the type of results that emerge.

The work of the US Task Force illustrates both many strengths and weaknesses of such large organizational endeavors. To begin with such efforts are to be lauded for their sustained work over many years; sustained resources for such efforts in changing organizational and political climates are always noteworthy. However, this sustainability comes at great financial cost and the employment of many staff and associated experts over a long period of time. Such an effort can only be sustained through renewed government support and political commitment. This sustainability is obviously subject to the vagaries of leadership support that affect any large institution. The scope and size of the tasks taken on by the guide is wide as is befits a group examining a complex field such as public health interventions to promote health. It also implies that a staff must consist of experts with a broad knowledge of public health, preventive medicine, and health promotion. In addition, they should be independent from overt influence, both political and ideational, by the institution in which they are based. These are complicated requirements that illustrate the challenges that face any effort to carry out a systematic, long-term review and assessment of a large body of interventions in many fields that are pertinent to public health interventions. In conducting an evidentiary assessment of interventions hundreds of studies are reviewed, evaluated, and examined by a team of many abstractors using a standardized evaluation protocol. An enormous weeding out effort is undertaken. Nonetheless, this search for evidence is still largely limited to published literature accessible to data retrieval systems and generally only reviewed when in English and conducted in industrialized advanced economies. Fortunately in recent years Internet search engines of great power have made this search more inclusive. Despite many limitations the guide's work has produced a large body of findings of value to those concerned with the evidence and causality question.

In the European region there have been a number of organizationally based efforts to assess the evidence of effectiveness of interventions. One such effort was the IUHPE report to the European Commission that took an approach to evidence more rooted in health promotion ideology. An advisory group, consisting of 13 senior persons in the health promotion field, 15 authors, and a "witness group" of some 25 "political experts," produced a report for the European Commission (EC) on the evidence of health promotion effectiveness (IUHPE 1999). The great value of this report is that it identifies a considerable body of evidence pointing to the value of health promotion and attesting to its effectiveness. The report was also clear to recommend those areas where more research was needed, as well as those open to debate about effectiveness. Some areas of health promotion activity stand out. One often cited example is the evidence of a strong inverse relationship

between price and use of tobacco. Therefore, health-promoting efforts that lead to price increases of tobacco should lead to less use of tobacco. This finding mirrors that from the CDC group working on tobacco for the Community Guide (Zaza et al. 2005). Thus there is an accumulating international evidence base that supports global efforts to reduce tobacco consumption through pricing.

Despite all the difficulties with the notion of evidence, the writers of the IUHPE-EC report concluded that (1) comprehensive approaches using all five Ottawa strategies are the most effective; (2) certain "settings" such as schools, workplaces, cities, and local communities offer practical opportunities for effective health promotion; (3) people, including those most affected by health issues, need to be at the heart of health promotion action programs and decision-making processes to ensure real effectiveness; (4) real access to information and education, in appropriate language and styles, is vital; and (5) health promotion is a key "investment"—an essential element of social and economic development (IUHPE 1999). These findings ultimately led to the development of the idea for a more comprehensive global approach to evidence that became the IUHPE Global Programme on Health Promotion Effectiveness (GPHPE) (McQueen and Jones 2007).

In the UK the ongoing work of the National Institute for Health and Clinical Excellence (NICE) continues to provide guidance for public health interventions (NICE 2008). Their systematic work generally relies on a strong biomedical model of evidence and causality and tends to emphasize interventions addressed at individual risk factors for disease. Nonetheless, the comprehensive document on methods for the development of NICE public health guidance illustrates the complexity and sensitivity to the key methodological problems faced in carrying out this work (NICE 2009). Furthermore, the document extensively looks at the issues related to areas of keen interest regarding NCDs such as the social determinants of health and carefully considers value areas such as equity that are part of the understanding of health promotion interventions. In many ways NICE, though based in a setting interested mainly in health care and the clinical, provides welcome insight into the issues critical to assessing evidence in NCD and heath promotion interventions. The depth of this insight is revealed in a critical article by Kelly and Moore (2012) on the role of judgment in evidence-based medicine and technology assessment.

Challenges in Seeking Evidence of Causality and Summation

There are many challenges in seeking evidence of causality. Several have already been discussed. However, the list of challenges is very long. We have discussed at some depth the basic epistemological problems concerning evidence and causality. Most other discussions in the "evidence debate" have been along these lines (McQueen and Jones 2007). Many debates on the appropriateness of the RCT for assessing causality have occurred and continue to occur. A subtheme of the RCT debate is on a "hierarchy of evidence" where some believe that some types of "evidence" are superior to others. Often this debate occurs in terms of hard facts versus judgment in assessing causality. In any case this debate will continue because essentially there is not a satisfactory answer as to how to determine the evidence of causality in all the forms of interventions in the different types of context that characterizes so much of public health.

There are some challenges that are less discussed, but remain important. Perhaps one of the greatest is the problem of "insufficient evidence." This arises when, despite the best of efforts to examine all the interventions, examine all the relevant literature, make careful systematic analyses, and follow all the best and most appropriate guidelines, the result is that one cannot determine whether there is evidence or not, or even if there are some indications of causality operating, it cannot be specified in enough detail. This is a common outcome for systematic reviews; and it is not just a problem for those reviewing, it is a problem for those who would use the reviews. What is more important, this is the area where science bumps up against ethics. Many "ethically" sound

interventions may have no evidence of effectiveness, or the reverse (McQueen 2009).

Most organizational efforts find three rather distinct patterns that emerge after concerted work, namely, strong evidence, sufficient evidence, or insufficient evidence. Strong evidence is the ideal case and in some areas, e.g., smoking behavior and health effects, it tends to be a main finding, yet in others, e.g., the assessment of the effectiveness of programs to reduce individual smoking behaviors, the evidence is often merely sufficient, that is, yes, there is an effect, but it is neither strong nor simple. However, in many cases there is insufficient evidence, even in the smoking area. Why is insufficient evidence such a common occurrence? We have mentioned the epistemological reasons that might be active, but there are more prosaic reasons such as too few studies on which to base a conclusion, or worse still inconsistent results, and of course simply poor research and/or evaluation designs. In the area of interventions related to NCDs the problem of too few studies is rampant. Years of neglect, often by the very public health organizations making the evidence evaluation, to carry out a large number of interventions in NCDs and health promotion yields a costly price of failure with regard to judging evidence.

When one considers the ways to address insufficient evidence there are possibilities, but many are not simple, quick, or easy solutions. The additional interventions in NCDs and health promotion and their proper design and execution followed by an examination of the evidential causality in the interventions cannot be undertaken overnight and without considerably more resources than now appropriated. There are more radical approaches; one could simply only report evidence that is sufficient, a rather draconian measure and ethically questionable. A "softer" solution is to report in depth why evidence could not be found and offer strategies for resolving the situation to arrive at an appropriate "better" answer. Another option that suggests the precautionary principle is to make it clear that there is no evidence that any harm has been done by carrying out the interventions with insufficient evidence and that it is therefore possible to continue further similar interventions that continue to explore the area of insufficient evidence. This choice falls in that difficult category of addressing the need for more information. This choice is not so rare, because in the analysis of interventions there are many possibilities that might lead to an insufficient evidence outcome. One common finding in studies when they are grouped and appear to be similar is that they are not as similar as they would appear. In actually carrying out an intervention in the complexity and contextually different settings one sees many inconsistent findings when studies are compared.

There may be a bias when one observes consistent findings of evidence. Many interventions tend to group in clusters of interventions carried out by the same individuals or research groups that are highly related. These research clusters are common in academia and tend to reinforce each other. Further positive findings tend to be reported in multiple published sources. This type of bias is often repeated and reinforced by the prejudice in academic publishing against reporting negative or "uninteresting" findings. As a result, a common observation in large systematic reviews is the appearance of multiple studies that are carried out under this type of bias. This is not insignificant, as external users tend to reinforce this type of replicability in that external policy makers may make assessments of evidence on the basis of these biased reports and continue to fund dubious interventions as well as more research.

No single chapter can fully address the complicated world of evidence and causality on dealing with NCDs and health promotion. As will be seen in many subsequent chapters in this monograph causality and its implications are of fundamental concern for those working in public health whether research or practice. What is clear is that the need to develop, promote, fund, and carry out interventions that are effective to address the burden of NCDs and promote health is critical. Given the scare resources in public health dedicated to NCDs and health promotion, the argument on economic grounds is clear enough. However there is the equally critical ethical concern that interventions should be conducted that do not harm and in the best of cases improve the negative situation with regard to health outcomes. What becomes increasingly clear in the evidence debate is that judgment is important and that debate on the nature of evidence and causality will continue. It is also clear that complexity enters not only in terms of understanding causality in the interventions themselves but also as represented in the organizational efforts themselves to address the issues. Evidence of causality is dependent on all of these factors.

References

Berkman, L. F., & Breslow, L. (1983). *Health and ways of living: The Alameda County study*. New York, NY: Oxford Press.

Bertalanffy, L. V. (1969). *General system theory: Foundations, development, and applications (Revised)*. New York, NY: George Braziler.

Bhaskar, R. (1997). *A realist theory of science* (2nd ed.). New York, NY: Verso.

Black, D., Morris, J. N., Smith, C., & Whitehead, M. (1988). *Inequalities in health*. London: Penguin.

Box, G. E. P., & Draper, N. R. (1987). *Empirical model-building and response surfaces*. New York, NY: John Wiley & Sons.

Braveman, P. A., Cubbin, C., Egerter, S., Williams, D. R., & Pamuk, E. (2010). Socioeconomic disparities in health in the United States: What the patterns tell us. *American Journal of Public Health, 100*(S1), S186–S196.

Briss, P. A., (2000). Developing an evidence-based guide to community preventive services – Methods. *American Journal of Preventive Medicine, 18*(1), 35–43.

Cochrane, A. L. (1972). *Effectiveness and efficiency: Random reflections on health services*. London: Nuffield Provincial Hospitals Trust.

Diez Roux, A. V. (2007). Integrating social and biological factors in health research: A systems view. *Annals of Epidemiology, 17*, 569–574.

Groves, R. M., & Lyberg, L. (2010). Total survey error: Past, present, and future. *Public Opinion Quarterly, 74*(5), 849–879.

Harper, W. L., & Meerbote, R. (Eds.). (1984). *Kant on causality, freedom, and objectivity*. Minneapolis, MN: University of Minnesota Press.

Hill, A. B. (1965). The environment and disease: Association or causation? *Proceedings of the Royal Society of Medicine, 58*, 295–300 (cf. http://www.drabruzzi.com/hills_criteria_of_causation.htm)

Hofrichter, R. (Ed.). (2003). *Health and social justice: A reader on the politics, ideology, and inequity in the distribution of disease*. San Francisco, CA: Jossey-Bass.

Hollingshead, A., & Redlich, F. C. (1958). *Social class and mental illness: A community study*. New York, NY: Wiley.

Hume, D. (2007). *An enquiry concerning human understanding*. Oxford: Oxford University Press. P. Millican (ed. and intro.). First published 1748.

IUHPE. (1999). *The evidence of health promotion effectiveness*. A report for the European Commission by the International Union for Health Promotion and Education, ECSC-EC-EAEC, Brussels, Luxembourg.

Kant, I. (1781). The critique of pure reason. In J. M. D. Meiklejohn (Ed. & Trans), from Project Gutenberg, www.gutenberg.org/catalog/world/readfile?fk_files=2681870&pageno=1

Kelly, M. P., & Moore, T. A. (2012). The judgement process in evidence-based medicine and health technology assessment. *Social Theory and Health, 10*, 1–19.

Kirk, G. S., Raven, J. E., & Schofield, M. (1983). *The presocratic philosophers: A critical history with a selection of texts*. Cambridge: Cambridge University Press.

Krieger, N. (2011). *Epidemiology and the people's health*. New York, NY: Oxford University Press.

Kuh, D., Ben-Shlomo, Y., Lynch, J., Hallqvist, J., & Power, C. (2003). Life course epidemiology. *Journal of Epidemiology and Community Health, 57*, 778–783.

McQueen, D. V. (2001). Strengthening the evidence base for health promotion. *Health Promotion International, 16*(3), 261–268.

McQueen, D. V. (2002). The evidence debate. *Journal of Epidemiology and Community Health, 56*, 83–84.

McQueen, D. V. (2003). The evidence debate broadens: Three examples, Editorial. *Social and Preventive Medicine, 48*(5), 275–276.

McQueen, D. V. (2007). The evaluation of health promotion practice: 21st Century debates on evidence and effectiveness. In J. Douglas, S. Earle, S. Handsley, C. Lloyd, & S. M. Spurr (Eds.), *A reader in promoting public health: Challenge and controversy* (2nd ed., pp. 89–96). London: Open University.

McQueen, D. V. (2009). Ethics and evidence in health promotion. In A. Killoran & M. Kelly (Eds.), *Evidence-based public health: Effectiveness and efficiency* (pp. 27–40). Oxford: Oxford University Press.

McQueen, D. V., & Anderson, L. (2001) What counts as evidence? Issues and debates, Chapter 4. In I. Rootman, et al. (Eds.), *Evaluation in health promotion: Principles and perspectives* (pp. 63–83). Denmark: WHO. (Reprinted in *Debates and dilemmas in promoting health: A reader*, by M. Sidell, et al. Ed., 2002, 2nd ed., Milton Keynes: Open University Press)

McQueen, D. V., & Jones, C. M. (Eds.). (2007). *Global perspectives on health promotion effectiveness*. New York, NY: Springer Science & Business Media.

NICE. (2008). *Social value judgements: Principles for the development of NICE guidance* (2nd ed.). London: NICE, http://www.nice.org.uk/media/C18/30/SVJ2PUBLICATION2008.pdf

NICE. (2009). *Methods for the development of NICE public health guidance* (2nd ed.). London: NICE, http://www.nice.org.uk/aboutnice/howwework/developingnicepubli-chealthguidance/publichealthguidanceprocessand-methodguides/public_health_guidance_process_and_method_guides.jsp?domedia=1&mid=F6A97CF4-19B9-E0B5-D42B4018AE84DD51

Rosen, L., Manor, O., Engelhard, D., & Zucker, D. (2006). In defense of the randomized controlled trial for health promotion research. *American Journal of Public Health, 96*(7), 1181–1186.

Sackett, D. L., Rosenberg, W. M. C., Gray, J. A. M., Haynes, R. B., & Richardson, W. S. (1996). Evidence based medicine: What it is and what it isn't. *British Medical Journal, 312*, 71–72.

Suppe, F. (Ed.). (1977). *The structure of scientific theories* (2nd ed.). Urbana, IL: University of Illinois Press.

Syme, S. L., Hyman, M. M., & Enterline, P. E. (1964). Some social and cultural factors associated with the occurrence of coronary heart disease. *Journal of Chronic Diseases, 17*, 277–289.

Tones, K. (1997). Beyond the randomized controlled trial: A case for "Judicial Review". *Health Education Research, 12*(2), 1–4.

USDHHS. (2010). *How tobacco smoke causes disease: The biology and behavioral basis for smoking-attributable disease: A report of the surgeon general*. Atlanta, GA: U.S. Department of Health and Human Services, Centers for Disease Control and Prevention, National Center for Chronic Disease Prevention and Health Promotion, Office on Smoking and Health.

Venkatapuram, S. (2011). *Health justice: An argument from the capabilities approach*. Cambridge, UK: Polity Press.

WHO. (1986). *Ottawa charter for health promotion*. Geneva: WHO.

WHO, EURO. (1998). *Health promotion evaluation: Recommendations to policymakers*. Copenhagen: WHO (cf. http://whqlibdoc.who.int/euro/1998-99/EUR_ICP_IVST_05_01_03.pdf)

WHO. (2009). *Milestones in health promotion: Statements from global conferences*. WHO: Geneva (cf. http://www.who.int/healthpromotion/Milestones_Health_Promotion_05022010.pdf)

WHO, EURO. (1984). *Health promotion: A discussion document on the concepts and principles*. Copenhagen: WHO.

WHOCSDOH. (2008). *Closing the gap in a generation. Health equity through action on the social determinants of health*. Geneva: WHO.

Zaza, S., Briss, P., & Harris, K. (Eds.). (2005). *The guide to community preventive services*. Oxford: Oxford University Press.

Further Reading

Allison, K., & Rootman, I. (1996). Scientific rigor and community participation in health promotion research: Are they compatible? *Health Promotion International, 11*(4), 333–340.

Anderson, L., & McQueen, D. V. (2010). Informing public health policy with the best available evidence,

Chapter 30. In A. Killoran & M. Kelly (Eds.), *Evidence-based public health: Effectiveness and efficiency* (pp. 436–447). Oxford: Oxford University Press.

Butcher, R. B. (1998). *Foundations for evidence-based decision making* (Evidence and information, Canada health action: Building on the legacy, Vol. 5). Quebec: Editions MultiMondes.

Campbell, D. T., & Stanley, J. C. (1966). *Experimental and quasi experimental designs for research*. Chicago, IL: Rand McNally.

CDC. *Internet site for the community guide*. http://www.health.gov/communityguide

Davidson, K., (2003). Evidence-based behavioral medicine: What it is and how do we achieve it? *Annals of Behavioral Medicine, 26*(3), 161–171.

Doyle, J., Waters, E., Yach, D., McQueen, D., De Francisco, A., Stewart, T., et al. (2005). Global priority setting for Cochrane systematic reviews of health promotion and public health research. *Journal of Epidemiology and Community Health, 59*, 193–197.

Finegoood, D. T., (2012). Complexity and systems theory in oxford bibliographies in public health. http://www.oxfordbibliographies.com/view/document/obo-9780199756797/obo-9780199756797-0049.xml

Juneau, C. E., Jones, C. M., McQueen, D. V., & Potvin, L. (2011). Evidence-based health promotion: An emerging field. *Global Health Promotion, 18*(1), 79–89.

Kelly, M. P., & Moore, T. A. (2010). *Making a difference: Using the NICE public health guidance and embedding evaluation*. London: IDEA.

Kelly, M. P., Morgan, A., Ellis, S., Younger, T., Huntley, J., & Swann, C. (2010). Evidence based public health: A review of the experience of the national institute of health and clinical excellence (NICE) of developing public health guidance in England. *Social Science & Medicine (1982), 71*, 1056–1062.

Killoran, A., Swann, C., & Kelly, M. (2006). *Public health evidence: Tackling health inequalities*. Oxford: Oxford University Press.

Millican, P. (2007). *Introduction to Hume's enquiry concerning human understanding*. Oxford: Oxford University Press.

Pawson, R. (2006). *Evidence based policy: A realist perspective*. London: Sage.

Rootman, I., Goodstadt, M., McQueen, D., Potvin, L., Springett, J., & Ziglio, E. (Eds.). (2000). *Evaluation in health promotion: Principles and perspectives*. Copenhagen: WHO (EURO).

Task Force on Community Preventive Services. (2000). Introducing the guide to community preventive services: Methods, first recommendations and expert commentary. *American Journal of Preventive Medicine, 18*(1S), 1–142.

Surveillance for NCDs and Health Promotion: An Issue of Theory and Method

Stefano Campostrini

Introduction (Why a Chapter on Surveillance)

Surveillance has been for long time a core issue for infectious diseases, and it is still one of the main focuses for those working in public health. In the recent years, parallel to the rising importance of NCDs, we have seen a growing demand for information, particularly on the "causes" of NCDs, the risk factors, and the other determinants of NCDs and chronic diseases (WHO 2002). Initially it has been thought that the usual health (cross-sectional) surveys were sufficient to offer information on changes and trends over time of risk factors and other related variables, but soon (although not obviously for many decision makers and practitioners) it has been clear that:

(a) Behaviors such as smoking and physical activity can change much more rapidly than expected, and also in short times—within a year—dramatic changes can happen (often in response to public health and health promotion actions).

(b) To observe trends and changes is not enough: There is a need for understanding why attitudes and behaviors are changing, and there is an increasing need for answers to questions such as "changes have happened because of secular trends or because of interventions?" Or, "what are the mechanisms that generate changes and trends?"

Most of the existing health survey systems (typically carried out yearly or even every 3–5 years) were not capable to answer these questions, from this the need, also for NCDs, of real surveillance systems. In this chapter we address some fundamental issues, both from a theoretical and methodological point of view, about NCD surveillance (and more specifically about behavioral risk factor surveillance) starting from a historical excursus and ending with highlighting some of the critical challenges that this peculiar surveillance is addressing now or will have to address in the next future. Trying to focus on the major issues in showing the state of the art of surveillance, we are much less worried in answering necessarily all the challenges raised: this type of surveillance has such a brief history and has benefited from so little funding (in comparison with other health fields) that we can, without too many worries, for future research, work, and studies reflect on these challenges.

Surveillance: A Brief Historical Excursus

The roots of surveillance go back in the past. First historical traces come from the Venetian Republic that in 1348 kept a register of infectious diseases for their control in a nation in which

S. Campostrini (✉)
University Ca' Foscari Venice, S.Sebastiano -
Dorsoduro 1686, 30123, Venice, Italy
e-mail: stefano.campostrini@unive.it

trade was bringing, besides wealth, new and dangerous diseases (Declich and Carter 1994). For similar reasons, the Rhode Island colony in 1741 approved an act requiring taverns to report contagious diseases among their customers (Thacker 2000). Since then, surveillance moved in steps to a systematic registration of infectious diseases, first in Europe (Italy in 1881, the UK in 1890) and then in the USA (1893–1901). Until the mid-twentieth century, surveillance remained mainly related to infectious diseases, while morbidity and mortality data started to be regularly collected in several countries. It has been only since 1968, with the World Health Assembly, that a broader concept of surveillance (named at that time "epidemiological surveillance") emerged, not solely linked to infectious diseases.

In few years surveillance became a global practice, and serving to health systems with level of complexity always increasing that asked for an even broader concept of surveillance, the so-called *public health surveillance* (Thacker et al. 2012; Smith et al. 2012; Meriwether 1996).

Definition of Surveillance(s)

The World Health Organization (WHO) defines *public health surveillance* as "the continuous, systematic collection, analysis and interpretation of health-related data needed for the planning, implementation, and evaluation of public health practice. Such surveillance can:

- Serve as an early warning system for impending public health emergencies
- Document the impact of an intervention, or track progress towards specified goals
- Monitor and clarify the epidemiology of health problems, to allow priorities to be set and to inform public health policy and strategies" (http://www.who.int/topics/public_health_surveillance/en/)

Other definitions given from other organizations and literature are very similar. "Systematic and continuous collection, analysis, and interpretation of data, closely integrated with the timely and coherent dissemination of the results and assessment to those who have the right to know so that action can be taken"—it is written in the Dictionary of Epidemiology (Porta 2008). The US Centers for Disease Control (CDC) official documents and Web site share a very similar definition (Teutsch and Churchill 2000).

There are three major characteristics (covered later in this chapter) coming from these definitions:

- Systematic and continuous data collection/ analysis/interpretation
- Data assessment and consolidation
- Diffusion of the results to those responsible for action

It is important to consolidate these points, to better understand the theory, the methods, and the role itself of surveillance. But, these general definitions embrace all public health, and, consequently, several sectors of interest, which ask for different data and information, and, eventually, different specific kinds of surveillance. For instance, in infectious disease (ID) surveillance, the timely, accurate, and complete (on all interested cases) data are essential characteristics. The role of surveillance in ID is fundamentally that of an alarm system, helping to raise attention in the case of an insurgence of an epidemic, monitoring it, and assess effectiveness of possible interventions.

If many characteristics are shared by any surveillance system, some are particular. In NCD surveillance, timely and accurate data continue to be important, but the definition of "timely" or "complete" is certainly different from that given in ID surveillance. This consideration is important to define in this chapter: following the purpose of the present book, we will focus on those particular forms of surveillance that are related to NCDs and even more specifically to NCDs and health promotion (HP).

First, consider the general aspects of surveillance. From a theoretical point of view, looking at the different definitions, it appears quite clearly that the concept of surveillance is, in some way, twofold. It can be seen as a *system*, particularly an information system (Wysocki and Young 1990; Bellini et al. 1994), or a health information system (Thacker and Stroup 1994; Haux 2006; Campostrini and McQueen 2005), because of the presence of several components (data collection, assessment, analysis, interpretation, diffusion), and the importance given to the relationship among them. But it can be seen also as a *function*: the aim of surveillance is quite specific in the health information system panorama, and certainly quite different from that of a simple series of surveys, and much more than merely "a system to release information." It is more specific and advanced: it is to support with the information the action needed for a particular setting, problem, etc. In this respect surveillance is quite far from research: it is not looking for new information, previously unknown relationships, or some innovation. Surveillance is focused on offering *useful* and *timely* information to decision makers on *specific issues* considered of *major importance* for *public health action*. This does not imply that in *using* surveillance systems and their data one cannot carry on research and studies: the richness of data collected over time offers unique possibilities for research and studies, but this is not the first aim of surveillance. Nor does this mean that surveillance does not need research and innovation, quite the contrary: for the complexity of surveillance asks for the best and most advanced informative systems (data gathering, analyses, communication, etc.). However, the research and innovation are *external* to the surveillance systems. Thus it is important to emphasize surveillance as a specific *function* in the broader health information system that is the integrated effort to collect, analyze, and report health data, information, and knowledge to support decision making in public health action (AbouZahr and Boerma 2005; Lippeveld 2001).

The duality of the surveillance concept could be misleading, as sometimes surveillance is viewed as merely a set of offices that gather data and release information, or only as a general purpose that can be fulfilled by any informative source, losing the need for a systematic (and consequently dynamic) organization behind this to offer actively answers for this, not general, but very specific purpose. It is important for the success of a surveillance system to concentrate on both aspects: never losing the main track, surveillance has a specific *function* in supporting public health action, and, to serve properly to this function, surveillance must be well rooted into a *surveillance system*.

NCD and HP Surveillance

Taking into consideration the HP perspective in NCD surveillance narrows the field of general public health surveillance, further specifying it as surveillance of not only NCDs but also NCDs *and* HP. As mentioned, different fields imply different roles and types of surveillance. In this relatively limited NCD and HP field there may be different types of surveillance serving different purposes, but one could assert that essentially there are two major NCD surveillances: one concerned mainly with diseases and the other with risk factors. The first, disease surveillance, reports mainly on NCD morbidity and mortality to inform decision making concerning health care organization and priorities, but also, particularly when brought at local level, NCD surveillance becomes important in informing on environmental health. The major sources for this type of surveillance are registries (cancer registry, etc.), hospital records and notifications, and vital registrations (Birkhead and Maylahn 2000). Although statistics from this surveillance are fundamental to give a framework for HP objectives at national and local level, this type of surveillance rarely helps directly in HP actions.

The evidence that several NCDs were related with specific (changeable) behaviors implied that we needed systems capable of collecting and analyzing data and providing information useful for public health action on NCD-related risk factors. Therefore, in the 1980s the first so-called *behavioral risk factor surveillance* (BRFS) system was developed. Although, as we will see, the focus will remain over the years on the risk factors, and the name of this form of surveillance remains, typically, in this form of surveillance several types of information are collected, analyzed, and communicated. It is this combination that makes this surveillance a valuable and unique source for HP (Campostrini 2007).

During the process of risk factor surveillance development an important, fundamental link between HP and surveillance emerged. The possibility, ability, capability, and, eventually, effectiveness (McQueen and Jones 2007) of HP (particularly in tackling NCDs) emerged as an area to be informed by BRFS offering critical data and sometimes the only possible type of *evidence* needed for HP credibility (McQueen 2009; Campostrini 2007). Thus, surveillance not only helps to set the targets (priorities) for HP action but also offers unique opportunities for monitoring and evaluating its results, and provides fundamental information about the *context* in which the HP activity takes place. HP deals with changes at the societal level that eventually produce changes on risk behaviors, access to services, attitudes, and beliefs often measured by BRFS. This is why HP, among the choices of types of surveillance and surveillance tools available in public health, is mainly interested in BRFS.

Development of BRFS

Probably the earliest and most fully developed system has been the US behavioral risk factor surveillance system (BRFSS, www.cdc.gov/brfss/). Since 1984, the BRFSS has collected millions of interviews in the US states and territories, offering a unique monthly time series of estimates of the main risk factors and many other variables. That such a system has remained intact for nearly three decades is a tribute to the importance of political stability and government support over a long time period. Such stability and support are rare and arguably necessary for the maintenance of ongoing surveillance of those factors related to health and disease.

The history of the development of the BRFSS is noteworthy and valuable as a lesson in developing and establishing a new approach to such surveillance. The system started, mainly, as an efficient way of gathering data related to risk factors for chronic diseases (notably the word "surveillance" was added later). Initially the result diffusion process was only a small part of the many aspects of the system. Over time the importance of a strong link to public health action emerged as one of the main characteristics of the

system, bringing also considerable changes in the questionnaire adopted by the US states joining the system. Interestingly, besides the well-established questions concerning the main risk factors (around the leading "big four" smoking, physical inactivity, unhealthy diet, and alcohol consumption), other questions regarding beliefs, attitudes, and access to preventive services have been added to the questionnaire, as well as other important aspects to inform not only the priorities of public health action but also the use for deciding "how to" deliver these actions and evaluate their effectiveness.

The history of BRFSS is reported very briefly here in part to justify the terminology of this specific kind of surveillance as is commonly used now. In point of fact the range of information collected and analyzed goes well beyond behavioral "risk factors." Although such risk factors remain at the core of questions asked and internationally this surveillance is generally known as "risk factor surveillance," the reality is that in most countries, as well as in the USA, the systems now offer much broader information and involve questions on many areas related to public health and health promotion. Recognizing that BRFS is only one component in the complex panorama of public health surveillance (Parrish and McDonnell 2000) and sources of information available in the broader *health information system* (AbouZahr and Boerma 2005), and given the purpose of this chapter, we concentrate our attention on BRFS, and from now on when we will generically refer to surveillance, we refer to this specific kind of surveillance, often simply called BRFS. BRFS has developed considerably globally in the past two decades. In general the approaches have modeled themselves on the American CDC experience, the WHO approach (http://www.who.int/chp/steps/en/), an independent approach, or a mixture of these approaches.

The International Union for Health Promotion and Education (IUHPE) supports a coordinating process that started informally in 1999 with biannual Global Conferences (McQueen and Puska 2003; Choi et al. 2008) realized in partnership with CDC and agencies of several other countries (with a first conference held in Atlanta, in the USA, and following events hosted in Finland, Australia, Uruguay, Italy, and Canada). In 2008 this informal network was formally recognized as an IUHPE global working group, under the name of World Alliance for Risk Factor Surveillance (WARFS, Campostrini et al. 2009). WARFS supports the development of BRFS as a tool for evidence-based public health, acknowledging the importance of this information source to inform, monitor, and evaluate disease prevention and health promotion policies, services, and interventions (http://www.iuhpe.org/?page=497&lang=en).

WARFS has the following aims:

- To integrate surveillance as a tool into the mainstream of health promotion work
- To finalize the definition and conceptual framework of BRFS that can be shared and discussed globally
- To serve as a reference for researchers, BRFS practitioners, and countries that are developing BRF surveillance
- To share findings and results and experiences with IUHPE community to facilitate the discussion regarding the role of BRFS

The "Theory" of BRFS

To discuss the main aspects of the theory of surveillance we will start from the global view given by the WARFS experience, since it has recently produced, thanks to the work of members from several countries, a white paper, which provides a conceptual framework to BRFS-type surveillance (http://www.iuhpe.org/uploaded/Activities/Scientific_Affairs/GWG/WARFS_white_paper_draft_may_2011.pdf).

This document defines what are considered the main, systemic, BRFS characteristics:

1. Data collection, analysis, and use are *continuous*.
2. The system is *population based*.
3. The individual (respondent) is *not* the focus.
4. A *social survey* is the "instrument" for the collection of data.
5. *Time* is a critical variable.
6. *Change over time* is central.

7. *Technical and structural* aspects are critical and equitably weighted.
8. A coherent *theoretical base* underlies the system.

Time and Continuity

In the study of causation, after the works of Konrad Lorenz, as in many, many fields of scientific research, the examination and study of dynamic phenomena are fundamental, and most scientific disciplines now take advantage of the recent development in technology (for measurement purposes), computer sciences (for dealing with great amounts of data), and mathematics and statistics (to carry on suitable and sophisticated analyses) to perform advanced research for better understanding of changes and development over time. Surveillance is no exception. Health promotion and public health deal with (social) changes, trends, and dynamic aspects of populations and thus the need for observing, studying, and examining events *over time* is crucial, whatever definition of surveillance one chooses. There is an evident need for surveillance to catch as much "time" as possible, i.e., to be *continuous* in its action. This is perhaps one of the most contentious issues in the surveillance of socio-behavioral risk factors: the notion of a continuous system.

Returning to the general notion of surveillance, in ideal surveillance, whether the monitoring of the Earth's geological movements in a seismograph or the use of a surveillance camera in a shop, the data collection should be continuous. For example, one would not think of turning on a seismograph only whenever convenient; obviously an earthquake may occur at a most inconvenient time and there would be no continuous record of the event as it occurred. Similarly a surveillance camera in a shop is only of use if it is on during the time a burglary occurs. While this may be self-evident to the point of absurdity the notion of continuity breaks down when it comes to calling something a surveillance system in public health practice; routinely public health practitioners will use the word "surveillance" to describe data collection survey efforts that are not in the field collecting data most of the time, but only periodically. Thus similar appearing surveys that occur every few months or even years apart will often be described as a surveillance system. Even if systematic, they do not meet the fundamental logical requirement of continuous data collection. The idea of a *continuous system* also implies that data collection, analysis, and use are also occurring continuously.

Of course, the notion of a continuous system must be practically defined. The reality is that, even if one were to collect data "continuously" he/she would not collect in a day every hour, in an hour every minute, in a minute every second, and so forth. The notion of continuity, from a practical (measurement) point of view is relative to the dynamic process one is observing. So, in order to catch the action in a football match cameras collect "data" several times every second, and to control a shop for safety purposes usually cameras take pictures every few seconds, enough to catch the "action" of a burglar and identify his/her face. That is, data also in surveillance are collected routinely on a highly regular basis, preferably on a daily basis, with standardized time periods each day. This would still be an ideal case. The ability to collect data on such a rigorous plan approximating a "continuous" data stream is conditioned on the instrument and data collection methodology available. In our case the instrument is the questionnaire-survey and it has limitations. But it is important to note that all instruments have limitations. The shop surveillance camera is actually not collecting images continuously, but, rather like a motion picture, recording multiple single images over a fixed unit of time. The seismograph is subject to the random perturbations and movement caused by man-made disturbances occurring in the range of detection. But these two instruments simply reflect types of errors that accrue to the instrument, not flaws in the theoretical basis for the use of the instrument to collect continuous data. Therefore we postulate a *definition of continuity* useful for surveillance, accepting the relativity discussed above. Surveillance requires continuous observation with time intervals

sufficiently close one to the others to catch all the important actions (changes) on the variables under observation.

Time and Change as Theoretically Central Concepts: It Is all About Dynamics

The central notion of socio-behavioral risk factor surveillance is that it tracks changes in behaviors in the population over time. This is in sharp distinction to point in time surveys, which are concerned with the magnitude of behaviors in the population at a fixed point in time. In public health we are interested in both the magnitude of a behavior and its change over time; however, it is not easily possible nor appropriate to measure both at once. This aspect is theoretically analogous to the Heisenberg uncertainty principle that states that certain pairs of physical properties, like position and momentum, cannot both be known to precision. That is, the more precisely one property is known, the less precisely the other can be known. Thus if one wants to know the exact percentage of smokers in a population at a given point in time, then a census of the population must be undertaken; if one wants a close estimate, a large sample survey would suffice. However, the exact percentage of smokers in a population varies over time and if you want to understand that variation over time you have to conduct surveillance. Obviously, to use the smoking example, there are many reasons why smoking patterns may change in a population over time, including demographic changes, deaths, illness, taxation, economic downturns, custom, and popularity, to name just a few. It is quite clear, given all the changing influences, that it is very unlikely that the percentage of smokers would be the same at any two points in time over a period of months or years. For public health policy, the concern is mostly on increases and decreases of smoking behaviors.

Particularly from a health promotion perspective, continuing the smoking example, the precise measure of smokers is not so relevant, neither in a general surveillance perspective: there is no threshold over which some alarm bell should sound. The "ideal" percentage of smokers, as we all well know, is zero, but this, so far, has never been realized in any country. So, while it could be important to know how far in our intervention area we are from the ideal 0 % (but, note, to support action we do not need this information to have such precision), it is even more important to know *if* it is changing, *if* there are increasing or decreasing trends, and eventually if all the health promotion and public health action has produced an effect. This is the information that surveillance can and should offer.

Smoking is again a good example to clarify the concept of continuity and why we need this. One could reasonably (and correctly) claim that the usual cross-sectional annual or 3–5-year health surveys are capable to estimate the trend of smokers among a population. For instance these surveys have shown the decline of smokers in most of the Western countries since the years in which all Hollywood stars were pictured with a cigarette. But this is the *secular trend*: quite often behaviors follow a clear path that for a set of concurring causes brings a steady decline (or increase—take the example of obesity). We certainly do not need surveillance to estimate these. But public health action (and particularly health promotion) deals with secular trends, and specifically aims to produce changes much more rapidly. Let us follow the smoking example: we have seen in recent years among the young population and particularly among the female young population a (possible) shift in this secular trend, with girls picking up smoking instead of giving it up. So public health policy makers ask questions. "Is this happening also in my country?" "If so, has my action averted, as hoped, this tendency?" "Is my territory changing more rapidly than others?" "Who is changing?" "Are there differences that can lead to inequalities?" "Is my public health campaign changing anything?" These are the critical questions that a comprehensive, systematic, timely BRFSS-type surveillance system can answer. That implies that one *needs* a surveillance system.

If health promotion is all about *social change*, this implies that to support (in terms of offering information useful to programming, monitoring, and evaluating) health-promoting actions we need to better understand the dynamics of change (Tuma and Hannan 1984). To better understand the dynamics of (social) change, we certainly need dynamic tools. This is why BRFS must be set and planned as a *dynamic system*. To better understand the evolution of the variables of interest we need a surveillance that implements a dynamic observation (to detect the evolution) and models (theoretical and statistical) capable of *understanding* the mechanisms behind the observed evolution of change.

It is clear that the dynamic reality of surveillance introduces complexity and that is one of the theoretical characteristics of surveillance that distinguishes it from other informative approaches and presents unique challenges to data analysis and interpretation. While many data collection approaches (e.g., surveys, registries) tend to move towards data analyses that are reductionist, surveillance data cannot so easily be reduced to single-variable analyses. The reality of surveillance is that all the measured variables are changing over time in some observable relationship to each other. Thus, any analytic approach must be very dynamic. Fortunately modern statistical approaches exist to address that dynamism.

Time and the Systemic Approach

The dynamic issue described above implies that if we want to answer practical questions we need an efficient and *systematic* approach. We have already mentioned that surveillance can be seen as an *Information System* inside the bigger health information system. We have stated that surveillance must be dynamic. But, what does this all mean, in terms of how surveillance (for the moment) from a theoretical point of view be organized? In order to help answer this question Campostrini and McQueen (2005) have proposed a surveillance system as a learning system (Argyrols and Scion 1996) that dynamically performs its major action (data collection, data analysis, interpretation, and data use); doing so it produces knowledge that is always the starting

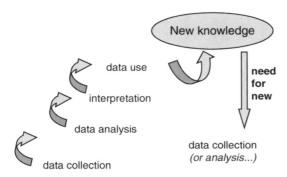

Fig. 4.1 The "spiral" of surveillance: Surveillance elements are linked dynamically and surveillance itself can be seen as a learning system (Campostrini and McQueen 2005)

point of surveillance. But every time this knowledge is a *new* starting point: it is a learning system (Fig. 4.1). Notably, the surveillance system *learns* not only from the knowledge produced by its own system but also from any other source of the health system. Data collected in a surveillance system are collected to support public health action, and so are collected because someone has defined certain priorities for action and because (quite often somewhere else) it has been provided some *evidence* for to support that action.

The systematic approach is the only one that allows for starting, keeping together, and maintaining the dynamicity necessary for a surveillance system. So, those willing to build up a surveillance system must take care of the "usual" social research and epidemiological aspects (sampling, questionnaire, data gathering and analysis, etc.) as much as they need to pay attention to the *elements* and *procedures* constituting the architecture of the system.

The "Instrument" of Surveillance Data Collection: The Survey Approach and Questionnaire

That the "instrument" for data collection in BRFS is based on a survey methodology is a critical point that is often not considered theoretically because it is simply assumed to be the basis for risk factor surveillance. In fact, the survey

approach is rather recent and highly tied to the social sciences, notably sociology, and to the rise of computing and calculating devices able to handle large numbers. Fundamentally a social survey is not a method to investigate a single individual; it is theoretically tied to a population statistics approach. Many assume that the "instrument" is the questionnaire that is used in a survey, but it is more appropriate to conceive of the whole survey package (from sampling to data analysis) as the "instrument." Thus the survey is a conceptual "structure" that houses components that are questions based on variables that relate to socio-behavioral concepts that relate to health. The theory underlying a survey is complex (see, for instance, Bickman and Rog 1998; Groves et al. 2004; Moser and Kalton 1989). In essence it is based on a complex modeling approach that assumes that through a patterned number of questions the socio-behavioral patterns of populations of respondents can be modeled. Once modeled the results are entered into a population frame as an entity. The result of many such models being aggregated at a point in time reveals an estimated point in time picture of social behavior in the population. Like all instruments the survey has many possibilities for error (Groves 1989; Biemer et al. 1991) and those practicing the art of surveillance spend an inordinate amount of time trying to get the instrument to work as well as possible. Those who work with surveys refer to problems with concepts such as reliability, validity, error, and other terms. But, as with all instruments, when allowed to run over a long period of time the problems, the errors, become understood and therefore manageable. This is one of the most important points of "continuous" data collection—as the instrument, the survey, is used day in and day out, and its operating characteristics, positive and negative, become better understood by the operators of the system. This is a unique aspect of true surveillance; it is a learning system (also from an error standing point of view). The same cannot be said for the occasional population survey.

Both the social survey and surveillance are rooted in a population-based, statistical approach. That is they yield results about the characteristics of the population in which individuals are actors. It is a common error to assume that the social survey tells one about an individual in a population when in fact the individual, the respondent, is in actuality merely an informant on behaviors in the population and at the same time an informant on the social structural characteristics of the population. Thus in a socio-behavioral risk factor surveillance system one is not monitoring changes in individuals, but changes in behaviors in the population. The individuals do not own the behaviors. Perhaps because of the initial epidemiological, individual, medically based orientation of many who work in public health and use surveillance data this remains puzzling. In considering social surveys on economic and labor-type variables and their change over time we easily attribute the results from a population perspective and do not seem to be driven to anthropomorphisms when discussing the data.

Another major aspect of the survey approach is the reliance on a stimulus–reaction (question and answer) process that is in many ways has been recognized as an "art" since its very beginning (Payne 1951). Here we will not linger over the many interesting and challenging aspects of the social surveys; we would like only to point out that the output of this stimulus–reaction process is always an indicator, i.e., not the *actual measure* of the target variables (phenomena), but a *proxy* of it. This must be kept in mind, particularly when someone claims that there are better measures around … possible, but quite often unimportant, since these will be in any case indicators and not actual measures, and I would never give up one indicator for a potentially better one if this means to lose possibility for comparison over time. Certainly we all want reliable, valid indicators but the importance of an indicator lies in its (shared) use, more than in its technical aspects. And this is peculiar in a surveillance system. We ask as major characteristic to our indicators to be sensitive to changes, since that is what we want, not the perfect actual measure (quite often impossible to obtain) but a reliable source of information about changes when these occur. When driving a car, we do not need the perfect measure of the pressure of the oil in the engine; we need only an *indicator* that lights up when this is dangerously dropping suggesting us a stop at the first garage.

While we have explored some underlying theoretical dimensions of surveillance there are many that remain. Implicit in the idea of socio-behavioral changes over time are many assumptions about the "causes" of these changes. Herein one enters the world of ideas and theories about individual and societal change over time. One may classify these theories of causality into what may be termed little theories, mainly at the individual behavioral level, and big theories that operate at the societal level. Among the former are ideas, such as risk behaviors, lifestyle concepts, personal behaviors, and many others, which stem from a rich sociopsychological literature on human behavior. Among the big theories are broad concepts such as globalization, urbanization, religion, values, and other broad societal perspectives that change in the population over time but which may not be uniform within the population or predictable. The issue with such theories for those engaged in surveillance is how to incorporate these ideas into the "instrument" of surveillance and, lacking the ability to do that in some cases, how to analyze the data we have in a way that incorporates theoretical explanations from these many causes. To give a concrete example, take the phenomenon of obesity whose trajectory in the West has been so well documented by existent surveillance systems. Clearly there has been a proportionate change in the weight of the population over time, but what are the causes? Some of the answers must be in the data that have been collected, and in many cases not discovered because of lack of analyses. This point leads us from theory to methods.

Methodological Aspects

Continuous Survey Approach

As mentioned earlier, ideally the observation process should be continuous (as defined above). Here we will try to examine this issue from a methodological, practical point of view. Let us go back to the example of security cameras. For security purposes, one would always desire the surveillance camera switched on for not losing what is going on in the area under control. Nevertheless, even in this example, security control cameras do not register each second of action, but, to save hard disk space, collect one photogram, say, every 2–3 s: enough for not losing the relevant information about who, when, and how someone got into the area. If for disease surveillance continuity is defined differently depending on the different sources (quite often registers and hospital records collect information on each case, so neither problem of sampling nor problem of continuity are questioned), in BRFS continuity must be properly addressed both from the theoretical point of view (is it sufficiently continuous?) and from the methodological one to provide sufficiently reliable information about trend and changes.

While the first aspect has been already addressed in previous paragraphs, the second poses several methodological problems that here we would like to mention and briefly discuss. As it is the state of the art in several countries, BRFS is performed through a series of repeated surveys on the same population with independent samples drawn at fixed time. As in the security camera example, the frequency of the samples is determined trying to combine parsimony and the need for reliable and sufficiently precise estimates. Let us clarify the last point. If for a cross-sectional survey the precision is determined (mainly) by the *sample size*, for a time series (such are surveillance data when one wants to observe trends or detect changes) the number of observations over time is as much important as the sample size (of each observation). The big question could be "how many points of observation do we need?" And a simple answer could then be "as many as possible." But, to be a little more precise, we will try to explain why one should have as many observations as possible. All depends on two factors: the purpose of the study and the variability in the evolution of the variable considered. Of course for a very steady variable we need less information to determine its evolution, while for a very

unstable one, we need much more information to know if the possible change observed is a structural one or simply a random effect. But also the purpose is important: if one is studying secular trends then frequent observations are not as necessary as when one wants to estimate short-time trend or changes, as in evaluation studies. If seasonal aspects are to be considered, obviously we need sufficient information about the "seasons." That is why in many countries in which a BRFS proper system is developed, a quite common standard for data collection is the monthly observation (it is the case, to name some quite developed surveillance systems in Australia, Brazil, Canada, Italy, and the USA). Drawing an independent sample every month allows for a suitable number of observations to start to estimate trends in few years from the starting of the system, sufficiently precise estimates of changes in the trends (if any occur), to study seasonal effects, and to perform evaluative studies (Campostrini et al. 2006; Taylor et al. 2010).

Sampling and the "Aggregate Over Time or Over Space" Game

In surveillance, setting the frequency of observations does not end the issues in sampling design. Sample size and sampling strategies remain important issues in surveillance as in any system based on random sampling surveys. As already mentioned if the frequency of observation is important, a time series in which all the point estimates are based on small sample size offers little information about the evolution of the variables under study. Quite often then, surveillance systems must address another problem: if typically systems are organized at state/national level, information is ideally needed also for more local levels. We mentioned as constituent characteristic of surveillance that of bringing information for public health action. Action, quite often, is at local level. If, as we will briefly explain later, statistics can help in offering better estimates for small areas, there is nothing miraculous: if data are not collected thinking of possible use at local level, there will be very little to do in the analysis phase. So it is highly recommendable when drawing the sample design for surveillance to take into consideration the local level.

This is also for the unique possibility that surveillance data offer to play the game of "aggregate over time or over space." If the sampling design has considered the local level, i.e., has collected perhaps a very limited number of cases for each observation and for *each* local entity, it is always possible in the analysis to pool aggregate data over time to have sufficiently precise estimates to publish also at local level. And the "sufficiently" can be defined according to the size of the local level and the purpose of the study. So, in a surveillance system we could have monthly estimate for the state, quarterly for the province/region, annual for some local entity, and, say, every 3 years for the county level. Similarly (this is the other "game"), when we need information on the evolution, time frequency is important, and we will pool together data *over space*, aggregating samples from adjacent areas (as when we need information for local areas we pooled data *over time*), aggregating the, say, monthly samples until we have sufficiently precise estimates. This "game," then, in the phase of analysis can be even improved through the use of suitable statistical tools that enhance the precision of local estimate (small area statistics—see for example Rao 2003 or Pfeffermann 2007).

The System's Challenge for Sustainability

Collecting data every month could seem much more difficult than a yearly collection. Experience proves that this is not true and that a day-in day-out data collection is much more efficient than systems that collect data at large interrupted intervals of time, since the start-up costs are, quite often, the most relevant ones. But a surveillance system, as claimed here, is much more than data collection: it is made of a complexity of persons, procedures, networks, communication activities, etc. that in some way must be funded and sustained over time. The "over time" is quite often the problem. Politicians typically prefer to invest on projects

capable of showing results in the short term (before next election), while one can really only appreciate the value of a surveillance system after few years (when trend and change analyses start to be meaningful). So, while the trigger for a surveillance system to start lies in its capability to offer unique (and quite often the only possible) answers to several public health questions, as we discussed at the beginning of this chapter, it is something else that keeps a system alive.

From the experience collected now in several countries, two major aspects appear necessary for the maintenance of a surveillance system:

- The institutionalization of the surveillance in the broader health information system (HIS)
- The networking of the surveillance system

To *institutionalize* means to settle the system in a way that it has the capacity to sustain itself over a long period of time and have a future (Campostrini and McQueen 2005). Institutionalization is often seen as essentially a problem of financial resources, but such resources are only sustained once a system is institutionalized and legitimized as part and parcel of the underpinning expectations of a public health system. It is a matter of developing relationships, networking, and, most critically, facilitating the use of data and information. If surveillance plays a peculiar role in the HIS, as we mentioned before, this role must be affirmed, recognized, and actively continued using all possible means (normative, structural, networking, etc.)

Quite often in the past too little attention has been paid to these aspects of institutionalization, and the dissemination of information from surveillance ended after the production of an official report. Now we recognize that if we want a surveillance system to be effective, it must include elements such as networking, social marketing, and information brokering. In general, a surveillance system must include a marketing strategy that is designed to proactively inform "consumers" and stakeholders. Then, the importance of *networking* for a surveillance system cannot be overemphasized. Legitimization, institutionalization, and, eventually, sustainability rest with the capability of the system to produce effective networks.

Data Analysis: Each Purpose Has Its Own Tool

We could not end the methodological part without a reference to data analysis. Just naming all the possible methods, approaches, and techniques for surveillance data analysis is practically impossible and in any case far from the purpose of this chapter. Here it is important to underline how data analysis to properly fit a surveillance system should be capable to answer all the questions that a surveillance system poses. So, if it is certainly important to produce regularly simple reports, the bread and butter of a surveillance system, possibly in such a communicative way to allow for readability and easiness to use, it is also important that the data analysis system is capable of detecting those changes and trends for which a surveillance system is unique and incomparable with respect to other health survey-based systems.

Going back to the bread and butter issue, it is important to notice how "readability and easiness to use" should be spelled in the data analysis language. The time of crosstabs has ended; the public now requires to really use data, maps, graphs, and interactive systems that allow not only to "read the data" but are also capable to offer at a quick glance a reasonable interpretation of the findings. Mapping, for instance, has been proven to be a very effective way to communicate geographical differences, but also how these change over time: it is acknowledged that the American general public really understood the obesity epidemic only when media reported the graphs from the BRFSS showing the map of the US states going more uniformly colored and darker over the years as the percentage of obese persons steadily increased in all the states.

And now let us address the main, and more advanced from a statistical point of view, issues of data analysis with surveillance data: trend and changes. It took a while to see trend analyses produced by surveillance systems; the reason was essentially cultural: epidemiologists and health data analysts did not have in their working bag appropriate tools for this. Time series analysis was considered something for economists or statisticians applied to other fields, and, although the system was providing good monthly estimates, data were yearly aggregated to show, using crosstabs, "changes over the years." What a waste of information!

Now sophisticated statistical tools are available to most analysts, and also in surveillance it is becoming common to see trend graphs that use all the available information and in a proper way. Without going into technicalities far from the purpose of this book, let us try to answer the fundamental question on trend analysis: "Why we need 'proper' statistical analyses? Cannot we simply plot our data on a scatter plot and calculate a regression line to show the trend?"

The answer to the latter question is no. Here are the reasons:

- Time affects the time series (e.g., the observed prevalence of one risk factor over time) differently, with different effects.
- Some of these could hide the actual effects, and, particularly, bring to considerations about the significance (of trends or changes) far from the truth.

When analyzing a time series the researcher wants to detect, separate, and estimate the different effects of time. It is like what we see in some TV series where police listen to telephone conversations, trying to isolate (using machines that in the real life perform statistical analysis similar to those we are referring here) different sounds to recognize some of peculiar interest ("yes, this is the sound that cars make when passing over the bridge on 34th street" …). Similarly, researchers analyzing a time series want to get rid of the "noises" to recognize peculiarities such as seasonality, trends (linear and cycles), and changes. If considered all together (the simple regression), like with the conversation intercepted by police, one could overcome the others, or the interactive effects could make significant something that, once isolated, is not significant at all. So, it is important to use the right tools for different purposes. And this is also in relation to the sophistication of the analysis: quite often complex problems require complex analysis. That is, if one wants to analyze the simple trend of a single variable, once appropriate test for "other effects" of time is run (such as the Durbin–Watson test), and also a simple regression is sufficient, while for forecasting or estimating the effect of an intervention ARIMA models and the so-called interrupted time series models (Box and Jenkins 1976; McDowall et al. 1980) can be reasonably applied. Furthermore, in looking at more complex problems, such as multivariate trends, or in analyzing if and how the relationship among some variables has changed over time, other statistical models are more appropriate. Quite often, for the latter, it is not easy to find in the surveillance literature examples of application, giving the relative novelty of such surveillance and the cultural gap we mentioned above. So, it is up to the researcher to "import" these methods and models from other fields of application (Campostrini 2003).

Communication and Data Use

We have already noted in the data analysis section the importance of a communicative "style" in producing simple data analysis reports. But this is not enough to assure a real use of surveillance data and information (and consequently its sustainability and existence). This goes back to the issue of surveillance as a system. Among the different *functions* of such a system, there is that of communication. If we want our surveillance data to be used, we must be capable of communicating them in a usable way. We learn from social marketing (see, for instance, Kotler et al. 2002) how important, for an effective communication, are aspects such as communication planning, careful definition of messages and how these can be delivered, and the application of suitable strategies customized to the specific audience one wishes to reach. We already mentioned that a surveillance system cannot work properly if it has not built a network around itself. Data use is an effect of the network. As much effective is the networking of the surveillance system as much its data will be used, and the system will be legitimized. If these concepts are fairly simple and almost self-evident, more reflection is required to better understand what is about this networking process and who are the major actors of this.

Networking relies in building relationships among individuals and institutions for exchanging purposes. In our case the exchange concerns mainly information. From the surveillance system perspective, these are incoming or outgoing.

Incoming information and requests: Surveillance lives (as learning system) on the evidence produced elsewhere, and consequently much attention must be paid to shared results coming from the literature (evidences), not only in choosing the variables to survey but also in how questions are worded. Then, if we want our data used, we must pay attention to the stakeholders' needs; those conducting surveillance must see how the data collected and information released are used and by whom. Since not all the possible questions can be asked for clear matters of parsimony (and burden for the respondents), prioritization should be made mainly on the bases of the priorities for public health and health promotion, as they emerge from the evidence provided in the literature and from the requests (needs) of the stakeholders.

Outgoing information: Surveillance must rely on a proper dissemination system, with organized (and not seldom) networking activities (such as newsletters, meeting on specific subjects, etc.). Particular attention must be paid to the form of communication and to the outputs: results cannot be presented in the same way to the media and to the general public or to some academic or professional society potentially interested.

Typical stakeholders: All public health and health promotion decision makers (local, regional/provincial, national), media, NGOs, and particularly "single diseases society" (cancer association, etc.). The dialogue with stakeholders is fundamental; it is important to listen and understand their needs, and to share the message that surveillance is not by itself property of those who run it, but for users, it belongs to everyone, and it is a common good.

Finally, there is one thing to keep always in mind: sustainability of a surveillance system is all in its data use. The most reluctant politician under a spending review fever (there are quite a few around nowadays) will think twice to switch off a system in which data are used everywhere, and particularly if they are also used in official documents; it will not take more than a second, instead, if data are disseminated only through recognized and highly rated scientific literature (very few will notice, and very few will protest...).

Surveillance and Social Determinants of Health

Why dedicate a paragraph to surveillance and the social determinants of health (SDH). Why not surveillance and gender, surveillance and healthy setting, or surveillance and physical activities? Certainly we could linger over many aspects of surveillance and public health, NCDs, and health promotion to fill in more than a book, and all these could be really relevant. But, today, particularly in relationship with NCDs, none can be more important than SDH. The first reason, certainly well discussed in other chapters of this volume, is that today, to tackle NCDs, social determinants cannot be ignored. And this is not (only) for ethical reasons, or for shared values that tell us that equity is something to aspire to and inequity something to avoid. SDH are quite often the mechanisms for which NCDs are increasing in most of the world; they are, quoting Marmot and Rose (Marmot 2005; Rose 1992), the "causes of the causes." So it is far too limited to carry on surveillances on risk factors without considering SDH; it cannot provide sufficient information to really address NCD problems. Consequently, and this perhaps is the most important and sensitive issue, if we are looking for answers on how to better address NCDs in our country, region, and territory, we necessarily need to better understand how SDH are changing over time, and how these changes are affecting NCDs. Public health is facing new challenges and certainly much more complexity than in the past (Hanlon et al. 2011).

If medical research tells us that one NCD (say cardiovascular diseases—CVDs) is *caused* by one risk factor (say obesity), it is only surveillance that can tell us how and why this risk factor is increasing/decreasing among certain strata of the population. And if, as it is quite often the case, there are inequalities in CVDs, to know how and why certain strata of the population are becoming more obese is fundamental to tackle CVDs (and its inequalities). It is even more relevant for health promotion. How can we run a health promotion program, let us stay with the example, to reduce obesity among a certain population and particularly aimed to reduce obesity among those at higher risk (that we found more present in the less educated and poorer strata of the population) without information on:

– The changing relationship among SDH and obesity in our target area.
– The changing SDH in our target area.
– How previous interventions have affected obesity and linked behaviors/attitudes, and how much these have increased/decreased SDH effects?

I do not see any other source of data, but surveillance, to offer this fundamental information.

Now, it must be said that existing surveillance systems are already quite well equipped to answer several questions regarding SDH (Campostrini et al. 2011): all the several variables collected on the "causes" of NCDs can be related to some SDH such as education or income, regularly collected in most of the existing BRFS (Minardi et al. 2011). Nevertheless, a lot is still to do. SDH are not circumscriptive only to education and income, and, for a deeper understanding of the mechanisms by which SDH cause the causes of NCDs, more information is needed. Some can be reasonably gathered directly through BRFSs, and others can be acquired through data linkage with other sources (e.g., information on urban aspects, housing, etc.). For this much research is still needed to inform the "surveillance learning system."

In these research issues, we can see some additional difficulties. And, again, they are cultural. Research on NCD, surveillance, and SDH is asked to understand and study complex social models. To do this, necessarily, research must leave the biomedical roots, common to most researchers working on NCDs, to adopt some sociological view of the research, more accustomed to these kinds of problems. Only in this way will it be possible to find new ways, new measures, and new approaches capable to bring new light on the complex relationship between NCDs, the causes (risk factors), and the causes of the causes (SDH).

The introduction of NCDs and HP into surveillance is part of the "natural" evolutionary process of surveillance. If, for instance, parallel surveys that took into account also physical measures were fundamental at the infant stage of surveillance, for validation purposes, to understand limit and potentiality of self-reported data (Nelson et al. 2001; Oswald and Wu 2010), now, from my view, this belongs to the past. And the fact that with some questions we under- or overestimate a prevalence is not any more a problem, since the task assigned to surveillance is not that of producing the most precise estimates, but that of "ringing alarm bells" if an indicator (that is never the actual measure) is going too up or too down; the task is to inform about changes (for whom, where, and how these happen). Certainly there are, also in recent official documents, those who claim that physical measures are still needed for good surveillance, and unfortunately some of these occupy position in some recognized international organization, but they are wrong, they belong to the past, and they are not listening to the evidence coming from "real" BRFS. So much information has been produced without the need of costly physical measures: we knew that obesity was becoming an epidemic without weighting significant samples of Americans (and then of Europeans, etc.); we found that smokers were decreasing without taking samples of saliva from people; and now we know that there are important differences in risk factors among the less educated and poorer strata of the population without any physical measures, any test to prove the educational level, or any survey on the actual wealth of individuals.

Some Final Remarks, Looking Forward to a Development of NCD and HP Surveillance

After this excursus on several aspects of surveillance, it is difficult to summarize the many important points discussed. As final remarks, we, instead, would like to have a look forward and try to briefly examine the challenges that this particular type of surveillance is facing, and will likely face in the immediate future. Some of these are technical-methodological; some are more political-structural. Though for descriptive purposes we will present them separately, the two challenges quite often go together, and the ability to strengthen the methodological challenges puts more pressure on efforts to solve political issues, and the other way round.

Challenges in Data Collection

Both economically developed and developing countries are facing major problems in data collection. If the latter, often in the high-burden area for NCDs, suffer for lack of adequate structure for surveillance (Alwan et al. 2010), in many high- and middle-income countries the problem is related to the survey methodology usually applied (telephone surveys) for surveillance that is experiencing (a) a continuing decline in the response rate (Schneider et al. 2012) and (b) a shift in large parts of the population from the easy-to-reach landline phones to cellular phones (Mokdad 2011). For the developed countries the problems are mainly political (and cultural as we will see later on), for the latter are from one side methodological (if we want to maintain the telephone survey structure) and on the other side structural, if we want to look to future and more advanced ways of collecting data. The lack of information given from low response rates and the possible biases introduced by dual-mode ways of collecting data (landline and cell phones) poses mainly statistical problems and asks for more advanced statistical tools (Mokdad 2011; Pierannunzi et al. 2012) to produce reliable prevalence estimates. But, taking a broader view, telephone surveys have been an innovation started in the 1960s/1970s that took place in many countries only in the 1990s and now, perhaps, is declining. Well, there will or could be some other innovation (from the Web, the smart phones, the social networks, etc.) that perhaps in few years, as happened for telephone surveys, will become the standard. So, surveillance research must pay attention to new ways of collecting data and information to be ready to shift (partially and then totally) to new ways of data collection. But this is not all. As BRFS is developing in many countries we can see some successful stories, also with regard to response rate and cell phones. It is the case of the Italian surveillance system PASSI (Baldissera et al. 2011) that is performing an amazing steady 80 % response rate over, now, 5 years of experience. What is the secret? Go local. Interviews are administered by nurses of the Local Health Units (LHU); if any problem or questions, respondents can call the LHU or their general practitioners, who help also in providing numbers (typical cell phones) if the person selected in the sample does not have a telephone number listed in the LHU archives. Certainly this is a peculiar model not immediately exportable to other countries; still, it can be a lesson for those developing surveillance systems about the importance of involving the local authorities/organizations.

Data Linkage and Information Networking

As mentioned earlier, with regard to SDH, surveillance cannot collect all the possible data and information, because of the time limit of an interview and because some important data (typically ecological) are not collectable through surveys on individuals. And if some of these data are already collected or collectable by other means, the problem is that quite often one does not need only this information, but have to put it in relationship with others, typically produced by surveillance system, i.e., to have them in a single data file. This is, theoretically, quite easily solvable through data linkage: it is sufficient to have one data in common (e.g., the county, the district, etc.) and the link is possible. Still this is rarely done, for several reasons. The first, again, is cultural, or at least derives from cultural aspects. Quite often researchers and those responsible for data gathering develop an idea (value) of "data property"; those working with data often believe that the data is personally theirs and that they are important because they have a lot of data. This is

really far from the present world in which the most powerful global companies are those that do not possess any data, but have the ability to connect with data/information from elsewhere. Still, mentalities are difficult to change, and many are reluctant in agreeing that the value of data is in its use, its sharing. Related to this problem, there is another one, more technical (and consequently easier to solve): the difficulties in the linkage determined by data that are not thought to be linked (e.g., do not have many variables to help the linkage). One example for all: geo-reference. It is now, not in some far future, that a lot of our activities have some geo-reference: our car, our phones, and our bills are all geo-referenced with precise coordinates that enable to find and plot the activity on a map with an error of less than 10 m. Surveillance data, in best cases, have county-level geo-reference. Today this level is perhaps enough for data linkage, tomorrow certainly will not be; the possibilities for ecological studies offered by geo-referencing are so many; think only of the possibilities of linking risk factors, or perceived health with geographical information related to availability of services, urban aspects, presence of dangerous activities, etc.

Another major problem with data linkage is that of *privacy*. Often (particularly when hospital records are involved) privacy is the word that closes any door for possible interesting data linkage. Governments and privacy authorities should understand that when information is applied for public health action, this should be considered as much important as medical interventions (for which, typically, all sorts of exception for privacy are adopted). Secondly, privacy can be always easily assured: now the most common tools for data linkage can assure 100 % privacy (destroying the personal information used for linkage at the same time of the linkage process). So in reality privacy is not the problem, again mentality and regulations are; it is just a matter of pushing for advanced regulations that allow, and at the same time fix the rules for, "proper" data linkages.

Finally, let us go back to the cultural issue. If we really want to share data and information, besides data linkage, or better to facilitate data linkage processes, the network is, again, important. Networking, in this case, means fixing channels and procedures that allow and facilitate data exchange. And when the network has been built, this will last and be useful for several data exchanges and data linkages. Perhaps in simplifying data linkage one should look to "information networking."

Surveillance Capacity

It is a fact: "real" (as defined above) NCD/HP surveillance systems have been developed only in few countries. Certainly we can hide beside the (relative) novelty of a (real) surveillance approach to NCDs and related risk factors. Then, one could argue that only recently NCDs (and risk factors) have been posed on the global political agenda. One could even claim that among the general population perception (and politicians and resources follow quite closely this) objects as risk factors, or chronic diseases, have very little appeal and create very little attention, even if they involve (globally) millions of deaths and billions of "lost healthy years." When one compares the apparent appeal of perhaps few hundred or even few individuals that die from a strange communicable disease that (perhaps with a probability of less than 1 over a million) also *you* could get, the NCDs seem to lose importance. (We remain prejudiced and cannot easily liberate ourselves from the fear of plagues that have affected so profoundly our history for centuries and centuries.) This is all very true, still not a complete justification for such scarce development of NCD surveillance. But the reality today is that, with the exceptions of a few great successful stories, there is a profound lack of capacity to carry out and maintain NCD/HP surveillance. This is for several reasons, and here we will try to mention a few.

Stability and resources: Already mentioned, surveillance produces interesting results only in the long run, and must be funded for years and years, something not too appealing for contemporary politicians and decision makers, and particularly problematic for low- and middle-income countries. Nevertheless, we have seen how the major investments required to set up a system and the

lesser investments to keep it running yield innovative ways not only to collect data, but that the ongoing operation of the system facilitates both the institutionalization and the efficiency of the system.

Cultural aspects: Surveillance (BRFS) is an innovation in the health world, and the evolutionary process has just started, requiring for instance to go behind the biomedical research model (for reasons discussed above), and this means that time is required to carry on the innovation, to allow for mentality changes, and to solve many related problems, such as the *need for training in public health* (particularly when we are proposing something culturally far from previous experiences) or the problem of involving *national and international institutions*, which, by "nature," think to survive only by adopting *conservative policies* (no matter if this is in reaction to a world changing more and more rapidly), and consequently are always reluctant to support innovations. In this regard, at personal level there is very little to do, but wait while organizations (NGOs, academic societies, networks, etc.) accept the need to advocate for "real" surveillance development.

What Next? (A Personal Note)

I thought the answer to this question would have been the perfect end for this chapter. The only problem is that I do not know the answer, or *all* the possible relevant answers. Certainly after 20 years from when I finished my Ph.D. thesis on the methodological problems of surveillance, several aspects of the challenges have been acquired. Some, particularly linked to data analysis, are still open to exploration. Few are absolutely new and not on the radar screen 20 years ago. So, from my perhaps limited but privileged (thanks only to the contacts with few BRFSs around the globe) observatory, I can see that there is still a lot of thinking to do. But after all, infectious disease surveillance developed over decades with massive financial support, and NCD/HP surveillance in the last two decades made so many progresses, relying on so little that I cannot end without an optimistic view. Now that NCDs are on the first places of many political agendas, and now that HP and SDH are coming back in relevant position for public health, perhaps some good minds will see that, also in time of economic crises, money invested in informing how to tackle the causes and the causes of the causes are well invested and can save a lot of money, producing much better health; well, I am pretty sure that surveillance will rapidly develop also where it has not (and it is most needed) and many of the problems and challenges here only mentioned will be solved in much less than two decades.

Acknowledgments With my colleague David McQueen, we have discussed dynamics and continuity in observation since 1989; at that time he was running one of the first pilot "real" BRFS-type systems in the world at the University of Edinburgh. Since then, we have continued to discuss these issues, and what is written here would not be without this intellectual debate. Many other colleagues have contributed to develop and spread these ideas around the globe, among these Bernard Choi, Vivian Lin, Stefania Salmaso and the Italian PASSI network, Anne Taylor, and many others. To all of them my gratitude, but all the responsibility for what is written is only mine, and in any case never of the institutions I am representing.

From the Web

WHO

Definition of Surveillance
http://www.who.int/topics/public_health_surveillance/en/

Political declaration of the High-level Meeting of the General Assembly of the United Nations on the Prevention and Control of Non-communicable Diseases (September 2011)—http://www.un.org/ga/search/view_doc.asp?symbol=A%2F66%2FL.1&Lang=E

A comprehensive global monitoring framework including indicators and a set of voluntary global targets for the prevention and control of NCDs (discussion paper)—http://www.who.int/entity/nmh/events/2012/discussion_paper2_20120322.pdf

WHO commission on Social Determinants of health – Closing the gap in a generation: Health equity through action on the social determinants of health—http://whqlibdoc.who.int/publications/2008/9789241563703_eng.pdf

Rio Political Declaration on Social Determinants of Health – World Conference on Social Determinants of Health (Rio de Janeiro, Brazil, 21 October 2011)—http://www.who.int/entity/sdhconference/declaration/Rio_political_declaration.pdf

International Union for Health Promotion

White Paper on Surveillance
http://www.iuhpe.org/uploaded/Activities/Scientific_Affairs/GWG/WARFS_white_paper_draft_may_2011.pdf

IUHPE Call for Action on Health Promotion Approaches to Non-communicable Disease Prevention

- *Short version*: http://www.iuhpe.org/uploaded/Activities/Advocacy/IUHPE_KeyMessagesNCDs_WEB.pdf
- *Longer version*: http://www.iuhpe.org/uploaded/Activities/Advocacy/IUHPE%20Key%20Messages%20_LONG_WEB.pdf

IUHPE Position Statement on the Social Determinants of Health

http://www.iuhpe.org/uploaded/Activities/Scientific_Affairs/GWG/IUHPEPosition%20paper_SDH_DRAFT_ENG.pdf

IUHPE Key Messages on the Social Determinants of Health (in Folder)

CDC

Evaluation of Public Health Surveillance Systems
http://www.cdc.gov/mmwr/preview/mmwrhtml/rr5013a1.htm

Behavioral Risk Factor Surveillance System

http://www.cdc.gov/BRFSS

References

AbouZahr, C., & Boerma, T. (2005). Health information systems: The foundations of public health. *Bulletin of the World Health Organization, 83*, 578–583.

Alwan, A., Maclean, D. R., Riley, L. M., d'Espaignet, E. T., Mathers, C. D., Stevens, G. A., et al. (2010). Monitoring and surveillance of chronic noncommunicable diseases: Progress and capacity in high-burden countries. *Lancet, 366*, 1861–1868.

Argyrols, C., & Scion, D. (1996). *Organizational learning II: Theory, method and practice*. Reading, MA: Addison Wesley.

Baldissera, S., Campostrini, S., Binkin, N., Minardi, V., Minelli, G., Ferrante, G., et al. (2011). Features and initial assessment of the Italian Behavioral Risk Factor Surveillance System (PASSI), 2007–2008. *Preventing Chronic Disease, 8*(1), 1–8.

Bellini, P., Campostrini, S., Balestrino, R., & Masselli, M. (1994). Public statistical information systems: Definition aspects and architectural issues. *Statistica Applicata, 6*(3), 239–248.

Bickman, L., & Rog, D. J. (Eds.). (1998). *Handbook of applied social research methods*. Thousand Oaks, CA: Sage.

Biemer, P. P., Groves, R. M., Lyberg, L. E., Mathiowetz, N. A., & Sudman, S. (1991). *Measurement errors in survey*. New York, NY: John Wiley & Sons.

Birkhead, G. S., & Maylahn, C. M. (2000). State and local public health surveillance. In S. M. Teutsch & R. E. Churchill (Eds.), *Principles and practice of public health surveillance*. New York, NY: Oxford University Press.

Box, G. E. P., & Jenkins, G. M. (1976). *Time series analysis: Forecasting and control*. Oakland, CA: Holden-Day.

Campostrini, S. (2003). Surveillance systems and data analysis. In D. V. McQueen & P. Puska (Eds.), *Global behavioral risk factor surveillance* (pp. 47–55). New York, NY: Kluwer.

Campostrini, S. (2007). Measurement and effectiveness. Methodological consideration, issues and possible solutions. In D. V. McQueen & C. Jones (Eds.), *Global perspective on health promotion effectiveness* (pp. 305–326). New York, NY: Springer.

Campostrini, S., Holtzman, D., McQueen, D. V., & Boaretto, E. (2006). Evaluating the effectiveness of health promotion policy: Changes in the law on drinking and driving in California. *Health Promotion International, 21*, 130–135.

Campostrini, S., & McQueen, D. V. (2005). Institutionalization of social and behavioral risk factor surveillance as a learning system. *Sozial- und Präventivmedizin, 50*, s9–s15.

Campostrini, S., McQueen, D. V., & Abel, T. (2011). Social determinants and surveillance in the new Millennium. *International Journal of Public Health, 56*, 357–358.

Campostrini, S., McQueen, D. V., & Evans, L. (2009). Health promotion and surveillance: The establishment of an IUHPE working group. *Global Health Promotion, 16*(4), 58–60.

Choi, B. C. K., McQueen, D. V., Puska, P., Douglas, K. A., Ackland, M., Campostrini, S., et al. (2008). Enhancing global capacity in the surveillance, prevention, and control of chronic diseases: seven themes to consider and build upon. *Journal of Epidemiology and Community Health, 62*(5), 391–397.

Declich, S., & Carter, A. O. (1994). Public health surveillance: Historical origins, methods and evaluation. *Bulletin of the World Health Organization, 72*(2), 285–304.

Groves, R. M. (1989). *Survey errors and survey costs*. New York, NY: John Wiley & Sons.

Groves, R. M., Fowler, F. J., Jr., Couper, M. P., Lepkowski, J. M., Singer, E., & Tourangeauet, R. (2004). *Survey Methodology*. New York, NY: John Wiley & Sons.

Hanlon, P., Carlislea, S., Hannahb, M., Reillyc, D., & Lyond, A. (2011). Making the case for a 'fifth wave' in Public Health. *Public Health, 125*(1), 30–36.

Haux, R. (2006). Health information systems— past, present, future. *International Journal of Medical Informatics, 75*, 268–281.

Kotler, P., Roberto, N., & Lee, N. R. (2002). *Social marketing: Improving the quality of life*. Thousand Oaks, CA: Sage Publications.

Lippeveld, T. (2001). Routine health information systems: The glue of a unified health system. In The RHINO workshop on issues and innovation in routine health information in developing countries. The Bolger Center, Protomac, MD, USA 14–16 March 2001 (pp. 13–27). Arlington, VA, USA: MEASURE Evaluation, JSI Research and Training Institute.

Marmot, M. (2005). Social determinants of health inequalities. *Lancet, 365*, 1099–1104.

McDowall, D., McCleary, R., Meidinger, E. E., & Hay, R. A., Jr. (1980). *Interrupted time series analysis*. Beverly Hills, CA: Sage Publications.

McQueen, D. V. (2009). Ethics and evidence in health promotion, Chapter 3. In A. Killoran & M. Kelly (Eds.), *Evidence-based public health: Effectiveness and efficiency* (pp. 27–40). Oxford: Oxford University Press.

McQueen, D. V., & Jones, C. M. (Eds.). (2007). *Global perspectives on health promotion effectiveness*. New York, NY: Springer Science & Business Media.

McQueen, D. V., & Puska, P. (Eds.). (2003). *Global behavioral risk factor surveillance*. New York, NY: Kluwer.

Meriwether, R. A. (1996). Blueprint for a national public health surveillance system for the 21st century. *Journal of Public Health Management and Practice, 2*(4), 16–23.

Minardi, V., Campostrini, S., Carrozzi, G., Minelli, G., & Salmaso, S. (2011). Social determinants effects from the Italian risk factor surveillance system PASSI. *International Journal of Public Health, 56*, 359–366.

Mokdad, A. H. (2011). The behavioral risk factor surveillance system: Past, Present and Future. *Annual Review of Public Health, 30*, 43–54.

Moser, K., & Kalton, G. (1989). *Survey methods in social investigation* (2nd ed.). Aldershot: Gower.

Nelson, D. E., Holtzman, D., Bolen, J., Stanwyck, C. A., & Mack, K. A. (2001). Reliability and validity of measures from the Behavioral Risk Factor Surveillance System (BRFSS). *Sozial- und Präventivmedizin, 46*(Suppl 1), S3–S42.

Oswald, A. J., & Wu, S. (2010). Objective confirmation of subjective measures of human well-being: Evidence from the U.S.A. *Science, 327*, 576–579.

Parrish, G. B., II, & McDonnell, S. (2000). Sources of health related information. In S. M. Teutsch & R. E. Churchill (Eds.), *Principles and practice of public health surveillance* (2nd ed., pp. 76–94). New York, NY: Oxford University Press.

Payne, S. L. (1951). *The art of asking questions*. Oxford, England: Princeton U. Press.

Pfeffermann, D. (2007). Small area estimation-new developments and directions. *International Statistical Review, 70*, 125–143.

Pierannunzi, C., Town, M., Garvin, W., Shaw, F. E., & Balluz, L. (2012). Methodologic changes in the behavioral risk factor surveillance system in 2011 and potential effects on prevalence estimates. *Morbidity and Mortality Weekly Report, 61*(22), 410.

Porta, M. (Ed.). (2008). *Dictionary of epidemiology. International Epidemiological Association* (5th ed.). New York, NY: Oxford University Press.

Rao, J. N. K. (2003). *Small area estimation*. New York, NY: Wiley.

Rose, G. (1992). *Strategy of preventive medicine*. Oxford: OxfordUniversity Press.

Schneider, K. L., Clark, M. A., Rakowski, W., & Lapane, K. L. (2012). Evaluating the impact of non-response bias in the Behavioral Risk Factor Surveillance System (BRFSS). *Journal of Epidemiology and Community Health, 66*, 290–295.

Smith, F. P., Hadler, J. L., Stanbury, M., Rolfs, R. T., & Hopkins, R. S. (2012). "Blueprint Version 2.0": Updating public health surveillance for the 21st century. Journal of Public Health Management Practice, doi:10.1097/PHH.0b013e318262906e.

Taylor, W. A., Campostrini, S., Gill, K. T., Herriot, M., Carter, P., & Dal Grande, E. (2010). The use of chronic disease risk factor surveillance systems for evidence-based decision-making – physical activity and nutrition as examples. *International Journal of Public Health, 55*(4), 243–249.

Teutsch, S. M., & Churchill, R. E. (Eds.). (2000). *Principles and practice of public health surveillance* (2nd ed.). New York, NY: Oxford University Press.

Thacker, S. B. (2000). Historical development. In S. M. Teutsch & R. E. Churchill (Eds.), *Principles and practice of public health surveillance* (2nd ed., pp. 1–16). New York, NY: Oxford University Press.

Thacker, S. B., Qualters, J. R., & Lee, L. M. (2012). Public health surveillance in the United States: Evolution and challenges. *Morbidity and Mortality Weekly Report, S-61*, 3–9.

Thacker, S. B., & Stroup, D. F. (1994). Future directions for comprehensive public health surveillance and health information systems in the United States. *American Journal of Epidemiology, 140*(5), 383–397.

Tuma, B. N., & Hannan, M. T. (1984). *Social dynamics: Models and methods*. New York, NY: Academic.

WHO. (2002). *Reducing risks, promoting healthy life: World Health Report 2002*. Geneva: World Health Organization.

Wysocki, R. K., & Young, J. (1990). *Information systems. Management principles in action*. New York, NY: John Wiley & Sons.

Section II

Lenses for Understanding NCDs

Learning from the Social Sciences in Chronic Diseases Health Promotion: Structure, Agency and Distributive Justice

Katherine L. Frohlich

The role that the social sciences can play in chronic disease health promotion is such a vast endeavour that it could be the subject of a book on its own. I choose in this chapter, instead, to focus on two major "hot topics" within the last 10 years in the discussion of chronic diseases and health promotion. These two topics, how to understand how and why people change their health behaviours and how to understand the inequitable distribution of these behaviours, are intimately related. In describing the relationship between these two issues, our discussion will bring us to the input that sociology, ethics and political philosophy could have on the development of chronic disease health promotion in the years to come.

The Role of Sociology

Social science has played a major, even cathartic, role in developing the current range of concepts used within health promotion. Sociology and psychology in particular have made significant contributions, positing theories of behaviour related to health by reference to social constructs. Social psychological reasons for morbidity and individual health action have been put forward by

some, whilst explanations referring to social structures and macro-processes as determinants of health have been emphasised by others. These social sciences have drawn the interest of other disciplines in health promotion, most notably education, economics and communication theory. Along with sociology, psychology and epidemiology may be called primary feeder disciplines in that they have made a major and direct contribution to health promotion theory and practices but are increasingly supported by secondary feeder disciplines whose contribution is at present less than obvious. These would include, I would argue, ethics and political philosophy. These primary and secondary disciplines consolidate what for many has been a growing, even irritating, feeling that the bio-medical model of health promotion no longer offers an adequate explanation of why people think and behave in the way they do (Bunton and Macdonald 2002).

The seeking out of social scientific theories, concepts and methods for health promotion coincides with the reduction of infectious diseases as the main causes of morbidity and mortality in the early twentieth century. This led to increasing epidemiologic attention being focused on identifying the determinants of chronic diseases associated with an aging population and modern living conditions (Hansen and Easthope 2007). Among the main contributors to these chronic diseases were cancer, cardiovascular disease and diabetes. By the mid 1970s, epidemiological evidence gathered on the determinants of these diseases pointed increasingly towards health-related

K.L. Frohlich (✉)
Département de médecine sociale et préventive,
Université de Montréal, 7010 Avenue du Parc,
Montréal, QC, Canada H3C 3J7
e-mail: katherine.frohlich@umontreal.ca

behaviours such as regular exercise, safe sex, not smoking, reducing alcohol consumption, using unleaded petrol, rejecting pharmacotherapy drugs in favour of herbal or alterative medicines, eating organic foods and participating in screening tests for blood pressure and cholesterol.

This etiologic research was followed by the development of public health interventions that focused specific attention on these health risk behaviours. These interventions, such as the MRFIT, COMMIT and other programmes (MRFIT 1981, 1982; COMMIT 1995), targeted the segment of the population with the highest level of risk exposure determined by their health-related behaviours. The assumption was that the high prevalence of chronic diseases was the result of unhealthy behaviours or lifestyle, both of which were viewed to be chosen and under an individual's control. Consequently, particular emphasis in these interventions was placed on personal responsibility and individuals' ability to make personal change towards better health and health behaviours, largely through increased education regarding the dangers of "poor" behaviours. This approach was championed by the Lalonde Report of 1974 in which Lalonde insisted on the importance of intervening on populations "at risk", populations composed of individuals all showing elevated risk for some specific disease based on their behavioural profile. This focus, Lalonde argued, would lead to the greatest public health impact (Lalonde 1974).

The Lalonde approach was challenged early on from within health promotion, beginning with the Ottawa Charter (WHO 1986). The authors of the Charter questioned Lalonde's assumptions based on results from numerous "at-risk" population interventions that had largely failed to change the behaviours of those they had targeted (MRFIT 1981, 1982). The disappointing outcomes of large-scale expensive and labour-intensive interventions gave researchers reason to pause. Behaviour change, they realised, was difficult to achieve and sustain for individuals (despite intense intervention efforts). Part of the difficulty of changing behaviour, researchers surmised, was that individuals were being asked to change omnipresent behaviours. Individuals

were expected to reduce their smoking, change their eating patterns and exercise more in environments where many, if not most, people smoked, ate poorly and exercised little. In sum, they were being asked to change in a direction away from the norm. In addition, even if the targeted individuals were to change their behaviour (which they largely did not), these interventions had no influence on the behaviour of the rest of the population not deemed "at risk", despite the fact that many of these people are also later affected by chronic diseases and their associated risk factors (Syme 1994).

The challenges brought forward in the Ottawa Charter pointed towards the neglect from within health promotion with regard to the "structure" of lifestyle, that is, the social conditions of daily life conduct (Frohlich et al. 2001; Kickbusch 1986; Ruetten 1995; WHO 2008). Two fundamental aspects of sociological thinking are at the root of this challenge. First, sociology views health, well-being and behaviour of individuals as being affected by the social milieu within which they live; individual health-related outcomes and behaviours are a function of shared social dynamics.

This assumption has come to be attributed in public health to Emile Durkheim's work, the most famous of which is found in his work on suicide (Durkheim 1897). In *Suicide*, Durkheim demonstrates the social patterning of suicide, an intimate, highly individual act. He elegantly details how suicide in the nineteenth century across several European countries was patterned by religious denomination, marital status, country of origin and other social categories. He also noted that suicide rates in countries and across social groups exhibited a patterned regularity over time, even though the individuals in these groups would change. He concluded that society is not just the sum of individuals, and that well-being cannot be reduced simply to individual risk factors; collective characteristics of groups shape individual and group outcomes with regard to health.

A second sociological assumption attributed to Max Weber (as well as current discussions regarding the relationship between structure and agency) focuses on the relationship between individual behaviour and the social structure. Max Weber's work in this area draws on the notion of "Lebensführung" (Weber 1978). Weber focused on life conduct to explain how individuals actively contribute to the social reproduction of status group distinctions through their behaviours (dress codes, marriage patterns, eating habits, etc.). He argued that people's choices with regard to their everyday behaviours are constrained by the material resources and normative rules of the community or status group they belong to, thereby acknowledging the role of structure in shaping group behaviour. These resources and rules are all components of what Weber referred to as life chances, what we now refer to as the social structure (Abel 1991; Ruetten 1995). Life chances thus refer to the structurally anchored probabilities of achieving one's goals (Cockerham et al. 1997). Weber was concerned with the social processes that link structural constraints and opportunities (life chances) on the one hand, and people's re-active or proactive behaviours (life choices), on the other. This issue has been at the root of the sociological discourse on lifestyles from both a Weberian and a Bourdieusian perspective (Abel and Frohlich 2012; Bourdieu 1980; Cockerham et al. 1997) and has been taken up by more recent writing in sociology such as that of Margaret Archer (Archer 2003). It is Weber's dualism of structure-based life chances and people's choice-based life conduct, however, that provides the basis for thinking in terms of a duality of structure and agency with regard to chronic disease health promotion and behaviour change.

Both of these sociological concerns have clear relevance for chronic disease health promotion which is today in the business of facilitating change at two levels: that of the individual and that of organizations or the social structure. This has become particularly salient given the relative failure of health promotion to change people's behaviours, on a large scale, using individual-level techniques such as education or counselling alone. The evidence for taking a structural level approach for intervention is incontrovertible and has led to innovations in health promotion such as the Healthy Cities initiatives as well as the

settings approach (Davies and Kelly 1993; Poland et al. 2000).

One of the seminal tensions between a health education or a psychological approach to behaviour change and that upheld by sociologists of health surrounds this Weberian notion of choice. Traditionally under the rubric of health education, individuals are viewed to be responsible for making their own healthy choices. It is assumed that once in possession of the information, clarified norms and values and the decision-making skills, and with sociocultural barriers removed, any rational person could not help but make the healthy choice. Under such conditions healthy behaviour is seen by health education to be synonymous with rational behaviour.

Modern sociology would question confounding informed populations with rational populations or the assumption that there is a causal link between being informed and acting rationally. Here again Weber's ideas are useful to move the discussion about individual rationality in another direction. What Weber and others underscore is that people have different abilities to use resources, such as information, in a health-promoting way. This, he would argue, is a function of life chances: chances that are beyond the control of any individual. One's ability to act as an individual and one's choices are prescribed by one's position within the class structure.

Social Inequities in Health and the Important Roles of Ethics and Political Philosophy

These same sociological issues of choice and chance were confronted (albeit unconsciously) in the legendary 1978 epidemiological article entitled *Employment grade and coronary heart disease in British civil servants* (Marmot et al. 1978). Spearheaded initially by Sir Geoffrey Rose, and passed on to Sir Michael Marmot, the Whitehall I Study, begun in 1967, was a prospective cohort study examining over 18,000 male civil servants within the British civil service. Originally the Whitehall researchers sought out to investigate the social determinants of health, and specifically, cardiorespiratory disease prevalence and mortality rates among these civil servants between the ages of 20 and 64. The initial Whitehall study found, as has the subsequent Whitehall II Study, a strong association between grade levels of civil servant employment and morbidity and mortality rates from a range of causes. For instance, men in the lowest grade (messengers, doorkeepers, etc.) had a mortality rate three times higher than that of men in the highest grade (administrators). Importantly, this gradient was only very partially explained through health behaviours. For instance, pack-a-day smokers at the top ends of the social hierarchy were less ill and less likely to die than those at the bottom ends. This phenomenon has become known as the gradient effect, in opposition to the binary relationship between being rich and healthy and poor and sick that had previously been seen as the norm. Empirically the Whitehall study demonstrated that for each level of the Whitehall social hierarchy, for which there are five, the ascending level was healthier, and lived longer, than the one below, and this in an incremental fashion.

The results from Whitehall created a flurry of excitement in the nascent world of social epidemiology (and eventually in health promotion as well). From the 1980s onwards studies began to replicate this gradient effect, an effect which turned out to be robust across cultures, time and space. The focus of these studies remained, however, on the outcome side of the equation; much emphasis was (and still is) given to describing how unequal people are with regard to their health behaviours, morbidity and mortality outcomes, with less attention being paid to the inequitable processes leading to these health inequalities. This is not entirely surprising given that epidemiology is the study of the determinants and distribution of disease, and not an area of inquiry that seeks to understand *why* the gradient exists (this being the work of sociologists interested in social stratification). Unfortunately, while the Ottawa Charter set social justice and equity as one of its fundamental conditions and resources for health (WHO 1986), a rigorous discussion with regard to theories of distributive justice in health promotion has since been wanting, leading to some important oversights.

Some of these oversights are debated in the day-to-day work of political philosophers and ethicists. These thinkers discuss issues of social inequality under the purview of equity and choice. Political philosophers concerned with issues of social inequality, for instance, have considered the problem of focusing on the voluntariness or otherwise of behavioural choices. Many of them have argued that by doing so this clouds an important consideration in the normative analysis of these "choices", the unequal background conditions against which individuals from different social groups make decisions about what they do. These suggest that a host of external factors affects whether or not individuals start to, for instance, smoke, whether or not they attempt to quit and whether or not any quit attempts are successful (Viehbeck et al. 2011).

The issue of choice brings us to a fundamental distinction often neglected in health promotion and epidemiology, the difference between (in)equality and (in)equity. Health inequality has been defined by Margaret Whitehead (1992) as "measureable differences in health experience and health outcomes between different population groups—according to socioeconomic status, geographical area, age, disability, gender or ethnic group". Health inequity, on the other hand, has a moral and ethical dimension. It refers to differences in health which are unnecessary and avoidable and in addition, are also considered unfair and unjust. Inequities include differences in opportunity for different population groups which result in inequitable: life chances; access to health services; nutritious food; adequate housing, etc. These differences are judged to be unfair and unjust.

But judgements on which situations are unfair will vary from place to place and time to time. One widely used criterion, however, is the degree of choice involved. Where people have little to no choice in living and working conditions, the resulting health conditions are likely to be considered particularly unjust. Social inequities, of course, can make certain choices easy and accessible for some, but costly and difficult for others. Even if we think that individuals' choices can, in principle, justify unequal health outcomes, we must still ask whether different people's choices were made against roughly equal background conditions (Viehbeck et al. 2011). This sense of injustice increases for groups where disadvantages cluster together and reinforce each other, making them even more vulnerable to ill health (a theme that is returned to at the end of this chapter under the rubric of vulnerable populations).

Because epidemiologists focus on the outcome side of the gradient effect, they only really place emphasis on the unfairness of the outcome. By turning the lens from the issue of inequality to one of equity, we could begin to ask why some people are not able to be healthy while others are. For instance, why is it that for the equivalent amount smoked those civil servants higher up in the social hierarchy were still healthier than those at the bottom? They are equal in their smoking. So where is the problem?

Precisely these issues are what Marmot and the Whitehall researchers missed until they began to consider issues of distributive justice largely through the influence of Amartya Sen (who, not coincidentally, was a Commissioner on the WHO Commission on Social Determinants of Health that Sir Michael Marmot chaired). With the WHO Report on the Social Determinants of Health (2008), Amartya Sen's capability theory was given official recognition within public health rhetoric. In what follows I will explore the importance of integrating discussions regarding distributive justice in our chronic disease health promotion work in order to improve both research and intervention and to help shift the current focus from health inequality to health equity.

Distributive Justice and Health Promotion

An engagement with theories of distributive justice in chronic disease health promotion would assist in placing the focus of our research and intervention on the issue of fair opportunities, that is, equity of primary goods, choice and agency, rather than on equality of outcomes alone. The focus on the equity of fair opportunities could also assist health promotion in moving the discussion away from inequities in chronic disease outcomes to discussions with regard to the processes through which people become unequally susceptible and ill from chronic diseases. Before we do so, however, it is crucial to understand the differences between two of the most influential theories of distributive justice (utilitarianism and egalitarianism) and their relationships to choice, freedom and outcomes.

One of the leading frameworks of normative ethics, particularly in health studies, is utilitarianism, originally associated with British philosophers John Stuart Mill and Jeremy Bentham. Utilitarian frameworks require allocations that maximise social utility: the greatest good to the greatest number. Rights, choice, freedom and need are not in the forefront of concern in utilitarianism as the focus rests on the overall utility maximisation, generally evaluated now in health research using cost–utility analysis (Ruger 2010). As such, the moral worth of an action is determined only by its resulting outcome (much like epidemiology).

In distinction from utilitarianism, egalitarian perspectives of justice focus on equal opportunity, welfare and resources. John Rawls, one of the greatest philosophers of the twentieth century and himself an egalitarian philosopher, developed the foundational idea that justice has to be understood in terms of the demands of fairness. Central to Rawls' idea of fairness was the avoidance of bias through impartiality. Rawls developed the idea of the "original position", central to this theory of justice as fairness (Rawls 1971). The original position is an imagined situation of equality where the individuals involved have no knowledge of their personal identities or their respective vested interests within the group as a whole. Under these conditions, entitled the "veil of ignorance", individuals choose the principles of justice that are the most fair for the collective (as they do not know where they will fall and therefore have their own interests to consider).

Rawls argued that the following two principles of justice would emerge with unanimous agreement from the original position (Rawls 1993, p. 291):

(a) Each person has an equal right to a fully adequate scheme of equal basic liberties which is compatible with a similar scheme of liberties for all.

(b) Social and economic inequalities are to satisfy two conditions. First, they must be attached to offices and positions open to all under conditions of fair equality of opportunity and second, they must be to the greatest benefit of the least advantaged members of society.

Rawls' analysis of equity in the distribution of resources calls upon what he calls "primary goods", which are the means to achieve a variety of ends. These primary goods include such things as rights, opportunities, liberties, income, wealth, and self-respect. By focusing on primary goods Rawls gives indirect acknowledgement to the importance of human freedom in giving people real opportunity to do what they would like with their lives.

What Rawls' theory fails to take into account, however, is the wide variation existing in people's abilities to convert primary goods into the ends they desire (whether this be happiness, prosperity or health), what we referred to earlier as freedom. The conversion of primary goods into the capability to do various things that a person may value doing can vary enormously based on life chances. In order to adequately integrate a concern with the variation in life chances with the variation in primary goods, one must actually assess freedoms and capabilities (Sen 2009). And this is precisely what Amartya Sen's capability theory sets out to do.

Aristotle's theory of the good is drawn on significantly by Sen to raise the issue of capability— what humans are able to do and be and what is possible for them. If the good is a desirable outcome of society, then our social obligations involve enabling all to live flourishing lives, a key goal, non-coincidentally, of the Ottawa Charter. In the Aristotelian theory of the good the political goal is defined in terms of "the capability to function well if one so chooses" (Nussbaum 1990, p. 165). This formulation also distinguishes between achievement and the freedom to achieve. By focusing on the capability to achieve valuable functionings, the theory secures differential allotments of goods and circumstances needed to produce capabilities and also respects the central

importance of freedom and reason in enabling humans to make their own choices (Ruger 2010). This is again consonant with the Ottawa Charter by recognising the importance of respecting humans' abilities for practical reason and choice. Once capabilities are assured, people must be free to make the choices they like.

Freedom is important to distributive justice and equity issues for Sen for at least two different reasons. First, more freedom gives us more opportunity to pursue our objectives. It helps, for example, in our ability to decide to live as we would like and to promote the ends that we may want to advance. This aspect of freedom is concerned with our ability to achieve what we value, no matter what the process is through which that achievement comes about (Sen 2009). To draw on the earlier sociological language used in this chapter, this aspect of freedom focuses on life chances, the ability to make choices according to how one wishes to live. Second, we may attach importance to the process of choice itself. We may, for example, want to make sure that we are not being forced into behaviour, or not able to behave in the way we wish, because of particular constraints.

Sen distinguishes between two types of freedom: opportunity and process (Sen 2009). Again, drawing on the earlier sociological literature with regard to structure and agency when describing opportunity freedom, Sen draws on the structural constraints and opportunities that people have to make choices. The ability to be a certain way and live a certain life is confined, or not, by the options that are available for people to choose from. The process aspect, on the other hand, focuses on the "true" agency that people have to make their choices.

To use a contemporary example, the introduction of a bike path in a neighbourhood may have different results depending on each individual's opportunity and process freedoms. Person A may not have a bicycle, or even know how to ride one. Person B may not have the time to ride a bike, therefore requiring her to use a car for expediency purposes. Person C may choose to ride her bike on the path because she feels it is good for her physically and mentally. Person D may choose to ride his bike for environmental reasons.

And lastly, person E may be forced to ride her bike on the path to get around as she is too poor to afford a car and public transport.

The freedom to use the bike path is ostensibly the same for all persons; the bike path has been put into place, it is free and open to all. But the opportunities and choices available to each of these persons differ according to the structural choices within which they find themselves, leading them not only to use, or not, the bike path but also to use it for very different reasons (which might even have differential effects on their health). Persons A and B confront structural constraints, and are therefore not able to profit from the bike path. Persons C and D have no structural constraints and can profit fully from their agency by choosing to use the bike path for the reasons they deem important. Person E, while using the bike path, has not "chosen" to use the bike path, but must as this is her only mode of transport.

The focus of the capability approach is thus not just on what a person actually ends up doing (or achieving) but also on whether or not she chooses freely to make use of that opportunity and what her overall options are. The focus is therefore on the ability of people to choose to live different kinds of lives within their reach, rather than confining attention only to what may be described as the culmination—or aftermath—of choice. In this sense, freedom is both structured (having collective/shared aspects) and individual. This seems to be precisely what the Ottawa Charter sought out to do when it put its focus on increasing people's control over their health, through access to resources as well as the ability to use these resources to convert them into health (WHO 1986).

Essentially Sen argues that equality as an abstract idea does not have much cutting power. The real work begins for him with the specification of what it is that has to be equalised, that is, equality of what. With regard to health in particular, Sen's theory points to inequality as being the lack of opportunity that some may have to achieve good health because of inadequate social arrangements. He eloquently argues that health equity cannot only be concerned with inequality of either health or health care, and must take into account how resource allocation and social arrangements link health with other features or states of affairs. The health equity discussion must grapple with the larger issues of fairness and justice in social arrangements, including economic allocations, paying appropriate attention to the role of health in human life and freedom. Fundamentally, health equity is not just about the distribution of health (Sen 2002).

Jennifer Prah Ruger has recently extended Sen's more general capability theory to the particular case of health (Ruger 2010). She views health capability theory to encompass three essential concepts: health agency, health capability and health functioning (health as an outcome). She views health agency to be a key component to this theory and as a more specific form of human agency relating specifically to health. She defines it as the ability to engage with and navigate one's environment to prevent mortality and morbidity and to meet health needs.

Health capabilities, on the other hand, represent the ability of individuals to achieve certain health functionings as well as the freedom they have to achieve these functionings. The difference between health capabilities and health functionings is the difference between an achievement and the freedom to achieve, as health functionings do not fully represent autonomy and freedom. If we think back to the example given earlier with regard to bike paths, the individual who was too poor to afford a car or a public transport may have been using the bike path, but she had not freely chosen to.

This tri-partite theory of social justice, in relation to health, has the advantage of both assessing justice in terms of health outcomes (what health is actually achieved) and what health outcomes people are able to achieve while at the same time accommodating liberal and political considerations of choice and health agency. Health capabilities appeal to theories of choice by shedding light on the choices and options that individuals have, or do not have, at their disposal in achieving health outcomes.

This theory could be an interesting focus for the work of health promotion concerned with inequities in chronic diseases. Rather than focusing strictly on the outcome side (the tendency for epidemiology), or on the choice side (the tendency of health education and some psychology), health promotion could instead focus on removing barriers to freedom that leave people with little choice to exercise their reasoned agency. In this way an emphasis would be given to the actual opportunities available to people (their life-chances) as well as the freedom of action and decision-making available to people (their life choices).

Bringing It All Together: The Special Case of Vulnerable Populations

I end this chapter with a discussion of the inequality paradox and vulnerable populations, both of which highlight the importance for chronic disease health promotion to address issues of social structure, agency and distributive justice. Increasing evidence has demonstrated that public health interventions targeting the determinants of chronic diseases may unintentionally be widening social inequities in the very same behavioural outcomes they sought to reduce (Frohlich and Potvin 2008; Lorenc et al. 2013; Smith et al. 2009). The debate on this inequality paradox has been particularly fierce with regard to population-level interventions, interventions closely associated with the thinking of Sir Geoffrey Rose (Rose 1992). Rose was directly inspired by Durkheim's idea of a "social reality", that the behaviour and health of individual members of society are profoundly influenced by its collective characteristics and social norms (Rose 1992, p. 62). Rather than focusing on individuals at high risk, as Lalonde had proposed, Rose suggested that interventions target the social context of chronic disease-related behaviour and their population determinants. In this way, Rose moved the focus away from an agent-based approach to public health and brought in some understanding of the structural influences on health and behaviour. Population approaches to intervention based on these ideas have involved mass environmental control methods and interventions that attempt to alter some of society's behavioural norms,

such as the denormalisation of smoking through public bans.

While Rose's ideas and population-level interventions have played an important role in the recent history of chronic disease health promotion and public health in general, Rose overlooked an important equity concern. Population-level interventions, based on his theory, are presumed to affect every member of the population to the same extent; everyone's risk exposure in the distribution is supposed to be reduced by the same amount, regardless of one's initial position in the risk exposure distribution. It appears from empirical observation, however, that certain population groups are less able to positively respond to population-approach interventions. This "inverse care law" states that those with the most resources at hand to adapt to new situations will be the first to derive maximum benefits from population-approach interventions (Victora et al. 2001; Phelan and Link 2005), leaving those with fewer resources behind.

As discussed with regard to Sen's capability theory, the focus on human heterogeneity in capability theory provides reasons for treating individuals differently (read equitably), not equally, as Rose proposes. Individual and social variations in people's capabilities affect the relationship between the resources provided by the population intervention and the ability to profit from the intervention. So for instance, conditions such as handicaps (which reduce capabilities) can make it harder to convert income into good health. Returning back, once again, to our example of bike paths, Persons A, B and E were not able to profit from the bike paths as much as Persons C and D due to their inability to convert the bike path (the population health intervention) into a pleasurable, health-enhancing activity. Recently these and similar problems have begun to be discussed in public health circles under the rubric of population and public health ethics (Viehbeck et al. 2011) and, more specifically, with regard to vulnerable populations (Frohlich and Potvin 2008).

Vulnerable populations, as described by Frohlich and Potvin, are a subgroup or subpopulation who, because of shared social characteristics, are at higher risk of risks. The notion of vulnerable populations refers to groups who, because of their position in the social structure, are commonly exposed to contextual conditions that distinguish them from the rest of the population. As a consequence, a vulnerable population's distribution of risk exposure has a higher mean than that of the rest of the population. In Canada, for example, vulnerable populations are people of Aboriginal descent, those with an income lower than the poverty threshold, and those who have not completed secondary education. The unintended adverse consequence for vulnerable populations of applying Rose's approach is, as we saw earlier, an inattention to equity issues, but also a lack of attention to issues of structure and agency. Vulnerable populations have fewer life chances, and have less freedom to make healthy life choices, due to their disadvantaged position in society. Population health interventions do not take into account differentials in life chances and choices; they treat everyone as though they can react to the intervention in an equivalent amount.

One way to ensure that vulnerable populations are not left behind in chronic disease health promotion endeavours is to design public health strategies that use both population and vulnerable population approaches to interventions. Many national jurisdictions have adopted policy recommendations that couple the reduction in health disparities with the improvement of overall population health. Such policies can be found in various reports, such as "Integrated Pan-Canadian Healthy Living Strategy" (Secretariat for the Healthy Living Network 2005), the Swedish "Health on Equal Terms Public Health Policy" (Hogstedt et al. 2004) and "Tackling Heath Inequalities: A Program for Action" in the United Kingdom (Tackling health inequalities: A program for Action 2003).

Conclusion

Essentially a chronic disease health promotion concerned with both equity and diminishing overall chronic disease might do well to consider the social scientific ideas and theories discussed in this chapter. Health education and psychological techniques, while playing an important role in health promotion, are unable to change behaviour on a large scale, do not help to change social norms and are rarely able to benefit those whose life chances preclude them from fully profiting from their related interventions. Here agency, as we discussed, is not always driven by rationality; people have different capabilities to act and these capabilities are often shaped by levels of marginalisation (life chances). Population-level interventions are also incomplete given the assumption that people act equally when exposed to structural change (McLaren et al. 2010). Population-level interventions draw on a notion of distributive justice akin to egalitarian ethics; if everyone is given the same exposure to the intervention then each should be able to benefit by the same amount. As we discussed, however, this is unfortunately not the case. Differential capabilities preclude everyone enjoying the change towards health that population-level interventions hope to offer. What is worse, given these differentials in capabilities, vulnerable populations stand to become further disadvantaged given the inequalities in health resulting from these interventions.

In an ethics of the social determinants of health a major goal of the health capability paradigm would be to reduce inequities in individuals' ability to achieve health-related functionings. We have an obligation to enhance the central health capabilities of all individuals, and the means and resources by which we are able to do so may very well go beyond the reach of health policies, extending into the realm of other policy domains.

References

Abel, T. (1991). Measuring health lifestyles in a comparative analysis: Theoretical issues and empirical findings. *Social Science & Medicine, 32*(8), 899–908.

Abel, T., & Frohlich, K. L. (2012). Capitals and capabilities: Linking structure and agency to reduce health inequalities. *Social Science & Medicine, 74*(2), 236–244.

Archer, M. (2003). *Structure, agency and the internal conversation*. Cambridge: Cambridge University Press.

Bourdieu, P. (1980). *Le sens pratique*. Paris: Les Editions de Minuit.

Bunton, R., & Macdonald, G. (2002). *Health promotion: Disciplines, diversity and developments* (2nd ed.). London: Routledge.

Cockerham, W. C., Ruetten, A., & Abel, T. (1997). Conceptualizing contemporary health lifestyles: Moving beyond Weber. *The Sociological Quarterly, 38*, 321–342.

COMMIT Research Group. (1995). Community intervention trial for smoking cessation (COMMIT), I: Cohort results from a four-year community intervention. *American Journal of Public Health, 85*, 183–192.

Davies, J. K., & Kelly, M. P. (1993). *Healthy cities. Research and practice.* London: Routledge.

Durkheim, E. (1897/1951). *Suicide: A study in sociology.* Glencoe, IL: Free Press.

Frohlich, K. L., Corin, E., & Potvin, L. (2001). A theoretical proposal for the relationship between context and disease. *Sociology of Health & Illness, 23*(6), 776–797.

Frohlich, K. L., & Potvin, L. (2008). The inequality paradox: The population approach and vulnerable populations. *American Journal of Public Health, 98*(2), 216–221.

Hansen, E., & Easthope, G. (2007). *Lifestyle in medicine.* London: Routledge.

Hogstedt, C., Lundgren, B., Moberg, H., Pettersson, B., & Ågren, G. (2004). Forward. *Scandinavian Journal of Public Health, 32*, 3.

Kickbusch, I. (1986). Life-styles and health. *Social Science & Medicine, 22*(2):117–124.

Lalonde, M. (1974). *A new perspective on the health of Canadians.* Retrieved October 4, 2012, from http://www.phac-aspc.gc.ca/ph-sp/pdf/perspect-eng.pdf

Lorenc, T., Petticrew, M., Welch, V., & Tugwell, P. (2013). What types of interventions generate inequalities? Evidence from systematic reviews. *Journal of Epidemiology and Community Health, 67*(2), 190–193.

Marmot, M. G., Rose, G., Shipley, M., & Hamilton, P. J. (1978). Employment grade and coronary heart disease in British civil servants. *Journal of Epidemiology and Community Health, 32*(4), 244–249.

McLaren, L., Macintyre, L., & Kirkpatrick, S. (2010). Rose's population strategy of prevention need not increase social inequalities in health. *International Journal of Epidemiology, 39*(2), 372–377.

Multiple Risk Factor Intervention Trial Research Group. (1981). Multiple risk factor intervention trial. *Preventive Medicine, 10*, 387–553.

Multiple Risk Factor Intervention Trial Research Group. (1982). Multiple risk factor intervention trial: Risk factor changes and mortality results. *Journal of the American Medical Association, 24*, 1465–1476.

Nussbaum, M. (1990). Nature, function, and capability: Aristotle on political distribution. In: G. Patzig (Ed.), *Aristotles' Politik Gottingen: Vandenhoeck and Ruprecht* (pp. 152–186).

Phelan, J., & Link, B. (2005). Controlling disease and creating disparities: A fundamental cause perspective. *Journal of Gerontology, 60*, 27–33.

Poland, B. D., Green, L. W., & Rootman, I. (2000). *Settings for health promotion: Linking theory and practice.* Thousand Oaks, CA: Sage Publications.

Rawls, J. (1971). *A theory of justice.* Cambridge, MA: Belknap Press of Harvard University Press.

Rawls, J. (1993). *Political liberalism.* New York, NY: Columbia University Press.

Rose, G. (1992). *The strategy of preventive medicine.* Oxford: Oxford University Press.

Ruetten, A. (1995). The implementation of health promotion: A new structural perspective. *Social Science & Medicine, 41*(12), 1627–1637.

Ruger, J. P. (2010). *Health and social justice.* Oxford: Oxford University Press.

Secretariat for the Healthy Living Network. (2005). *The integrated pan-Canadian healthy living strategy.* Retrieved October 4, 2012, from http://www.phac-aspc.gc.ca/hl-vs-strat/pdf/hls_e.pdf

Sen, A. (2002). Why health equity? *Health Economics, 11*, 659–666.

Sen, A. (2009). *The idea of justice.* Cambridge, MA: The Belknap Press.

Smith, P., Frank, J., & Mustard, C. (2009). Trends in educational inequalities in smoking and physical activity in Canada: 1974–2005. *Journal of Epidemiology and Community Health, 63*(4), 317–323.

Syme, S. L. (1994, Fall). The social environment and health. *Daedalus, 12*, 79–86.

UK Department of Health. (2003). *Tackling health inequalities: A program for action.* London: Author.

Victora, C. G., Barros, F. C., & Vaughan, J. P. (2001). The impact of health interventions on inequalities: Infant and child health in Brazil. In D. Leon & G. Walt (Eds.), *Poverty, inequality and health* (pp. 125–136). Oxford: Oxford University Press.

Viehbeck, S., Melnychuk, R., McDougall, C. W., Greenwood, H., & Edwards, N. C. (2011). Population and public health ethics in Canada: A snapshot of current national initiatives and future issues. *Canadian Journal of Public Health, 102*(6), 410–412.

Weber, M. (1978). *Economy and society: An outline of interpretive sociology.* Berkeley, CA: University of California Press.

Whitehead, M. (1992). The concepts and principles of equity and health. *International Journal of Health Services, 22*, 429–445.

WHO. (1986). *Ottawa charter for health promotion.* Ottawa, ON: World Health Organization, Health and Welfare Canada, Canadian Public Health Association.

WHO. (2008). *Closing the gap in a generation: Health equity through action on the social determinants of health.* Final report of the commission on social determinants of health. Geneva: World Health Organization.

Contextual Factors in Health and Illness

6

David V. McQueen

At first glance it would seem that health and illness are clearly understood and defined ideas. At closer inspection one observes that many preconceived ideas, opinions, and prejudices that underpin these ideas are apparent. The WHO has defined health as "a state of complete physical, mental and social well-being and not merely the absence of disease or infirmity" (WHO 1946). Such a definition, while concise and easy to state, raises many questions and practically every word is subject to further discussion, definition, and subjective interpretation. Illness also presents difficulties and is often simply defined as being the opposite of healthy. Sometimes it is defined biomedically as the subjective experience of disease or the absence of health. In any case, there are many variants of the definition of health and illness and in most cases the definitions reveal the background of the definer as much as any revelation of truth as to meaning. Still, most persons, whether professionals in public health or lay observers of life, have a broad view of these two terms and know that they are generally two distinct states for any individual experiencing them.

The problem that provides such a challenge for those in public health is not how an individual knows whether they are "healthy" or "ill," but what are the factors outside of the individual that relate to, correlate with, or actually cause

D.V. McQueen (✉)
2418 Midvale Court, Tucker, GA 30084, USA
e-mail: davidmcqueen07@gmail.com

health and illness at the population level. There are multiple ways to approach this problem and several will be discussed in this chapter. As a generic terminology we will consider all of these ways as "contextual" in health and illness. By "contextual" is meant that we are concerned primarily with those causal factors related to health and illness that are external to the individual. Thus, individual factors such as the genetic makeup of an individual or their own phylogeny are outside of the purview of this chapter. In making such a distinction it is important to recall that no causal phenomenon can be so simply isolated and that genetic characteristics of an individual or a group are not free from contextual (environmental) effects. It is merely to note that the topic of contextual factors in health and illness is an enormous area of consideration. This chapter seeks to give a general perspective, while other chapters in this section will be more specific.

A note on the word "factor" is in order. It is also a problematic word. It is a word that often implies causality, and is used often to describe a variable in a scientific model. It often implies agency, that is it acts on other components in any model. In short its meaning is quite interpretable. It is used here because it is widely used and it is a "softer" word than determinant with respect to causality, a subject discussed in more detail in Chap. 3. The term "determinant" implies a greater certainty of causality and rigor of proof that can rarely, if ever, be met in public health discussions. The term "factor" does convey a notion of complexity and a degree of uncertainty that is appropriate in most of the discussions related to context and health and illness. More critically, it conveys an image of an important relationship between context and health and illness. The existence of this relationship is hardly new to public health.

A Brief History of Contextual Factors in Public Health

While some may believe that the concern with NCDs, the social, and health is recent, it is actually ancient. In addition, the concern with the contextual is ancient, though not expressed in that modern word. A rereading of George Rosen's classic *A History of Public Health* (1958) is very illuminating and recommended for anyone interested in the role of the social context of public health. Rosen reminds us that housing, sanitation, and clean water are part and parcel of the social context of public health. Actions on these dimensions of public health are political and social and generally the result of good governance. Today many of these dimensions of public health practice are part of the general management of bureaucratic government, generally unseen by the lay public and unassociated with health, perhaps as a consequence of the medicalization of public health in the twentieth century. Those present-day politicians and citizens who argue that such areas as urbanization, governance, the environment, social determinants, and poverty are outside of the scope of public health, clearly are ignorant of the history of public health. What is more, it is arguably the most profound and successful part of public health. Rosen reminds of this in detail tracing this effort from the Greco-Roman world, where water supply and sanitation efforts reached great heights, to the accomplishments of the period of industrialization with the critical efforts to deal with poverty and with laws to protect the poor. He also details the critical rise of social medicine and the responsibility of the state to provide comprehensive public health services to all. "Virchow, for example, conceived the scope of public health as broadly as possible, indicating that one of its major functions was to study the conditions under which various social groups lived and to determine the effects of these conditions on their health. On the basis of this knowledge, it would then be possible to take appropriate action. Finally, the principle that follows from this is that steps taken to promote health and to combat disease must be social as well as medical" (Rosen, pp. 254–55). This thinking led to the Public Health Law in 1849 Germany and reflected the emergence and strengthening of the idea of political economy affecting all areas of life. The absolute modernity of this law and the public health actions resonate with the efforts of those in twenty-first century public health who are concerned with health promotion. It is unfortunate that these strong efforts of the mid- and late nineteenth century lost steam through much of the twentieth century and had little impact on public health efforts in low- and middle-income countries. Some current efforts are reviving this enthusiasm for a broad-based public health, but these efforts are still a small component of present-day public health efforts.

Historically, contextual factors in health were not just the focus of those in the medical world. In the social sciences there were the significant writings of Durkheim, Weber, Parsons, Goffman, Koos, Zola, and Dubos to name just a few. Émile Durkheim's classic on *Suicide* (1951) demonstrated with methodological rigor the importance of the modern concept of coherence in defining how certain religious and cultural groups differed in suicide practices in their context. In addition, in the 1890s, he introduced in detail the notion of a social fact as a "way of acting, fixed or not, capable of exercising on the individual an external constraint; or again, every way of acting which is general throughout a given society, while at the same time existing in its own right independent of its individual manifestations" (Durkheim 1964, p. 13). The great German sociologist Max Weber further developed this contextual notion and his theory continues to influence this contextual approach (cf. Abel and Frohlich 2012; and Chaps. 2 and 5 in this book). Many other great anthropologists, sociologists, and psychologists contributed to the development of a contextual approach.

But also those from different professions did as well. One such notable was René Dubos who influenced public health thinking in the 1960s and 1970s with his work that emphasized the importance of addressing contextual factors, especially environmental, ecological, and economic factors as critical in understanding global health issues (1968). He championed the notion of thinking globally, acting locally as an approach to public health action. There are many others who could be brought into this brief historical discussion, but a litany is not the point. The point is that contextual thinking about health and illness has a distinguished history; there is a record of careful and concerted thought to be relished. That such thinking goes in and out of favor in public health, often in relation to political movements of the time, is the subject of further historical insight.

How Contextual Factors Are Conceptualized

Before entering into a discussion of all the various contextual factors it is useful to consider some basics of their conceptualization. First, most contextual factors are conceived as complex variables. For example, a basic variable such as social class, while it may often be represented by a simple measure that ranges from low to high, or 1–5, is actually a very complex notion. The identification of the concept of class, since its early development in the writings of Marx (1967) and Weber (1947) has largely been conceptualized as an idea related to the means of production, Marx, or related a theory of structural-functionalism as in the case of the Weberian heritage. It is not the point here to delve into the incredible complexity and intricacies of this concept as it has been developed in the social sciences, but to simply point out that when one simply refers to such notions such as upper, middle, and lower classes when thinking about class that it is a gross under-representation of the complexity found within the concept of class. However, in much of the extant work in public health this complexity is generally represented by an even more complex variable SES of social economic status. It is inherent in

most research and work carried out that the use of the scientific method and its measurement demands results in a highly reductionist notion of this very complex variable. The contradiction of the complexity of the SES concept by its generally naïve usage in twentieth-century public health is the subject of another analysis.

Second, while a variable may be complex, there is another critical dimension of variability. Variability is really the extent that the concept can vary over time either in an individual or in a society. For example, for an individual, his or her SES may vary over a lifetime, starting as a working-class person and rising to the upper class, or vice versa. This lifetime trip for the individual is greatly dependent, in most cases, on other contextual variables. For example a wealthy upper-class person living in Europe or America through the period of the great depression might experience great diminishment of class. In sociological terms this would be expressed as going through status inconsistency, a notion which itself is a powerful variable. In a similar fashion whole societies or countries can have their class components vary over time.

Third, there is another key consideration in contextual variables. Some variables are descriptors of the situation at a point in time and they do not have any notion of change built into them; that is they are static. Class, for example, is a descriptor that holds at a point in time. It can change over time, but it has no built-in action component. Thus it is seen as a structural type variable. Some structural variables, such as ethnicity, gender, cultural background, are fixed and have little or no variation over time and cannot be changed. Other contextual variables of interest in the understanding of health and illness are different; they have a more verbal characteristic, what some would term "agency" (cf. Chap. 5). Many of these will be discussed later, but they fall into a grouping that has an underlying notion that they are agents of change. Examples are notions of governance, equity, social justice, and power, to name a few that appear often as contextual factors in models related to health and illness.

The fact that models of contextual factors mix these various types of variables has its challenges and problems. The chief problem of course is the impact on addressing causality and the championed causal relationships implied in the model. This has been discussed in Chap. 3 in more detail. However, there are also profound measurement problems in mixing types of variables. First is the problem of measurement level. Many social factors are ordinal measures at best; SES is a good example of an ordinal-level measure. Some, such as gender, are generally viewed as dichotomous. Many variables are at best nonparametric and these include many that are of keen interest. These are largely the highly conceptual variables such as social justice, capability, equity, power, governance, to name just a few. In methodological terms most of these variables present major challenges of construct validity.

Major Contextual Variables

Despite the many theoretical and methodological challenges found with studying contextual variables, there is little choice but to proceed with efforts to use and understand them. That is the nature of research, to explore where uncertainty still remains. Fortunately, after over a half-century of effort to understand the richness of the relationship between contextual variables and health and illness, a general understanding of this complexity is beginning to emerge. While it is difficult to argue that there is absolute proof of many of the observed relationships, the weight of decades of research, using sophisticated techniques to unravel these relationships has yielded consistent and profound findings. It is clear that contextual variables play a powerful role in understanding the relationship between the social and health and illness. Some variables, for example SES, have been explored in far more depth than others, for example religiosity. The socioeconomic type variables are explored more than the sociocultural in the public health literature. For those seeking elaborate and comprehensive reviews and analyses of the role of contextual, social, behavioral, economic, cultural, and ecological factors in health and illness the following documents are highly recommended.

Classics: A Personal Selection

1. The handbooks of medical sociology over the years, from the earliest to the latest editions give good overviews of the growth of the field with regard to contextual factors. Most illustrative is the second edition (Freeman et al. 1972) and in that edition the chapter by Graham and Reeder (pp. 63–107) on social factors in the chronic illnesses and the chapter by Kind (pp. 148–168) on social-psychological factors in illness. These types of chapters were repeated in the following editions, but notably in the fifth edition (Bird et al. 2000) a whole section of the handbook was devoted to the "social contexts of health and illness." This section introduced many areas including, causal explanations for social disparities in health, the importance of culture, race, ethnicity and health, political economy of health and the environment. By the latest edition (Bird et al. 2010) this area had morphed into a clear concern for social contexts and health disparities (pp. 3–146).

2. Over the years there has been a rich literature on the mix of the social, psychological, and biological factors underlying the context of disease. One comprehensive view of this was illustrated early on in Herbert Weiner's book *Psychobiology and Human Disease* (1977). Although largely medical with an emphasis on psychosomatic causes of chronic disease, it is remarkable the attention given to the social context; socioeconomic factors are discussed at length in addition to the emphases on stress-related factors. The growing literature in this area was examined in further and comprehensive detail by the NAS Committee on Health and Behavior: Research, Practice and Policy in 2001 (NRC 2001) This Report is most instructive and reinforces many of the issues already discussed above; a chief finding was: *Health and disease are determined by dynamic interactions among biological, psychological, behavioral, and social factors. These interactions occur over time and throughout development. Cooperation and interaction of multiple*

disciplines are necessary for understanding and influencing health and behavior (p. 16). It is notable that the report found many questions that have yet to be fully explored and answered by research to date. That finding still stands in the second decade of the twenty-first century.

3. A broad perspective on context is taken in the classic monograph *Sickness and Society* by Duff and Hollingshead (1968). This work emphasized the context of the medical care system and its relationship to external social factors, moving away from the idea of medical institutions as simply agents of biomedical care free from external social influences. The work also showed the power of the case study description in revealing social complexity. This monograph is illustrative of an area that spawned a large body of context-related work over the years that has led to a very different understanding of the role of hospitals and formal care institutions and ultimately an emergent area of health promoting hospitals (cf. Chap. 29).

4. The long concern with illness and health from an anthropological perspective could be illustrated by many earlier works. For example one should read the writings of Benjamin Paul. He is regarded as the founding father of medical anthropology and edited the influential work *Health, Culture and Community: Case Studies of Public Reactions to Health Programs* (1955). The breadth of these case studies, ranging from chapters on health programs among Zulus to nutritional research programs in Guatemala foreshadows the global health promotion actions and activities of today. Some 20 years later Horacio Fabrega published *Disease and Social Behavior: An Interdisciplinary Perspective* (1974) extending this perspective into the ecological and interdisciplinary realm.

5. Finally a most critical and influential work was by Lisa Berkman and Lester Breslow. While this work was carried out in Alameda County, California in the 1960s and 1970s the culminating monograph is the 1983 publication *Health and Ways of Living: The Alameda County Study.* What is critical from a contextual perspective is the elaboration and clarification of the role of social networks and how they relate to health and illness. The implications of this work for present-day social epidemiology and health promotion perspectives is profound as it established both an epidemiological approach and a strong emphasis on the community as a focus of long term research.

Many other works beyond these "classics" could have been cited and other authors would have their own personal list, however this selection illustrate the broad thinking about the role of contextual factors in health illness that was already well developed before the present day. They also illustrate that the great ancient heritage of concern with the social has continued in the twentieth century and been championed by epidemiologists and social scientists alike. Further they illustrate the complexity that such thinking must entail. Each field of endeavor, whether clinical medicine or contemporary sociology must now see the factors involved in health and illness as not only contextual and complex, but not contained in any single discipline. It is partly this aspect that has led to the emergence of a distinctive field of action called health promotion, a broad-based response to the needs of contextual understanding.

Present Day

1. A critical background to the dimensions of the NCD concept is provided by the notion of disease burden. The "burden" of noncommunicable diseases is and has been seen as a particular challenge for public health across the globe. In the mid-1990s seminal work was carried out and published jointly by the World Health Organization, Harvard University and the World Bank. Of particular note was volume one in this series of ten entitled *The Global Burden of Disease: A Comprehensive Assessment of Mortality and Disability from Diseases, Injuries, and Risk Factors in 1990 and Projected to 2020*, edited by Christopher Murray and Alan Lopez (1996). This work

lays out in detail the methodology and critical findings of this large study. Many other documents follow on from this study. Suffice it to say that this effort set out a comprehensive effort, not without critics of the particular methodology that remained a foundation for ongoing efforts to enhance the importance of NCDs in public health. Recently (The Lancet 2012) devoted an entire issue (http://www.thelancet.com/themed/global-burden-of-disease), to the update of this effort which both reinforced the original findings as well as to slightly alter the present view of the burden of NCDs. One should refer to this special issue to understand the wide variation in disease outcomes globally, however a summary statement is that "Since 1970, men and women worldwide have gained slightly more than ten years of life expectancy overall, but they spend more years living with injury and illness." In brief the newer findings add to the complex nature of NCDs and to any understanding of their causality.

2. Without doubt the most comprehensive collection of work related to contextual factors available currently has been provided by the work of the WHO Commission on the Social Determinants of Health. This is an exhaustive study. With the publication of the WHO Commission on the social determinants of health (WHOCSDOH 2008) and the accompanying work of the nine knowledge networks on early childhood development, globalization, health systems, measurement and evidence, urbanization, employment conditions, social exclusion, priority public health conditions, and women and gender equity the field of social epidemiology was greatly enhanced. These documents are readily available on the Internet. They illustrate boldly the vast accumulation of knowledge and synthesis of evidence on the relationship between contextual factors and disease. In many ways they illustrate how far descriptive social epidemiology can go in providing an encyclopedic description of contextual factors. What is lacking is a health promoting perspective on what actions need to be taken to address these contextual factors.

3. For a spirited discussion and consideration of the contextual factors from the viewpoints of income inequality, equity, and social justice there are three publications of note. The first is *Social Determinants of Health: Canadian Perspectives* (2004) a reader edited by Dennis Raphael who is the author of Chap. 7. Another reader of interest is that edited by Richard Hofrichter titled *Health and Social Justice: Politics, ideology, and inequity in the distribution of disease* (2003). This is a large document, with well-known authors contributing their views on a wide variety of contextual factors in health and illness. Finally a third monograph is that of Richard Wilkinson and Kate Pickett (2009) entitled *The Spirit Level: Why More Equal Societies Almost Always Do Better*. This work builds on the extensive influential work of the authors in the UK and addresses the notion of inequity in detail at the societal level; a topic that is gaining increased attention.

4. On the topic of societal-level issues in the contextual factors, three recent offerings are notable that look into this in detail. The first is *Successful Societies: how institutions and culture affect health,* edited by Peter Hall and Michele Lamont (2009). Second is an article by Johan P. Mackenbach on "The persistence of health inequalities in modern welfare states: The explanation of a paradox," in *Social Science and Medicine* (2012) that explores carefully three hypotheses. Most important of all is the recent, (2013), publication of the National Research Council and Institute of Medicine of the National Academies document entitled "U.S. Health in International Perspective: Shorter Lives, Poorer Health." This monograph, prepared by a panel of experts, documents carefully the role of contextual factors that result in less longevity and poorer health in the wealthiest country in the world and one that spends the most, both in terms of dollars and percentage of GNP on health care. It is both an indictment of the American way of dealing with health and illness but also a powerful statement of why sociocultural contextual

factors are so critical in understanding negative health outcomes. What is more, the comparisons with other wealthy OECD countries is most telling and a powerful illustration that health and illness is not simply a factor of spending money, but that many other factors play a powerful and convincing role.

5. Given that contextual factors that impact disease causation and health success spring greatly from non biological factors, social epidemiology, clearly one of the foundation sciences of modern public health has moved significantly away from traditional epidemiology. This movement and its importance is definitively laid out and comprehensively reviewed in Nancy Krieger's *Epidemiology and the People's Health: theory and context* (2011). It provides a very well referenced summation of the development over the past few decades and provides careful analyses of the major social epidemiological perspectives now extant.

As with my illustration of the "classics" the present-day citations are a purposive selection, obviously reflecting personal biases based upon four decades of academic and government work in public health. Others would undoubtedly offer a different package, but the growth of conceptual ideas in this area of public health has remained clear over the years. There is a persistent observation and finding that health and disease outcomes are not simply products of biology. There is a persistent finding that above the individual level, at the level of groups, collectives, and societies, that health differences are explained by factors that lie outside the medical arena. It is also clear that this context is complex and not given over to easy solutions or understanding. This fact alone makes simple and quick solutions to causality impossible. As Mencken wrote in 1917: *Explanations exist; they have existed for all times, for there is always an easy solution to every human problem—neat, plausible, and wrong* (Mencken 1949, p. 443). The growth of health promotion as an approach to public health is a recognition of this complexity challenge (cf. Chap. 22).

Missing Contextual Components

It is remarkable how far the social aspects of context have developed in recent years and the present-day citations noted above are a testimony of this advancement. It has become as commonplace to discuss areas such as social justice and equity as it once was to discuss individual behavioral risk factors or SES. The acceptance of the social is in contrast to the limited acceptance of the cultural among many of the same researchers and practitioners. This part of the contextual remains somewhat outside of the health and illness discussion. Some values and beliefs that may be critical in understanding the contextual factors in health and illness are given scant attention. Perhaps the most flagrant variable area missing in this research is religion. It is not that there has been total absence, after all the role of religion in suicide dates back to the classical work of Durkheim and has been pursued over time by scholars such as Steven Stack (2000) and others. In addition religion has been seen as having a place in developing participatory approaches to preventive interventions as for example in diabetes interventions among Afro-Americans (Samuel-Hodge et al. 2006). But the point is that is has been much less used and examined in a causal framework in the sense that SES has been used as a predictor of health and illness outcomes in populations. Similarly values, especially broad ones that have been asserted as culture specific, for example American "rugged individualism," have barely been mined in a causal framework. When considering some key findings such as that of the afore mentioned NRC/IOM report on the large discrepancy between advanced economic countries in health outcomes, the "cultural" factor of American individualism can only be speculated because of the lack of solid research examining its role. This is not to assert that it has such role, but only to note that as a "cultural variable" its potential role in explanation has been relatively unexamined. Undoubtedly the reader may be able to assert other missing contextual variable areas that may still lead to a better understanding of contextual factors in health and illness.

Organizations and Context

It should be noted that the whole discussion of contextual factors and their role in health and illness cannot easily be separated from the role of the organizations and institutions that deal with this area. These organizations themselves are in themselves contextual variables that affect how research is conceptualized, carried out, and funded. How contextual factors are viewed and understood by those who work in these institutions shapes the way research gets done. In the academic discipline-based sciences within universities much depends on how the departments emphasize the biomedical world. So, for example, medical sociology, which itself is a sizable component of the work in sociology departments highly reflects the mother discipline in its interests. That is there is much emphasis on the institution of medicine, professional care, health policy, and medical care. The medical sociology section of the American Sociological Association has been a major section for many years, reaching a peak of membership in 1980s, but still never comprising more than 9 % of ASA membership. In a similar way the fields of medical/health psychology and medical anthropology have been consistently a part of the mother discipline, but picking up discipline-related fields as their work. While these did include work on social, cultural, and contextual factors, as has been discussed above, the work was very bounded by the fields and the academic rewards bounded by the disciplines. Similar patterns emerged for the economics and political science areas. It is difficult to know if and how this academic disciplinary isolation affected the lack of sociologists, psychologists, anthropologists, political scientists, and the like in governmental public health organizations, but these disciplines are represented in very small numbers in such institutions globally.

Where this work was and continues to be carried out to scale is in professional schools of public health, mainly in departments of epidemiology, social and behavioral sciences, health education and promotion, medical care and hospitals, and international health. But it is probably safe to say that epidemiology is the underpinning science and methodology that addresses these contextual factors. Furthermore, the tradition in epidemiology has been biomedical with the medical degree as the foundation; of course, this has changed, with the emergence over the past few decades of more and more Ph.D. epidemiologists with more background in social science disciplines. Gradually this has changed the scope of the understanding of NCDs and health promotion and the role of contextual factors in health and illness. This change is reflected in many of the chapters of this handbook. Change in scope in academia does not quickly translate into change in the politically based public organizations of public health. It is not the topic of this chapter to detail this transition but only to note that the reader should peruse the organizational structures and funding disbursements of the great public institutions, from WHO to CDC to Ministries of Health throughout the world, to see what a relatively small emphasis is placed on understanding the contextual factors in health and illness, and the even more relatively small percentage of funds allocated to the prevention of NCDs and the promotion of health.

Conclusion

It is probably safe to speculate that most researchers and practitioners in public health recognize the role of contextual factors in NCDs; furthermore many would recognize that the broad field of health promotion is an important and useful approach to altering those contextual factors in a manner that would improve population health. Nonetheless, taking actions that would alter the role of these contextual factors remains problematic from both a scientific and a political perspective.

Scientifically one may view public health research as conservative. Methodological innovativeness does not occupy a prime role either in public health institutions or in public health academia. Therefore it is not surprising that complex models of causality are undertreated with complex methodologies. When contextual factors are considered it is far easier to work with proximal variables and close variables in time. It is far easier to show a correlation coefficient with high certainty when two variables are conceptually close in a model. Thus it is far easier to show the relationship between smoking behavior and lung cancer than between agricultural policy and lung cancer. The biomedical model underpinning the science of epidemiology rests comfortably with single measurable behaviors and biological outcomes. Further, the biostatistics taught most students in public health provide appropriate methods for such descriptive statistics. Of course there are sciences that use more complex mathematical and statistical models, but few in public health are trained in these areas. The social sciences, notably sociology and economics, do use more complex statistical approaches, but it is notable that these social sciences are not well represented in modern public health institutions. Health promotion as a field has often taken approaches regarded by many as soft science. For example, the area of participatory research, which is one of many health promotion intervention approaches, may be regarded by many in the field of public health as only quasi-scientific. These are aspects of modern public health that many in the field would recognize; they are part of the prejudicial scientific baggage that goes with the field. Fortunately this picture is changing. Unfortunately, the understanding of contextual factors scientifically is not free of these views that slow the progress of understanding contextual factors.

While one can easily propose solutions to the scientific problems through improved training, support of broader curricula in schools of public health, and through enlightened leadership in public health institutions, it is more difficult to address the political challenges faced by public health research and practice. To begin with many of the fundamental contextual factors are far upstream from the asserted population health outcome. As a simple example, agricultural policy, whether in terms of subsidies for the production of animal fats, or tobacco, or the lack of subsidies for fruits and vegetables, seems outside the realm of public health. Of course, many in public health now endorse thinking in terms of

health in all policy areas, but that does not mean that those in public health either know how to or have influences on the policies in other sectors. Furthermore, this very quickly gets into political controversy. A notorious example is the seeming inability, despite the epidemiologically well-documented deadly use of firearms contributing to shorter American life expectancy, for any meaningful political action to be taken on firearm control. Such action challenges many beliefs held by influential citizens. An easy solution is the claim that this is not a public health problem; but this denies the contextual role in health and illness.

The role of contextual factors in health and illness remains central to the concern with NCDs and the practice of health promotion in public health. Despite the complexity, the scientific and political challenges, those in public health have little choice but to embrace the reality that NCDs are a global burden and that health promoting interventions are a critical approach to reducing this burden. As reported above, this global burden has changed slightly in character, but it is barely reduced. The hopeful statement is that the efforts of public health in the past decades have retarded this burden and kept it from getting worse. Ultimately, this is not the optimal choice for public health.

References

Abel, T., & Frohlich, K. L. (2012). Capitals and capabilities: Linking structure and agency to reduce health inequalities. *Social Science & Medicine, 74*(2), 236–244.

Berkman, L. F., & Breslow, L. (1983). *Health and ways of living: The Alameda County study*. New York, NY: Oxford University Press.

Bird, C. E., Conrad, P., & Fremont, A. M. (2000). *Handbook of medical sociology* (5th ed.). Upper Saddle River, NJ: Prentice Hall.

Bird, C. E., Conrad, P., Fremont, A. M., & Timmermans, S. (2010). *Handbook of medical sociology* (6th ed.). Nashville, TN: Vanderbilt University Press.

Dubos, R. J. (1968). *Man, medicine, and environment*. New York, NY: Praeger.

Duff, R. S., & Hollingshead, A. B. (1968). *Sickness and society*. New York, NY: Harper & Row.

Durkheim, E. (1951). *Suicide: A study in sociology*. New York, NY: The Free Press.

Durkheim, É. (1964). *The rules of sociological method* (8th ed.). New York, NY: The Free Press.

Fabrega, H. (1974). *Disease and social behavior: An interdisciplinary perspective*. Cambridge, MA: The MIT Press.

Freeman, H. E., Levine, S., & Reeder, L. G. (1972). *Handbook of medical sociology*. Englewood Cliffs, NJ: Prentice-Hall, Inc.

Hall, P. A., & Lamont, M. (Eds.). (2009). *Successful societies: How institutions and culture affect health*. New York, NY: Cambridge University Press.

Hofrichter, R. (Ed.). (2003). *Health and social justice: A reader on the politics, ideology, and inequity in the distribution of disease*. San Francisco, CA: Jossey-Bass.

Krieger, N. (2011). *Epidemiology and the Peoples Health*. New York, NY: Oxford University Press.

Mackenbach, J. P. (2012). The persistence of health inequalities in modern welfare states: The explanation of a paradox. *Social Science & Medicine, 75*, 761–769.

Marx, K. (1967). *Capital: A critique of political economy. Vol. 1. The process of capitalist production [1867]* (F. Engels, Ed., S. Moore & E. Aveling, Trans.). New York, NY: International Publishers.

Mencken, H. L. (1949). *A Mencken Chrestomathy*. New York: Alfred Knopf. In an essay titled "The Divine Afflatus." (Originally published in the *New York Evening Mail*, November 16, 1917).

Murray, C., & Lopez, A. (Eds.). (1996). *The global burden of disease: A comprehensive assessment of mortality and disability from diseases, injuries, and risk factors in 1990 and projected to 2020* (Vol. 1). Cambridge, MA: Harvard University Press.

National Research Council. (2001). *Health and behavior: The interplay of biological, behavioral, and societal influences*. Washington, DC: The National Academies Press.

National Research Council and Institute of Medicine. (2013). *U.S. Health in international perspective: Shorter lives, poorer health* (S. H. Woolf & L. Aron, Eds.). Panel on understanding cross-national health differences among high-income countries. Committee on Population, Division of Behavioral and Social Sciences and Education, and Board on Population Health and Public Health Practice, Institute of Medicine. Washington, DC: The National Academies Press.

Paul, B. D. (Ed.). (1955). *Health, culture, and community: Case studies of public reactions to health programs*. New York, NY: Russell Sage Foundation.

Raphael, D. (Ed.). (2004). *Social determinants of health: Canadian perspectives*. Toronto, ON: Canadian Scholars' Press, Inc.

Rosen, G. (1958). *A history of public health*. New York, NY: MD Publications.

Samuel-Hodge, C. D., Keyserling, T. C., France, R., Ingram, A. F., Johnston, L. F., Davis, L. P., et al. (2006). A church-based diabetes self-management education program for African Americans with type 2 diabetes. *Preventing Chronic Disease* [serial online]. Retrieved from http://www.cdc.gov/pcd/issues/2006/jul/05_0085.htm

Stack, S. (2000, Summer). Suicide: A 15-year review of the sociological literature part I: Cultural and economic factors. *Suicide and Life Threatening Behavior, 30*(2), 145–162.

The Lancet. (2012) *Global burden of disease study 2010. Special Issue*. Retrieved December 13, 2012, from: http://www.thelancet.com/themed/global-burden-of-disease

Weber, M. (1947). *The theory of social and economic organization* (T. Parsons, Ed.). New York, NY: The Free Press.

Weiner, H. (1977). *Psychobiology and human disease*. New York, NY: Elsevier.

WHO. (1946). *Preamble to the Constitution of the World Health Organization as adopted by the International Health Conference*, New York, 19–22 June, 1946; signed on 22 July 1946 by the representatives of 61 States and entered into force on 7 April 1948.

WHOCSDOH. (2008). *Closing the gap in a generation. Health equity through action on the social determinants of health*. Geneva: WHO.

Wilkinson, R. G., & Pickett, K. (2009). *The spirit level: Why more equal societies almost always do better*. London: Allen Lane.

Further Reading

Allison, K., & Rootman, I. (1996). Scientific rigor and community participation in health promotion research: Are they compatible? *Health Promotion International, 11*(4), 333–340.

Braveman, P. A., Cubbin, C., Egerter, S., Williams, D. R., & Pamuk, E. (2010). Socioeconomic disparities in health in the United States: What the patterns tell us. *American Journal of Public Health, 100*(S1), S186–S196.

Black, D., Morris, J. N., Smith, C., & Whitehead, M. (1988). *Inequalities in health*. London: Penguin.

Diez Roux, A. V. (2007). Integrating social and biological factors in health research: A systems view. *Annals of Epidemiology, 17*, 569–574.

Drummond, M., Weatherly, H., Claxton, K., Cookson, R., Ferguson, B., Godfrey, C. et al. (2007) *Assessing the challenges of applying standard methods of economic evaluation to public health interventions. Public Health Research*. http://phrc.lshtm.ac.uk/papers/PHRC_D1-05_Final_Report.pdf.

McQueen, D. V., & Siegrist, J. (1982). Sociocultural factors in the etiology of chronic disease. *Social Science and Medicine, 16*(4), 353–367.

Syme, S. L., Hyman, M. M., & Enterline, P. E. (1964). Some social and cultural factors associated with the occurrence of coronary heart disease. *Journal of Chronic Diseases, 17*, 277–289.

USDHHS. (2010). *How tobacco smoke causes disease: The biology and behavioral basis for smoking-attributable disease: A report of the Surgeon General*. Atlanta, GA: U.S. Department of Health and Human Services, Centers for Disease Control and Prevention, National Center for Chronic Disease Prevention and Health Promotion, Office on Smoking and Health.

The Social Determinants of Non-communicable Diseases: A Political Perspective

Dennis Raphael

Introduction

It is profoundly paradoxical that, in a period when the importance of public policy as a determinant of health is routinely acknowledged, there remains a continuing absence of mainstream debate about the ways in which the politics, power, and ideology that underpin it influence people's health (Bambra et al. 2005, p.1).

One of the most intriguing issues facing the health care and public health sectors around the globe is the gap between governmental authorities and health officials' general acknowledgement of the importance of the social determinants of health (SDH) and the application of this concept in the cases of specific non-communicable chronic diseases (Raphael et al. 2003; Raphael and Farrell 2002). Cardiovascular disease (CVD) in all its forms and Type 2 diabetes mellitus (T2DM) are just two examples of these chronic diseases—there are many others—as their incidence and prevalence within a jurisdiction as well as their ensuing complications including mortality are related to the experience of SDH across the life span (Chaufan 2008; Davey Smith 2003; Hux et al. 2002; Naylor and Slaughter 1999). Surprisingly, the professional literature

and governmental and agency pronouncements of means of preventing and managing these and other chronic diseases show little acknowledgement of these links and their implications for public policymaking (Raphael et al. 2008).

SDH are the living and working conditions that shape health (World Health Organization 2008). Since these conditions are distributed unequally amongst populations they are also social determinants of health inequalities (Blas et al. 2008). These distributions are shaped by public policies that result from decisions made by governing authorities on how to distribute economic and social resources (Bryant 2009). And these decisions themselves are driven by political ideologies concerning the nature of society and the roles governments should play in providing citizens with the resources necessary for health and well-being (Raphael 2011b, c, 2012).

This chapter examines how the politics of a society shapes the distribution of the SDH of chronic diseases such as CVD and T2DM with a focus upon the wealthy developed nations of the Organization for Economic Cooperation and Development (OECD). It takes seriously the World Health Organization's conclusion that "This unequal distribution of health-damaging experiences is not in any sense a 'natural' phenomenon but is the result of a toxic combination of poor social policies and programmes, unfair economic arrangements, and bad politics" (World Health Organization 2008, p. 1). This chapter identifies how the unequal distribution of the SDH shapes the incidence and prevalence as well

D. Raphael, Ph.D. (✉)
York University, 4700 Keele Street, Room 418,
HNES Building, Toronto, ON, Canada M3J 1P3
e-mail: draphael@yorku.ca

D.V. McQueen (ed.), *Global Handbook on Noncommunicable Diseases and Health Promotion*,
DOI 10.1007/978-1-4614-7594-1_7, © Springer Science+Business Media, LLC 2013

as outcomes of chronic diseases such as CVD and T2DM within nations.

It also explores the hypothesis that the quality and distribution of the SDH can illuminate some of the differences in incidence, prevalence, and outcomes of chronic diseases that occur between nations. By linking chronic diseases' incidence and prevalence as well as their management to broad public policy decisions made by governing authorities, it places these issues within a broader political economy perspective that addresses issues of influence, power, and the willingness of governmental authorities to provide citizens with the means of achieving health and avoiding illness.

Social Determinants of Health

The poor health of the poor, the social gradient in health within countries, and the marked health inequities between countries are caused by the unequal distribution of power, income, goods, and services, globally and nationally, the consequent unfairness in the immediate, visible circumstances of people's lives—their access to health care, schools, and education, their conditions of work and leisure, their homes, communities, towns, or cities—and their chances of leading a flourishing life (World Health Organization 2008, p. 1).

SDH refer to the societal factors—and the unequal distribution of these factors—that contribute to both the overall health of a population and the presence of health inequalities (Graham 2004). With the publication of the Commission on Social Determinants of Health's final report and those of its knowledge hubs, the SDH concept has achieved a prominence that makes it difficult for policymakers, health researchers, and professionals to ignore (World Health Organization 2011). A variety of SDH frameworks are available but what they all have in common is their concern with the living and working conditions which a society provides for its members (Centers for Disease Control and Prevention 2006; Raphael 2009; Whitehead 1985; World Health Organization 2008).

The specific experiences of living and working conditions such as income and wealth, education,

employment and working circumstances, housing and food security, and access to health and social services shape the incidence of chronic diseases as well as their management once they appear. Much research has gone into how these experiences across the life span get under the skin to shape the incidence of chronic disease and then go on to influence their management (Brunner and Marmot 2006; Raphael et al. 2012). But of equal if not more importance is examining the extent of existing inequalities in the experiences of these SDH and the sources of these inequalities. Such examination naturally leads to concern with the public policies that shape these distributions (Bambra 2011; Graham 2007; Raphael 2010). Analysis also becomes necessary of the economic and political forces that underlie these public policies (Bryant 2010; Navarro et al. 2006; Navarro and Shi 2002; Raphael 2012). Rather than simply examine the health effects of the SDH, inquiry becomes focused on the social determinants of health inequalities, the public policies that spawn them, and the societal forces that shape these health-enhancing or health-threatening public policies (Raphael 2011a).

This increasing concern with the SDH has certainly been evident in Canada where the SDH figure prominently in health policy documents produced by the Federal government (Public Health Agency of Canada 2007), the Chief Health Officer of Canada (Butler-Jones 2008), the Canadian Senate (Senate Subcommittee on Population Health 2008), numerous public health and social development organizations and agencies and research-funding agencies (Health Council of Canada 2010). Even the business-oriented Conference Board of Canada has established an initiative focused on the social and economic determinants of health (Conference Board of Canada 2008).

This has also been the case for many other OECD nations (Hogstedt et al. 2009; Raphael 2012). Reducing health inequalities through action on the SDH is a key policy objective of the European Union (Equity Action 2012) and has been a mainstay of the health promotion concept since the mid-1980s (World Health Organization 2009). But surprisingly, the importance of addressing SDH—that is, the living and working conditions and their unequal distribution—at a conceptual level frequently fails to find traction in discussions about reducing the incidence and prevalence—as well as promoting the successful management—of chronic diseases such as CVD and T2DM (Blas and Kurup 2010).

Social Determinants of Chronic Disease

As one example, consider how Canadian authorities address the prevention and management of chronic disease in general and CVD and T2DM in particular. The Canadian example is illustrative as it demonstrates the wide gap between rhetoric and action on the SDH. Canada had long been considered as a leader in advancing health promotion and population health concepts that take into account broader living and working conditions (Restrepo 2000). But Canada is now clearly seen as a SDH laggard in applying these concepts through public policy activity (Bryant et al. 2011; Hancock 2011). Other nations do a much better job of making the links between living and working conditions and health outcomes but even then the links of living and working conditions with chronic disease incidence, prevalence, and management are not usually made explicit (Raphael 2012).

This is surprising as there is now an extensive empirical literature that documents how experiences associated with the SDH—especially the material deprivation associated with low income—across the life span contributes to the onset and management of a variety of chronic diseases during adulthood (Davey Smith 2003; Kuh et al. 2004; Lynch and Kaplan 2000; Raphael 2011d). The evidence for CVD and T2DM is especially persuasive (Brunner and Marmot 2006; Chaufan 2008; Cruickshank et al. 2001; Davey Smith et al. 2002; Raphael et al. 2003; Raphael and Farrell 2002; Riste et al. 2001).

The mechanisms that link CVD and T2DM with material deprivation during early life begin with adverse experiences during intrauterine development and continue over the course of the life span; body systems responses to psychosocial stress associated with the experiences of these adverse SDH; and the adoption of health-threatening coping responses such as take-up of tobacco and carbohydrate-rich diets (Brunner and Marmot 2006; Davey Smith 2003; Lynch et al. 1997; Lynch and Kaplan 2000; Raphael 2011d).

In regard to managing CVD and T2DM and preventing adverse outcomes, adverse SDH contribute to difficulties acquiring opportunities for physical activity and adequate diet (Chaufan et al. 2012; Clark et al. 2009; Raphael et al. 2003, 2012; Raphael and Farrell 2002). Much of these difficulties result from the experience of material and social deprivation and the stresses associated with such deprivation (Chaufan 2008; Chaufan et al. 2012, 2013; Pilkington et al. 2010; Raphael et al. 2012).

In Canada, however, federal and provincial governments—supported by agencies such as the national and provincial Heart and Stroke Foundations and Diabetes Associations—develop and implement CVD and T2DM prevention and management strategies and programmes that appear to be oblivious to these findings (Kabir 2010). These strategies and programmes focus on modifying risk behaviours associated with the incidence and management of CVD and T2DM such as tobacco and alcohol use, poorly chosen diets, excess weight, and lack of physical activity with any mention of the SDH relegated to background status (Raphael et al. 2012). That is, these SDH are seen as providing a means of understanding how these risk factors are more prevalent among certain populations with rather less attention to their direct effects upon health and the importance of improving their quality and making their distribution more equitable through public policy action.

This relegation of the SDH concept to background status can be illustrated through an examination of varying discourses associated with the SDH concept. Table 7.1 presents eight different manners by which the distribution of chronic disease can be conceptualized together with their implications.

Approaches 1–3 dominate thinking about chronic disease in Canada and elsewhere with

Table 7.1 SDH approaches directed towards chronic disease issues

Social determinants interpretation	Key SDH concept	SDH practice approach	Practical implications
1. Chronic disease results from genetics and biological dispositions which interact with SDH.	Chronic disease can be reduced by identifying the triggers for genes and the physiological processes that cause disease.	Carrying out of more and better epigenetic research.	Medicalization of chronic disease issues and endorsement of the societal status quo.
2. Chronic disease results from differences in access and quality of health and social services.	Chronic disease can be reduced and better managed by strengthening health care and social services.	Creation of higher quality hospitals, clinics, and social service agencies.	Focus limited to promoting the health of those already experiencing or at risk for chronic disease.
3. Chronic disease results from differences in important modifiable medical and behavioural risk factors.	Chronic disease can be reduced by enabling people to make "healthy choices" and adopt "healthy lifestyles."	Development and evaluation of healthy living and behaviour modification programs and protocols.	Healthy lifestyle programming ignores the material basis of chronic disease and may widen existing inequalities.
4. Chronic disease results from differences in material living conditions.	Chronic disease can be reduced and management improved by improving material living conditions.	Community development and participatory research that enables people to gain control over their health.	Assumption that governmental authorities are receptive to and will act upon community voices and research findings.
5. Chronic disease results from differences in material living conditions that are a function of group membership.	Chronic disease and can be reduced and management improved by improving the material living conditions of particular disadvantaged groups.	Targeted development and research activities among specific disadvantaged and cultural groups to improve material living conditions.	Assumption that governmental authorities are receptive to such activities and anticipated outcomes.
6. Chronic disease results from differences in material living conditions shaped by public policy.	Chronic disease can be reduced and management improved by advocating for healthy public policy that reduce disadvantage.	Analyze how public policy decisions impact health (i.e., health impact analysis).	Assumption that governments will create public policy on the basis of its effects upon health.
7. Chronic disease results from differences in material living conditions that are shaped by economic and political structures and their justifying ideologies.	Chronic disease can be reduced and management improved by influencing the societal structures that create chronic disease.	Analysis of how the political economy of a nation creates chronic disease identifies avenues for social and political action.	Requirement that health workers engage in the building of social and political movements that will reduce chronic disease.
8. Chronic disease results from the power and influence of those who create and benefit from health-threatening social inequalities.	Chronic disease can be reduced by increasing the power and influence of those who experience the inequities that create chronic disease.	Critical analysis empowers the disadvantaged to gain understanding of, and means of increasing, their influence and power.	Requirement that health workers engage in the building of social and political movements that increase the power of the disadvantaged.

an obvious neglect of the role material living conditions—and the public policies that spawn these—play in the incidence and prevalence, and management of these diseases. More recently, an approach that may be described as Approach $3^{1/2}$ is seen where there is recognition that material living conditions may shape the presence of risk behaviours, the focus of Approach 3—what

Nettleton describes as the *Holy Trinity of Risk* of poor diet, lack of exercise, and tobacco use (Nettleton 1997)—but there is little if any recognition that material living and working conditions have a direct link to chronic disease through pathways of material deprivation and psychosocial stress nor is there explicit concern with modifying adverse living conditions through public policy action.

One example of such an approach is seen in a recent edited volume where the presence of four key behavioural risk factors, diet, tobacco use, physical activity, and alcohol use is placed within a sophisticated perspective with no mention of the direct effects upon chronic disease incidence and management of material deprivation and the stresses associated with such deprivation (Stuckler and Siegel 2011). Instead, the presence of these behavioural risk factors is seen as the prime cause of the major chronic diseases of cardiovascular disease, cancer, chronic respiratory disease, and diabetes around the globe with an extensive political economy analysis directed solely to explaining the prevalence of these behavioural risk factors.

This neglect of the role of the factors identified in the discourses of Approach 4 and beyond occurs despite the extensive efforts to raise these issues by the World Health Oganisation's Commission on Social Determinants and the accumulating research literature. Attention in the chronic disease practice literature to SDH such as early child development, income and wealth, and food security that have been shown to be potent predictors of the incidence and successful management of CVD and T2DM is sporadic at best (Raphael et al. 2012).

A particular blind spot in these governmental and institutional approaches to CVD and T2DM prevention and management is the deleterious direct influence of material deprivation associated with living in poverty (Chaufan and Weitz 2009; Raphael et al. 2003; Raphael and Farrell 2002). Material deprivation is problematic as there is extensive evidence that the experience of poverty is an important precursor to CVD and T2DM and a barrier to its successful management (Chaufan 2008; Chaufan et al. 2012; Choi and Shi 2001; Dinca-Panaitescua et al. 2012; Raine 2002; Riste et al. 2001).

In Canada, there is evidence that declines in supports for those living in poverty are fuelling increasing rates of mortality from T2DM in low income neighbourhoods (Wilkins 2007). And since policy directions taken by governments determine the incidence and experience of poverty (Raphael 2011b), it is imperative to consider how public policy fits into the chronic disease incidence, prevalence, and management pictures (Raphael et al. 2003).

These issues require moving beyond approaches that simply describe the behavioural and socioeconomic factors correlated with the incidence and prevalence as well as the management of chronic disease to one that analyzes (a) the public policy decisions that shape material living conditions (Approach 6 in Table 7.1); (b) the economic and political structures and the political ideologies that shape these public policy decisions (Approach 7), and (c) the means by which specific societal groups such as the business and corporate community unduly shape public policy in such a manner as to create the conditions under which these chronic diseases appear and are unsuccessfully managed (Approach 8).

The following sections identify the processes and forces that shape the quality and distribution of the SDH of chronic diseases—e.g., CVD and T2DM—such as income and wealth, employment and working circumstances, housing and food security, and health and social services, among others (Mikkonen and Raphael 2010). These social determinants of health are not themselves health outcomes, but they are rather good predictors of the incidence, prevalence, and management of these chronic diseases. These SDH are not simply predictors of behavioural risk factors such as poor diet, lack of physical activity, and alcohol and tobacco use, they are direct determinants of the incidence and management of chronic disease such as CVD and T2DM whose effects operate through pathways of material deprivation and the experience of health-threatening stress.

Social Inequalities and Chronic Disease

Social injustice is killing people on a grand scale (World Health Organization 2008, p. 1).

Important to this analysis is consideration of how differences in experiences of SDH can be explained. It is the position taken in this chapter—and amply supported by accumulated evidence—that differences in chronic disease incidence and prevalence, and management are primarily due to social inequalities in living and working circumstances. In Canada and elsewhere, wealthy, high-income individuals enjoy better health and are less likely to experience CVD and T2DM, and when they do experience it, have better outcomes because their living and working circumstances are better than those experienced by others.

These social inequalities in living and working circumstances and their manifestation in chronic disease occur all the way from the top to the bottom of the socioeconomic ladder. These differences are important to health as they are closely related to experiences with the SDH: *Social inequality can refer to any of the differences between people (or the socially defined positions they occupy) that are consequential for the lives they lead, most particularly for the rights or opportunities they exercise and the rewards or privileges they enjoy* (Grabb 2007, p. 1). Therefore these differences in exposures to the social determinants of health are not simply risk factors or risk conditions; they are fundamental statements about one's life situation. And it is increasingly clear that these living situations are shaped by public policies that determine the distribution of SDH.

The Social Determinants of the Incidence and Management of Chronic Disease: A Canadian Example

What is the evidence concerning the SDH and their distribution and their relationship to chronic disease within and between nations? The evidence is rather clear as to the relationship of the SDH to the incidence, prevalence, and management of chronic diseases such as CVD and T2DM within nations and this is especially the case in Canada, the UK, and the USA (Chaufan 2008; Clark et al. 2009; Raphael et al. 2012; Riste et al. 2001).

Recent studies from a team of Canadian researchers identify how the SDH structure the incidence and prevalence, and management of T2DM. To investigate these issues, a two-pronged study was carried out. First, the researchers analyzed data from the Canadian Community Health Survey (CCHS) (cycle 3.1) and the National Population Health Survey (NPHS) (Dinca-Panaitescua et al. 2011, 2012). The CCHS is a very large cross-sectional survey of over 105,000 Canadians. The researchers predicted that (a) low income would be a strong predictor of T2DM; and (b) once income was known, risk factors would not tell much more about the distribution of T2DM. The NPHS is a longitudinal survey and it was predicted that living on low income would anticipate people developing T2DM. This relationship would also be independent of the presence of behavioural risk factors.

Findings from the Canadian Community Health Survey

Approximately 8,200 respondents reported a diagnosis of T2DM and of those 95.8 % or 7,806 were identified as having type 2 diabetes (Dinca-Panaitescua et al. 2011). Having T2DM was strongly related with income and these differences increased with age (Fig. 7.1). Lower-income older Canadians were twice as likely to have T2DM as wealthy older Canadians. The important question is whether these differences between lower income and wealthier Canadians could be accounted for by differences in factors such as education, body mass index (BMI)—overweight or obese—and lack of physical activity, the mainstay of most chronic disease epidemiological research.

For men, being of very low income (annual income <$15,000) doubles the risk of T2DM (2.07) as compared to the wealthiest group of Canadians (>$80,000). Once education level,

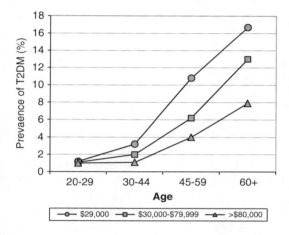

Fig. 7.1 Prevalence of T2DM among Canadians by age and annual family income, 2005. *Source*: Statistics Canada Canadian Community Health Survey

BMI, and physical activity are taken into account—reducing risk by only 6 %—the risk is still very close to double (1.94).

For the next group of lower income Canadian males ($15,000–$30,000), the increased risk of 1.72 is only reduced to 1.66—only 2 %—when these other factors are taken into account. Income plays a stronger role in T2DM for women. Even after risk is reduced by 22 % for the lowest income group (from 3.57 to 2.75) and 19 % for the next lowest income group (2.58–2.1) by controlling for the risk factors of education, BMI, and physical activity, the role income plays in T2DM continues to be stronger for very low income females (2.75–2.07) and low income females (2.1–1.66) than for men.

Findings from the National Population Health Survey

All seven cycles of Statistics Canada's NPHS survey from 1994/1995 to 2006/2007 were used to trace 17,276 respondents and observe who developed T2DM over the cycles (Dinca-Panaitescua et al. 2012). A total of 690 respondents developed T2DM over the course of the study (about 100 during each 2 year cycle). The rate at which new cases of T2DM were diagnosed slightly increased from 6.54 per 1,000 person-years in

1996/1997 to 7.41 per 1,000 persons-years in 2006/2007.

Those identified as living on low incomes were living in a household of one or two persons with less than $15,000 annual income, less than $20,000 for a household with three or four persons, and less than $30,000 for a household with five or more persons. The researchers then calculated the risk of developing T2DM as a function of living on low incomes during the period just prior to developing T2DM and the risk of developing T2DM as a function of having ever lived on low income during the course of the study. Data were combined for men and women because of the relatively small number of Canadians in the survey developing T2DM during the study.

Living on low income provides an increased risk of developing T2DM of 24 % over a 2 year period. Ever having lived on low income during the study period returns a similar figure. These increased risks of developing T2DM are not affected by being obese or lack of physical activity. A final analysis examined whether living for longer periods of time on low income increased the risk of T2DM.

The researchers found those living more often on low incomes over the 12-year study had a 41 % greater chance of developing T2DM (risk of 1.41). Taking into account obesity and lack of physical inactivity only reduced this greater risk from 41 to 36 %, a reduction of only 12 % of the original poverty-related risk (risk of 1.36). These findings are consistent with an expanding literature as to the effects of varying exposures to the SDH across the lifespan upon the development of T2DM during adulthood (Chaufan 2008; Kuh et al. 2004; Lawlor et al. 2002).

Similar findings concerning the effects of SDH are available for CVD (Davey Smith et al. 2002; Stansfeld and Marmot 2002). There is also extensive evidence as to how degrees of advantage and disadvantage during child are potent predictors of the onset of both CVD and T2DM during adulthood (Raphael 2011d). A recent review concluded:

> The experience of poverty during childhood is a potent predictor of a variety of adverse health outcomes during middle and late adulthood. Children who live in poverty are more likely as adults than

their peers to develop and die earlier from a range of diseases. These effects are especially strong for cardiovascular disease and type II diabetes. Most disturbingly, these effects appear in large part to be biologically embedded such that later improved life circumstances have only a modest ameliorative effect (Raphael 2011d) (abstract).

In addition, these same factors—material advantage or disadvantage across the life span— are also related to the likelihood of developing arthritis, respiratory disease, and some cancers during adulthood (Davey Smith 2003; Raina et al. 2000). Additionally, though not as extensively researched as CVD and T2DM, there is evidence that the same kind of relationship between SDH that reflect material deprivation and adverse health outcomes holds for such diverse chronic diseases as allergies, hypertension, and a range of psychiatric disorders (Kuh et al. 2004). In addition, since social class during adulthood is related to greater incidence of numerous other adult disorders such as arthritis, osteoporosis, and Alzheimer's disease, and adult social class is itself strongly predicted by childhood social class, the possibility of a SDH link to these other chronic afflictions seems likely.

Findings from Interviews with 60 Low-Income Individuals with T2DM

In terms of management of chronic diseases, there is an emerging literature that moves beyond traditional explanations of lack of access to health care and lack of knowledge to link adverse outcomes with material and social deprivation and the stress that results from such deprivation. This is the case for T2DM and CVD (Chaufan et al. 2012, 2013; Clark et al. 2009; Clark and Thompson 2008; Raphael et al. 2012).

As an example, the same research project that identified the precursors of T2DM among Canadians also found that the living conditions of 60 low income Canadians with T2DM were so impoverished as to make it almost impossible for 72 % of these individuals to acquire the diet necessary to prevent the adverse outcomes associated with T2DM (Raphael et al. 2012). While

they received excellent health care through local community health centres, their lives appeared to be a "daily struggle to survive in the face of multiple challenges" presented by having to manage not only their diabetes but also the various hardships that arise when living on a low income (Pilkington et al. 2010).

What was most striking was their description of their lives as a "constant juggling act" required to survive on a limited income. A common situation was having to decide whether to buy good quality food, or diabetes medication, or pay the rent (Pilkington et al. 2010). These findings are remarkable similar to the experiences of low-income people in the USA with T2DM (Chaufan et al. 2012, 2013).

The Social Determinants as Explanations of Differences in Chronic Disease Incidence and Management Among Nations

Findings are less clear concerning the power of the SDH and their distribution to explain differences between nations. Wilkinson and Picket have documented how income inequality is a good predictor of national indicators of health such as life expectancy, infant mortality rates, and obesity (Wilkinson and Pickett 2009). Inequalities in income is one of the best indicators between what have been termed differing forms of the welfare state.

Numerous researchers have documented the profound differences in economic and social security as well as income inequality and poverty rates that exist between the well developed social democratic welfare states of Denmark, Finland, Norway, and Sweden with those of the less developed liberal welfare states of Canada, Ireland, UK, and USA (Bambra 2005, 2011; Blas et al. 2008; Navarro and Shi 2002; Raphael 2011b, c). The conservative welfare states of Germany, France, Belgium, and Netherlands fall midway between the social democratic and liberal welfare states.

There are differences among these nations in health indicators such as infant mortality and low

Table 7.2 Variations in health indicators among differing welfare states, 2009

Welfare state type	Nation	Life expectancy	Premature years of life lost F	M	Infant mortality/1,000	Low birthweight/100
Social democratic	Denmark	79.0	2,493	4,311	3.1	6.1
	Finland	80.0	2,208	4,696	2.6	4.3
	Norway	81.0	2,063	3,518	3.1	5.2
	Sweden	81.4	1,916	3,081	2.5	4.1
	Mean	80.3	2,170	3,901	2.8	4.9
Conservative	Belgium	80.0	2,500	4,585	3.4	7.6
	France	81.0	2,202	4,459	3.9	6.6
	Germany	80.3	2,123	3,824	3.5	6.9
	Netherlands	80.6	2,235	3,114	3.8	5.5
	Mean	80.5	2,265	3,995	3.6	5.3
Liberal	Canada	80.7	2,554	4,168	5.1	6.0
	Ireland	80.0	2,302	4,239	3.2	4.8
	UK	80.0	2,479	3,988	4.6	7.4
	USA	78.2	3,555	6,133	6.5	8.2
	Mean	79.8	2,722	4,632	4.8	6.6

Source: Organization for Economic Co-operation and Development. (2011). *Health at a Glance: OECD Indicators 2011* Edition. OECD: Paris

birthweight rates, the latter of which has been shown to be a good predictor of CVD and T2DM during adulthood (Barker et al. 2001; Fall et al. 1995; Kuh et al. 2004) (see Table 7.2). Social democratic welfare states fare better than the liberal welfare states (Bambra 2011; Organization for Economic Co-operation and Development 2011a). Conservative states fall midrange. Are these identifiable differences of societal approaches to the provision of economic and social security to citizens related to the incidence and prevalence as well as success in managing chronic diseases such as CVD and T2DM?

There are some differences among the most distinctly different nations—the liberal welfare states of USA, Canada, UK and Ireland, and the social democratic welfare states of Norway, Finland, Sweden, and Denmark in overall health indicators. These are not apparent in terms of life expectancy, where Sweden and Norway have the longest, followed by Canada, UK, Finland, Ireland, Denmark, and the USA (Table 7.2). They are more apparent where Sweden, Norway, and Finland have fewer potential years of life lost than Canada, UK, Ireland, and the USA. Denmark falls just behind Ireland and the UK.

Differences are more apparent in infant mortality and low birth weight rates (Organization for Economic Co-operation and Development 2011a). These indicators are important as infant mortality rate is a sensitive indicator of overall population health and low birth weight is a strong predictor of the appearance of CVD and T2DM later in life (Raphael 2011d). More specifically, each of the four social democratic welfare states have lower infant mortality rates than the liberal welfare states and except for the case of Ireland these differences are of rather strong magnitude (Organization for Economic Co-operation and Development 2011a). The same is generally the case in terms of low birthweight rate. Sweden, Finland, and Norway have rather lower rates than Canada, the USA, and UK, with Ireland being just above Norway.

Norway and Denmark have lower mortality rates for ischemic disease than all four liberal nations but Finland's highest rates and Sweden's moderate rates make generalizations risky (Table 7.3). Of interest is the finding that the conservative welfare states present the most favourable picture. No pattern emerges for mortality from stroke however. All cancer mortality rates are

Table 7.3 Variations in chronic disease mortality among differing welfare states, 2009

Welfare state type	Nation	Ischemic heart disease		Stroke		Cancers		Lung cancer	
		F	M	F	M	F	M	F	M
Social democratic	Denmark	49	93	45	56	173	237	42	62
	Finland	74	170	38	50	105	165	13	41
	Norway	42	87	31	42	126	185	24	42
	Sweden	58	118	36	45	125	165	22	29
	Mean	56	117	38	48	132	188	26	43
Conservative	Belgium	42	94	38	45	122	226	17	75
	France	19	50	22	31	111	221	14	57
	Germany	56	110	32	39	121	193	18	50
	Netherlands	27	62	32	35	144	226	30	65
	Mean	36	79	31	38	124	217	20	62
Liberal	Canada	61	123	29	34	143	205	36	60
	Ireland	65	137	n/a	n/a	143	218	27	50
	UK	50	110	39	42	141	199	30	48
	USA	68	129	29	32	130	185	36	57
	Mean	61	125	32	36	139	201	32	54

Source: Organization for Economic Co-operation and Development. (2011). *Health at a Glance: OECD Indicators 2011* Edition. OECD: Paris

Table 7.4 Variations in chronic disease among differing welfare states, 2009

Welfare state type	Nation	Diabetes/ prevalence	Cancers/ incidence
Social democratic	Denmark	5.6	321
	Finland	5.7	250
	Norway	3.6	298
	Sweden	5.2	260
	Mean	5.0	282
Conservative	Belgium	n/a	309
	France	6.7	300
	Germany	8.9	282
	Netherlands	5.3	290
	Mean	7.0	295
Liberal	Canada	9.2	297
	Ireland	5.2	317
	UK	3.6	269
	USA	10.3	300
	Mean	7.1	295

Source: Organization for Economic Co-operation and Development. (2011). *Health at a Glance: OECD Indicators 2011* Edition. OECD: Paris

lowest in Sweden and Finland with the ranking being Sweden, Finland, USA, Norway, UK, Canada, Ireland, and Denmark. Lung cancer mortality rates are lowest in Sweden followed by Finland and Norway and then UK, Ireland, USA,

and Canada. Denmark has the highest rates among these nations. In terms of prevalence of diabetes (both type 1 and 2), the social democratic welfare states have markedly lower rates than Canada and the USA and as a group, somewhat lower cancer incidence rates than other nations (Table 7.4).

In terms of obesity and the behavioural risk factors of tobacco and alcohol use which is of such concern among chronic disease researchers, a clear pattern for overweight and obesity is evident. Norway, Sweden, Denmark, and Finland have lower obesity rates than do Ireland, UK, Canada, and the USA. In the case of the first three social democratic welfare states—Norway, Sweden, and Denmark, these differences are rather wide. Tobacco and alcohol use provides a more mixed picture with no differences apparent between these two groups of nations (Table 7.5).

These are admittedly very rough comparisons and finer analyses into the relationship of income and wealth distribution and provision of other forms of citizen security are required. The scarcity of research into the political economy of differences among nations in incidence and prevalence, and management of chronic diseases suggests a real need for further research.

Table 7.5 Variations in risk behaviours among differing welfare states, 2009

Welfare state type	Nation	Obesity adults	Overweight children		Tobacco use	Alcohol (litres/capita)
			F	M		
Social democratic	Denmark	13.4	15.2	14.1	19.0	10.1
	Finland	20.2	19.1	23.6	18.6	10.0
	Norway	10.0	14.7	12.9	21.0	6.7
	Sweden	11.2	19.5	17.0	14.3	7.4
	Mean	13.7	17.2	16.9	18.2	8.6
Conservative	Belgium	13.8	n/a	n/a	20.5	9.7
	France	11.2	14.9	13.1	26.2	12.3
	Germany	14.7	17.6	22.6	21.9	9.7
	Netherlands	11.8	17.9	14.7	22.6	9.4
	Mean	12.9	16.8	16.8	22.8	10.3
Liberal	Canada	24.2	26.1	28.9	16.2	8.2
	Ireland	23.0	n/a	n/a	29.9	11.3
	UK	23.0	26.6	22.7	21.5	10.2
	USA	33.8	35.9	35.0	16.1	8.8
	Mean	26.0	29.5	28.9	20.9	9.6

Source: Organization for Economic Co-operation and Development. (2011). *Health at a Glance: OECD Indicators 2011* Edition. OECD: Paris

As one interesting example, Offer, Pechley, and Ulijaszek make the argument that the higher obesity rates—perhaps leading to greater incidence and prevalence of chronic diseases—found in liberal welfare states is a reflection of maladaptive means of coping with greater competition, uncertainty, and inequality than is seen in non-liberal social democratic and conservative (see below) welfare states (Offer et al. 2010).

A similar analysis by Komlos and Baur explores how Americans have gone from being the "tallest to the fattest" among those living in wealthy developed nations during the twentieth century (Komlos and Baur 2004). Even less is known concerning how differing forms of the welfare states influence successful management of chronic diseases. This would require inquiry into the organization and delivery of health care services across the socioeconomic spectrum.

Public Policy and the Social Determinants of Health

This unequal distribution of health-damaging experiences is not in any sense a "natural" phenomenon but is the result of a toxic combination of poor social policies and programmes, unfair economic arrangements, and bad politics (World Health Organization 2008, p. 1).

It is the argument advanced here that these factors that shape the incidence, prevalence, and management of chronic disease within nations—and possibly among them—are a reflection of how governmental authorities choose to distribute economic and social resources amongst the population. This area is commonly defined as the domain of public policy analysis.

Defining Public Policy

The quality and distribution of the social determinants of health are shaped by public policy decisions. Public policy concerns courses of action or inaction taken by public authorities—usually governments—to address a given problem or set of problems (Briggs 1961). Governments constantly make decisions about a wide range of issues, such as national defence and the organization and delivery of health, social, and other services. The decisions that are the special concern of this chapter concern those that determine how economic and social resources are distributed among the population, the implication being that these shape the distribution of the incidence and prevalence as well as the management of chronic diseases such as CVD and T2DM.

Governments influence the distribution of the SDH by establishing tax levels, setting the nature and quality of employment, wages, and other benefits and how workers' employment conditions and working benefits are negotiated. Governments are also responsible for establishing housing policies, maintaining the social safety net, enacting labour regulations and laws, and providing training related to employment and education.

This broader approach recognizes the important role material living circumstances play in producing health inequities but then goes on to consider how these circumstances are shaped by public policy decisions made by governing authorities. The importance of public policy in creating health inequalities is becoming increasingly apparent but remains relatively unspoken of among many chronic disease researchers and workers. In many ways this approach states the obvious: *The distribution of economic and social resources that influence the presence of and management of chronic diseases result from public policy decisions made by governing authorities*. This is most obvious when examining the key drivers of health inequalities: the differences among individuals, groups, and residents of different communities and regions in access to the SDH.

The World Health Organization states this conclusion rather more strongly in the quote provided above: "This unequal distribution of health-damaging experiences is not in any sense a 'natural' phenomenon but is the result of a toxic combination of poor social policies and programmes, unfair economic arrangements, and bad politics" (World Health Organization 2008, p. 1). In this analysis, the presence of health inequalities is shaped by access to material resources such as income, housing, food, and educational and employment opportunities, among others. These resources are related to employment security, wages, and the quality of individuals' working circumstances and availability of quality, regulated childcare, all of which are shaped by public policy decisions (Raphael 2009).

Theories of Public Policy

How is public policy made and why does it frequently appear to be at odds with promoting health? The first explanation of governing authorities producing health-threatening public policy is inadequate knowledge translation from research to policymaking. This view is consistent with what political scientists term the pluralist approach to public policy making. In this model, policy development is driven primarily by the quality of ideas in the public policy arena such that those judged as beneficial and useful will be translated into policies by governing authorities (Brooks and Miljan 2003). More research and publications such as this one can be brought to the attention of policy makers who will evaluate their potential contribution and then act on it.

The pluralist approach suggests the need for further research, knowledge dissemination, and public policy advocacy with the aim of convincing policymakers to enact health-supporting public policies. And the implementation of this analysis can be seen in Canada and other nations by increasing funding of health inequality-related research, prolific governmental and institutional reporting of the importance of health inequalities research, and involvement with a variety of inequality related organizations and institutions such as the SDH Commission and its knowledge networks. The problem is that in Canada and other liberal nations such as the USA, these activities have so far had little impact in terms of policy action to address the SDH. This is less the case in other nations (Raphael 2012).

In contrast, the alternative explanation of how nations approach public policy that shapes the quality and distribution of the SDH is what political scientists term the materialist analysis of public policy making (Brooks and Miljan 2003). In this model, policy development is driven primarily by powerful interests who assure their concerns receive rather more attention than those not so situated. In wealthy developed nations these powerful interests are usually based in the private sector and have powerful partners in the political arena (Navarro 2009; Scambler 2002). The materialist model suggests the need for developing strong social and political movements with the aim of forcing policymakers to enact health-supporting public policy.

Key Areas of Public Policy Relevant to the SDH of Chronic Disease

Public policies that influence the SDH of chronic disease and make their distribution more equitable take various forms. The focus in this chapter is on broad macro-level public policy approaches that involve the distribution of economic and social resources rather than specific programmes directed at those perceived as being in need. One public policy area that has been neglected by the health promotion literature in general and the chronic disease literature in particular is that of the rights of citizens to collective employment bargaining, sometimes through the facilitation of workplace unionization, at other times through employer provision of employment security and benefits (Organization for Economic Co-operation and Development 2004).

This neglect is puzzling as the extent of collective bargaining agreements has been associated with lower rates of poverty and income inequality, and generally stronger provision of economic and social security (Swank 2005) all of which have been found to be strongly related to health outcomes (Navarro et al. 2004). Working under a collective agreement is certainly related to higher wages and employment security as well as receipt of benefits in Canada (Jackson 2010). Closely related to this is the percentage of workers who are members of unions. This latter indicator provides a measure of power balance between workers and owners and managers of the economy (Olsen 2010). Raphael recently examined extent of collective bargaining and found strong relationships between collective bargaining rates and union density in infant mortality rates among wealthy developed nations (Raphael 2011c). Similar findings are apparent for low birth weight rate (Organization for Economic Co-operation and Development 2011a).

Another important public policy area is that of investing in the population through provision of benefits, supports and services that provide the prerequisites of health (Raphael and Bryant 2006). These investments involve spending on universal programmes that benefit virtually all citizens such as early child education and care, employment training, pensions, and provision of community-based health care and social services (Hemrijck 2002). At other times this spending involves provision of adequate benefits to those who are unable to work because of illness, disability, or unemployment due to the loss of jobs in a changing economy (Organization for Economic Co-operation and Development 2003, 2011b). These expenditures are especially important with regard to families with children (Esping-Andersen 2002; Innocenti Research Centre 2005, 2007). A similar pattern is seen between these expenditures and indicators of health such as infant mortality and low birthweight rates (Innocenti Research Centre 2007; Raphael 2011c)

A shorthand way of thinking about these potential relationships between public policy indicators and chronic health outcomes is that nations that provide SDH that support health ensure that the meeting of citizens needs of adequate income, housing and employment, health, and social services does not fall by the wayside against the needs of those who manage the economy. This usually involves State intervention in the operation of the market economy (Esping-Andersen 1985, 2009). Such a balance is seen in the Scandinavian and European Continental nations but is rather less apparent among English-speaking nations such as the UK, Ireland, Canada, and USA (Alesina and Glaeser 2004; Micklewright 2004; Olsen 2010; Pontusson 2005). This leads to an examination of what has been termed the political economy of the welfare state.

The Political Economy of the Welfare State

The social democratic welfare states are distinguished by their strong commitments to State provision of citizen economic and social security—a concept that appears closely related to provision of the prerequisites of health—while the liberal welfare states generally rely upon the economic marketplace to distribute economic and social resources (Raphael 2011b).

Recent literature has considered differences in broad public policy approaches within a "worlds of welfare" framework that distinguishes between differing forms of the welfare state (Bambra 2007; Eikemo and Bambra 2008). In this framework, varied public policy components fit together to define a specific welfare state regime. Esping-Andersen identifies three regimes of welfare capitalism: social democratic, conservative, and liberal to which Saint-Arnaud and Bernard (2003) add a fourth Latin type (Esping-Andersen 1990, 1999). Bambra (2007) identifies no less than 12 different welfare state typologies but virtually all make a distinction between liberal or residual welfare states and social democratic or encompassing types with a mid-level type that usually corresponds to what is called the conservative form. The Scandinavian, Continental, and English-speaking nations mentioned above appear to correspond to social democratic, conservative, and liberal political economies, respectively. Esping-Anderson sees these differing regimes as resulting from distinctive political and social histories (Esping-Andersen 1990).

The social democratic welfare states (e.g. Finland, Sweden, Denmark, and Norway) emphasize universal welfare rights and provide generous benefits and entitlements. Their political and social history is one of political dominance by social democratic parties of the left, a result of political organization of initially industrial workers and farmers, and later the middle class. Through universal provision of a range of benefits, these regimes have been able to secure the loyalties of a significant proportion of the population (Esping-Andersen 1990, 1999).

Conservative welfare states (e.g. Belgium, France, Germany, and Netherlands) also offer generous benefits but provide these based on social insurance plans associated with employment status with emphasis on primary male wage earners. Their political and social history is one of political dominance by Christian Democratic parties where traditional Church concerns with supporting citizens merges with traditional approaches towards maintaining status differences and adherence to authority (Esping-Andersen 1990, 1999).

These tendencies sometimes manifest in corporatist approaches (e.g. Germany) where business interests are major influences or in Statist approaches (e.g. France) where the State plays a key role in provision of citizen security (Pontusson 2005).

Liberal welfare states (e.g. Australia, Canada, UK, and USA) provide modest benefits and the State usually steps in with assistance only when the market fails to meet citizens' most basic needs. Their political and social history is one of dominance by business interests that has led the population to give its loyalty to the economic system rather than the State as a means of providing economic and social security (Esping-Andersen 1990, 1999). These liberal welfare states are the least developed in terms of provision of citizen economic and social security. A key feature is their use of means-tested benefits that are targeted only to the least well-off. Latin welfare states (e.g. Greece, Italy, Spain, and Portugal) are identified by Saint-Arnaud and Bernard (2003) as less developed family oriented versions of the conservative welfare regime.

Figure 7.2 identifies key elements of each of these four forms of the welfare state. There are clear affinities between the provision of health supporting SDH and aspects of these differing forms of the welfare state. The liberal welfare state with its emphasis on minimizing State intervention in the operation of the marketplace and provision of minimal benefits appears to be the least likely to produce public policy that prevents chronic disease and promotes its management. The social democratic and conservative welfare states—with their emphasis on promoting equality in the former case and solidarity in the latter—should be more likely to implement public policies that do so.

Little has been written about how the Latin welfare states may provide the prerequisites of health except to point out their relatively undeveloped nature and their emphasis upon the family as providing the primary means of support (Navarro and Shi 2002; Saint-Arnaud and Bernard 2003). Therefore, they may be expected to provide to a lesser extent the prerequisites of health than the social democratic and conservative welfare states.

Evidence exists that this is the case. State provision to citizens of economic and social supports

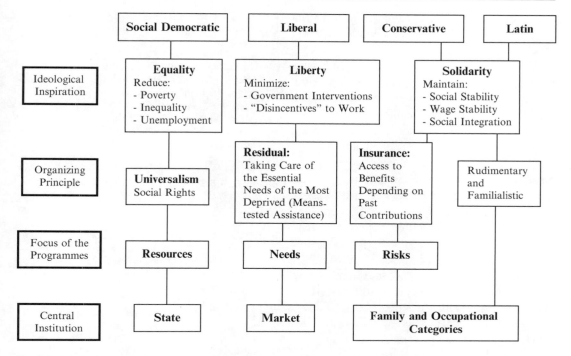

Fig. 7.2 Ideological variations in forms of the welfare state. *Source*: Saint-Arnaud, S., & Bernard, P. (2003). Convergence or resilience? A hierarchical cluster analysis of the welfare regimes in advanced countries. *Current Sociology, 51*(5), 499–527, Figure 2, p. 503

appears to lag among liberal welfare states with the greatest differences seen between the social democratic and liberal welfare states (Bambra 2006; Navarro et al. 2004; Navarro and Shi 2002). But to date there has been little systematic research and analysis of how these issues shapes the profile of chronic disease such as CVD and T2DM among others. There are some suggestive research inquiries that support the importance of doing so but as the overwhelming proportion of inquiries focus on identification and modification of individual risk factors.

The Politics of Chronic Disease Prevention and Management: What Is to Be Done?

Over two hundred years of anecdotal, epidemiological, and experimental evidence indicate that poverty breeds disease, and that socioeconomic differences cause systematic differences in disease and death rates (hereafter, health inequalities), even as the major types of diseases and the particular

mechanisms linking inequalities in their distribution with socioeconomic factors have changed over time. Moreover, there has been no scarcity of theories attempting to explain this relationship, in the past and in our day (Chaufan et al. 2013).

There are two main directions for chronic disease researchers and workers to take concerning the politics of chronic disease. The first is redirecting research activities to take seriously the view that living and working conditions shape the incidence and prevalence as well as the management of chronic disease. This involves moving beyond the focus on behavioural risk factors of diet, physical activity and alcohol and tobacco use to examination of material and social conditions and the stress associated with such experiences. There is ample evidence that within jurisdictions material and social conditions—and the stress associated with these conditions—have direct effects upon the incidence and prevalence, as well as the management of chronic diseases. The overwhelming proportion of research activity is directed towards the relationship between behavioural risk factors and chronic disease incidence and prevalence. Research in this vein has been presented in regards to CVD and T2DM. Much more needs to be done.

The second avenue of research is to undertake investigation of the public policies and the economic and political structures and accompanying ideologies that shape the circumstances that spawn chronic disease and influence their management. This involves the development of a political economy of chronic disease that move beyond a focus on behavioural risk factors towards one of linking these broader issues with concrete manifestation and outcomes of chronic diseases. In terms of explaining these effects within nations, an extensive literature is now available (Davey Smith 2003) and needs to be strengthened with a political economy analysis. In terms of explaining how these broader forces explain differences in chronic disease incidence and prevalence as well as management among nations, the articles by (Offer et al. 2010) and (Komlos and Baur 2004) offer a template for such inquiries.

The idea that the understanding of disease can be furthered by the study of society is not new. It is time for those concerned with preventing and managing chronic diseases to take seriously Virchow's statement: *Do we not always find the diseases of the populace traceable to defects in society?* (Virchow 1848/1985). Beginnings have been made in these areas but more need to be done.

References

Alesina, A., & Glaeser, E. L. (2004). *Fighting poverty in the US and Europe: A world of difference*. Toronto, ON: Oxford University Press.

Bambra, C. (2005). Cash versus services: Worlds of welfare and the decommodification of cash benefits and health care. *Journal of Social Policy, 34*(2), 195–213.

Bambra, C. (2006). Health status and the worlds of welfare. *Social Policy and Society, 5*, 53–62.

Bambra, C. (2007). Going beyond the three worlds of welfare capitalism: Regime theory and public health research. *Journal of Epidemiology and Community Health, 61*(12), 1098–1102.

Bambra, C. (2011). Health inequalities and welfare state regimes: Theoretical insights on a public health 'puzzle'. *Journal of Epidemiology and Community Health, 65*, 740–745.

Bambra, C., Fox, D., & Scott-Samuel, A. (2005). Towards a politics of health. *Health Promotion International, 20*(2), 187–193.

Barker, D., Forsen, T., Uutela, A., Osmond, C., & Eriksson, J. (2001). Size at birth and resilience to effects of poor living conditions in adult life: Longitudinal study. *British Medical Journal, 323*(7324), 1273–1276.

Blas, E., Gilson, L., Kelly, M. P., Labonté, R., Lapitan, J., Muntaner, C., et al. (2008). Addressing social determinants of health inequities: What can the state and civil society do? *The Lancet, 372*(9650), 1684–1689.

Blas, E., & Kurup, A. (Eds.). (2010). *Equity, social determinants and public health programmes*. Geneva: World Health Organization.

Briggs, A. (1961). The welfare state in historical perspective. *European Journal of Sociology, 2*, 251–259.

Brooks, S., & Miljan, L. (2003). Theories of public policy. In S. Brooks & L. Miljan (Eds.), *Public policy in Canada: An introduction* (pp. 22–49). Toronto: Oxford University Press.

Brunner, E., & Marmot, M. (2006). Social organization, stress, and health. In M. Marmot & R. G. Wilkinson (Eds.), *Social determinants of health* (2nd ed., pp. 6–30). Oxford: Oxford University Press.

Bryant, T. (2009). *An introduction to health policy*. Toronto: Canadian Scholars' Press.

Bryant, T. (2010). Politics, public policy and health inequalities. In T. Bryant, D. Raphael, & M. Rioux (Eds.), *Staying alive: Critical perspectives on health, illness, and health care* (2nd ed., pp. 239–265). Toronto: Canadian Scholars' Press.

Bryant, T., Raphael, D., Schrecker, T., & Labonte, R. (2011). Canada: A land of missed opportunity for addressing the social determinants of health. *Health Policy, 101*(1), 44–58.

Butler-Jones, D. (2008). *Report on the state of public health in Canada 2008: Addressing health inequalities*. Ottawa, ON: Public Health Agency of Canada.

Centers for Disease Control and Prevention. (2006). *Social determinants of health*. Retrieved March 1, 2009, from http://www.cdc.gov/sdoh/

Centre, I. R. (2005). *Child poverty in rich nations, 2005. Report Card No. 6*. Florence: Innocenti Research Centre.

Centre, I. R. (2007). *An overview of child well-being in rich countries: A comprehensive assessment of the lives and well-being of children and adolescents in the economically advanced nations*. Florence: Innocenti Research Centre.

Chaufan, C. (2008). What does justice have to do with it? A bioethical and sociological perspective on the diabetes epidemic. *Bioethical Issues, Sociological Perspectives, 9*, 269–300.

Chaufan, C., Constantino, S., & Davis, M. (2012). "It's a full time job being poor." Understanding barriers to diabetes prevention in immigrant communities in the USA. *Critical Public Health, 22*, 147–158.

Chaufan, C., Constantino, S., & Davis, M. (2013). "You must not confuse poverty with laziness": A case study on the power of discourse to reproduce diabetes inequalities. *International Journal of Health Services, 43*(1), 143–166.

Chaufan, C., & Weitz, R. (2009). The elephant in the room: The invisibility of poverty in research on type 2 diabetes. *Humanity and Society, 33*, 74–98.

Choi, B. C. K., & Shi, F. (2001). Risk factors for diabetes mellitus by age and sex: Results of the National Population Health Survey. *Diabetologia, 44*(10), 1221–1231.

Clark, A. M., DesMeules, M., Luo, W., Duncan, A. S., & Wielgolz, A. (2009). Socioeconomic status and coronary heart disease: Risks and care implications. *Nature Reviews Cardiology, 6*(11), 712–722.

Clark, A. M., & Thompson, D. R. (2008). The future of management programmes for heart failure. *The Lancet, 372*(9641), 784–786.

Conference Board of Canada. (2008). *Healthy people, healthy performance, healthy profits: The case for business action on the socio-economic determinants of health*. Ottawa, ON: Author.

Cruickshank, J., Mbanya, J., Wilks, R., Balkau, B., McFarlane-Anderson, N., & Forrester, T. (2001). Sick genes, sick individuals or sick populations with chronic disease? The emergence of diabetes and high blood pressure in African-origin populations. *International Journal of Epidemiology, 30*(1), 111–117.

Davey Smith, G. (Ed.). (2003). *Inequalities in health: Life course perspectives*. Bristol: Policy Press.

Davey Smith, G., Ben-Shlomo, Y., & Lynch, J. (2002). Life course approaches to inequalities in coronary heart disease risk. In S. A. Stansfeld & M. Marmot (Eds.), *Stress and the heart: Psychosocial pathways to coronary heart disease* (pp. 20–49). London: BMJ Books.

Dinca-Panaitescua, S., Dinca-Panaitescu, M., Bryant, T., Daiski, I., Pilkington, B., & Raphael, D. (2011). Diabetes prevalence and income: Results of the Canadian Community Health Survey. *Health Policy, 99*, 116–123.

Dinca-Panaitescua, S., Dinca-Panaitescu, M., Raphael, D., Bryant, T., Daiski, I., & Pilkington, B. (2012). The dynamics of the relationship between the experience of low income and type 2 diabetes: Longitudinal results. *Maturitas, 72*(3), 229–235.

Eikemo, T. A., & Bambra, C. (2008). The welfare state: A glossary for public health. *Journal of Epidemiology and Community Health, 62*(1), 3–6.

Equity Action. (2012). *European portal for action on health inequalities*. Retrieved February 7, 2012, from http://www.health-inequalities.eu/HEALTHEQUITY/EN/home/

Esping-Andersen, G. (1985). *Politics against markets: The social democratic road to power*. Princeton, NJ: Princeton University Press.

Esping-Andersen, G. (1990). *The three worlds of welfare capitalism*. Princeton, NJ: Princeton University Press.

Esping-Andersen, G. (1999). *Social foundations of post-industrial economies*. New York, NY: Oxford University Press.

Esping-Andersen, G. (2002). A child-centred social investment strategy. In G. Esping-Andersen (Ed.), *Why we need a new welfare state* (pp. 26–67). Oxford: Oxford University Press.

Esping-Andersen, G. (2009). *The unfinished revolution: Welfare state adaptation to women's new roles*. Cambridge: Polity Press.

Fall, C. H. D., Vijayakumar, M., Barker, D. J. P., Osmond, C., & Duggleby, S. (1995). Weight in infancy and prevalence of coronary heart disease in adult life. *British Medical Journal, 310*(6971), 17–20.

Grabb, E. (2007). *Theories of social inequality* (5th ed.). Toronto: Harcourt Canada.

Graham, H. (2004). Social determinants and their unequal distribution: Clarifying policy understandings. *The Milbank Quarterly, 82*(1), 101–124.

Graham, H. (2007). *Unequal lives: Health and socioeconomic inequalities*. New York, NY: Open University Press.

Hancock, T. (2011). Health promotion in Canada: 25 years of unfulfilled promise. *Health Promotion International, 26*(Suppl 2), ii263–ii267.

Health Council of Canada. (2010). *Stepping it up: Moving the focus from health care in Canada to a healthier Canada*. Toronto: Author.

Hemrijck, A. (2002). The self-transformation of the European model. In G. Esping-Andersen (Ed.), *Why we need a new welfare state* (pp. 173–214). Oxford: Oxford University Press.

Hogstedt, C., Moberg, H., Lundgren, B., & Backhans, M. (Eds.). (2009). *Health for all? A critical analysis of public health policies in eight European nations*. Stockhom: Swedish National Institute for Public Health.

Hux, J., Booth, G., & Laupacis, A. (2002, September 18). *The ICES practice atlas: Diabetes in Ontario*. Retrieved September 2002, from http://www.ices.on.ca/

Jackson, A. (2010). *Work and labour in Canada: Critical issues* (2nd ed.). Toronto: Canadian Scholars' Press.

Kabir, S. (2010). *Social determinants of health approach to reduce the prevalence of type-2 diabetes in Canada*. Unpublished MA Major Research Paper, York University, Toronto.

Komlos, J., & Baur, M. (2004). From the tallest to (one of) the fattest: The enigmatic fate of the American population in the 20th century. *Economics and Human Biology, 2*(1), 57–74.

Kuh, D., Ben Shlomo, Y., & Susser, E. (Eds.). (2004). *A life course approach to chronic disease epidemiology* (2nd ed.). Oxford: Oxford University Press.

Lawlor, D., Ebrahim, S., & Smith, G. D. (2002). Socioeconomic position in childhood and adulthood and insulin resistance: Cross sectional survey using data from British women's heart and health study. *British Medical Journal, 325*(12), 805–807.

Lynch, J., & Kaplan, G. A. (2000). Socioeconomic position. In L. F. Berkman & I. Kawachi (Eds.), *Social epidemiology* (pp. 13–35). New York, NY: Oxford University Press.

Lynch, J., Kaplan, G., & Salonen, J. (1997). Why do poor people behave poorly? Variation in adult health behaviours and psychosocial characteristics by stages of the socioeconomic lifecourse. *Social Science & Medicine, 44*(6), 809–819.

Micklewright, J. (2004). *Child poverty in English-speaking countries*. Bonn: Institute for the Study of Labour.

Mikkonen, J., & Raphael, D. (2010). *Social determinants of health: The Canadian facts*. Retrieved November 1, 2010, from http:/thecanadianfact.org

Navarro, V. (2009). What we mean by social determinants of health. *Global Health Promotion, 16*(1), 5–16.

Navarro, V., Borrell, C., Benach, J., Muntaner, C., Quiroga, A., Rodrigues-Sanz, M., et al. (2004). The importance of the political and the social in explaining mortality differentials among the countries of the OECD, 1950–1998. In V. Navarro (Ed.), *The political and social contexts of health* (pp. 11–86). Amityville, NY: Baywood Press.

Navarro, V., Muntaner, C., Borrell, C., Benach, J., Quiroga, A., Rodríguez-Sanz, M., et al. (2006). Politics and health outcomes. *The Lancet, 368*, 1033–1037.

Navarro, V., & Shi, L. (2002). The political context of social inequalities and health. In V. Navarro (Ed.), *The political economy of social inequalities: Consequences for health and quality of life* (pp. 403–418). Amityville, NY: Baywood.

Naylor, C. D., & Slaughter, P. M. (Eds.). (1999). *Cardiovascular health and services in Ontario: An ICES atlas*. Toronto: Institute for Clinical Evaluative Sciences.

Nettleton, S. (1997). Surveillance, health promotion and the formation of a risk identity. In M. Sidell, L. Jones, J. Katz, & A. Peberdy (Eds.), *Debates and dilemmas in promoting health* (pp. 314–324). London: Open University Press.

Offer, A., Pechey, R., & Ulijaszek, S. (2010). Obesity under affluence varies by welfare regimes: The effect of fast food, insecurity, and inequality. *Economics and Human Biology, 8*(3), 297–308.

Olsen, G. (2010). *Power and inequality: A comparative introduction*. Toronto: Oxford University Press.

Organization for Economic Co-operation and Development. (2003). *Transforming disability into ability: Policies to promote work and income security for people with disabilities*. Paris: Author.

Organization for Economic Co-operation and Development. (2004). *OECD employment outlook 2004*. Paris: Author.

Organization for Economic Co-operation and Development. (2011a). *Health at a glance: OECD indicators 2011 edition*. Paris: Author.

Organization for Economic Co-operation and Development. (2011b). *Society at a glance 2011, OECD social indicators*. Paris: Author.

Pilkington, F. B., Daiski, I., Bryant, T., Dinca-Panaitescu, M., Dinca-Panaitescu, S., & Raphael, D. (2010). The experience of living with diabetes for low income Canadians. *Canadian Journal of Diabetes, 34*(2), 119–126.

Pontusson, J. (2005). *Inequality and prosperity: Social Europe versus liberal America*. Ithaca, NY: Cornell University Press.

Public Health Agency of Canada. (2007). *Canada's response to WHO Commission on Social Determinants of Health*. Retrieved March 1, 2008, from http://www.phac-aspc.gc.ca/sdh-dss/bg-eng.php

Raina, P., Wong, M., Chambers, L. W., Denton, M., & Gafni, A. (2000). *Describing disability among high and low income status older adults in Canada*. Retrieved August 2002, from http://netec.mcc.ac.uk/adnetec-cgi-bin/get_doc.pl?urn=RePEc:mcm:qseprr:351&url=http%3A%2F%2Fwww.socsci.mcmaster.ca%2F~qsep%2Fp%2Fqsep351.PDF

Raine, K. (2002). Poverty, ethnicity and type 2 diabetes. *International Diabetes Monitor, 14*(4), 15–16.

Raphael, D. (Ed.). (2009). *Social determinants of health: Canadian perspectives* (2nd ed.). Toronto: Canadian Scholars' Press Incorporated.

Raphael, D. (2010). *About Canada: Health and illness*. Winnipeg: Fernwood Publishing.

Raphael, D. (2011a). A discourse analysis of the social determinants of health. *Critical Public Health, 21*(2), 221–236.

Raphael, D. (2011b). The political economy of health promotion: Part 1, national commitments to provision of the prerequisites of health. *Health Promotion International*. doi:10.1093/heapro/dar084.

Raphael, D. (2011c). The political economy of health promotion: Part 2, national provision of the prerequisites of health. *Health Promotion International*. doi:10.1093/heapro/dar058.

Raphael, D. (2011d). Poverty in childhood and adverse health outcomes in adulthood. *Maturitas, 69*, 22–26.

Raphael, D. (Ed.). (2012). *Tackling inequalities in health: Lessons from international experiences*. Toronto: Canadian Scholars' Press Incorporated.

Raphael, D., Anstice, S., Raine, K., McGannon, K., Rizvi, S., & Yu, V. (2003). The social determinants of the incidence and management of Type 2 Diabetes Mellitus: Are we prepared to rethink our questions and redirect our research activities? *Leadership in Health Services, 16*, 10–20.

Raphael, D., & Bryant, T. (2006). Maintaining population health in a period of welfare state decline: Political economy as the missing dimension in health promotion theory and practice. *Promotion and Education, 13*(4), 12–18.

Raphael, D., Curry-Stevens, A., & Bryant, T. (2008). Barriers to addressing the social determinants of health: Insights from the Canadian experience. *Health Policy, 88*, 222–235.

Raphael, D., Daiski, I., Pilkington, B., Bryant, T., Dinca-Panaitescu, M., & Dinca-Panaitescu, S. (2012). A toxic combination of poor social policies and programmes, unfair economic arrangements and bad politics: The experiences of poor Canadians with Type 2 diabetes. *Critical Public Health, 22*(2), 127–145.

Raphael, D., & Farrell, E. S. (2002). Beyond medicine and lifestyle: Addressing the societal determinants of cardiovascular disease in North America. *Leadership in Health Services, 15*, 1–5.

Restrepo, H. E. (2000). *Health promotion: An anthology*. Washington, DC: Pan American Health Organization.

Riste, L., Khan, F., & Cruickshank, K. (2001). High prevalence of type 2 diabetes in all ethnic groups, including

Europeans, in a British inner city. Relative poverty, history, inactivity, or 21st century Europe? *Diabetes Care, 24*, 1377–1383.

Saint-Arnaud, S., & Bernard, P. (2003). Convergence or resilience? A hierarchial cluster analysis of the welfare regimes in advanced countries. *Current Sociology, 51*(5), 499–527.

Scambler, G. (2002). *Health and social change: A critical theory*. Buckingham: Open University Press.

Senate Subcommittee on Population Health. (2008). *A healthy, productive Canada: A determinant of health approach*. Ottawa, ON: Government of Canada.

Stansfeld, S. A., & Marmot, M. (Eds.). (2002). *Stress and the heart: Psychosocial pathways to coronary heart disease*. London: BMJ Books.

Stuckler, D., & Siegel, K. (Eds.). (2011). *Sick societies: Responding to the global challenge of chronic disease*. New York, NY: Oxford University Press.

Swank, D. (2005). Globalisation, domestic politics, and welfare state retrenchment in capitalist democracies. *Social Policy and Society, 4*(2), 183–195.

Virchow, R. (1848/1985). *Collected essays on public health and epidemiology*. Cambridge: Science History Publications.

Whitehead, M. (1985). *The concepts and principles of equity and health*. Copenhagen: WHO Regional Office for Europe.

Wilkins, R. (2007). *Mortality by neighbourhood income in urban Canada from 1971 to 2001*. Ottawa, ON: Statistics Canada, Health Analysis and Measurement Group.

Wilkinson, R. G., & Pickett, K. (2009). *The spirit level— why more equal societies almost always do better*. London: Allen Lane.

World Health Organization. (2008). *Closing the gap in a generation: Health equity through action on the social determinants of health*. Geneva: Author.

World Health Organization. (2009). *Milestones in health promotion: Statements from global conferences*. Geneva: Author.

World Health Organization. (2011). *Rio political declaration on social determinants of health*. Retrieved March 9, 2012, from http://www.who.int/sdhconference/declaration/Rio_political_declaration.pdf

Risk Factors: Tobacco

8

Michael Eriksen and Carrie Whitney

Introduction

Noncommunicable diseases (NCDs), including heart attacks and strokes, cancers, diabetes, and chronic respiratory disease kill more than 36 million people annually and account for over 63 % of worldwide deaths (WHO 2011f, g). Tobacco use is the only shared risk factor for the four leading NCDs (see Fig. 8.1), and globally tobacco use kills nearly as many people annually as the other three risk factors combined (WHO 2008, 2011f). Cigarettes, the primary cause of the world's most damaging NCDs, are the most deadly artifact in human history (Proctor 2012a). Tobacco use was responsible for 100 million deaths in the twentieth century, and if current trends continue, approximately one billion people will die from tobacco use during the twenty-first century (Peto and Lopez 2000).

Harm from Tobacco and Secondhand Smoke Exposure

> When individuals inhale cigarette smoke, either directly or secondhand, they are inhaling more than 7,000 chemicals: hundreds of these are hazardous, and at least 69 are known to cause cancer. (U.S. Department of Health and Human Services 2010)

M. Eriksen, Sc.D. (✉) • C. Whitney, M.P.H.
Institute of Public Health, Georgia State University, P.O. Box 3995, Atlanta, GA 30302-3995, USA
e-mail: meriksen@gsu.edu; cwhitney8@gsu.edu

Active Smoking

At the beginning of the twentieth century, lung cancer, nearly always caused by cigarette smoking, was considered rare, and Dr. Isaac Adler, a pioneer in lung cancer research, noted its rarity in 1912, saying:

> On one point, however, there is nearly complete consensus of opinion, and that is that primary malignant neoplasms of the lungs are among the rarest forms of the disease. This latter opinion that the extreme rarity of primary tumors has persisted for centuries (Adler 1912).

During the twentieth century, the evidence establishing the causal link between smoking and cancer continued to develop. Through experimental research, in the early 1930s Angel Roffo demonstrated that cancers developed along the "smoking highway" (lips, tongue, throat, cheek, bronchial passages, etc.) wherever the tissue was exposed to tars during the act of smoking (Proctor 2006). Today, clinical observation, experimental research, and epidemiological research have overwhelmingly established the causal relationship between smoking and cancer.

The fact that smoking causes so much cancer, and so little is done to prevent it, is a worldwide tragedy and embarrassment. Tobacco use results in almost six million deaths globally each year, and smoking causes cancers of the lung, larynx, oral cavity, pharynx, esophagus, pancreas, bladder, kidney, cervix, stomach, and can cause acute leukemia (US DHHS 2004; WHO 2012a). Each year, approximately one and a half million people

D.V. McQueen (ed.), *Global Handbook on Noncommunicable Diseases and Health Promotion*,
DOI 10.1007/978-1-4614-7594-1_8, © Springer Science+Business Media, LLC 2013

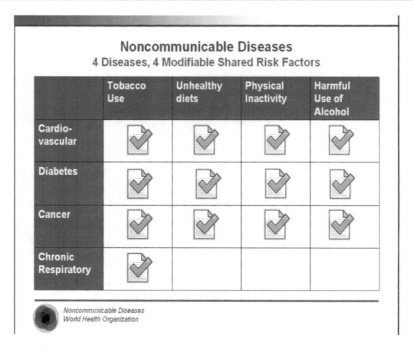

Fig. 8.1 Noncommunicable diseases and risk factors. Reproduced with permission by WHO. Credit: WHO

die from lung cancer throughout the world, and nearly 80 % of male and almost 50 % of female lung cancer deaths are the result of smoking (Ezzati and Lopez 2003). The smoking and cancer link is so severe that since 1980, middle-aged men in Poland were more likely to die from smoking-related cancers than from all other causes of cancer combined (see Fig. 8.2) (IARC 2007a). In 2012 in the USA, estimates indicate that more Americans will die from lung and bronchus cancer (160,340) than from the next four leading causes of cancer combined (colon: 51,690, breast: 39,510, pancreas: 37,390, and prostate: 28,170) (ACS 2012). Due to the delayed disease burden of smoking, global lung cancer rates and deaths are expected to continue to rise and an estimated two million people will die annually from lung cancer during the next few decades (Proctor 2012b).

In addition to causing lung and other cancers, tobacco use is a cause of death for the other leading NCDs, and the number of individuals impacted is expected to increase globally in the coming decades. Cardiovascular disease is the leading global cause of death, and smoking is a risk factor for cardiovascular diseases, such as coronary heart disease and stroke (US DHHS 2004; WHO 2011a). Smoking increases illness and death among diabetics by exacerbating common diabetes-related complications among the 346 million individuals who have diabetes worldwide (Haire-Joshu et al. 1999; WHO 2011c). Smoking is the primary cause of chronic respiratory illnesses, such as chronic obstructive pulmonary disease, which inflicts over 64 million people globally and is not curable (US DHHS 2004; WHO 2011b).

The harm associated with tobacco use is a function of nicotine addiction and the desire to obtain nicotine as quickly and efficiently as possible. Combustion, or burning tobacco leaves, is the traditional way of absorbing nicotine. In addition to delivering nicotine efficiently to the bloodstream, combustion creates carbon monoxide, nitrosamines, other tobacco-specific carcinogens, and a variety of other toxic substances resulting in a myriad of health effects and problems to the cardio-respiratory system, such as

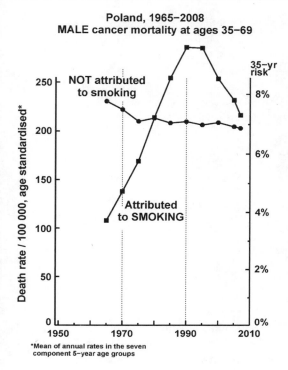

Poland, 1965–2008
MALE cancer mortality at ages 35–69

Fig. 8.2 Smoking-attributed cancers in males in Poland result in more deaths than all other cancers combined. Reproduced with permission by Tobacco Control. Credit: Tobacco Control

lung cancer, emphysema, and heart disease. When tobacco is used orally, it causes mouth cancer and other harm to the oral mucosa. When human tissue is exposed to the carcinogens in tobacco smoke or products, major harm results to all areas exposed, hence Roffo's "smoking highway" of the 1930s (Proctor 2006).

Globally, tobacco use is responsible for approximately 16 % of deaths among men and 7 % of deaths among women age 30 and older, with the highest mortality rates occurring in high- and middle-income countries (see Table 8.1) (WHO 2012c). Tobacco-related deaths are concentrated in these populations because sufficient time has passed since the significant uptake of cigarette smoking within the population, and the countries are now experiencing the delayed illness and mortality caused by smoking (Thun et al. 2012). For example, in the USA approximately 400,000 smokers die each year as a result of

smoking, and an additional eight million current and former smokers are living with a chronic condition caused by smoking (Hyland et al. 2003).

The harm from tobacco use varies as a function of how the nicotine is delivered. For example, if nicotine is absorbed as part of nicotine replacement therapy (NRT) provided by pharmaceutical companies to assist with smoking cessation, the harm is minimal. These NRT products undergo rigorous premarket testing to assure their safety and efficacy. If nicotine is absorbed through some of the many novel nicotine delivery systems that are currently being introduced, such as snus, electronic cigarettes (e-cigarettes), dissolvables, and orbs, the risk is unknown due to the lack of research and regulation of these new products (see Global Types of Tobacco: Novel Nicotine Products). If nicotine is absorbed orally through smokeless tobacco, the damage tends to be located in the oral cavity. If nicotine is absorbed through combusted tobacco products, the harm is inflicted throughout the body, but particularly in the cardio-pulmonary areas. The use of tobacco to obtain nicotine is harmful whether the products are smoked, chewed or inhaled, and subsequently there is no safe way of using tobacco. Additional research is needed to determine if there are safer ways to obtain nicotine, such as NRT, and novel products need to be evaluated for safety and efficacy before being allowed on the commercial market.

Secondhand Smoke

Secondhand smoke, also known as passive smoking, involuntary smoking, or "forced smoking," harms individuals who have made the conscious decision not to smoke or who are unable to remove themselves from exposure to someone else's smoke. Nonsmokers exposed to secondhand smoke inhale the same carcinogens inhaled by smokers (mainstream smoke), as well as the unfiltered smoke that comes from the burning end of the cigarette (sidestream smoke), and the associated health effects of chronic exposure have been a public health concern for decades. Documentation of the increased lung cancer risk from secondhand smoke began to emerge in the

Table 8.1 Countries with the highest proportion of tobacco-attributable mortality among males and females

Country	Male percent (%)	WHO region	Country income category
Turkey	38	European	Middle
Kazakhstan	35	European	Middle
Armenia	33	European	Middle
Poland	31	European	High
Belgium	31	European	High
Hungary	30	European	High
Bosnia and Herzegovina	30	European	Middle
Country	Female percent (%)	WHO region	Country income category
Maldives	25	South-East Asia	Middle
USA	23	American	High
Ireland	22	European	High
Denmark	21	European	High
Canada	20	American	High
United Kingdom	20	European	High
Iceland	20	European	High

early 1980s based on epidemiological analyses in Greece, Japan, and the USA (Trichopoulos et al. 1981; Hirayama 1981; Garfinkel 1981). The level of public health concern rose substantially in 1986 when three organizations issued studies linking the risk of lung cancer and exposure to secondhand smoke. The International Agency for Research on Cancer (IARC), the U.S. National Research Council, and the U.S. Surgeon General all concluded that involuntary exposure to secondhand smoke causes increased cancer risk (IARC 1986; National Research Council 1986; U.S. Department of Health and Human Services 2006). In 1992, the U.S. Environmental Protection Agency concluded that secondhand smoke was a human lung carcinogen and responsible for 3,000 lung cancer deaths annually in U.S. nonsmokers (EPA 1992). The 2006 Surgeon General's Report on Involuntary Smoking confirmed the causal relationship between secondhand smoke and lung cancer, estimating a 20–30 % increased risk of lung cancer for a nonsmoker living with a smoker (US DHHS 2006).

There is no safe level of exposure to secondhand smoke, and the act of breathing secondhand smoke immediately harms the respiratory and cardiovascular systems (US DHHS 2006). The 2006 U.S. Surgeon General's report on involuntary smoking documented the dangers

of secondhand smoke exposure and found sufficient[1] and suggestive[2] evidence of many diseases and illnesses among adults and children exposed to secondhand smoke. Exposure to secondhand smoke over the long term can result in lung cancer and coronary artery disease in adults. Expectant mothers, fetuses, and infants are at particular risk of negative health consequences when exposed to secondhand smoke. Infants and children who are exposed to secondhand smoke can experience low birth weight, respiratory problems, and behavioral and learning issues, and exposure contributes to Sudden Infant Death Syndrome (SIDS) (US DHHS 2006).

Nearly 40 % of children and a third of nonsmoking adults worldwide were exposed to secondhand smoke in 2004 (Öberg et al. 2011). Each year, 600,000 individuals die from secondhand smoke, and 75 % of these deaths occur among women and children (Öberg et al. 2011). In China, approximately 95 % of women do not smoke and are more likely to die from chronic exposure to secondhand smoke from their

---

[1] Sufficient evidence indicates a strong suggestion of a causal relationship.

[2] Suggestive evidence suggests an indicative but not causal relationship.

spouses or workplaces than they are to die from active smoking themselves (Gan et al. 2007). Deaths caused by exposure to secondhand smoke are involuntary and entirely preventable, and tobacco control measures should be taken to protect nonsmokers from "forced smoking" and prevent these needless deaths

Global Types of Tobacco

> Snus is less dangerous than cigarettes, for sure, but it is very hard to find anything more dangerous than cigarettes … [T]here is no natural law that says 30 percent of the population should be nicotine addicts. Goran Pershagen, professor at Stockholm's Karolinska Institute, 2007 (Hundley 2007)

Tobacco products and their use vary greatly around the world, with combusted cigarettes as the primary means for consuming nicotine. Smokeless tobacco, also commonly referred to as oral tobacco, is widely popular, especially in certain regions of the world.

Relatively new to the tobacco market are novel nicotine products. New products are emerging regularly, particularly from the tobacco industry under the guise of reducing health risks, and this will only increase the variation in the number and type of nicotine products available to consumers. The result of novel nicotine products might mean that individuals use new products, such as snus, nicotine lozenges, dissolvables, and e-cigarettes, instead of traditional means of consuming tobacco, or they may use these novel products in addition to their traditional means of using tobacco, resulting in the dual use of tobacco products, and even higher levels of exposure to nicotine and other potentially harmful compounds.

Smoking Tobacco

Tobacco is most commonly consumed through the combustion of manufactured cigarettes, although cigars, pipes, waterpipes, kreteks, and bidis are other common forms of smoking tobacco. Through combustion, tobacco leaves are burned at high temperatures and the smoke is then inhaled. This method is the most efficient way for the brain to receive nicotine, and nearly six trillion cigarettes are manufactured and consumed annually, with the highest consumption occurring in high- and middle-income countries (ERC 2010). Manufactured cigarettes contain more than 7,000 ingredients and additives, approximately 69 of which are proven to cause cancer (USDHS 2012). While manufactured cigarettes are the most popular tobacco product worldwide, other smoking tobacco products dominate in various regions. For example, bidis, which are created by hand rolling tobacco in a temburni leaf, are the most heavily consumed smoked tobacco product in India, accounting for more than 80 % of the country's tobacco market (Gilmore 2012). Kreteks, or clove cigarettes with exotic flavorings, dominate the tobacco market in Indonesia. Hookah, or water pipes through which tobacco is smoked, is most common in North Africa, the Mediterranean, and parts of Asia, but its popularity is spreading worldwide.

Smokeless Tobacco

Smokeless tobacco is a nonhomogenous group of tobacco-containing products that are primarily used orally, but sometimes used nasally. Globally, smokeless tobacco products/preparations range from those containing only cured tobacco to complex products including a range of chemical ingredients (sweetener, flavorings, moisteners, alkaline agents, etc.) and, in some cases, nontobacco plant material (betel leaf, areca nut, tonka bean, etc.) (IARC 2004, 2007b; Stanfill and Stepanov in press; Stanfill et al. 2011). In terms of form and consistency, smokeless tobacco are available in a variety of forms, including, but not limited to, ground tobacco, dry tobacco, twisted tobacco leaves, loose tobacco, tars, pastes, tobacco-containing chewing gum, dissolvable tablets, pressed cakes, pellets, powders, and mixtures of tobacco with other materials (IARC 2004, 2007b; SCENIHR 2008). Some products are manufactured, but many are hand-prepared for sale or personal use. In all there are approximately 35 distinct product/preparation types documented to date and the number continues to grow as new ones, many from remote areas, are characterized (Stanfill et al. 2011; IARC 2004, 2007b; SCENIHR 2008). Key ingredients, which impact addictiveness and toxicity among various smokeless tobacco products, include tobacco (can vary in type and species), alkaline agents (that boost free nicotine levels), areca nut (a known carcinogen) and other plant materials that can add additional toxicants.

The prevalence of smokeless tobacco varies by region. Approximately 8.1 million individuals in the USA and 258 million individuals in Southeast Asia use oral tobacco (Stanfill et al. 2011). In a recent global study of 53 products from nine countries, it was found that total nicotine concentrations in smokeless tobacco products varied from 0.16 to 34.1 mg/g (Stanfill et al. 2011). Even higher total nicotine concentrations (up to 95 mg/g) have been reported in nass from Uzbekistan (Brunnemann et al. 1985). By comparison, cigarettes contain approximately 13.9 mg per cigarette and smokers ultimately absorb 1–2 mg per cigarette (Connolly et al. 2007; ACS 2011). Over 30 carcinogens, including the potent tobacco-specific N-nitrosamines, are found in various oral tobacco products, and the carcinogenic content varies by product and region (IARC 2004, 2007b; SCENIHR 2008; Stanfill et al. 2011).

Novel Nicotine Products

Novel nicotine products are being created by tobacco companies and entrepreneurs in an effort to keep individuals addicted to nicotine, and to possibly reduce the toxic exposure and disease that occurs from traditional cigarette and oral tobacco use. New products that have been created by the tobacco industry include noncombustible cigarettes (e.g., Eclipse, Accord, Premier) and oral tobacco or dissolvables (e.g., lozenges, strips, snus, sticks, orbs). In 2012, Altria Group, the parent company of Philip Morris USA, decided to test market a new disc-like product that does not contain tobacco. The product, Verve, is made from a polymer, nontobacco cellulose fibers with mint flavoring and nicotine (Blackwell 2012). In 2010, 10 % of British American

Tobacco's sales came from new products, and almost half of those products were not available the year before (Gilmore 2012). Tobacco companies are expanding product lines and interests in order to maintain their status as the primary means for people to receive nicotine.

Entrepreneurs have entered the nicotine and tobacco market with products such as nicotine water, gels, wafers, candy, inhalers, and electronic nicotine delivery systems (ENDS), such as e-cigarettes. ENDS first appeared in 2004 and have grown significantly in popularity since that time. Creators of e-cigarettes believe they are effective at delivering nicotine and are more acceptable than regular cigarettes, and thus should be used as a replacement product for cigarettes (Henningield and Zaatari 2010). Tobacco companies are becoming more involved in new tobacco products and technology, causing the tobacco markets to converge. In 2011 Philip Morris International bought patent rights to a technology that delivers nicotine-infused aerosol (Kesmodel and Korn 2011). In 2012 Lorillard acquired Blu Cigs, an electronic cigarette company, allowing Lorillard to enter the e-cigarette market previously held by entrepreneurs (Lorillard 2012).

Novel nicotine products, sold by both tobacco companies and entrepreneurs, are largely unregulated and the risks associated with their use are mostly unknown. While some products are defined as "potential reduced-exposure products" (PREPS), there is little research about these products and a 2001 U.S. Institute of Medicine report noted that the public health impact of PREPS is unknown, acknowledging that these products could potentially have an overall negative effect on population health (Stratton et al. 2001). The use of novel nicotine products is concerning as it might result in dual use (usage of cigarettes and other nicotine products) and could ultimately mean individuals are exposed to higher levels of nicotine than when smoking cigarettes alone. Additionally, the use of novel nicotine products could mean individuals use alternate products rather than quitting nicotine altogether. The 2012 U.S. Surgeon General Report on tobacco and youth notes that one-third of female high school students and one-half of male high school students used more than one tobacco product, making this age group a target for the dual use of tobacco products (US DHHS 2012). While tobacco products vary worldwide, the emerging novel nicotine delivery systems will increase this variation while potentially leading to new addiction and health issues.

As outlined, there is a proliferation of novel nicotine delivery products on the market. The gradual movement away from combusted products, particularly in developed countries, has major implications for global tobacco use and the fundamental issue of nicotine addiction. When and if nicotine can be delivered safely, we must ask ourselves if it is sound public policy to allow for widespread nicotine addiction from the many products now available. There are many health, social, and economic implications of nicotine addiction, and due to the novelty of these products, the full impact of novel nicotine use and addiction is not yet known.

Prevalence of Cigarette Use

> Nobody should cry because of lower consumption of a product that kills half the people who use it.
> Danny McGoldrick, Vice President of research at the Campaign for Tobacco-Free Kids, 2007 (Cauchon 2007)

In most high-income countries, men and women smoke at roughly the same rates, although men smoke slightly more than women. However, in many parts of the world, particularly in emerging markets, it is not uncommon for men to smoke ten times more than women (Eriksen et al. 2012). Worldwide, there are one billion adult smokers, equaling nearly 20 % of the world's adult population (Eriksen et al. 2012). Several high-income countries and regions have documented declining daily smoking rates for males and females combined (see Table 8.2) (Australian Institute of Health and Welfare 2011; Centers for Disease Control and Prevention 2011a; Health Canada 2011; Mercado 2011; Ministry of Health, Singapore 2010; Organization for Economic Co-Operation and Development 2011a, b). These declining rates show that tobacco control measures are effective and that it is feasible to expect and work towards daily smoking rates in the single digits.

Table 8.2 Selected locations with low daily smoking rates for males and females

Country	Daily smoking total (%)
Hong Kong	11.1
Canada	13.0
Iceland	14.3
Singapore	14.3
Sweden	14.3
Australia	15.1
USA	15.1

Tobacco Epidemic

Over the course of a century, smoking patterns and the resultant disease, reflects an epidemic curve, with a rapid onset, plateau, and a more gradual decline. While smoking is often referred to in "epidemic" terms when considering the long view (over the course of a century), in the short term, smoking can be viewed as being "endemic" in that it is a risk factor that is present in every country of the world and that changes in smoking rates occur rather slowly. The global tobacco problem, as documented in high-income populations, plays out over the course of a century and can be segmented into four stages: the beginning of the epidemic, the significant increase in smoking prevalence, a decline in smoking prevalence, and then several decades later a spike in smoking-related illnesses and diseases (Lopez et al. 1994; Thun et al. 2012). In general, countries in stage one have smokers who are wealthy, educated, and referred to as "innovators." While these individuals tend to quit sooner, their behavior is imitated by individuals in lower education and income groups. These individuals are more likely to continue the habit, have a harder time quitting, and have fewer resources available for dealing with the harm caused by smoking. Although countries may have similar smoking prevalence rates, each country's stage in the tobacco epidemic is important. For example, two countries may have the same smoking prevalence rate, but the two countries may be in different stages of the epidemic. One country may be in the early stages of the epidemic and experience different challenges, with increased smoking rates and the morbidity and mortality that results from tobacco use still yet to come. Another country in the latter stages, may have already experienced the peaking of smoking rates and is still confronted with the morbidity and mortality resulting from tobacco use.

Adult Male Prevalence

Almost 800 million men throughout the world smoke cigarettes, and over 80 % of these smokers live in low- and middle-income countries (Eriksen et al. 2012; WHO 2011h). The 2010 weighted average of smoking prevalence among males in high-income countries is 30 %, 34 % in middle-income countries, and 21 % in low-income countries (Eriksen et al. 2012).[3] The smoking prevalence rate for men in most high-income countries has leveled out and in some cases is decreasing (Thun et al. 2012). Smoking prevalence rates for men in middle- and low-income countries vary, but these rates are typically increasing and have not yet reached a plateau. Among adults, men generally smoke more than women, and there are nearly 50 countries where men's smoking rates are at least ten times as high as women's smoking rates (Eriksen et al. 2012).

Adult Female Prevalence

Nearly 200 million adult women throughout the world smoke cigarettes (Eriksen et al. 2012). Over the past few decades, the highest female smoking rates have been concentrated in high-income countries, and half of the world's female smokers live in these countries (Eriksen et al. 2012; WHO 2011h). The 2010 weighted average of smoking prevalence among women in high-income countries is 19 %, 5 % in middle-income countries and 3 % in low-income countries

(Eriksen et al. 2012).[4] The female smoking rates in many high-income countries are nearly equal with male smoking rates, and there are two countries (Nauru and Sweden) where women smoke more than men (Thun et al. 2012; Swedish National Institute of Public Health 2009; WHO 2011h). The lower prevalence rates among females in middle- and low-income countries demonstrate the potential for female smoking rates to skyrocket in these areas. Changes in women's rights, economics, cultural norms, and political influence may result in increased smoking rates among women in middle- and low-income countries (Thun et al. 2012). If these rates increase to meet the rates of male smokers, a public health catastrophe would occur that will lead to decades of future illness, an increase in noncommunicable diseases, and ultimately an increase in tobacco-related mortality.

Youth Prevalence

While smoking rates among adult males and females vary greatly, there is less variance in rates among boys and girls between the ages of 13–15. The smoking rates among boys and girls differ by less than 5 percentage points in almost half of the world's countries, and there are at least 25 countries where girls smoke more than boys (see Table 8.3) (CDC 2011b, c). It is unclear if current youth smoking patterns among girls will lead to more adult female smokers. But it is clear that if this pattern continues, there will be an increase in female tobacco-related illness and disease. The vast majority of smokers begin the habit during their youth, and tobacco companies have long viewed youth as a target market for their products. A 1984 document from R.J. Reynolds noted that "younger adults are the only source of replacement smokers" (Reynolds 1984). Tobacco control measures need to be implemented that curb youth smoking rates and

---

[3]Data derived from the following sources: WHO Report on the Global Tobacco Control 2011, UN Population Estimates, World Bank Income Categorizations.

[4]Data derived from the following sources: WHO Report on the Global Tobacco Control 2011, UN Population Estimates, World Bank Income Categorizations.

Table 8.3 Selected locations where substantially more girls than boys smoke cigarettes

Country	Girls (%)	Boys (%)	Difference
Chile (Santiago)	39.9	28.0	11.9
Sweden	13.0	5.0	8.0
Slovenia	23.0	15.2	7.8
Bulgaria	31.6	24.4	7.2
Uruguay	22.9	16.4	6.5
Argentina	27.3	21.1	6.2
New Zealand	20.6	14.5	6.1
Cuba	13.1	8.7	4.4
Brazil (Sao Paulo)	13.2	9.2	4.0

Subnational data used for Chile and Brazil

prevent youth uptake of tobacco while regulating the tobacco industry from marketing to youth. Only these actions can save future generations from tobacco-related illness and death.

Smoking and Social Factors

While tobacco use is a behavioral risk factor for illness and disease, many social factors influence tobacco use. There is a direct correlation between income level and education (Riordan 2012). In the USA in 2010, 28.9 % of adult smokers were living below the poverty level compared to 18.3 % of adult smokers who were living at or above the poverty level (CDC 2011d). In terms of the correlation between education and smoking, 25.1 % of adults who did not graduate from high school smoked, 9.9 % of adults who had a college degree smoked and 6.3 % of adults with a graduate degree smoked (CDC 2011d). These statistics support the idea that increased education and income levels are associated with lower smoking rates. The tie between smoking and social factors, such as education and income, is true in high-income countries, demonstrated by the above examples from the USA, but these patterns also prove true in some middle- and low-income countries as well. A cross-national sample of 50 low-, middle-, and high-income countries found that increased education was linked to lower smoking rates in males and that males working in nonmanual positions were less likely to smoke than those in agricultural or manual work positions (Pampel

and Denney 2011). The results of the study indicate that social and economic patterns of cigarette use among individuals in low- and middle-income countries seems to follow the same patterns previously seen in high-income countries and that increased smoking prevalence in low- and middle-income countries will widen the disparities in smoking-related mortality in these countries (Pampel and Denney 2011). Due to tobacco's tie with social factors, certain subpopulations are disproportionately impacted by tobacco. In the USA, minority populations are more at-risk for lower educational attainment and income, and these populations often smoke at higher rates and maintain the habit over time, exacerbating existing health disparities. In addition to racial and ethnic groups, other U.S. populations that experience higher smoking rates are the mentally ill, single-mothers, the homeless, and the long-term unemployed (David et al. 2010).

Global Tobacco Industry

Tobacco use is unlike other threats to global health. Infectious diseases do not employ multinational public relations firms. There are no front groups to promote the spread of cholera. Mosquitoes have no lobbyists. Report on the Committee of Experts on Tobacco Industry Documents (Zeltner Report), 2000

Economics

Smoking has strong business and economic dimensions, and in general, the tobacco industry acts in a collusive manner with the ultimate goal to benefit the companies, irrespective of the harm caused to its customers. The tobacco industry is dominated by six main tobacco manufacturers who market, manufacture, and politic in a similar manner. In 2010, the value of the global tobacco market was around half a trillion dollars,[5] similar

---

[5]The value of the global tobacco market varies between $375 and $650 billion USD depending on where in the distribution channel (retail vs. manufacturing) the value is measured.

Table 8.4 2010 revenue and profits for the six leading tobacco companies 2010 value in billions (USD)

Tobacco company	Gross revenue	Profit/net income
Philip Morris International	$67.70	$7.50
Altria/Philip Morris USA	$24.40	$3.90
British American Tobacco	$58.12	$4.16
China National Tobacco Corporation	$91.70	$16.00
Imperial Tobacco	$38.35	$2.02
Japan Tobacco International	$65.90	$1.50
Total	$346.17	$35.08

to the gross domestic product of Poland and Sweden (ERC 2010; Euromonitor 2011; The World Bank 2011). The top six cigarette companies include China National Tobacco Corporation, Philip Morris International, Japan Tobacco Company, British American Tobacco, Imperial Tobacco and Altria/Philip Morris USA. In 2010, the combined revenue of these six companies was $346.2 billion and their combined profit totaled $35.1 billion, which was equal to the combined profits of Coca-Cola, Microsoft, and McDonald's in the same year (see Table 8.4) (Altria 2010; British American Tobacco 2010; Businessweek 2010a, b, c; Imperial Tobacco 2010; Japan Tobacco 2010; Philip Morris International 2010; Wang 2011).

China National Tobacco Corporation (CNTC), the largest tobacco company in the world, is a state-owned monopoly. Therefore, tobacco control in China is balanced between the economic benefits from government production and sale of tobacco, the collection of taxes from tobacco sales on one hand, and the health of the public on the other. China leads the world in tobacco production, farming, and consumption. In 2008, China manufactured more than two trillion of the world's six trillion cigarettes (ERC 2010). The country grew 43 % of the world's tobacco in 2009, more than the other top nine tobacco-consuming countries combined (FAO 2009b). China also leads the world in cigarette consumption, with more than a third of the world's cigarettes being smoked by Chinese men (ERC 2010). In 2011 the tobacco industry in China contributed approximately 8 % of the central government's revenue (Netscribes 2012). China's statistics

related to population size, smoking prevalence, and the industry's size and influence makes this country central to the topic of global tobacco.

Tobacco Marketing

Tobacco companies have long used marketing techniques to advance their products, and the first U.S. tobacco advertisement, which promoted snuff, ran in 1789 by the company now known as Lorillard Tobacco (James 2009). The tobacco industry claims that the goal of its tobacco advertising is to encourage adult smokers to switch brands or maintain their current brand status. In fact, tobacco advertising is often aimed at securing new consumers, especially youth. The 2012 U.S. Surgeon General's report on youth smoking found that the "evidence is sufficient to conclude that there is a causal relationship between advertising and promotional efforts of the tobacco companies and the initiation and progression of tobacco use among young people" (US DHHS 2012, p. 6). In 2010, tobacco companies in the USA spent $8.05 billion marketing cigarettes and an additional $444 million marketing smokeless tobacco (FTC 2012a, b). Over $23 million is spent each day in the U.S. by tobacco companies on cigarette and smokeless tobacco advertising and promotions (FTC 2012a, b). Cigarette marketing is 48 % higher and smokeless tobacco marketing is 277 % higher than it was in 1998, the year of the U.S. Master Settlement Agreement (US DHHS 2012). Tobacco companies focus their advertising spending on price discounts, coupons, and retail-value added promotions (such as buy-one get-one free offers), effectively lowering the cost of smoking to the consumer. These cost-reduction promotions account for 81 % of cigarette marketing expenditures in the U.S. (FTC 2012a).

Despite increasing marketing restrictions, tobacco companies promote their products in any manner possible, and this practice occurs globally. In advance of a proposed Health Ministry ban on marketing cigarettes in Russia, cigarette company Donskoy Tabak introduced an advertisement of a female teen licking an ice cream cone. The caption read "If you're not allowed it, but you really want

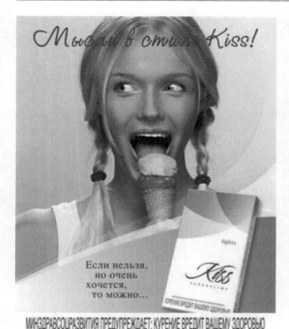

Fig. 8.3 Russian example of current tobacco advertising. Reproduced with permission. Credit: Katarina Radovic

it, then you can have it" (see Fig. 8.3) (Okorokova 2011). When Cambodia banned tobacco advertising and sponsorship in 2011, tobacco company Korean Tobacco & Ginseng (KT&G) changed its name to Korean Tomorrow & Global, likely in an effort to allow the company to keep its recognized initials and tobacco association without violating advertising regulations (Kong and Assunta 2012). Shanghai Tobacco Company created a specialty brand of cigarettes called "Love China" and displayed the text on generic billboards supposedly to promote patriotism and love of country, but that in effect, were bypassing marketing restrictions and advertising a specific cigarette brand (see Fig. 8.4) (Live China 2011). As technology and social media progress, tobacco companies are utilizing new media options for brand placement and promotion (James 2009). It is essential that tobacco control advocates understand the changing influence and role of new media technology, use it to their advantage and learn how tobacco companies are and could use new media to circumvent marketing restrictions.

Undue Influence

Tobacco companies spend millions of dollars annually to influence politics, legislation and business, and this practice is common worldwide. The undue influence of these companies occurs through direct political influence, legislative action, indirect influence, and corporate social responsibility (e.g., charitable giving among other activities). In 2010 in the USA, 168 lobbyists were employed by companies with tobacco interests, and a total of $16.6 million was spent directly on influencing U.S. political decisions (Opensecrets. org 2011). Tobacco companies commonly use legislation as a tool to protect their products. A recent and monumental example is the court action British American Tobacco, Philip Morris, Imperial, and Japan Tobacco brought against the Australian government when it passed plain packaging laws in 2011. Indirect influence occurs through partnerships the tobacco industry has made with organizations such as convenience store owners, advertising associations, and farmers' associations. Additionally, tobacco companies commonly fund front groups who in turn promote the agendas of the tobacco companies. Corporate social responsibility includes charitable donations that conveniently promote the image of tobacco companies. For example, China National Tobacco Corporation has sponsored more than 60 elementary schools, and pro-tobacco messages, such as "Genius comes from hard work/ Tobacco helps you to be successful" are posted on the school grounds (NTD Television 2010). Tobacco companies work to maintain their image and client base, and this is done through both obvious and more covert measures.

Growing Tobacco

Tobacco is grown in at least 124 of the world's countries on 4.2 million hectares of agricultural land (FAO 2013a; Australian Institute of Health and Welfare 2011). In 2009, 7.5 million tonnes of tobacco were produced globally (FAO 2013a, b). Most tobacco is grown in low- and middle-income

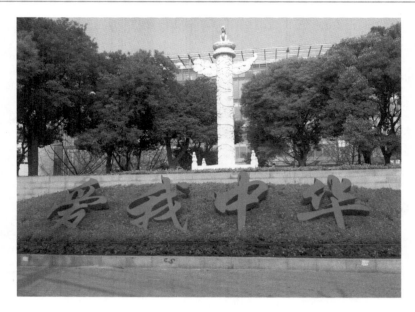

Fig. 8.4 "Love China" picture. Reproduced with permission. Credit: Michael Eriksen

countries, and growing tobacco contributes to a cycle of poverty for farmers and laborers. Farmers are required to purchase infrastructure and equipment from tobacco companies, often going into debt, with little or no profit remaining. Tobacco workers are exposed to pesticides and nicotine which result in neurological damage and green tobacco sickness (WHO 2004). Additionally, land used to grow tobacco cannot be used for growing other food, which can contribute to undernourishment in countries already experiencing food and hunger problems. For example, Malawi is a top tobacco producing country with an undernourishment rate of 27 %. In 2008, Malawi grew 1 tonne of tobacco per hectare, but could have grown 14.6 tonnes of potatoes on the same hectare of land (FAO 2008a, b, c; FAO 2011a, b).

Global Tobacco Control

Defendants have marketed and sold their lethal products with zeal, with deception, with a single-minded focus on their financial success, and without regard for the human tragedy or social costs that success exacted. U.S. District Judge Gladys Kessler's Final Opinion: Summary of Findings Against the Tobacco Industry, August 2006

WHO Framework Convention on Tobacco Control and Global Resources

While a thorough discussion of global tobacco control is beyond the scope of this chapter, there are several resources and interventions aimed at global tobacco control. The World Health Organization's Framework Convention on Tobacco Control (WHO FCTC) provides an evidence-based treaty that addresses the global tobacco epidemic (WHO 2011e). The treaty is one of the most rapidly embraced treaties with 176 parties as of 2013 (WHO 2012b). Additionally, mounting global resources and dedication to the topic of tobacco control is of paramount importance. Since 2006, Michael Bloomberg, philanthropist and Mayor of New York City, has pledged a total of $600 million for global tobacco projects, primarily focused on low- and middle-income countries. This former smoker turned tobacco control advocate, made his most recent pledge of an additional $220 million at the 15th World Conference on Tobacco OR Health in March 2012 in Singapore (Lopatto 2012). Bloomberg's contributions, combined with the efforts of the Bill & Melinda Gates

Foundation, lend a combined $725 million in global tobacco control. This monumental support leads the way for further attention and resources for global tobacco control efforts.

Legal Challenges and Litigation

Under the U.S. Master Settlement Agreement of 1998, seven major tobacco companies agreed to pay 46 States approximately $206 billion in revenue over a 25-year period. The tobacco companies also agreed to change their marketing strategies, open previously closed documents, and finance a multi-billion anti-smoking campaign (National Association of Attorneys General 1998). While the lawsuit was intended to prevent youth smoking and reimburse states for healthcare costs of smokers, the agreement did not mandate that revenues be dedicated to tobacco prevention or cessation initiatives (National Association of Attorneys General 1998). The CDC *Best Practices for Comprehensive Tobacco Control* recommended in 2007 that the States spend a combined total of $3.7 billion annually on evidence-based state tobacco control programs (CDC 2007). In 2010, the total state and federal expenditures for tobacco control totaled $641.1 million (CDC 2012). In addition to the payments from the Master Settlement Agreement, states also collect excise taxes on cigarette sales, totaling almost $24 billion combined for all states in 2010 (CDC 2012). In contrast, in 2010 the states spent only 2.4 % of total state tobacco revenues on tobacco control programs (CDC 2012).

Other countries have launched law suits against tobacco companies in an effort to recover healthcare costs for smokers. In mid-2012, Quebec launched a $60 billion lawsuit against tobacco companies, joining the ranks of four other Canadian Provinces (Ontario, British Columbia, New Brunswick, and Newfoundland). Quebec's lawsuit is significant in that it means half of the country's provinces have now sued the tobacco industry, and Quebec's $60 billion in reparations is the highest amount being sought in damages by any of the provinces that have sued thus far (The Canadian Press 2012).

Industry Accountability

In furthering global tobacco control, the tobacco industry must be held accountable for the damage and harm their products cause worldwide. This requires increased discovery into the industry and their inner workings. This can occur, in part, through further mandates for the release and disclosure of industry documents and methodology. Individuals must learn firsthand how the tobacco industry employs manipulation to further their own gain. With this knowledge, it will hopefully no longer be socially acceptable to support tobacco companies, their products, or initiatives.

Cessation Interventions

Tobacco control initiatives vary globally, and interventions such as those outlined in the WHO FCTC may need to be implemented differently depending on each country's prevalence of tobacco use, types of tobacco used, and social norms. Despite the variability in countries, some tobacco control methods are universal, such as the use of tobacco taxes and quitlines. Economics have shown that as price increases, consumption decreases. While this varies slightly depending on the elasticity of products, it has been shown globally that increased tobacco taxes result in decreased consumption (Chaloupka et al. 2012). Easily accessible and free quitlines are an effective tobacco cessation method, yet slightly more than a quarter of the world's countries have quitlines available (WHO 2011h). Other aspects of tobacco-control, such as cessation interventions, vary globally. For example, pharmacologic products have been successful in assisting in cessation among smokers in the U.S., and approximately half of all smokers attempt quitting each year (Zhu et al. 2012). Other countries, such as China, will benefit more from population-based interventions that build self-efficacy and demonstrate the feasibility of quitting.

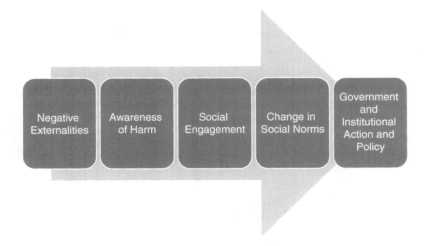

Fig. 8.5 Process of social change. Permission not needed

Graphic Warning Labels and Plain Packaging

Graphic health warnings were first introduced on cigarette packages by Canada in 2000. As of early 2012, at least 49 countries have graphic warning labels and approximately 30 countries and jurisdictions met the WHO FCTC criteria of graphic warning labels covering at least 30 % of the package (Campaign for Tobacco-Free Kids 2011; Physicians for a Smoke-Free Canada 2012). The effectiveness of warning labels must be apparent to tobacco companies as they have sued countries implementing these policies, and in the case of New Zealand, have found ways to counter the warning labels, such as including adhesive seals or stickers in their Dunhill cigarettes. The stickers, which read "exclusively Dunhill," conveniently can be placed to cover the majority of the pack's warning labels (Simpson 2012).

Australia led the world in 2011 by passing the first plain packaging legislation and requiring that all cigarettes be sold in plain, brown packages starting in December 2012 (Parliament of Australia 2011). The goal of plain packaging is to decrease the appeal of tobacco products to consumers, primarily to youth, to increase the effectiveness and noticeability of the health warnings, to decrease the ability of packaging to mislead consumers, and to ultimately help curb smoking

rates (Australian Government Department of Health and Ageing 2011). Despite Big Tobacco's claims that plain packaging will not work, four major tobacco companies have mounted law suits against the Australian government, thus indicating their concern over the possible impacts of plain packaging. Additionally, Honduras and Ukraine have filed complaints with the World Trade Organization (WTO) citing that plain packaging violates trade agreements, and it is likely that the plain packaging debate will be decided by the WTO (Miles 2012). The world is anxiously watching and anticipating the results of this strong tobacco control law and its potential impact on cigarette users and tobacco companies.

Changing Social Norms

In order to further tobacco control, global advocates must continue to change social norms in a manner similar to what has occurred with second-hand smoke in developed countries (see Fig. 8.5). At its most basic level, smoking creates second-hand smoke, which harms those forced to breathe it. This involuntary exposure on those who have chosen not to smoke is a "negative externality" and has resulted in unprecedented citizen mobilization and action in many high-income countries. The harm and annoyance caused by involuntary exposure and the resultant mobilization for action was confirmed and validated through research and reports, such as the Surgeon General Reports in the U.S. Once sufficient evidence was gathered and accepted, individuals demanded social action and protection from secondhand smoke. As social norms changed, public smoking became unacceptable and ultimately smoking was seen as a "deviant" behavior. Once the social norm changed, the government and institutions began to change their rules and policies to comply with the social norm and to protect nonsmokers from negative externalities. A 2006 study found that increased social unacceptability of smoking is nearly as effective at reducing cigarette consumption as increasing tobacco taxes. The study found that if the social unacceptability of smoking in the USA increased by 40 %, there would be a 15 % decrease in consumption. This decrease in consumption could also be achieved by a tax increase of $1.17 per pack, indicating the effectiveness of changing social norms in order to decrease tobacco consumption (Alamar and Glantz 2006). This process of changing social norms that has occurred first in developed countries must be replicated throughout the world so that changes in the social unacceptability of smoking is accelerated and that citizens demand policies and regulations that protect them from the harm caused by involuntary exposure to secondhand smoke.

Tobacco Control as a Lesson for Other Risk Factors

Tobacco control has been one of the central focuses of public health for the past few decades, resulting in evidence-based guidelines, interventions, and frameworks. Many of the tobacco control measures, such as price increases, marketing restrictions, changes in labeling and product information have implications for the other risk factors of unhealthy diets, physical inactivity, and alcohol use. The topic of how tobacco control lessons relate to unhealthy diets, and particularly preventing childhood obesity are outlined as an example of this relationship between tobacco control and other NCDs. Some of these lessons may also be relevant to the risk factors of physical inactivity and alcohol use, but are not explored in detail in this chapter.

Comparison of Risk Factors: Tobacco and Unhealthy Diets

There are many similarities, but also differences, in reducing tobacco use and improving dietary behavior. The most important difference is that food is necessary for survival and tobacco is completely unnecessary. Another difference lies in the fact that the tobacco industry, with their subversive advertising, manipulation, deception, and secrets, is a significant part of the tobacco control problem. On the other hand, the food industry has the potential to be a part of the obesity solution, although whether they will be so or not has yet to be determined.

The lessons learned through tobacco control about product and ingredient labeling can be successfully applied to preventing unhealthy diets. In terms of product and ingredient labeling, the tobacco industry attempted to mislead consumers by marketing products as "light" or "low tar." These terms led consumers to mistakenly believe that using these products was a "healthier" choice than smoking regular cigarettes, but this is not the case and consumers of these products experience the same negative health effects as those who smoke regular cigarettes. Similarly, product labeling on food and drinks can be confusing and misleading, as it is relatively unregulated and the industry and companies can choose how to label products and what information to include on front-of-label packaging (Brownell and Koplan 2011). An example of a confusing aspect of the U.S. nutrition labeling system is the fact that information is presented on one serving, yet often a bag of chips or soft drink contain multiple servings and consumers may not notice the serving information and recognize the full amount of calories and fat that are being consumed (Lyn et al. 2012). Food products can benefit from more intuitive and consistent labeling that will help consumers make informed choices. The U.S. Food and Drug Administration announced in 2009 that it will make recommendations that manufacturers must meet for front-of-package labeling and shelf labels, and since this announcement two major food-industry trade associations have formed an industry-created front-of-package labeling system called "Nutrition Keys."

(US DHHS 2009; Brownell and Koplan 2011). Some grocery store chains have implemented their own point-of-purchase labels, such as the Guiding Stars program found in a grocery store chain in the northeastern part of the U.S. This three-tiered star icon is placed on shelves and rates food and beverage products. The clear and simple message of the stars appears to be effective in changing food purchases among consumers (Sutherland et al. 2010). The United Kingdom and Australia have considered traffic-light labeling that uses the colors red, yellow, and green to show which nutrients in the food should be consumed in low, medium, or high levels (Australian Medical Association 2011). In general, front-of-label packaging and nutrition labels should be based on research and science and should be presented in a clear, easy to understand, and consistent method.

Both food consumption and tobacco consumption are influenced by marketing, and the lessons learned from tobacco control can be applied to help prevent obesity. The goal of marketing is to promote, sell, or distribute a particular service or product, and thus tobacco and food marketing aims at getting consumers to purchase particular tobacco or food products, and hopefully become returning customers. The tobacco industry has taken marketing to an extreme and has successfully managed to sell a product that kills half of all long-term users (WHO 2011d). Tobacco marketing is aimed at getting new smokers, maintaining brand loyalty, and convincing other smokers to switch. Tobacco marketing takes place through advertisements, social media, sponsorships, promotions, give-aways, and discounts. Youth are particularly influenced by tobacco marketing and therefore the WHO FCTC has proposed global tobacco marketing bans and restrictions. Food marketing occurs through similar channels as tobacco and business marketing. Consumers are inundated with brand names and messages through traditional media (e.g., mail, commercials, point-of-sale advertisements, billboards), social media, as well as promotions (e.g., coupons, sales, and giveaways). Youth are exposed to additional marketing at school through product placement in vending machines and specific brand foods in cafeterias (Lyn et al. 2012).

Tobacco companies also utilize Corporate Social Responsibility (CSR) programs to further their image. For example, in 2010 Philip Morris International contributed $25 million in donations to global nonprofits and initiatives. In reality, this was less than 1 % of the company's net profits of $7.5 billion, but it helped further their image and name recognition (Philip Morris International 2011). A comparison has been drawn between the use of CSR by big tobacco and the soda industry. Since sugary beverages are often implicated in the global tobacco crisis, beverage companies have launched extensive CSR campaigns (Dorman et al. 2012). Like the CSR campaigns of big tobacco, the soda industry focuses their campaigns on individual responsibility and choice, increasing product popularity, and preventing regulation (Dorman et al. 2012). A unique difference between the CSR campaigns of big tobacco and the soda industry is that the soda industry can openly focus on young audiences and they initiated their campaigns quickly following the backlash about soda's contribution to the obesity epidemic (Dorman et al. 2012).

While the tobacco control movement can provide a helpful model for obesity prevention, there are several important differences between the prevention models for these two risk factors. For example, the global tobacco control model focuses on population-based initiatives to curb smoking and deter new smokers. Alternatively, obesity programs often focus on individual-level interventions and programs. Tobacco has proven to be a price-sensitive commodity and price increases result in decreased consumption. It is unclear how taxation of certain food products will impact consumers, and there is some concern that low-income groups could be disproportionately affected (Lyn et al. 2012). While taxing food products is a somewhat new concept, several countries are taking the first steps to see if this is an effective method to prevent obesity. Some countries, such as Hungary, Denmark, and France have implemented "fat taxes" on unhealthy foods or sweetened drinks (Mytton et al. 2012). A 2012 study found that these types of taxes must be at 20 % or more of the food value to have an impact on consumption (Mytton et al. 2012). New York has proposed a ban on soft drinks that are 16 ounces or larger (CBS News 2012). While the New York ban is highly controversial and debated, a 2012 study found that a penny-per-ounce tax on sugar-sweetened beverages would be effective in reducing consumption of sugary beverages by 15 % among adults ages 25–64. If this tax were implemented during the study period (between 2010 and 2020), it would result in a savings of $17 billion in medical costs and would generate approximately $13 billion in annual tax revenue, indicating that taxing unhealthy products might be an effective method in curbing the obesity epidemic (Wang et al. 2012).

The above examples compare the tobacco control lessons to obesity prevention. Many of the lessons learned from tobacco control can also be applied to physical inactivity and alcohol consumption, although the research is less established in these areas. For example, a 2012 study found that a 25-cent per drink increase on alcohol would be effective at reducing excessive drinking (Stuckler et al. 2012; Daley et al. 2012). There is emerging research on the impact that global producers have on increasing the consumption of unhealthy foods, alcohol, and tobacco (Stuckler et al. 2012). Unhealthy diets, physical inactivity, and alcohol consumption, along with tobacco use, are risk factors for the world's most damaging NCDs. The risk factor of tobacco use has been and continues to be addressed globally, and the other risk factors can be addressed using some aspects of the tobacco control model. All three risk factors can benefit from the global recognition and recommendations provided by overarching organizations. For example, the World Health Organization's Framework Convention on Tobacco Control (WHO FCTC) is the world's most rapidly embraced treaty that provides guidelines and recommendations for addressing tobacco-related issues. WHO offers guidelines and recommendations about diets, physical inactivity, and alcohol consumption through the WHO Global Strategy on Diet, Physical Activity and Health and through the WHO Global Strategy for Reducing the Harmful Use of Alcohol. A global health treaty, currently referred to as the Framework Convention on Global Health has been proposed by the Joint Action and Learning Initiative on National and Global Responsibilities for Health (JALI). The Framework Convention on Global Health has been endorsed by the UN Secretary-General, and this type of global framework would help improve global health and reduce inequalities (Gostin 2012). While these global strategies are not binding like the WHO FCTC is for those countries that have ratified it, they represent a global recognition of the importance of these risk factors, their influence on global health, and the need for unified and proven methods to address these risk factors.

Conclusion

We've come a long way, bullies. We will not be fazed by your harassment. Your products kill nearly 6 million people each year. You run a killing and intimidating industry, but not in a crush-proof box. Tobacco industry: the number and fortitude of your public health enemies will damage your health. Margaret Chan, Director-General of the World Health Organization at the World Conference on Tobacco OR Health, 2012

Tobacco and its use have evolved considerably over the past decades. Society has moved from a complete absence of understanding about the dangers of tobacco to a full awareness of the extent of harm it causes. Despite this knowledge, more than a billion adults still currently smoke cigarettes. It is now known that tobacco use results in morbidity and mortality, but that individuals can successfully quit this damaging addiction. The tobacco industry, which remains highly secretive, has finally been held partially accountable for their fraudulent and damaging ways. Smoking rates in many high-income countries have hit a plateau and some have even declined, but these countries have paid high direct and indirect costs for the tobacco-related illness and death they have and continue to experience. Unfortunately, the harm caused by today's tobacco use will extend decades into the future as today's smokers, especially young smokers, will undoubtedly develop tobacco-related illness and diseases (Thun et al. 2012). The world is at a unique juncture as high-income smoking rates have started to level out and global tobacco control is now in a position to prevent smoking rates (and thus illness and disease rates) in middle- and low-income countries, especially among women, from ever reaching the levels seen in high-income countries. Country leaders and tobacco control advocates must take seriously the possibility that female and youth smoking rates have the potential to increase, and all must do everything in their power to prevent further death from tobacco use. Tobacco needs to be treated commensurate with the harm it causes, and we must take drastic measures to stop tobacco use from killing one person every 6 seconds (WHO 2011d).

Acknowledgments Special acknowledgments to Stephen B. Stanfill, Research Chemist, Centers for Disease Control and Prevention, National Center for Environmental Health for his assistance with the smokeless tobacco section.

For more information on tobacco visit the comprehensive Web site www.tobaccoportal.org.

References

Adler, I. (1912). *Primary malignant growths of the lungs and bronchi: A pathological and clinical study.* London: Longmans, Green and Co.

Alamar, B., & Glantz, S. A. (2006). Effect of increased social unacceptability of cigarette smoking on reduction in cigarette consumption. *American Journal of Public Health, 96*(8), 1359–1363.

Altria Group Inc. (2010). *2010 annual report.* Retrieved August 9, 2011, from http://investor.altria.com/phoenix.zhtml?c=808.

American Cancer Society. (2011). *Learn about cancer: Cigarette smoking.* Retrieved July 3, 2012, from http://www.cancer.org/Cancer/CancerCauses/TobaccoCancer/CigaretteSmoking/cigarette-smoking-tobacco.

American Cancer Society. (2012). *Cancer facts & figures 2012.* Atlanta, GA: American Cancer Society. Retrieved March 27, 2012, from http://www.cancer.org/acs/groups/content/@epidemiologysurveilance/documents/document/acspc-031941.pdf.

Australian Government Department of Health and Ageing. (2011). *Public consultation on plain packaging of cigarettes.* Retrieved 29 March, 2012, from http://www.yourhealth.gov.au/internet/yourhealth/publishing.nsf/Content/plainpack-tobacco#.T3RxzXnYEUg.

Australian Institute of Health and Welfare. (2011). *2010 National Drug Strategy Household Survey Report.* Retrieved October 5, 2011, from http://www.aihw.gov.au/publication-detail/?id=32212254712.

Australian Medical Association. (2011, November 30). *Traffic light food labelling.* Retrieved July 3, 2012, from http://ama.com.au/traffic-light-labelling.

Blackwell, J. R. (2012, May 23). *Altria to test market new nicotine product in Virginia. Richmond Times-Disptach.* Retrieved July 3, 2012, from http://www2.timesdispatch.com/business/virginia-news/2012/may/23/tdbiz01-altria-to-test-market-new-nicotine-product-ar-1935376/.

British American Tobacco. (2010). *Annual report 2010.* Retrieved August 9, 2011, from http://www.bat.com/servlet/SPMerge?mainurl=%2Fgroup%2Fsites%2Fuk__3mnfen.nsf%2FvwPagesWebLive%2FDO52AK34%3Fopendocument%26amp%3BSKN%3D1.

Brownell, K. D., & Koplan, J. P. (2011). Front-of-package nutrition labeling—an abuse of trust by the food industry. *The New England Journal of Medicine, 346*(25), 2373–2375. Retrieved July 3, 2012, from http://www.nejm.org/doi/full/10.1056/NEJMp1101033.

Brunnemann, K. D., Genoble, L., & Hoffmann, D. (1985). N-Nitrosamines in chewing tobacco: An international comparison. *Journal of Agricultural and Food History, 33,* 1178–1181.

Businessweek. (2010a). *McDonalds Corporation: 2010 financials.* Retrieved August 9, 2011, from http://investing.businessweek.com/research/stocks/financials/financials.asp?ticker=MCD:US.

Businessweek. (2010b). *Microsoft Corporation: 2010 financials.* Retrieved August 9, 2011, from http://investing.businessweek.com/research/stocks/financials/financials.asp?ticker=MSFT:US.

Businessweek. (2010c). *The Coca-Cola Company: 2010 financials.* Retrieved August 9, 2011, from http://investing.businessweek.com/research/stocks/financials/financials.asp?ticker=KO:US.

Campaign for Tobacco-Free Kids. (2011). *Pictoral warning labels by country and jurisdiction.* Retrieved April 10, 2012, from http://global.tobaccofreekids.org/files/pdfs/en/WL_examples_en.pdf.

Cauchon, D. (2007). Smoking declines as taxes increase. *USA Today.* Retrieved April 12, 2012, from http://www.usatoday.com/news/health/2007-08-09-1Alede_N.htm.

CBS News. (2012, June 12). *Mayor Bloomberg's soda ban proposal to be submitted to NYC health board today.* Retrieved June 30, 2012, from http://www.cbsnews.com/8301-504763_162-57451372-10391704/mayor-bloombergs-soda-ban-proposal-to-be-submitted-to-nyc-health-board-today/.

Centers for Disease Control and Prevention. (2007, October). *Best Practices for Comprehensive Tobacco Control Programs—2007.* Atlanta: U.S. Department of Health and Human Services, Centers for Disease Control and Prevention, National Center for Chronic Disease Prevention and Health Promotion, Office on Smoking and Health; Reprinted with corrections.

Centers for Disease Control and Prevention. (2011a). *Current smoking, adults, early release.* Retrieved November 2, 2011, from http://www.cdc.gov/nchs/data/nhis/earlyrelease/201106_08.pdf.

Centers for Disease Control and Prevention. (2011b). *Global tobacco surveillance system: Global School-Based Health Survey.* Retrieved October 15, 2011, from http://www.cdc.gov/gshs/ and via personal communication.

Centers for Disease Control and Prevention. (2011c). *Global tobacco surveillance system: Global Youth Tobacco Survey.* Retrieved October 15, 2011, from http://nccd.cdc.gov/gtssdata/Ancillary/Documentation. aspx?SUID=1&DOCT=1 and via personal communication.

Centers for Disease Control and Prevention. (2011d). *Vital signs: Current cigarette smoking among adults aged ≥ 18 years—United States, 2005–2010.* Retrieved June 21, 2012, from http://www.cdc.gov/mmwr/preview/mmwrhtml/mm6035a5.htm?s_cid=mm6035a5_w.

Centers for Disease Control and Prevention. (2012). *State tobacco revenues compared with tobacco control appropriations—United States, 1998–2010.* Retrieved July 3, 2012, from http://www.cdc.gov/mmwr/pdf/wk/mm6120.pdf.

Chaloupka, F. J., Yurekli, A., & Fong, G. T. (2012). Tobacco taxes as a tobacco control strategy. *Tobacco Control, 21*(2), 172–180.

Chan, M. (2012). *The changed face of the tobacco industry—Keynote address at the 15th World Conference on Tobacco OR Health.* Retrieved April 12, 2012, from http://www.who.int/dg/speeches/2012/tobacco_20120320/en/.

Connolly, G. N., Alpert, H. R., Wayne, G. F., & Koh, H. (2007). *Trends in smoke nicotine yield and relationship to design characteristics among popular U.S. cigarette brands 1975–2005.* A report of the Tobacco Research Program, Division of Public Health Practice, Harvard School of Public Health. Retrieved July 3, 2012, from http://www.hsph.harvard.edu/nicotine/trends.pdf.

Daley, J. I., Stahre, M. A., Chaloupka, F. J., & Naimi, T. S. (2012). The impact of a 25-cent-per-drink alcohol tax increase. *American Journal of Preventive Medicine, 42*(4), 382–389.

David, A., Esson, K., Perucic, A., & Fitzpatrick, C. (2010). Tobacco use: Equity and social determinants. In E. Blas & A. S. Kurup (Eds.), *Equity, social determinants and public health programmes* (pp. 199–207). Geneva: World Health Organization.

Dorman, L., Cheyne, A., Friedman, L. C., Wadud, A., & Gottlieb, M. (2012). Soda and tobacco industry corporate social responsibility campaigns: How do they compare? *PLoS Medicine, 9*(6), e1001241. doi:10.1371/journal.pmed.1001241.

ERC. (2010). *World cigarette reports 2010.* Suffolk: ERC Group Ltd.

Eriksen, M., Mackay, J., & Ross, H. (2012). *The tobacco atlas* (4th ed.). Atlanta, GA: American Cancer Society.

Euromonitor International. (2011). *Passport database.* Retrieved October 1, 2011.

Ezzati, M., & Lopez, A. (2003). Estimates of global mortality attributable to smoking in 2000. *The Lancet, 362,* 847–852.

Federal Trade Commission. (2012a). *Cigarette report for 2009 and 2010.* Retrieved May 21, 2013, from http://www.ftc.gov/os/2012/09/120921cigarettereport.pdf.

Federal Trade Commission. (2012b). *Smokeless tobacco report for 2009 and 2010.* Retrieved May 21, 2013, from http://www.ftc.gov/os/2012/09/120921tobaccoreport.pdf.

Food and Agricultural Organization. (2008a). *FAOSTAT data, tobacco unmanufactured: Area harvested, 2008.* Retrieved April 1, 2011, from http://faostat.fao.org/site/567/DesktopDefault.aspx?PageID=567.

Food and Agricultural Organization. (2008b). *FAOSTAT data, tobacco unmanufactured: Production quantity, 2008.* Retrieved April 1, 2011, from http://faostat.fao.org/site/567/DesktopDefault.aspx?PageID=567#ancor.

Food and Agricultural Organization. (2008c). *FAOSTAT data, potatoes: Production quantity, 2008.* Retrieved April 1, 2011, http://faostat.fao.org/site/567/DesktopDefault.aspx?PageID=567#ancor.

Food and Agricultural Organization. (2011a). *Hunger statistics: 2005–2007.* Retrieved April 1, 2011, from http://www.fao.org/hunger/en/.

Food and Agricultural Organization. (2011b). *Hunger map 2010: Prevalence of undernourishment in developing countries (2005–2007).* Retrieved April 1, 2011, from http://faostat.fao.org/site/563/default.aspx.

Food and Agricultural Organization. (2013a). *FAOSTAT data, tobacco unmanufactured: Area harvested, 2011.* Retrieved May 21, 2013, from http://faostat.fao.org/site/567/DesktopDefault.aspx?PageID=567.

Food and Agricultural Organization. (2013b). *FAOSTAT data, tobacco unmanufactured: Production quantity, 2011.* Retrieved May 21, 2013, from http://faostat.fao.org/site/567/DesktopDefault.aspx?PageID=567.

Gan, Q., Smith, K., Hammond, K., & Hu, T. (2007). Disease burden of adult lung cancer and ischaemic heart disease from passive tobacco smoking in China. *Tobacco Control, 16*(6), 417–422.

Garfinkel, L. (1981). Time trends in lung cancer mortality among nonsmokers and a note on passive smoking. *Journal of the National Cancer Institute, 66*(6), 1061–1066.

Gilmore, A. B. (2012). Understanding the vector in order to plan effective tobacco control policies: An analysis of contemporary tobacco industry materials. *Tobacco Control, 21*(2), 119–126.

Gostin, L. O. (2012). A framework convention on global health: Health for All, Justice for All. *Journal of the American Medical Association, 307*(19), 2087–2092. doi:10.1001/jama.2012.4395.

Haire-Joshu, D., Glasgow, R. E., & Tibbs, T. L. (1999). Smoking and diabetes. *Diabetes Care, 22*(11), 887–1898.

Health Canada. (2011). *Canadian Tobacco Use Monitoring Survey: Summary of annual results for 2010.* Retrieved October 5, 2011, from http://www.hc-sc.gc.ca/hc-ps/tobac-tabac/research-recherche/stat/_ctums-esutc_2010/ann_summarysommaire-eng.php.

Henningield, J. E., & Zaatari, G. S. (2010). Electronic nicotine delivery systems: Emerging science foundation for policy. *Tobacco Control, 19*(2), 89–90.

Hirayama, T. (1981). Non-smoking wives of heavy smokers have a higher risk of lung cancer: A study from Japan. *British Medical Journal (Clinical Research Ed.), 282*(6259), 183–185.

Hundley, T. (2007, September 16). Snuffing out smokes. *Chicago Tribune.* Retrieved August 2, 2011, from http://articles.chicagotribune.com/2007-09-16/

business/0709150068_1_snus-smokeless-tobacco-tobacco-product/2.

Hyland, A., Vena, C., Bauer, J., Li, Q., Giovino, G.A., Yang, J., et al. (2003). Cigarette smoking-attributable morbidity—United States, 2000. *Morbidity and Mortality Weekly Review*. Atlanta, GA: Centers for Disease Control and Prevention.

Imperial Tobacco. (2010). *Annual report and accounts 2010*. Retrieved August 9, 2011, from http://www.imperial-tobacco.com/files/financial/reports/ar2010/index.asp?pageid=64.

International Agency for Research on Cancer (IARC). (1986). *IARC monographs on the evaluation of the carcinogenic risk of chemicals to humans: Tobacco smoking*. IARC 38. Lyon, France: IARC press

International Agency for Research on Cancer (IARC). (2004). *Monograph 85: Betel-quid and areca-nut chewing and some tobacco specific N-nitrosamines*. Retrieved June 5, 2012, from http://monographs.iarc.fr/ENG/Monographs/vol85/index.php.

International Agency for Research on Cancer (IARC). (2007a). *The hazards of smoking and the benefits of stopping: Cancer Mortality and overall mortality. IARC handbooks of cancer prevention* (Vol. 11, pp. 15–27). Lyon: IARC press.

International Agency for Research on Cancer (IARC). (2007b). Smokeless tobacco and some tobacco-specific N-nitrosamines. In: *IARC monographs on the evaluation of carcinogenic risks to humans* (Vol. 890. Lyon, France. Retrieved June 5, 2012, from http://monographs.iarc.fr/ENG/Monographs/vol89/index.php.

James, R. (2009, June 15). Cigarette advertising. *Time Magazine*. Retrieved April 1, 2012, from http://www.time.com/time/magazine/article/0,9171,1905530,00.html.

Japan Tobacco Inc. (2010). *Annual report 2010*. Retrieved August 9, 2011, from http://www.jti.com/documents/annualreports/Annualreport2010.pdf.

Kesmodel, D., & Korn, M. (2011, May 27). Philip Morris Looks to Nicotine Aerosol. *The Wall Street Journal*. Retrieved June 21, 2011, http://online.wsj.com/article/SB10001424052702304066504576347513991162274.html.

Kessler, G. (2006). *Final Opinion Civil Action No. 99-2496 (GK)*. United States District Court for the District of Columbia. Retrieved April 12, 2012, from http://www.tobaccofreekids.org/content/what_we_do/industry_watch/doj/FinalOpinion.pdf.

Kong, M., & Assunta, M. (2012). Worldwide news and comment—Cambodia: KT&G? 'Korean Tomorrow & Global', Of Course. *Tobacco Control, 21*(2), 82–86.

Live China. (2011, May 8). *Chinese Love "China Love" Cigarettes*. Retrieved July 3, 2012, from http://golivechina.com/newsitem/chinese-love-china-love-cigarettes/.

Lopatto, E. (2012, March 22). *Mayor Bloomberg donates $220 million to fight smoking abroad. Bloomberg*. Retrieved April 1, 2012, http://www.bloomberg.com/news/2012-03-22/mayor-bloomberg-donates-220-million-to-fight-smoking-overseas.html.

Lopez, A., Collishaw, N., & Piha, T. (1994). A descriptive model of the cigarette epidemic in developed countries. *Tobacco Control, 3*, 242–247.

Lorillard. (2012). *Lorillard, Inc. Reports First Quarter 2012 Results and Acquisition of blu ecigs*. Retrieved July 3, 2012, from http://investors.lorillard.com/phoenix.zhtml?c=134955&p=irol-newsArticle&ID=1687024&highlight.

Lyn, R., Moore, B. J., & Eriksen, M. (2012). The application of public health lessons to stemming the obesity epidemic. In S. R. Akabas, S. A. Lederman, & B. J. Moore (Eds.), *Textbook of obesity: Biological, psychological, and cultural influences* (pp. 58–83). Chichester: John Wiley & Sons.

Mercado, S. (2011). *World Health Organization*: Western Pacific Region Office, Personal communication.

Miles, T. (2012). *Honduras joins WTO complaint on Australia tobacco packaging*. Retrieved April 11, 2012, from http://www.reuters.com/article/2012/04/04/wto-australia-tobacco-idUSL6E8F4BQC20120404.

Ministry of Health, Singapore. (2010). *National Health Survey 2010, Singapore*. Epidemiology and Disease Control Division, Ministry of Health, Singapore. Retrieved April 9, 2012, from http://www.moh.gov.sg/content/dam/moh_web/Publications/Reports/2011/NHS2010%20-%20low%20res.pdf.

Mytton, O. T., Clarke, D., & Rayner, M. (2012). Taxing unhealthy food and drinks to improve health. *British Medical Journal, 344*, e2931. Retrieved July 5, 2012, from http://www.bmj.com/content/344/bmj.e2931.

National Association of Attorneys General. (1998). *Master settlement agreement*. Retrieved July 10, 2012, from http://www.naag.org/backpages/naag/tobacco/msa/msa-pdf/MSA%20with%20Sig%20Pages%20and%20Exhibits.pdf.

National Research Council, Committee on Passive Smoking. (1986). *Environmental tobacco smoke: Measuring exposures and assessing health effects*. Washington, DC: The National Academies Press.

Netscribes. (2012, February). *Tobacco market – China*. Netscribes Food & Beverage Industry Series.

NTD Television. (January 26, 2010). *Tobacco companies sponsor 69 elementary schools in China*. Retrieved July 3, 2011, from. http://english.ntdtv.com/ntdtv_en/ns_china/2010-01-26/907134456872.html.

Öberg, M., Jaakkola, M., Woodward, A., Peruga, A., & Prüss-Ustün, A. (2011). Worldwide burden of disease from exposure to secondhand smoke: A retrospective analysis of data from 192 countries. *The Lancet, 377*, 139–146.

Okorokova, L. (2011, August 25). Teenage cigarette scandal. *The Moscow News*. Retrieved August 28, 2011, from http://themoscownews.com/society/20110825/188961025.html.

OpenSecrets.org. (2011). *Tobacco*. Retrieved July 28, 2011, from http://www.opensecrets.org/industries/lobbying.php?cycle=2010&ind=A02.

Organization for Economic Co-Operation and Development (OECD). (2011a). *OECD health data 2011: Frequently requested data*. Retrieved November

29, 2011, from http://www.oecd.org/document/16/0,3 746,en_2649_37407_2085200_1_1_1_37407,00. html.

Organization for Economic Co-Operation and Development (OECD). (2011b). *Stat extracts: Health status*. Retrieved October 5, 2011, from http://stats. oecd.org/index.aspx?DataSetCode=HEALTH_STAT.

Pampel, F. C., & Denney, J. T. (2011). Cross-national sources of health inequality: Education and Tobacco Use in the World Health Survey. *Demography, 48*, 653–674.

Parliament of Australia. (2011). *Tobacco Plain Packaging Bill*. Retrieved March 29, 2012, from http://www. yourhealth.gov.au/internet/yourhealth/publishing.nsf/ Content/6B16D93A9E2CF9CECA2579540005F62D /$File/Tobacco%20Plain%20Packaging%20Bill%20 2011%20-%20Exposure%20Draft%20-%2031%20 March%202011.pdf.

Peto, R., & Lopez, A. (2000). *The future worldwide health effects of current smoking patterns*. Clinical Trial Service Unit & Epidemiological Studies Unit— University of Oxford. Updated via personal communication, June 2011. Retrieved December 3, 2011, from http://www.ctsu.ox.ac.uk/pressreleases/2000-08-02/ the-future-worldwide-health-effects-of-current-smoking-patterns.

Philip Morris International. (2010). *Annual report 2010*. Retrieved August 9, 2011, from http://investors.pmi. com/phoenix.zhtml?c=146476&p=irolreportsannual.

Philip Morris International. (2011). *Charitable contributions 2010*. Retrieved July 3, 2011, from http://www. pmi.com/eng/about_us/corporate_contributions/docu-ments/2010_charitable_contributions_total.pdf.

Physicians for a Smoke-Free Canada. (2012). *Picture based cigarette warnings*. Retrieved April 12, 2012, from http://www.smoke-free.ca/warnings/default.htm.

Proctor, R. (2006, June). Angel H Roffo: the forgotten father of experimental tobacco carcinogenesis. *Bulletin of the World Health Organization, 84*(6), 494–496.

Proctor, R. (2012a). *Golden holocaust: Origins of the cigarette catastrophe and the case for abolition*. Berkeley, CA: University of California Press.

Proctor, R. N. (2012b). The history of the discovery of the cigarette–lung cancer link: Evidentiary traditions, cor-porate denial, global toll. *Tobacco Control, 21*(2), 87–91.

Report on the Committee of Experts on Tobacco Industry Documents. (2000). *Tobacco company strategies to undermine tobacco control activities at the World Health Organization*. Retrieved August 12, 2011, from http://www.who.int/tobacco/en/who_inquiry. pdf.

Reynolds, R. J. (1984). *RJR report—young adult smokers: Strategies and opportunities*. Retrieved October 6, 2011, from http://legacy.library.ucsf.edu/tid/fet29d00/pdf.

Riordan, M. (2012). *Tobacco and socioeconomic status*. Campaign for tobacco-free kids. Retrieved June 21, 2012, from http://www.tobaccofreekids.org/research/ factsheets/pdf/0260.pdf.

Scientific Committee on Emerging and Newly Identified Health Risks (SCENIHR). (2008, February 6). *Opinion On Health Effects Of Smokeless Tobacco Products*. Taken from 22nd Plenary Meeting. Retrieved June 5, 2012, from http://ec.europa.eu/health/ph_risk/ committees/09_scenihr/scenihr_opinions_en.htm#5.

Simpson, D. (2012). Worldwide news and comment— New Zealand: Pack seal can cover warnings. *Tobacco Control, 21*(2), 82–86.

Stanfill, S. B., & Stepanov, I. (in press). Chapter 3. Global View of smokeless tobacco products: constituents and toxicity. *Smokeless tobacco and public health: A global perspective*.

Stanfill, S. B., Connolly, G. N., Zhang, L., Jia, T. L., Henningfield, J., Richter, P., et al. (2011). Surveillance of international oral tobacco products: Total nicotine, un-ionized nicotine and tobacco-specific nitrosamines. *Tobacco Control, 20*, e2. doi:10.1136/tc.2010.037465.

Stratton, K., Shetty, P., Wallace, R., & Bondurant, S. (Eds.). (2001). *Clearing the smoke: Assessing the sci-ence base for tobacco harm reduction*. Washington, DC: Institute of Medicine, National Academy Press.

Stuckler, D., McKee, M., Ebrahim, S., & Basu, S. (2012). Manufacturing epidemics. The role of global produc-ers in increased consumption of unhealthy commodi-ties including processed foods, alcohol, and tobacco. *PLoS Medicine, 9*(6), e1001235.

Sutherland, L. A., Kaley, L. A., & Fischer, L. (2010). Guiding stars: The effect of a nutrition navigation pro-gram on consumer purchases at the supermarket. *The American Journal of Clinical Nutrition, 91*(suppl), 1090S–1094S.

Swedish National Institute of Public Health. (2009). *Public health 2009: Open comparisons*. Retrieved August 25, 2011, from http://www.fhi.se/ PageFiles/9183/open-comparisons-2009.pdf.

The Canadian Press. (2012, June 8). *Quebec sues big tobacco companies for $60-billion, joining four other provinces in lawsuits*. Retrieved July 3, 2012, from http://news.nationalpost.com/2012/06/08/ quebec-sues-big-tobacco-companies-for-60-billion-joining-four-other-provinces-in-lawsuits/.

The World Bank. (2011). *Gross domestic product, 2010*. Retrieved June 21, 2011, http://siteresources.world-bank.org/DATASTATISTICS/Resources/GDP.pdf.

Thun, M., Peto, R., Boreham, J., & Lopez, A. D. (2012). Stages of the cigarette epidemic on entering its second century. *Tobacco Control, 21*(2), 96–101.

Trichopoulos, D., Kalandidi, A., Sparros, L., & MacMahon, B. (1981). Lung cancer and passive smoking. *International Journal of Cancer, 27*(1), 1–4.

U.S. Department of Health and Human Services. (2004). *The health consequences of smoking: A report of the Surgeon General*. Atlanta, GA: Department of Health and Human Services, Centers for Disease Control and Prevention, National Center for Chronic Disease Prevention and Health Promotion, Office on Smoking and Health.

U.S. Department of Health and Human Services. (2006). *The health consequences of involuntary exposure to tobacco smoke: A report of the Surgeon General*. Atlanta, GA: U.S. Department of Health and Human Services, Centers for Disease Control and Prevention, Coordinating Center for Health Promotion, National

Center for Chronic Disease Prevention and Health Promotion, Office on Smoking and Health.

U.S. Department of Health and Human Services. (2009). *Guidance for industry—letter regarding point of purchase food labeling.* U.S. Department of Health and Human Services, Food and Drug Administration, Center for Food Safety and Applied Nutrition. Retrieved July 3, 2012, from http://www.fda.gov/Food/GuidanceComplianceRegulatoryInformation/GuidanceDocuments/FoodLabelingNutrition/ucm187208.htm.

U.S. Department of Health and Human Services. (2010). *How tobacco smoke causes disease: The biology and behavioral basis for smoking-attributable disease: A report of the Surgeon General.* Atlanta, GA: U.S. Department of Health and Human Services, Centers for Disease Control and Prevention, National Center for Chronic Disease Prevention and Health Promotion, Office on Smoking and Health.

U.S. Department of Health and Human Services. (2012). *Preventing tobacco use among youth and young adults: A report of the Surgeon General—executive summary.* Atlanta, GA: U.S. Department of Health and Human Services, Centers for Disease Control and Prevention, National Center for Chronic Disease Prevention and Health Promotion, Office on Smoking and Health.

U.S. Environmental Protection Agency. (1992). *Respiratory health effects of passive smoking: Lung cancer and other disorders.* Washington, DC: U.S. Environmental Protection Agency, Office of Research and Development, Office of Air and Radiation.

Wang, Y. C., Coxson, P., Shen, Y. M., Goldman, L., & Bibbins-Domingo, K. (2012). A penny-per-ounce tax on sugar-sweetened beverages would cut health and cost burdens of diabetes. *Health Affairs, 31*(1), 199–207. doi:10.1377/hlthaff.2011.0410.

Wang, Ke-an. (2011). Think tank Beijing. Personal communication.

World Health Organization. (2004). *Tobacco and poverty: A vicious circle.* Retrieved April 25, 2011, from http://www.who.int/tobacco/communications/events/wntd/2004/en/wntd2004_brochure_en.pdf.

World Health Organization. (2008). *2008–2013 action plan for the global strategy for the prevention and control of noncommunicable diseases.* Retrieved August 16, 2011, from http://whqlibdoc.who.int/publications/2009/9789241597418_eng.pdf.

World Health Organization (2011a). *Cardiovascular diseases (CVDs).* Retrieved March 30, 2012, from http://www.who.int/mediacentre/factsheets/fs317/en/index.html.

World Health Organization. (2011b). *Chronic obstructive pulmonary disease (COPD).* Retrieved March 30, 2012, from http://www.who.int/mediacentre/factsheets/fs315/en/index.html.

World Health Organization. (2011c). *Diabetes.* Retrieved March 30, 2012, from http://www.who.int/mediacentre/factsheets/fs312/en/index.html.

World Health Organization. (2011d). *Fact Sheet Number 339—tobacco.* Retrieved July 28, 2011, from http://www.who.int/mediacentre/factsheets/fs339/en/index.html.

World Health Organization. (2011e). *Framework Convention on Tobacco Control.* Retrieved May 22, 2013, from http://www.who.int/fctc/en/.

World Health Organization. (2011f). *Noncommunicable diseases.* Retrieved March 30, 2012, from http://www.who.int/mediacentre/factsheets/fs355/en/index.html#.

World Health Organization. (2011g). *United Nations high-level meeting on Noncommunicable Disease Prevention and Control.* Retrieved March 30, 2012, from http://www.who.int/nmh/events/un_ncd_summit2011/en/.

World Health Organization. (2011h). *WHO report on the Global Tobacco Epidemic, 2011: warning about the dangers of tobacco.* Geneva: World Health Organization

World Health Organization. (2012a). *Cancer.* Retrieved March 30, 2012, from http://www.who.int/mediacentre/factsheets/fs297/en/.

World Health Organization. (2012b). *Parties to the WHO framework convention on tobacco control.* Retrieved May 22, 2013, from http://www.who.int/fctc/signatories_parties/en/index.html.

World Health Organization. (2012c). *WHO global report: Mortality attributable to tobacco.* Geneva: World Health Organization. Retrieved March 26, 2012, from http://whqlibdoc.who.int/publications/2012/9789241564434_eng.pdf.

Zhu, S. H., Lee, M., Zhuang, Y. L., Gamst, A., & Wolfson, T. (2012). Interventions to increase smoking cessation at the population level: How much progress has been made in the last two decades? *Tobacco Control, 21*(2), 110–118.

Physical Inactivity and Health Promotion: Evidence and Challenges

Alfred Rütten, Karim Abu-Omar, Annika Frahsa, and Peter Gelius

Introduction

Physical activity promotion has been labeled a "magic bullet" and a "best buy" (Munro et al. 1997). It has become a major public health topic in industrialized nations. This development might be partially explained by increasing rates of obesity and Type II Diabetes as well as the global spread of noncommunicable diseases (IDF 2009). For example, longitudinal data from the USA reveals a steady increase in the rate of obese adults since the mid-1980s, with some states reporting obesity prevalence among adults at 35 % in 2010 (National Center for Chronic Disease Prevention and Health Promotion 2011). Also, the global burden of noncommunicable diseases is expected to rise to 52 million annual deaths (United Nations 2011). Sedentary lifestyles have been identified as an important risk factor for obesity and a number of chronic diseases. The health benefits of physical activity include, among other things, positive effects on cardio-respiratory health, musculoskeletal health, functional health, cancer, mental health, and all-cause mortality (Physical Activity Guidelines Advisory Committee 2008).

Despite the known health benefits of physical activity, the prevalence of physical inactivity has remained rather high in most industrialized nations. For example, 39 % of European adults respond that they never engage in sport or exercise, and an additional 21 % state that they do so only rarely (European Commission 2010). In the USA, 85 % of those who did not complete high school, 78 % of those who completed high school, and 57 % of those with a college degree reported not engaging in regular leisure-time physical activity in 2007. These results showed no significant increases in leisure-time physical activity compared to the year 1997 (National Center for Health Statistics 2009).

The increased burden of diseases for which sedentary lifestyles are a major risk factor, paired with the comparably high prevalence of physical inactivity in industrialized nations, have made the identification of successful strategies to promote physical activity on the population level an important topic. To this point in time, numerous studies have investigated the effectiveness of different strategies to promote physical activity, and more and more reviews and even reviews of reviews have been devoted to this topic.

In this chapter, we review some of the existing evidence on the effectiveness of different physical activity promotion intervention strategies. We also address some of the challenges confronting

A. Rütten (✉) • K. Abu-Omar • A. Frahsa • P. Gelius
Institute of Sport Science and Sport, Friedrich-Alexander-University Erlangen-Nürnberg, Gebberststr. 123b, 91058, Erlangen, Germany
e-mail: alfred.ruetten@sport.uni-erlangen.de;
karim.abu-omar@sport.uni-erlangen.de;
annika.frahsa@sport.uni-erlangen.de;
peter.gelius@sport.uni-erlangen.de

D.V. McQueen (ed.), *Global Handbook on Noncommunicable Diseases and Health Promotion*,
DOI 10.1007/978-1-4614-7594-1_9, © Springer Science+Business Media, LLC 2013

research both from a theoretical perspective and with regard to the improvement of physical activity promotion policies and practice. In the first part, special attention is devoted to the challenges intervention studies and reviews face when setting out to evaluate the potential of interventions to be broadly transferred and disseminated; tasks which are frequently warranted from a public health perspective. In the second part, we introduce a theoretical model that might assist in overcoming some of the challenges faced by intervention studies that focus on physical activity promotion. This theoretical model attempts to specify distinct patterns that emerge in relation to the interplay between individual and/or collective action and societal and political structures at two different levels (operational and collective choice). Such a model might be of significant value, as reviews suggest that contextual determinants are extremely relevant when planning and promoting physical activity. In the third part, we use this model to investigate the challenges of promoting physical activity by referencing case examples from local and national/international levels.

Evidence on the Effectiveness of Different Intervention Strategies for Physical Activity Promotion from a Public Health Perspective

From a public health perspective, successful intervention strategies for the promotion of physical activity can be characterized by the following:

1. Effectiveness of the intervention strategy to increase physical activity levels over time. It is acknowledged, however, that some strategies for the promotion of physical activity (e.g., developing policies) do not easily lend themselves to evidence-based investigations of effectiveness.
2. Cost-effectiveness of the intervention strategy to be disseminated broadly and thus to potentially achieve public health impact. Here it is acknowledged that cost-effectiveness might be defined differently for "low-risk" versus "high-risk" population subgroups.

3. Effectiveness of the intervention strategy to reduce physical activity/health inequalities between population groups, or at least no evidence that the intervention strategy contributes to physical activity/health inequalities. It is important to keep in mind that certain intervention strategies target individuals directly, while others target the broader determinants of individual behavior.
4. Indications that the intervention strategy can be successfully transferred to other sites, nations, or cultural and political contexts. Here it is important to keep in mind that transfers to other sites, or cultural or political contexts might have impacts on overall intervention effectiveness.

The following section provides an overview of some of the more prominent physical activity promotion intervention strategies. It should be mentioned that current reviews dealing with this topic have had a primary focus on investigating the overall effectiveness of different intervention strategies. Additionally, while some studies have investigated the cost-effectiveness of different intervention strategies, very few studies have investigated the potential of different intervention strategies to reduce health inequalities or to be transferred and/or adapted within and across nations and cultural or political contexts.

Individual or Group-Based Interventions: These Promote Physical Activity by Offering Exercise Classes or Advising Target Groups to Exercise or Be Physically Active

Such interventions usually consist of regular exercise classes, active living encouragements (e.g., prompts to engage in regular walking or cycling) and/or psychological counseling for behavior modification. Often, these approaches are founded on models of behavior modification such as the Stages of Change Model (Prochaska and DiClemente 1983). In recent years, these approaches have increasingly attempted to incorporate internet- or telephone-based counseling techniques. Usually, the intervention period lasts between 3 and 12 months. The effectiveness of this type of intervention strategy is commonly investigated by controlled study designs including pre and post measurements of potential effects on various physical activity, fitness, and health parameters.

This type of intervention strategy has, in general, been identified as an effective means by which to promote physical activity. A Cochrane Review (Foster et al. 2005), and the CDC (Task Force on Community Preventive Services 2005) have concluded that it can result in increased levels of physical activity. There is some indication that interventions that fall in this category and that directly target individual behavior (e.g., by offering exercise classes) achieve greater effectiveness compared to interventions that target individual attitudes and knowledge regarding physical activity (Conn et al. 2011). For older people, it has been suggested that group-based exercise programs show greater effectiveness compared to home-based programs when it comes to increasing fitness levels. At the same time, home-based programs seem to achieve more sustained effects (Ashworth et al. 2005).

The cost-effectiveness of this type of intervention strategy has been investigated in some studies. Graves et al. (2009) investigated the cost-effectiveness of a telephone-delivered intervention that targeted physical activity and diet. The costs were estimated to be approximately $500 U.S. per year per person. Compared to existing practices, the intervention was deemed to be cost-effective (29.375 U.S.$ per Disability Adjusted Life-Year saved). Müller-Riemenschneider et al. (2009) estimated the cost of converting an adult who is sedentary to one that meets physical activity recommendations at about 1,000 U.S.$ per person per year. Wu et al. (2011) concluded that the cost-effectiveness of this intervention strategy type, compared to other intervention strategy types, is rather low, with annual costs of 1.1 million U.S.$ to reach 10,000 persons (Wu et al. 2011).

The potential of individual or group-based interventions to contribute to the reduction of health inequalities is difficult to assess. Some studies have demonstrated that physical activity counseling interventions are effective in minority populations (Coleman et al. 2012), but, for example, there is a lack of reviews that focus on inequalities in relation to individual and group access to behavior change interventions (Jepson et al. 2010).

Results from intervention studies suggest that multidimensional interventions that address individual, sociocultural, and environmental barriers to physical activity are more promising in their abilities to reach socially disadvantaged groups than one-dimensional interventions. Multidimensional interventions build upon tenets of participation and empowerment. They involve target groups in all aspects of interventions (Lowther et al. 2002; Taylor et al. 1998; Yancey et al. 2006); and they are culturally sensitive (Yancey et al. 2006), promote partnerships (Wang et al. 2006) and develop adequate and tailored recruitment strategies (Yancey et al. 2006).

Community-Based Interventions

These interventions commonly utilize various measures such as radio and newspaper postings, advertisements, mass events, and the development of adequate infrastructures to promote physical activity on the community level. While these interventions target physical activity behavior, they are often part of broader efforts to publicize other health issues like diet, smoking cessation, or cholesterol and cancer screenings. The Minnesota Heart Health Study (Luepker et al. 1994) serves as a good example of this type of intervention.

Commonly, community-based interventions last for several years. Potential effects are evaluated by nested cross-sectional and longitudinal study designs that rely mainly on self-reported health behavior at the individual level. In some studies, control communities were matched and assessed as part of the evaluation design. Due to the high diversity of intervention strategies implemented across studies in this category, it is difficult to rate the overall effectiveness of community-based interventions.

The CDC (Task Force on Community Preventive Services 2005), and WHO (2009) have asserted that community-based interventions are effective in increasing physical activity rates. The CDC has stated that such interventions might reduce the rate of sedentary adults by up to 4 %. A Cochrane Review, however, has recently questioned the effectiveness of community-based interventions in increasing physical activity rates. This review has argued that more rigorous evaluation methodologies would be needed in order to demonstrate the effectiveness of these interventions (Baker et al. 2011).

Regarding the cost-effectiveness of community-based interventions, Wu et al. (2011) found a large diversity in investigated trials, which makes it nearly impossible to provide a an estimate. Other cost-effectiveness studies such as Müller-Riemenschneider et al. (2009) have subsumed individual-level behavioral interventions under the category of community-based interventions, resulting in estimates that are somewhat misleading.

Mass Media Campaigns

These interventions rely predominantly on the promotion of physical activity by television or radio spots, billboards, or other informational means. In addition to advertising campaigns, some interventions support telephone counseling hotlines. Common intervention periods for these campaigns are 6–12 months. Evaluation efforts often include pre–post assessments of campaign awareness, knowledge about physical activity recommendations, and self-rated physical activity levels. Some studies have used other regions within the same country to control for secular trends.

In 2005, the CDC rated the effectiveness of mass media campaigns and concluded that there is a limited evidence-base for this type of intervention strategy (Task Force on Community Preventive Services 2005). More recently the WHO (2009) and one other review (Wakefield et al. 2010) have hinted that such interventions may result in moderate increases in physical activity. Especially motivated individuals who contemplate becoming more active might benefit from such campaigns. Most studies have been able to demonstrate changes in knowledge and attitudes about physical activity, but not necessarily changes in actual physical activity behavior.

The cost-effectiveness of mass media campaigns has been investigated in at least two studies. Cobiac et al. (2009) rate mass media campaigns as being among the more cost-effective physical activity promotion intervention. Wu et al. (2011) state that point-of-decision prompts (e.g., signs to encourage use of stairs) are the most cost-effective physical activity promotion strategies. However, in their study such strategies might contribute only an additional 0.2 % to overall physical activity levels of adults.

Interventions in the Health Care Setting

These interventions attempt to increase the awareness of patients about the importance of regular physical activity through counseling by medical practitioners during ambulatory or outpatient care. Interventions in this category range from brief counseling sessions with sedentary/at-risk adults to more elaborate activities that may include a number of face-to-face or telephone counseling sessions combined with innovative motivators like "green prescriptions," which refer patients to exercise classes or gyms. Interventions in this category often resemble individual or group-based interventions. Beyond the investigation of effectiveness on physical activity levels and health parameters, studies often assess effects of interventions on the utilization of medical services and health care costs.

In 2002 a review of interventions in the health-care setting concluded that the evidence for their effectiveness is limited (Eden et al. 2002). The British National Institute for Health and Clinical Excellence (NICE 2006) has hinted that these interventions might produce at least short-term effects on physical activity, and the WHO (2009) does recommend them, especially if patients are directed by "green prescriptions" to providers of exercise classes or gyms.

Regarding their cost-effectiveness, Cobiac et al. (2009) concluded that referrals and exercise prescriptions given to sedentary adults by general practitioners might be cost-effective, but are still considered more costly when compared to mass-media campaigns or interventions that distribute pedometers to individuals. Hagberg and Lindholm (2006) concluded that healthcare-based interventions might be cost-effective among high-risk groups, but not necessarily among groups whose only risk factor is that they are sedentary. Garrett et al. (2011) stated that interventions that are rather brief and make referrals to exercise groups that do not require highly qualified supervision/instruction are more likely to be cost-effective.

Policy and Environmental Interventions

Intervention strategies in this category are diverse. Most reviews on the subject incorporate interventions that create physical activity friendly policies and interventions that create physical activity friendly infrastructures into one category when investigating effectiveness. This approach may blur findings related to both intervention strategies.

In general, policy interventions develop and implement regulations or organizational rules in order to increase opportunities for individuals to be physically active (e.g., daily physical education lessons required by school curricula). These interventions are often performed within school or worksite settings, or at the community level. Environmental interventions are commonly aimed at building or providing access to infrastructures that support opportunities to engage in physical activity (e.g., building sidewalks, sports facilities). Building of such infrastructures also requires, at some point in the process, the making of policy decisions (e.g., devoting budget lines to built sidewalks) by different actors.

In general, the evaluation of effectiveness of interventions in this category leans on pre–post assessments of utilization or physical activity rates. In some instances, monitoring and documentation of utilized routines and practices have been used. Policy and environmental interven-

tions have been recommended as being effective in increasing physical activity by the CDC (Task Force on Community Preventive Services 2005), the WHO (2009), and NICE (2008). The WHO (2009) recommends this type of intervention, especially if infrastructures for physical activity at the community level are to be built.

To date, a limited amount of studies have investigated the cost-effectiveness of policy and environmental interventions. Müller-Riemenschneider et al. (2009) and Wu et al. (2011) give some indication that these interventions might be cost-effective. Guo and Gandavarapu (2010) have calculated that constructing sidewalks in an entire neighborhood would increase walking by 1.7 min per person per day, yielding a positive cost-to-benefit ratio of 1.87 over 10 years.

Overall, from a public health perspective, reported insights from reviews seem to be of limited help when attempting to identify promising intervention strategies to combat sedentary lifestyles. In our opinion, this might be due to two types of shortcomings: (1) those associated with the process of conducting intervention effectiveness studies and (2) those associated with the process of conducting systematic reviews of such studies. We propose that some of these shortcomings may be overcome if the following five activities are performed during various phases of intervention development, implementation, and evaluation:

1. Analyze and report the broader context within which an intervention study took place and how this context might have affected outputs and outcomes of the study.

   At this point in time, available literature on intervention studies devotes very little attention to the broader context under which studies were conducted. In our opinion, however, arriving at an understanding of context is of high importance in relation to evaluating the overall effectiveness and potential for transfer of interventions. Contextual determinants of effectiveness might operate on individual, social, organizational, community; or broader cultural, political, and environmental levels. Health behavior interventions, and especially interventions for the promotion of physical activity, might be very vulnerable to these contextual features. As such it might be of limited value to assess the effects of an intervention without a thorough understanding of the context within which it took place.

2. Provide a detailed description of dominant and subdominant intervention strategies and their political and environmental components.

At this point in time, available intervention studies and reviews of intervention studies utilize very different typologies to distinguish between different intervention strategies. Often, these typologies are composed of a mix of intervention strategies that focus on changing physical activity behavior, settings where interventions take place, and physical activity rates among target groups (e.g., WHO 2008a). This holds particularly true when it comes to policy and environmental approaches to physical activity promotion. In our opinion, there is an urgent need to develop a consistent typology that differentiates between commonly utilized intervention strategies. Such a typology must consider that each intervention strategy features at least some political and/or environmental components.

3. Conduct a broad evaluation of outputs and outcomes of the intervention strategy, with specific consideration of effects on health disparities and cost-effectiveness.

At this point in time, available intervention studies most often focus on reporting proximate outputs. This might be due to the fact that proximate outputs (e.g., increased levels of physical activity, increased aerobic capacity) are fairly easy to assess, given the time constraints that most studies face, in comparison to assessing more distal outputs (e.g., worksite continues to offer exercise classes to employees beyond study realm) and outcomes (e.g., health effects associated with participating in exercise classes). From a public health perspective, however, a focus on proximate outputs might limit insights into the potential of an intervention to be broadly disseminated. We would thus suggest, that intervention studies utilize available frameworks such as RE-AIM (Glasgow et al. 1999) to assess

broader outputs and outcomes. Importantly, applying such frameworks fosters analysis of the "reach" that interventions have and how that relates to their impacts on health inequalities and cost-effectiveness.

4. Analyse and report the potential of the intervention strategy to be disseminated and transferred broadly.

At this point in time, available intervention studies seem to devote little attention to the potential of a given intervention to be transferred to other sites and to be disseminated broadly. In our opinion, more detailed accounts of the contexts under which interventions take place, the dominant intervention strategies that are utilized, and a broad examination of the outputs and outcomes achieved by them might allow for more accurate assessments of their potential for transfer. Further, intervention studies need to address the issue of adapting interventions before being transferred. From a strict methodological viewpoint, adaptations of interventions automatically raise the issue of whether or not they are still effective. Also, adoption of interventions to other sites or settings without adjustments to different contextual factors might be, from a public health perspective, rather unrealistic. This is especially true for policy and environmental interventions, and improved insights about their transferability would be highly valuable.

5. Theory-based planning, implementation, and transfer of intervention strategies.

At this point in time, intervention studies rarely utilize theoretical models or frameworks that go beyond the individual level. In our opinion, there is an urgent need to develop and use theories that enable researchers to untangle the many determinants that might impact the effectiveness of a given intervention. The development of such theories would improve understanding of how contextual determinants might affect processes, outputs, and outcomes associated with interventions, which can result in improved intervention transferability. Such theories may also prove to be vital in assessing, for example, the potential of an intervention to be implemented as intended, to be sustained by an organization, or to be disseminated to other organizations or settings.

There are guidelines that stress the importance of using a broader public health perspective when evaluating the effectiveness of behavioral interventions (e.g., Armstrong et al. 2007). To our knowledge, however, such guidelines are rarely used when evaluating intervention studies for physical activity promotion, or drafting reviews on the subject. Giving consideration to the valuable potential that policy and environmental interventions have in promoting physical activity, we now present a model that can assist in analyzing different intervention strategies with respect to the relationship between their behavioral components on one hand and their policy and environmental components on the other.

Theoretical Model on the Interplay of Structure and Agency in Physical Activity Promotion

The emergence of the concept of HEPA (Health Enhancing Physical Activity, see e.g., Pate et al. 1995) in the mid-1990s sparked a new discussion about the focus of physical activity promotion. The new concept directed researchers' attention to "any form of physical activity that benefits health and functional capacity without undue harm or risk" (Foster 2000). Consequently, the scope of fields considered relevant to physical activity promotion was expanded beyond sport to include a number of broader domains, such as leisure-time, transportation, occupational/work and household. Endeavors to design adequate interventions (e.g., building bike lanes to promote human-powered transport) raised questions about how to foster environmental changes in physical activity promotion (Owen et al. 2004) and how to design policy interventions (Matsudo et al. 2004).

At the same time, in other areas of health promotion (in particular smoking prevention), the public health potential of policy and environmental approaches became quite evident, and the utilization of such approaches in physical activity promotion was highly recommended (King et al. 1995).

Besides stimulating investigations of the evidence base of policy and environmental approaches in the area of physical activity promotion (as mentioned above), this development also led to an increasing interest in putting traditional behavioral models of physical activity into broader social, environmental, and political contexts.

In particular, ecological health promotion models (e.g., Dahlgren and Whitehead 1992; Stokols 1992) became a frequently used frame of reference for demonstrating the relationship between physical activity behavior, environment, and policy (Sallis and Owen 1999). For example, Sallis et al. (2006, p. 300ff) developed a multilevel model of physical activity indicating "multiple levels of influences" between intrapersonal (e.g., biological) determinants, perceived environment (e.g., perceived crime rate), behavior (e.g., active transport), behavioral settings (e.g., neighborhood), policy environment (e.g., transport investments), and the natural, social-cultural, and information environment. Schmid et al. (2006) also followed ecological health promotion approaches but developed a more "simple model" in order to describe "relationships among policy, the environment, behavior, and health" (p. 20). According to Schmid et al. (2006, p. 21ff), their model—as well as other ecological models—can help to investigate a "causal chain" in which policy influences the built environment, which in turn influences behavior and, subsequently, health.

While the above-mentioned models aim at providing a framework for conceptualizing and organizing physical activity promoting policy interventions (Schmid et al. 2006, p. 23) or illustrating "the roles numerous disciplines can play in research on active living" (Sallis et al. 2006, p. 300), they are neither explicitly theory-based nor particularly focused on theory-building. Thus, there is a need to develop adequate theoretical models to further our theoretical understanding of the relationship between policy, the environment, and physical activity. In particular, such models should provide (1) a theory-based description of their distinct elements and (2) a theory-based description of the relationship between these elements. Moreover, in order to serve as a theory-based framework for physical activity promotion, it should provide (3) a sound explanation of how and why any given current relationship between policy, the environment, and physical activity might be subject to change. In the following sections, we describe such a theoretical framework, which is based on a comprehensive theory on the interplay between structure and agency in health promotion (Rütten and Gelius 2011). This framework builds on elements from different theories that are relevant to our multilevel model and explores potential relationships among these elements.

Theoretical Framework: Structure and Agency

In the social sciences, there has been a long-standing dispute between proponents of structuralist approaches and advocates of action theory. In public health, this controversy recently resurfaced in the discourse about the "inequality paradox," which, as some argue, is created by certain kinds of health promotion interventions (Allebeck 2008; Frohlich and Potvin 2008, 2010; McLaren et al. 2010). The debate also drew attention back to the most famous theoretical endeavor to link the concepts of "structure" and "agency": Anthony Giddens' theory of structuration (1984).

In his seminal work Giddens attempted to overcome the fundamental shortcomings of two opposing approaches in the social sciences: the structuralist approach, which tends to neglect the efficacy of human action in shaping structures, and the individualistic approach, which is prone to underestimate the efficacy of structures in shaping human action (e.g., Giddens 1984, 207ff).

According to Giddens' theory, human agency implies more than just "acting." It involves being knowledgeable about the rules that govern social interaction. By acting according to these rules, individuals contribute to the reproduction of the structures they live in. Structures, on the other hand, are "both the medium and the outcome" of the practices that constitute social systems (Giddens 1984, p. 25), i.e. they are both the result of human agency and the framework within which

human agency takes place. Giddens calls this twofold character the "duality of structure." He also underlines the point that structures do not always restrain people's actions. They can, in fact, also be enabling. As the mutual reinforcement of structure and agency is a process, Giddens terms his approach "theory of structuration."

Structure itself consists of two components: rules and resources, or "rule-resource sets" (Giddens 1984, p. 377). Rules are generalizable procedures in the reproduction of social life, composed of both formal regulations and informal conventions that govern everyday life. Resources are "sources of power" (Sewell 1992, p. 9), i.e. the means by which social interaction is executed. Resources may either be "authoritative" (power over people), or "allocative" (power over objects, Giddens 1984, p. 33).

As a matter of fact, both structural and agentic approaches are genuine perspectives inherent to health promotion. On the one hand, the very concept of health promotion is originally based on a fundamental critique of approaches focusing on individual lifestyles and health education. Instead, health promotion approaches emphasize the importance of the "structure" of lifestyle, i.e. the social conditions that affect individuals' daily life conduct (Anderson 1984; Kickbusch 1986; Rütten 1995; Wenzel 1983, pp. 1–18; also see the recent discussion on the social determinants of health, e.g., in WHO 2008b). On the other hand, the Ottawa Charter (WHO 1986) defines five key domains of health promotion in a way that clearly refers to agency (*building* healthy public policy, *creating* supportive environments, *strengthening* community action, *developing* personal skills, and *re-orientating* health care services).

Integrating a Concept of Structural Change

As authors such as Sewell (1992) and Archer (1995) have argued, one of the major drawbacks of Giddens' work is that he does not fully recognize the potential for structural change. Even though he emphasizes that structuration is a process, his main focus is on the constant reproduction of structures through agency, which leads to stasis rather than to change. But if there were nothing but constant reproduction, the implication for health promotion would be that any attempt to change "unhealthy" structures (e.g., related to unhealthy environments and policies or to unhealthy behaviors) would necessarily be futile.

In her "realist social theory," Archer (1995) presents an approach to conceptualizing processes of change related to structure and agency. Her critique focuses on the "central conflation" approach in Giddens's structuration model because of its reduced perspective on the "mutual constitution" (1995, p. 87) of structure and agency. Compared to the "limited time span" of conflation theories, Archer's own "morphogenetic approach" to structure and agency attempts to cover the full "timescale through which structure and agency themselves *emerge, intertwine* and *redefine* one another" (Archer 1995, p. 76). Thus, Archer's morphogenetic model has a particular focus on possibilities for change.

Sewell's (1992) critique is less fundamental and may, rather be conceptualized as a "reformulation" of Giddens's theory. Sewell's main interest is to integrate possibilities of change into the structure-agency model. After re-defining some of Giddens' concepts (including the substitution of the term "schemas" for Giddens' "rules"), he introduces five "axioms" to explain how the interaction of structure and agency can lead to structural change. Sewell's definition of "agency" goes beyond the reinforcement of existing structures and points to the ability of actors to draw on patterns of action they already know from other settings when trying to handle new situations. This *transposability* of schemas (e.g., of etiquette) is one opportunity for structural change. Transposability is closely connected to another axiom, namely the *multiplicity* of structures in which actors are embedded. Individuals act in various structures, e.g., in the family, at school, at the workplace, in the circle of their friends, in voluntary associations, and vis-à-vis public authorities. Change may also be brought about by the *unpredictability of resource accumulation*,

i.e. by the fact that transposing schemas from one structure to another may either lead to an increase or a loss of resources (Sewell 1992, p. 18). Another opportunity for structural change is related to the fact that structures do not simply exist side by side but often overlap. An example from everyday life for this *intersection* of structures could be an individual's school or workplace environment, which contains structures of formal education or of working relations as well as structures of private relations and friendships. Sewell's fifth axiom is the *polysemy of resources,* which holds that resources are subject to different interpretations by different agents. The prevailing interpretation will influence which schemas will be replicated and how the position of the agents involved may be altered.

Integrating the Policy Dimension

While there are references to policy in the discourse on structure and agency, this dimension has not been systematically integrated into the model. For example, in his considerations on the "forms of institutions," Giddens introduces a classification of institutional orders (1984, p. 31ff), allocating, among others, specific structures—and thus specific sets of rules and resources—to political institutions. However, he has general reservations about making clear-cut distinctions between the different institutional spheres and therefore remains rather vague on this point. Thus, he scarcely provides a starting-point for a concrete operationalization of the interplay between structure and agency in policy-making. This may also be one reason why this level has seldom been considered when applying Giddens' theory to health promotion. As has been suggested in the recent discourse on policy analysis in health promotion (Bernier and Clavier 2011; Rütten et al. 2011), using approaches from political science may be a fruitful way to conceptualize policy processes.

A particularly helpful multilevel theory of policy-making is Elinor Ostrom's (2007) "Institutional Rational Choice" or "Institutional

Analysis and Development" (IAD) framework. A crucial aspect of the IAD framework is the concept of different levels of action. The major levels identified by Ostrom are (1) the operational level (e.g., everyday life of individuals, working level of organizations), (2) the collective choice level, which includes more formal settings (e.g., legislatures, regulatory agencies, and courts) as well as informal arenas (e.g., gatherings, appropriation teams, and private associations) and (3) the constitutional level (with the potential addition of an even more basic metaconstitutional level, Ostrom 2007, p. 46). Of particular interest to the context of health promotion are the "collective choice level," where health promotion policy is made, and the "operational level," where individual health behavior occurs. In Ostrom's view, the different levels build upon each other, and more basic levels influence structures and actions on more specific levels by determining how their rules can be altered.

Ostrom (2007, p. 44) argues that there is a multiplicity of action arenas that are "nested" within each other (a notion similar to Sewell's idea of the multiplicity and intersection of structures), and that this nesting may occur either at the same level or between levels. For example, in their everyday lives, individual actors usually take part in multiple action arenas on the operational level (e.g., family, school, work), but at the same time, they may also be involved in action arenas on the collective-choice level (e.g., as voters in an election).

Upon closer examination, one can find several interesting links to Giddens in Ostrom's approach: Her notion of action arenas also combines structural and agentic aspects, although this link is not her major theoretical concern. There are also some interesting similarities between the concepts used by the two authors, for example concerning their notions of rules. On a general level, it might be rewarding to attempt to combine the two frameworks into a full-scale, unified approach that includes the duality of structure and the idea of action arenas. We outline some potential starting points for such an endeavor in the conclusion of this paper.

Based on these considerations, we present a multilevel model as shown in Fig. 9.1.[1] It uses the general framework provided by Giddens, with additions from Sewell and Ostrom. At the core are Giddens' dual, mutually reinforcing constructs of structure and agency. At the operational level, agency refers to actors' capabilities to engage in physical activity. We use the term "capabilities" here, which according to Giddens' original approach (1984, p. 14) means "to be able to 'act otherwise.'" This term is closely related to his concept of power as "transformative capacity" (p. 15) and of "resources" as "media through which power is exercised" (p. 16). "Structure" at the operational level refers (1) to (actors') "allocative resources," e.g., available environments, infrastructures, offers, and programs for physical activity practice, as well as to (actors') "authoritative resources," e.g., interpersonal or organizational support for physical activity practice. It is also relates to (2) "rules," e.g., rules of access and rules of conduct for physical activity practice. The arrows between structure and agency indicate that the two presuppose each other: This may be interpreted either in Giddens' original sense, i.e. that there is mutual reinforcement and thus structural stability, or following Sewell, for whom this duality provides several "entry lanes" for change.

---

[1]In a previous work (Rütten and Gelius 2011), we have outlined how our multi-level model on the interplay of structure and agency can be related to the central claims of the Ottawa Charter (WHO 1986), i.e. "build healthy public policy", "create supportive environments", "strengthen community actions", and "develop personal skills". This approach was helpful to demonstrate the specific fruitfulness of the model for health promotion theory development. But given the particular focus of this chapter it need to be advanced with respect to at least two aspects: (1) the central claims of the Ottawa Charter are not theory-based in a strict sense (i.e. they are not explicitly derived from theory). Therefore, an advanced model should use theoretical terms that are in line with our theoretical framework. (2) An adequate theoretical model for this the context of this book should consider specificities of physical activity promotion.

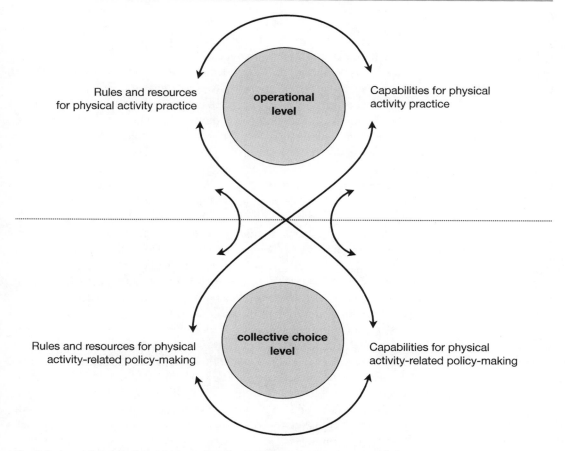

Fig. 9.1 A multilevel model of the interplay of structure and agency in physical activity promotion

To give an example, access rules to public gyms in Germany favor schools and sport clubs. Accordingly, physical activity practice in this context is characterized by physical education and institutionally organized sport activities produced and reproduced by sport club members. Those who are not members of these institutions—potentially because they prefer other forms of physical activity practice—are disadvantaged. However, they, too, are part of these mechanisms of production and reproduction, as their nonuse of these facilities stabilizes the status quo. Nonetheless, actors may also have transformative capabilities to change this situation. For example, nonmembers may be willing and able to become a member of a sport club and begin to benefit from the allocative and authoritative resources related to this status. Moreover, this might put them in a position to influence the rules of conduct within sport clubs practice by lobbying for their preferences. Other actors with transformative capacities may act "from without" and try to change rules of access to public gyms. However, any intended changes regarding the rules at the operational level automatically involve collective choice situations, which take us to the second level of the model.

On the collective choice level, agency refers to capabilities for policy-making, i.e. options of exercising power in collective choice situations that deal with operational rules and resources for physical activity practice. Again, such capabilities are related to structure, but in this case to those at the collective choice level, i.e. to rules and resources of policy-making. For example, certain rules of access and conduct may strictly prescribe which actors are allowed to participate in a collective choice process (e.g., in parliament) and how, exactly, decisions are made in this process. Allocative resources in this context may refer to goods and services, e.g., scientific advice that may be used by policy-makers, while authoritative resources reflect the political power of actors to be supported by other policymakers in order to determine decisions according to their own belief system.

For example, in Germany there exist certain access rules to public sport committees at local, regional, and national levels. Access to these important formal policy arenas is mainly limited to elected politicians, but especially in local contexts, representatives of sport clubs are also included. In addition, politicians who join public sport committees are often board members of sport clubs as well. Thus, the agenda of these committees and their rules of conduct are "biased" in favor of collective choice situations and decisions dealing with sport club affairs (e.g., rules for funding of sport clubs programs and infrastructures). Political capabilities of sport club representatives in public sport committees refer to *authoritative* resources (support by politicians), e.g., based on the political influence of sport club members as voters. In addition, sport club representatives exert political power in public sport committees through *allocative* resources, e.g., technical data on the use of sport facilities that may support political decisions in favor of certain operational rules. Consequently, in the face of the dominant role of sport clubs issues, operational rules, and resources related to other physical activity practices are often neglected, and respective stakeholders are not involved.

Again, the production and reproduction of collective choice processes as indicated in the examples above may be relatively stable over time, but nonetheless it is sensitive to change. Their transformative capabilities may allow some actors to become members of the collective choice processes, e.g., by getting elected as politicians or being nominated as sport club representatives, while other actors' capabilities may

focus on changing access rules. This, then, would refer to an additional, even more basic level of Ostrom's IAD model, the constitutional level.

Considering Ostrom's levels is important for two reasons. To begin with, as has been noted above, it allows for systematic consideration of the policy dimension, which is widely neglected by Giddens' original concept. We can thus theorize about physical promotion interventions that do not (or do not exclusively) take place at the operational level of physical activity behavior and the related environment but also in the field of policy-making (collective choice level). Second, we can now begin to see the connection between the two levels: Policies may reinforce or change structures at the operational level. For example, they may influence the rule-resource sets related to a specific context of physical activity and environment. Vice versa, the population's physical activity behavior may influence the rule-resource sets related to a specific policy context. For example, increased involvement in physical activity at the operational level may increase the participation of different stakeholders in the policy-making process. Moreover, such processes may ultimately result in changes in policy structures, i.e. modified procedures of policy-making and resource allocation.

It should be noted here that the idea of two clear-cut levels and only two action arenas is a radical simplification of *reality*. In the real world, there are usually multiple action arenas (e.g., parliament, policy-making of federal governments, physical activity promotion projects, and communities of people). In addition, the hierarchy in which these arenas are related to each other may be rather complex. Meanwhile, some might claim that our model is also a simplification of health promotion *theory*. As a matter of fact, there are theories more elaborate and detailed than any of the individual aspects of our model, e.g., the capabilities approach (Abel and Frohlich 2011; Sen 1985) or specific theories of the policy process (Rütten et al. 2011; Sabatier 2007). However, the strength of the model lies in its ability to connect all these categories with each other in a meaningful way, an issue that is not raised by other approaches. In addition, the model provides us with an effective link between Giddens' idea of the duality of structure, Sewell's account for the possibility of structural change, and Ostrom's levels of action. It also proposes a systematic way to theorize about how structure and agency at the various levels may interact in physical activity promotion to shape public health outcomes. In the following two sections, we will use two case examples to illustrate how structure and agency interact both on and between the operational and policy levels in different kinds of physical activity promotion interventions. The two cases also serve to point to some important differences between activities at the local and the regional/national level.

Case Study at the Local Level: BIG

"BIG—Movement as an investment for health" is an evidence-based approach to promoting physical activity with women in difficult life situations (Frahsa et al. 2011; Röger et al. 2011; Rütten et al. 2008, 2009, 2010). The BIG Project (BIG is the German acronym for "Movement as an Investment for Health") was originally a university-led health promotion action research project conducted in the German city of Erlangen between 2005 and 2008. It aimed to develop innovative means of physical activity promotion for women in difficult life situations (e.g., women with an immigrant background, recipients of social welfare, or single mothers), in three different settings (neighborhood, worksite, sports club). In 2009, the City of Erlangen took over responsibility for the project. Meanwhile, the project has also been transferred to other municipalities in Germany. Currently, each week more than 800 women in ten municipalities take part in BIG activities.

Instead of aiming at behavior change through ready-made interventions, BIG builds upon WHO's *Assets for Health* movement (Morgan et al. 2010; Morgan and Ziglio 2007) and uses a participatory approach called cooperative planning (Rütten 2001). Cooperative planning works with the principle of shared decision-making, which takes place in meetings facilitated and moderated by the research team. Women in difficult life situations, local policymakers, professionals, and researchers participate on equal footing in planning, implementing, sustaining, and evaluating physical activity promotion actions. Acknowledging the individual, educational, social, policy, and environmental dimensions of physical activity, BIG Erlangen implemented low-fee exercise classes that featured accompanying child care in a nearby neighborhood facility, women-only indoor pool hours, swimming classes for women-only, project offices to organize exercise classes run by the women themselves, a special exercise instructor training for women in difficult life situations, and the creation of a municipal coordination job position to sustain and institutionalize the BIG program. Evaluation of the project included assessments of the implementation of project activities (Rütten et al. 2008, 2010), the reach of project activities, potential changes in health behavior, potential health benefits, and potential social, political, and economical impacts. Consequently, being both a policy- and environmental-oriented approach and as one that aims at individual behavior modification and participants' empowerment, BIG is a good case example for the interplay of structure and agency at both the collective choice and operational levels.

The situation in Erlangen was characterized by stasis on both levels at the start of the project. On the operational level, many of the women in difficult life situations later involved in the project had predominantly inactive behaviors and were heavily focused on the structural barriers preventing a change of these behaviors. Women from the neighborhood were interested in engaging in affordable activities located within walking distance at familiar locations. They remained inactive, mainly because they had no adequate physical activity opportunities, especially due to a lack of access to sport facilities, affordable classes, and adequate childcare.

On the collective choice level, policy rules and resources were inappropriate. Women in difficult life situations tend not to form a coherent or even organized group of voters; they tend to be of minor relevance to most policymakers. Instead, local policy initiatives for physical activity promotion focused mainly on health sport offers of sport clubs. However, as most women of the BIG target group were not sport club members, their interests were not cared for. Representatives of sports clubs in municipal sport councils, etc., would (at best) try to integrate these women into existing sport club offers but would not want to give up their own privileges (access only for sport clubs to public school gyms in the afternoon and evening). Another issue might be that the women from the neighborhood who lobbied strongest for the elementary school to host BIG activities were women with a Muslim background. Usually, their men handle "public affairs," including interaction with the authorities, meaning that the women had not been able to voice their demand in the past.

The process of cooperative planning, however, created a new action situation in which the women involved were equal partners with community representatives (the mayor, the head of the sport authority, members of the city council, etc.). This new structure increased the women's capabilities to bring forth their requests. Mapping assets in the neighborhood at individual, organizational, and infrastructural levels was a crucial component of BIG (Rütten et al. 2009). The gym of the neighborhood elementary school was the most often mentioned and most discussed infrastructural asset by the cooperative planning group, representing a potentially supportive resource at the operational level. These discussions helped meeting participants understand current policy regulations associated with access to public spaces and how to bring about the changes required to be able to promote physical activity in the BIG Erlangen context, i.e. at the collective choice level through adjusted policy rules on access to sport facilities. The women themselves also represented a major asset. Participation in cooperative planning allowed their voices to be heard and their true needs to be understood by policymakers who had rarely interacted with these women in the past. The women continuously put issues of access to facilities in the neighborhood on the agenda of the cooperative planning meetings. However, plans to use the gym of the elementary school challenged existing policy regulations. City of Erlangen regulations restricted access to public sport facilities to institutional use by schools (during the day) and registered sports clubs (late afternoon, evening). The possibilities for other groups to make use of the elementary school sports facilities were therefore limited. To bring about the intended change of the environment, additional action on the policy dimension was necessary. Some of the policymakers, drawing on their experience from other policy issues (transposability of schemas), were able to overcome political resistance (e.g., in sport council). Through direct negotiations with professionals from the BIG sports club setting, they managed to create free hours at the gym. Additionally, they involved a different organization, the adult education center, in the hosting of BIG activities. The center represented a familiar (e.g., from language classes and family trainings) and affordable (course-based activities rather than annual membership fees) institution. By doing so, BIG participants from the political level did not overrule existing rules at the municipality but initiated a process of adapting them. They broadened regulations by allowing access to organizations other than sports clubs, i.e. the adult education center. This approach created less opposition than an attempt to abolish existing regulations would have caused and thus increased capacities for physical activity promotion.

Beyond the changes on the collective choice level, additional transfer back to the operational level took place for BIG participants. Women who had been involved in the planning process reported afterwards that they were now more self-confident when dealing with local authorities, e.g., going on errands at city hall themselves instead of sending their husbands (Röger et al. 2011). Another effect was the establishment of exercise classes at that gym, which, in turn, seems to have increased the participants' self-efficacy with respect to other forms of physical activity (for example, the women also reported an increase in walking and they demanded and participated in BIG classes to learn how to bicycle around the neighborhood).

Policymakers and professionals showed increased understanding of women's needs and obligations as well newly perceived competences in shared decision-making and intersectoral action (Frahsa et al. 2012). This fed back again to changing rules and resources for PA related collective choices, represented in a successful city council initiative by BIG policymakers to create an intersectoral position at the municipality to coordinate BIG Erlangen, providing increased and sustainable capabilities at the collective choice level as well.

BIG highlights that rules and resources as well as capacities for PA practices and PA related collective choice cannot be looked at from an additive perspective only. The interplay of structure and agency in BIG shows that a *resource for physical activity practice* (the elementary school gym) at the operational level in some cases can only be identified through *capabilities for PA practice* (women's demands to use that gym for their physical activities). However, only through interaction with the collective choice level could the resources be made accessible: *capabilities for PA policymaking* (represented through women's, policymakers' and professionals' agency in cooperative planning) were critical to changing existing rules for *PA related collective choices* (municipal access regulations with regard to public sport facilities). Only through these constant and repeating interactions, was the resource for physical active practice.(the gym), turned into a sustainable asset for women's physical activity in BIG Erlangen.

Case Study at the Regional Level: PASEO

The PASEO Project ("Building Policy Capacities for Health Promotion through Physical Activity among Sedentary Older People") was funded by the Health Programme of the European Union from 2009 to early 2011 (Rütten and Gelius, 2013). The project's intent was to build capacities for health promotion in 15 European nations, thus contributing to improved physical activity promotion for older people. The ADEPT model (Rütten et al. 2011) was used to conceptualize capacities. According to the model, capacities are comprised of goals, obligations, resources, and opportunities related to physical activity promotion.

The overall design of PASEO involved four main project phases based on the concept of cooperative planning (Rütten 2001). In each country, the scientific partner started by teaming up with a large NGO or governmental organization, thus adding "political" credibility to the project work and tapping additional resources for the ensuing planning process (e.g., communication channels, meeting venues). In the second phase, both partners approached relevant organizations from the sport, healthcare, social care, and other sectors in order to engage them as partners for the planned alliance. In the third phase, the alliances conducted a planning process, moderated by the scientific partner, to build new policy capacities. In the final phase of the project, alliance partners moved on to implement the measures developed in the planning phase. This would contribute to capacity building either directly (for example if measures tackle networking, goal definitions, resource allocation, and staff training) or indirectly (e.g., through pilot projects on specific topics, which in turn would improve capacities).

Across the 15 nations taking part in the project, PASEO involved more than 130 organizations from all sectors, including national and regional ministries from Finland, France, Bavaria, Extremadura, Flanders, and Vienna. One hundred fourteen specific measures were developed to improve capacities, including dissemination and networking activities, staff training, infrastructures, and pilot projects.

PASEO may serve as a point in case for the duality of structure and agency. At the same time, experience from the project sheds new light on the interaction between the operational level and the various collective choice arenas at regional, national, and international levels.

A comparison between the 15 countries participating in the project provides further insights for how the different political structures influenced how and at which level the alliances acted. While alliances were forged at the national level in more centralized states such as France, Norway, Sweden, Finland, and Lithuania, alliances in more federalist states such as Austria, Germany, Spain, and Belgium were established at the regional level. Likewise, the "developmental stage" of physical activity promotion for older people in the respective public health systems influenced the scope of the alliances' work: In Lithuania, where health enhancing physical activity (HEPA) policy is still in its infant stage, the alliance decided not to focus on the target group of older people alone but instead dealt with physical activity promotion for all population groups; in the Netherlands, where HEPA policy is well-advanced, the PASEO alliance was established as a sub-group to the existing "Fit for Life the Netherlands" alliance and focused on specific aspects of physical activity promotion for older people only.

By introducing a new form of practice (the cooperative planning process), PASEO influenced the interplay of structure and agency related to the organizations involved in the alliances. The practice involved both new rules (the concept as such) and resources (coordination activities of scientific partners and communication channels, venues, etc. provided by the collaborative partners). It brought together actors from different sectors (sport, healthcare, social care, tourism, etc.) that had not previously interacted concerning the issue of physical activity promotion for older people. A particularly interesting cooperation was the one between policy-makers and researchers, who were enabled by the cooperative planning concept to engage in a process of knowledge exchange and translation (see Rütten and Gelius, 2013; Rütten et al. 2013). Other important goals were to identify new resources for physical activity promotion among older people and to create new structures by turning the project alliances into sustainable institutions.

It is interesting to note, however, that both the process and the outputs/outcomes of the alliances differed significantly in all participating countries although all of them used the same structure of cooperative planning. Alliance sizes ranged from 3 (Portugal) to 20 (France), while the number of meetings held varied between 3 (France, Greece, Netherlands, Spain) and 7 (Belgium). Likewise, action plans varied significantly in length, scope, and kinds of measures taken. One important explanation for this is that different actors were involved in all countries, choosing different courses of action from the options they were given. Another factor are the different structures that surrounded PASEO, i.e. the national health promotion policy contexts (see Rütten et al. 2013). From this angle, PASEO may be viewed as a "natural experiment" (Yin 2009) in which the same intervention is implemented in varying contexts, leading to different outcomes.

The cooperative planning process influenced the interplay of structure and agency on the collective choice level in the participating countries. In Flanders, the regional Ministry of Health and the Ministry of Sport used the PASEO alliance as an instrument to coordinate all their activities in the field of physical activity promotion for older people. In Vienna and Finland, the respective Ministries of Health published the action plans of the PASEO alliances, thus establishing them as new players in the respective public health landscape. In Lithuania, the PASEO alliance became the first ever HEPA-related forum to be established in the country, and continues to influence policy-making on the subject, e.g., through initiatives in the national parliament.

The outputs of the planning process were directed both at the collective choice and the operational levels. Part of the measures developed were concerned with activities at the collective choice level, such as networking and lobbying, the development of guidelines and concepts, staff training, research or information gathering, and workgroups. Other measures, by contrast, targeted a change of physical activity behavior among older people directly, e.g., via campaigns and events, infrastructure development, or by developing new physical activity interventions. Another way in which PASEO alliances tried to bridge potential gaps between decisions at the collective choice level and impacts at the operational level was to develop local pilot projects as part of their action plans, with an option for future dissemination in the entire region/nation. In general, however, the comparison between BIG and PASEO underlines that there may always be a certain tradeoff between reach on the one hand and input from the target group and effect size on the other when deciding to work on the local or regional/national level, respectively.

Conclusion

The purpose of this chapter has been to give an overview of evidence on existing physical activity promotion strategies, contribute to the development of theories that expand our focus beyond the individual level, take into account the interaction between the environment, policy, and physical activity, and provide insights about such interactions based on actual research projects.

In the first section, we reviewed some of the existing evidence relating to physical activity promotion intervention strategies. We pointed out that beyond their effectiveness to increase physical activity levels, their cost-effectiveness, ability to reduce health inequalities, and their transferability, should also be considered. While we note that there is at least some evidence to support the effectiveness of all major intervention types (including individual and group-based interventions, community-based interventions, mass media campaigns, interventions in the health-care setting, and policy/environmental interventions), this evidence is far from comprehensive or conclusive. We have, therefore argued that future studies should include an in-depth analysis of intervention contexts as well as improved methodologies for describing interventions and evaluating their outputs, outcomes, and transferability. In addition, there is an urgent need to develop and utilize theories that go beyond dynamics that occur at the individual level and enable us to untangle the many determinants that influence the effectiveness of interventions.

The second part of this chapter presented a theoretical model that might help overcome some of the challenges researchers face when they conduct intervention studies for physical activity promotion. The model can also be used to help researchers understand the relationship between the environment, policy, and physical activity. Essentially, the model's multilevel design represents the integration of the concepts of structure and agency—two basic perspectives of health promotion. This approach is built on Giddens' theory of structuration but also draws on Sewell's additions, which more fully acknowledge and accept the possibilities where structural change is concerned. The model also incorporates Ostrom's notions of different levels of action, particularly the operational level (where physical activity practice occurs) and the collective choice level (where physical activity-related policy-making takes place).

In the third part of this chapter, we presented two case studies for purposes of illustrating the cross-level interplay between structure and agency in health promotion. Presenting an example of creating access to a local gym for women in difficult life situations, the BIG project illustrated how a new structure (in the form of a co-operative planning group) that was introduced to a particular community facilitated change at both the collective choice and operational levels. This approach also resulted in changes to structures (e.g., new access rules) and capabilities (agency) of those individuals involved in the process (e.g., increased self-confidence and physical activity levels). The PASEO case study provided insights from national and regional levels of policy-making. Resembling a natural experiment, it illustrated how a standardized action introduced at the collective-choice level (the alliances' planning process) was shaped by varying structures in 15 different countries. At the same time, the structures provided by the project influenced both the agency of actors involved (e.g., cooperations between researchers and policy-makers) and other structures at this level (e.g., national policies). Finally, the experience from PASEO indicates that while action initiated at more basic collective choice levels (regional, national) may have direct or indirect impacts at the operational level, the interaction between levels is more difficult than in local projects such as BIG, where the collective-choice level is not so far removed from the operational level, i.e. from people's daily lives and their physical activity behavior.

While the two case studies underline the multiple and complex interactions between the operational and the collective-choice level, it should be noted that evidence-based research concerning these two levels may have to follow fundamentally different logics.

Most current research that investigates physical activity promotion in terms of its existence a public health issue focuses on the operational level. Essentially, it deals with behavioral change that is brought about through a variety of measures, ranging from individual and small group interventions to environmental approaches (e.g., Oja and Borms 2004). Additionally, it considers the impact of the collective choice level on the operational level. For example, as outlined above, policy interventions are common features in reviews of evidence-based interventions. One primary goal of such research is to evaluate whether or not interventions are effective in promoting physical activity, either directly (behavioral changes caused by new legislation) or indirectly (through funding other evidence-based interventions, e.g., environmental approaches) (see Kahn et al. 2002; WHO 2009, etc.). This traditional perspective is very useful to explain the direct relationship between a policy intervention and its public health outcome (e.g., increased levels of physical activity). However, it is less well suited to explain why a certain policy intervention has been developed and implemented in case A but not in case B. To do so, one requires specific knowledge about the processes, contexts, and determinants of policy development and policy implementation.

Currently, there is a lack of this kind of knowledge and of research that directly focuses on processes that are related to the collective choice level. For example, a recent review (Breton and De Leeuw 2010) indicates that there is a shortage of policy-oriented research in public health in general and of theory-based research in particular. Moreover, the discussion of evidence may differ fundamentally between the operational and the collective choice level, i.e. "what works" in public health is different from "what works" in policy-making (Rütten 2011).

As we suggest elsewhere (Rütten et al. 2013), an example of how to conceptualize the initial steps of an *issue* into the world of *policy-making* is provided by Peters (2005) "policy problem" approach. It allows us to explain how the characteristics of physical activity promotion as a public health issue are related to (1) its definition as a policy problem, (2) the framing of the problem within policy processes and (3) its intended solution using different policy instruments. Thus, while the traditional perspective is helpful for explaining the public health effects of certain policy instruments and interventions, this new perspective is key for explaining the policy effects of the public health issue when translated into a policy problem.

A final point requiring attention is the question of whether or not the theoretical considerations and results presented in this chapter can be applied to countries around the globe (including middle and low income countries), or if, like the two case examples, their applicability remains limited to the region of Europe. On the one hand, we believe that several of our central findings are so generic that they may be universally applied. For example, when designing or choosing interventions for physical activity promotion, researchers and practitioners all over the world should bear in mind that criteria for the success of interventions go beyond their mere "effectiveness" at increasing physical activity levels. In addition, in any conceivable physical activity promotion environment, one has to bear in mind the complex interplay between structure and agency as well as the interplay between operational and collective-choice levels. Any intervention that only addresses one aspect or one level is prone to be flawed. On the other hand, it will be necessary to closely investigate national (and, where necessary, also regional and local) contexts and policy processes. As the case of PASEO demonstrates, efforts to implement the same policy instrument in 15 different countries in the same region may already lead to vastly different results. Variance may be expected to be even greater for other world regions or for countries with substantially different developmental statuses. Ultimately, selecting appropriate interventions and policies and adapting existing ones to new contexts (Glasgow et al. 1999; Bowen et al. 2010; Wang et al. 2006) are questions of central importance when thinking about physical activity promotion from a global perspective.

References

Abel, T., & Frohlich, K. (2011). Capitals and capabilities: Linking structure and agency to reduce health inequalities. *Social Science & Medicine.* doi:10.1016/j.socscimed.2011.10.028.

Allebeck, P. (2008). The prevention paradox or the inequality paradox? *European Journal of Public Health, 18*(3), 115.

Anderson, R. (1984). Health promotion: An overview. In L. Baric (Ed.), *European monographs in health education research, no. 6* (p. 4e126). Edinburgh: Scottish Health Education Group.

Archer, M. S. (1995). *Realist social theory: The morphogenetic approach.* Cambridge: Cambridge University Press.

Armstrong, R., Waters, E., Jackson, N., Oliver, S., Popay, J., Shepherd, J., et al. (2007). *Guidelines for systematic reviews of health promotion and public health interventions. Version 2.* Melbourne: Melbourne University.

Ashworth, N. L., Chad, K. E., Harrison, E. L., Reeder, B. A., & Marshall, S. C. (2005). Home versus center based physical activity programs in older adults. *Cochrane Database of Systematic Reviews,* (1), CD004017. doi: 10.1002/14651858.CD004017.pub2.

Baker, P. R. A., Francis, D. P., Soares, J., Weightman, A. L., & Foster, C. (2011). Community wide interventions for increasing physical activity. *Cochrane Database of Systematic Reviews,* (4), CD008366. doi: 10.1002/14651858.CD008366.pub2.

Bernier, N., & Clavier, C. (2011). Public health policy research: Making the case for a political science approach. *Health Promotion International, 26*(1), 109–116.

Bowen, S. K., Saunders, R. P., Richter, D. L., Hussey, J., Elder, K., & Lindley, L. (2010). Assessing levels of adaptation during implementation of evidence-based interventions: Introducing the Rogers-Rütten framework. *Health Education & Behavior, 37,* 815–830.

Breton, E., & De Leeuw, E. (2010). Political theory in health promotion policy development and analysis: A review. *Health Promotion International.* doi:10.1093/heapro/daq051.

Cobiac, L. J., Vos, T., & Barendregt, J. J. (2009). Cost-effectiveness of interventions to promote physical activity: A modeling study. *PLoS Medicine, 6*(7), e1000110.

Coleman, K. J., Farrell, M. A., Rocha, D. A., Hayashi, T., Hernandez, M., Wolf, J., et al. (2012). Readiness to be physically active and self-reported physical activity in low-income Latinas, California WISEWOMAN, 2006–2007. *CDC—Preventing Chronic Disease.* doi: http://dx.doi.org/10.5888/pcd9.110190

Conn, V. S., Hafdahl, A. R., & Mehr, D. R. (2011). Interventions to increase physical activity among healthy adults: Meta-analysis of outcomes. *American Journal of Public Health.* doi:10.2105/AJPH.2010.194381.

Dahlgren, G., & Whitehead, M. (1992). *Policies and strategies to promote equity in health.* Copenhagen: WHO Regional Office for Europe, Document ID: EUR/ICP/RPD 414(2) 9866n.

Eden, K. B., Orleans, C. T., Mulrow, C. D., Pender, N. J., & Teutsch, S. M. (2002). Does counselling by clinicians improve physical activity? A summary of the evidence for the U.S. Preventive Services Task Force. *Annals of Internal Medicine, 137,* 208–215.

European Commission. (2010). *Sport and physical activity. Special Eurobarometer 334.* Brussels: TNS Opinion & Social.

Foster, C. (2000). *Guidelines for health-enhancing physical activity promotion programmes.* Tampere: UKK Institute. Retrieved June 26, 2012, from http://www.panh.ch/hepaeurope/materials/Guidelines%20HEPA%20Europe.pdf.

Foster, C., Hillsdon, M., Thorogood, M., Kaur, A., & Wedatilake, T. (2005). Interventions for promoting physical activity. *Cochrane Database of Systematic Reviews,* (1). doi:10.1002/14651858.CD003180.pub2.

Frahsa, A., Rütten, A., Abu-Omar, K., & Wolff, A. (2011). Movement as investment for health: Integrated evaluation in participatory physical activity promotion among women in difficult life situations. *Global Health Promotion, 18,* 31–33.

Frahsa, A., Rütten, A., Röger, U., Abu-Omar, K., & Schow, D. (2012). *Enabling the powerful? Participatory action research with local policymakers and professionals for physical activity promotion with women in difficult life situations.* Health Promotion International. doi:10.1093/heapro/das050.

Frohlich, K., & Potvin, L. (2008). The inequality paradox: The population approach and vulnerable populations. *American Journal of Public Health, 98*(2), 216–221.

Frohlich, K., & Potvin, L. (2010). Commentary: Structure or agency? The importance of both for addressing social inequalities in health. *International Journal of Epidemiology, 39,* 378–379.

Garrett, S., Elley, C. R., Rose, S. B., O'Dea, D., Lawtonet, A. B., & Dowell, A. C. (2011, March). Are physical activity interventions in primary care and the community cost-effective? *British Journal of General Practice, 61*(584), e125–e133.

Giddens, A. (1984). *The constitution of society: Outline of the theory of structuration.* Berkely, CA: University of California Press.

Glasgow, R. E., Vogt, T. M., & Boles, S. M. (1999). Evaluating the impact of health promotion interventions: The RE-AIM framework. *American Journal of Public Health, 89,* 1322–1327.

Graves, N., Barnett, A. G., Halton, K. A., Veerman, J. L., Winkler, E., Owen, N., et al. (2009). Cost-effectiveness of a telephone-delivered intervention for physical activity and diet. *PLoS One, 4*(9), e7135.

Guo, J. Y., & Gandavarapu, S. (2010). An economic evaluation of health-promotive built environment changes. *Preventive Medicine, 50*, S44–S49.

Hagberg, L. A., & Lindholm, L. (2006). Cost-effectiveness of healthcare-based interventions aimed at improving physical activity. *Scandinavian Journal of Public Health, 34*, 641–653.

IDF. (2009). *IDF diabetes atlas* (4th ed.). Brussels: Author.

Jepson, R. G., Harris, F. M., Platt, S., & Tannahill, C. (2010). The effectiveness of interventions to change six health behaviours: A review of reviews. *BMC Public Health, 10*, 538.

Kahn, E. B., Ramsey, L. T., Brownson, R. C., Heath, G. W., Howze, E. H., Powell, K. E., et al. (2002). The effectiveness of interventions to increase physical activity. A systematic review. *American Journal of Preventive Medicine, 22*(4S), 73–107.

Kickbusch, I. (1986). Life-styles and health. *Social Science & Medicine, 22*, 117–124.

King, A. C., Jeffery, R. W., Fridinger, F., Dusenbury, L., Provence, S., Hedlund, S. A., et al. (1995). Environmental and policy approaches to cardiovascular disease prevention through physical activity: Issues and opportunities. *Health Education Quarterly, 22*, 499–511.

Lowther, M., Mutrie, N., & Scott, E. M. (2002). Promoting physical activity in a socially and economically deprived community: A 12 month randomized control trial of fitness assessment and exercise consultation. *Journal of Sports Sciences, 20*(7), 577–588.

Luepker, R. V., Murray, D. M., Jacobs, D. R., Mittelmark, M. B., Bracht, N., Carlaw, R., et al. (1994). Community education for cardiovascular disease prevention: Risk factor change in the Minnesota Heart Health Program. *American Journal of Public Health, 84*, 1383–1393.

Matsudo, V., Guedes, J., Matsudo, S., Andrade, D., Araujo, T., Oliveira, L., et al. (2004). Policy intervention: The experience of Agita São Paulo in using 'Mobile Management' of the ecological model to promote physical activity. In P. Oja & J. Borms (Eds.), *Health enhancing physical activity* (pp. 427–444). Oxford: Meyer & Meyer Sport.

McLaren, L., McIntyre, L., & Kirkpatrick, S. (2010). Rose's population strategy of prevention need not increase social inequalities in health. *International Journal of Epidemiology, 39*, 378–379.

Morgan, A., Davies, M., & Ziglio, E. (Eds.). (2010). *Health assets in a global context. Theory, methods, action.* New York, NY: Springer.

Morgan, A., & Ziglio, E. (2007). Revitalising the evidence base for public health: An assets model. *Global Health Promotion, 14*(Suppl. 2), 17–22.

Müller-Riemenschneider, F., Reinhold, T., & Willich, S. N. (2009). Cost-effectiveness of interventions promoting physical activity. *British Journal of Sports Medicine, 43*, 70–76.

Munro, J., Brazier, J., Davey, R., & Nicholl, J. (1997). Physical activity for the over-65s: Could it be a cost-effective exercise for the NHS? *Journal of Public Health Medicine, 19*, 397–402.

National Center for Health Statistics. (2009). Percentage of adults aged ≥25 years who reported regular leisure-time physical activity, by education level—National Health Interview Survey, United States, 1997 and 2007. *Morbidity and Mortality Weekly Reports, 58*(10), 261.

National Centerfor Chronic Disease Prevention and Health Promotion. (2011). *Obesity—healing the epidemic by making health easier.* Atlanta, GA: National Center for Chronic Disease Prevention and Health Promotion.

NICE (2006). *Four commonly used methods to increase physical activity: Brief interventions in primary care, exercise referral schemes, pedometers and community-based exercise programmes for walking and cycling.* Public Health Intervention Guidance no. 2. London: National Institute for Health and Clinical Excellence.

NICE. (2008). *Promoting and creating built or natural environments that encourage and support physical activity.* NICE Public Health Guidance 8. London: National Institute for Health and Clinical Excellence.

Oja, P., & Borms, J. (Eds.). (2004). *Health enhancing physical activity.* Oxford: Meyer & Meyer Sport.

Ostrom, E. (2007). Institutional rational choice: An assessment of the institutional analysis and development framework. In P. A. Sabatier (Ed.), *Theories of the policy process* (pp. 21–64). Boulder, CO: Westview Press.

Owen, N., Humpel, N., Salmon, J., & Oja, P. (2004). Environmental influences on physical activity. In P. Oja & J. Borms (Eds.), *Health enhancing physical activity* (pp. 393–426). Oxford: Meyer & Meyer Sport.

Pate, R. R., Pratt, M., Blair, S. N., Haskell, W, L., Macera, C, A., Bouchard, C., et al. (1995). Physical activity and public health: A recommendation from the Centers for Disease Control and prevention and the American College of Sports Medicine. *Journal of the American Medical Association, 273*, 402–407.

Peters, G. B. (2005). The problem of policy problems. *Journal of Comparative Policy Analysis: Research and Practice.* doi:10.1080/13876980500319204.

Physical Activity Guidelines Advisory Committee. (2008). *Physical Activity Guidelines Advisory Committee Report.* Washington, DC: U.S. Department of Health and Human Services.

Prochaska, J. O., & DiClemente, C. C. (1983). Stages and processes of self-change in smoking: Towards an integrated model of change. *Journal of Consulting and Clinical Psychology, 51*, 390–395.

Röger, U., Rütten, A., Frahsa, A., Abu-Omar, K., & Morgan, A. (2011). Differences in individual empowerment outcomes of socially disadvantaged woman: Effects of mode of participation and structural changes in a physical activity promotion program. *International Journal of Public Health, 56*(5), 465–473.

Rütten, A. (1995). The implementation of health promotion: A new structural perspective. *Social Science & Medicine, 41*, 1627–1637.

Rütten, A. (2001). Evaluating healthy public policies in community and regional contexts. In I. Rootman, M. Goodstadt, B. Hyndman, D. V. McQueen, L. Potvin, J. Springett, & E. Ziglio (Eds.), *Evaluation in health promotion: Principles and perspectives* (WHO Regional Publications, European series, Vol. 92). Geneva: World Health Organization.

Rütten, A. (2011). Evidence-based policy revisited: Orientation towards the policy process and a public health policy science. *International Journal of Public Health*. doi:10.1007/s00038-011-0321-1.

Rütten, A., Abu-Omar, K., Gelius, P., & Schow, D. (2013). Physical inactivity as a policy problem: applying a concept from policy analysis to a public health issue. *Health Research Policy and Systems*, 11:9.

Rütten, A., Abu-Omar, K., Frahsa, A., & Morgan, A. (2009). Assets for policy-making in health promotion: Overcoming political barriers inhibiting women in difficult life situations to access sport facilities. *Social Science & Medicine, 69*, 1667–1673.

Rütten, A., Abu-Omar, K., Levin, L., Morgan, A., Groce, N., & Stuart, J. (2008). Research note: Social catalysts in health promotion implementation. *Journal of Epidemiology and Community Health, 62*, 560–565.

Rütten, A., Abu-Omar, K., Seidenstücker, S., & Mayer, S. (2010). Strengthening the assets of women living in disadvantaged situations: The German experience. In A. Morgan, M. Davies, & E. Ziglio (Eds.), *Health assets in a global context. Theory, methods, action* (pp. 197–221). New York, NY: Springer.

Rütten, A., & Gelius, P. (2011). Interplay of structure and agency. *Social Science & Medicine, 73*, 953–959.

Rütten, A., & Gelius, P. (2013). *Building policy capacities: an interactive approach for linking knowledge to action in health promotion.* Health Promotion International. doi:10.1093/heapro/dat006.

Rütten, A., Gelius, P., & Abu-Omar, K. (2011). Policy development and implementation in health promotion-from theory to practice: The ADEPT model. *Health Promotion International, 26*(3), 322–329.

Sabatier, P. A. (Ed.). (2007). *Theories of the policy process.* Boulder, CO: Westview Press.

Sallis, J. F., Cervero, R., Ascher, W. W., Henderson, K., Kraft, M. K., & Kerr, J. (2006). An ecological approach to creating active living communities. *Annual Review of Public Health, 27*, 297–322.

Sallis, J. F., & Owen, N. (1999). *Physical activity and behavioral medicine.* Thousand Oaks, CA: Sage.

Schmid, T. L., Pratt, M., & Witmer, L. (2006). A framework for physical activity policy research. *Journal of Physical Activity and Health, 3*, S20–S29.

Sen, A. (1985). *Commodities and capabilities.* Amsterdam: Elsevier.

Sewell, W. (1992). A theory of structure: Duality, agency, and transformation. *The American Journal of Sociology, 98*(1), 1–29.

Stokols, D. (1992). Establishing and maintaining healthy environments. Towards a social ecology of health promotion. *American Psychologist, 47*(1), 6–22.

Task Force on Community Preventive Services. (2005). Chapter 2. Physical activity. In S. Zaza, P. A. Briss, K. W. Harris (Eds.) *The Guide to community preventive services. What works to promote health?* New York: Oxford University Press.

Taylor, W. C., Baranowski, T., & Young, D. R. (1998). Physical activity interventions in low-income, ethnic minority, and populations with disability. *American Journal of Preventive Medicine, 15*, 334–343.

United Nations. (2011). *Prevention and control of noncommunicable diseases. Report of the Secretary-General. Follow-up to the outcome of the Millennium Summit.* New York: Author, Document Reference No. A/66/83.

Wakefield, M. A., Loken, B., & Hornik, R. C. (2010). Use of mass media campaigns to change behaviour. *The Lancet, 376*, 1261–1271.

Wang, S., Moss, J. R., & Hiller, J. E. (2006a). Applicability and transferability of interventions in evidence-based public health. *Health Promotion International, 21*(1), 76–83.

Wang, Y., Tussing, L., Odoms-Young, A., Braunschweig, C., Flay, B., Hedeker, D., et al. (2006b). Obesity prevention in low socioeconomic status urban African-american adolescents: Study design and preliminary findings of the HEALTH-KIDS Study. *European Journal of Clinical Nutrition, 60*(1), 92–103.

Wenzel, E. (1983). *Lifestyles and living conditions and their impact on health: A report of a meeting* (European monographs in health education research, Vol. 5). Edinburgh: SHEG.

WHO (1986). *Ottawa charter for health promotion.* Geneva: World Health Organization. Document Reference No. WHO/HPR/HEP/95.1.

WHO. (2008a). *Inequalities in young people's health. HBSC international report from the 2005/2006 survey.* Geneva: Author.

WHO. (2008b). *Closing the gap in a generation: Health equity through action on the social determinants of health. Final report of the commission on social determinants of health.* Geneva: Author.

WHO. (2009). *Interventions on diet and physical activity: What works.* Geneva: Author.

Wu, S., Cohen, D., Shi, Y., Pearson, M., & Sturm, R. (2011). Economic analysis of physical activity interventions. *American Journal of Preventive Medicine, 40*, 149–158.

Yancey, A. K., Ortega, A. N., & Kumanyika, S. K. (2006). Effective recruitment and retention of minority research participants. *Annual Review of Public Health, 27*, 1–28.

Yin, R. K. (2009). *Case study research: Design and methods.* Los Angeles, CA: Sage.

NGOs Addressing NCDs Through a Health Promotion Lens

Marie-Claude Lamarre and Lauren Weinberg

Introduction

Non-governmental organizations are a heterogeneous group difficult to define and classify, and the term "NGO" is not used consistently (Wikipedia 2012a). What NGOs have in common is that they operate independently of government, usually to deliver resources or serve some social, environmental, cultural, or political purpose. The term NGO is also commonly used to describe non-state, not-for-profit, voluntary organizations (WHO/ Civil Society Initiative 2002a). There are many different classifications in use. The most common one uses a framework that includes orientation and level of operation. An NGO's orientation refers to the type of activities it takes on. These activities might include human rights, environmental, or development work. An NGO's level of operation indicates the scale at which an organization works, such as local, international or national (Vakil Anna 1997). NGOs exist for a variety of reasons, usually to further the political or social goals of their members or funders, in a flexible and independent manner. Examples include improving the state of the natural environment, encouraging the observance

of human rights, improving the welfare of the disadvantaged or representing a corporate agenda (Wikipedia 2012b). Their goals cover a broad range of political and philosophical positions. As a result, a long (and sometimes confusing or comical) list of additional acronyms has developed, including among many others:

- BINGO, short for "business-friendly international NGO" or "big international NGO".
- TANGO, "technical assistance NGO".
- DONGO: Donor organized NGO.
- INGO which stands for international NGO, like Oxfam, the Institute of Peace and Development or the International Union for Health Promotion and Education.
- CSO, short for civil society organization. These organizations draw from community, neighbourhood, work, social and other connections. CSOs have become an increasingly common channel through which people seek to exercise citizenship and contribute to social and economic change. They cover a variety of organizational interests and forms, ranging from formal organizations registered with authorities to informal social movements coming together around a common cause (WHO/Civil Society Initiative 2002b).
- ENGO, short for environmental NGO, such as Greenpeace and WWF.
- NGDO: Non-governmental development organization, etc. to cite a few (Wikipedia 2012c). Professor Peter Willetts, from the University of London, argues that the definition of NGOs can be interpreted differently by

M.-C. Lamarre (✉)
International Union for Health Promotion and
Education, 42, boulevard de la Libération, 93203,
Saint-Denis, France
e-mail: mclamarre@iuhpe.org

L. Weinberg
Ecole des Hautes Etudes en Santé Publique
Rennes, France

D.V. McQueen (ed.), *Global Handbook on Noncommunicable Diseases and Health Promotion*,
DOI 10.1007/978-1-4614-7594-1_10, © Springer Science+Business Media, LLC 2013

various organizations and depending on a situation's context. He defines an NGO as "an independent voluntary association of people acting together on a continuous basis for some common purpose other than achieving government office, making money or illegal activities" (Willetts 2012)

The Health Promotion Perspective on NCDs

Health is created when individuals, families and communities are afforded the income, education and power to control their lives; and their needs and rights are supported by systems, environments and policies that are enabling and conducive to better health (Shilton et al. 2011). This definition of health by the International Union for Health Promotion and Education was drafted in response to an article and editorial published in the British Medical Journal, in July 2011, challenging the validity, in the twenty-first century context, of the WHO definition of health (Huber et al. 2011). While agreeing with the authors that "adaptation" and "self-management" are important qualities, it was made very clear that a contemporary definition should extend to include health being both a human right protected by certain entitlements and a resource for life that is affected by social, political, economic and environmental factors (WHO 1986).

In the last decade, due to the threat that they represent for significant segments of the world populations and economies, NCDs have been allotted a very high priority on the global health agenda, exemplified by the UN General Assembly on the Prevention and Control of NCDs which took place in September 2011 and the WHO's Action Plan for the Prevention and Control of Non-Communicable Diseases 2008–2013. From these and other related meetings, a general consensus now exists that the rise in NCDs is due to a complex range of associated risk factors, causes and causes of the causes in social contexts that are highly varied and complicated to understand (McQueen 2011). These include early years' experiences, education, economic status, employ-

ment and decent work, housing and environment and effective systems of preventing and treating ill health. Action on these determinants, both for vulnerable groups and the entire population, is essential to create inclusive, equitable, economically productive and healthy societies.

Any policy to address health social inequalities, therefore those focusing specifically as well on NCDs, cannot rely exclusively on health policy institutions. The majority of public policies, each one in its domain, contributes to health and therefore must assess carefully any particular impacts of its action on various social groups. These include the development of adequate public transport, clearance of bad housing, reduction of pollution, improvement of urban infrastructure, equitable access and affordability of food, as well as public, stakeholder and industry engagement. As concepts, policy principles and governance practice, Health in All Policies and Health Impact Assessment have become increasingly important as governments come to recognise the achievements of health and well-being goals, such as the Millennium Development Goals and Health 2020, requiring a whole-of-government approach (Lin et al. 2012).

Public health action however remains essentially guided by a pathogenic biomedical perspective in many places around the world with severe limitations. Current NCD prevention and control efforts are no exception. It is however broadly recognised that rather than concentrating on a few specific diseases, or single-risk factors, governments and the international community should prioritise building systems that offer universal access to and the use of quality services that meet the multiple health needs of the population. To make meaningful differences for those who need them most, systems approaches to policy, legislation and environments—not just individual approaches to behaviours—are needed.

A key characteristic of health promotion is the planned articulation of a wide range of complementary actions in an organized context: academic, government or community. Its core activities include health literacy, health education and advocacy for horizontal policy approaches in all sectors of society which help to improve health, and, conversely, to prevent it from being threatened and undermined. The effectiveness of these activities is enhanced and underpinned by collaboration and alliance building among all sectors of society, applied research to improve the quality and effectiveness of health promotion and training people to help them acquire skills to engage effectively in health promotion work.

Health promotion implies a paradigm shift from a deficit model of health focused on disease to a socioecological model aimed at strengthening resilience and assets for health—in particular by addressing the social and economic determinants of health and the capabilities for health (Kickbush 2010a). Health promotion focuses upon the development and maintenance of health in everyday life and cultural factors play a crucial role in the fundamental structuring processes of societies (Abel 2007). A shift to a model of health promotion recognises the importance of the structural dimensions of a public health approach to health governance (Kickbusch 2007).

In a recent briefing paper about "Tackling Non-Communicable Diseases to Enhance Sustainable Development," the NCD Alliance recognises that efforts to address NCDs and their risk factors are closely linked to economic growth, social equity and environmental protection. It also recognises that the social dimensions of sustainable development have received less attention than the economic and environmental ones but they are critical for health development and poverty eradication, and sustainable development. When it states however that "if LMICs are to continue their upward trajectory towards better health and improved economic conditions, they must address the social conditions that expose their populations to NCDs and remove the barriers preventing access to health services," (Tackling Noncommunicable Diseases to Enhance Sustainable Development 2012) it fails to recognise the complexities and inconsistencies of our global political, economic and financial systems. As well described by Joseph Stiglitz (Stiglitz 2006), there is an incredible capacity of the world to live with and accept large-scale inequalities, as if it were part of a natural order, and yet, the origins of such inequalities are not biological but social, political

and economic. From a public health perspective, the lack of equity will only be reversed if we imagine and create political, social and economic will for fair trade to reduce inequalities whilst improving people's health and if we make this will a reality through concrete agreements. Consequently health promotion professionals from all countries, and especially from higher income countries, have the responsibility to question the impact of economic globalisation on health and to be successful in making it an absolute priority for public health in the twenty-first century.

Positioning human health and well-being as one of the key features of what constitutes a successful, inclusive and fair society is consistent with health promotion commitment to human rights at national and international levels.

Therefore an effective response to NCD prevention and control also needs to include multisectoral policies and actions for dealing with disease-related risk behaviours, environmental factors and their social and economic determinants in the entire population.

NCD efforts share a common perspective of social justice and should keep the role of the health system into proportion within the strategies of action that can be implemented when addressing the issue.

"The health system ends up owning the problems that result from the chronic disease epidemic and must deal with these. However, it does not own the ways of addressing the causes of the problems as the answers are not medical or clinical but environmental and social" (Kickbush 2010b).

According to Marmot (WHO 2009) (Marmot 2009), the Ottawa Charter (WHO 1986) states what is supposed to be done and how—the problem is it is not being done! It is not a question of not having the means and solutions; it is a question of not doing it. For example, there is a huge disconnect with what needs to be included in the global, forceful NCD risk factor monitoring systems to push programme development and implementation both in terms of types of surveillance data and the use of data. In recent years, the idea of surveillance has broadened to go beyond the mere collection of data to an evolving concern with analysis, interpretation and dissemination of the data as part of a system of surveillance, with activities ranging from recognising epidemiological parameters of disease to identifying the public health policies that could influence health and illness (Campostrini and McQueen 2011a). No evidence-based public health promotion programme can function well without some form of socio-behavioural surveillance system. Long-term health programs like NCD prevention and control need an evaluation in progress, to monitor, improve and potentially reorganize the interventions while they are carried out. Appropriate surveillance systems have to be designed in order to be able to provide the timely process information needed by decision makers to guide re-prioritisation of interventions and reallocation of resources (Campostrini and McQueen 2011b).

NGOs Addressing NCDs Through a Health Promotion Lens

NGOs addressing NCDs through a health promotion lens do not focus on specific diseases or risk factors but on the structural, organizational and environmental conditions for life. They focus on equity and the equitable distribution of wealth, resources and services as well as on the development of health-promoting policies, the creation of supportive environments for health and well-being, the strengthening of community action, the development of personal skills and the reorientation of health services, i.e. the essential foundation stones of health promotion as stated in the Ottawa Charter (Speller 2007). They focus upstream on reducing the causative factors of ill health and on creating the conditions for better health. Stress, social exclusion or deprivation, unemployment, inadequate food supply, access and affordability, or the lack of adequate public transport and poor habitat all have significant impacts on health which may lead to diabetes, high blood pressure, heart attack, stroke and other NCDs. NGOs addressing NCDs through a health promotion lens also focus on educational opportunities, urban planning and investment and

social equity, and on addressing the needs of disadvantaged groups. They value and explore participatory approaches founded on the sharing of knowledge among all stakeholders, the development of a collective vision, the empowerment of communities to take charge of their life and the transfer of best practices.

In terms of assets, health promotion NGOs also have in common their independence and capacity to advocate.

A few examples are given below:

The NCD Alliance

The NCD Alliance was founded by four international NGO federations representing the four main NCDs—cardiovascular disease, diabetes, cancer and chronic respiratory disease. Together with other major national and international NGO partners, the NCD Alliance unites a heterogeneous network of over 2,000 civil society organizations in more than 170 countries. The mission of the NCD Alliance is to combat the NCD epidemic by putting health at the centre of all policies.

The NCD Alliance uses targeted advocacy and outreach to ensure that NCDs are recognised as a major cause of poverty, a barrier to economic development and a global emergency. This is done by working with a wide range of partners and organizations, mobilising them to produce policy work on NCDs and building the evidence base, convening expert working groups on a range of topics and pressing governments to recognise that NCDs are a global development priority requiring an urgent response.

Recognising however the absence of genuine global coordination among stakeholders, the lack of multisectoral action at international and national levels, the inadequate involvement of organizations outside the health sector and the lack of mechanism to track progress of all sectors and stakeholders with regard to the implementation of the recommendations contained in the UN High Level Meeting Political Declaration, the NCD Alliance advocates for a global coordinating platform on NCDs which would align current efforts and bring together a diverse range of stakeholders including outside the health sector (NCD Alliance).

The International Union for Health Promotion and Education

The IUHPE is an independent expert and professional network for health promotion and education, gathering people and institutions from all over the world, working in all the different areas that health promotion encompasses—skilled advocacy, knowledge development and transferability, capacity building, partnership and alliance building, health-promoting environments, social determinants of health, surveillance, integration of health in all policies and health impact assessment of public policies that recognise the value of health in all sectors and are accountable for health impact. Forming a global network to strengthen dialogue and cooperation, it attempts to meet critical needs for health development in all parts of the world and to contribute to bridge the gap of inequalities. It is a medium and it is a network of professionals with which to share information and knowledge, to solicit the advice of peers, to benefit from their experience, to participate in an ongoing conversation and reflection about health promotion, and the evidence of its effectiveness, and to develop collaborations.

One goal of IUHPE is to serve as a ready platform to assist and conduct the research and practice its members identify as "cutting-edge" public health. Much of IUHPE's work concerns developing conceptual frameworks, tools, standards and guidelines to serve health professionals and practitioners across the world. Its niche is its approach in terms of effectively building learning systems, and developing tools and resources by a global, professional network for itself to serve its members as well as the broader health promotion community.

The IUHPE's advocacy to policy makers about the social determinants of health and their relation to NCD prevention and control is based on mobilising evidence and communicating examples of effective and scalable programmes and healthy public policy from around the world, and facilitating exchange between policy makers, researchers, practitioners and communities.

Like many other areas in the field of health and public health, health promotion has been influenced by the evidence-based movement. The IUHPE Global Programme on Health Promotion Effectiveness (GPHPE) has focused across the last 12 years on collecting and providing access to the evidence of approaches and interventions that work, and stimulating debate on the nature of evidence. It made clear that the nature of the assessment of evidence, effectiveness and evaluation was highly complicated and that health promotion had to draw on a broad set of methods from a wide set of disciplines (McQueen 2012). What distinguishes the GPHPE work to date has been the reliance on definitions of effectiveness that stem from practitioners who are working in the field while at the same time having a high degree of theoretical and methodological integrity in the pursuit of how to best define evidence and effectiveness for the field of health promotion. The GPHPE is now in the process of forming a Global Working Group of the IUHPE linked to others notably those on salutogenesis, social determinants of health and surveillance, to cite a few. The IUHPE has made NCD prevention and control one of its four priority areas of work for the period 2010–2016 and has published a call to action on health promotion approaches to NCDs that effectively calls for

1. An expanded role for comprehensive health promotion.
2. Coordinated actions that impact on the determinants that underpin NCD epidemic across populations.
3. Health systems to redirect resources to health promotion and prevention of NCDs and prioritise health promotion as an essential function of the Departments of Health.
4. An expansion of engagement with sectors outside health where many of the economic, social and environmental policy solutions to NCDs can be best advanced.
5. An increased investment in ensuring a health promotion workforce that is prominently placed and equipped with the core competencies to implement current knowledge, policies and practices.

6. A specific and considered approach to the three critical areas of healthy eating, physical activity and tobacco control, and an agreement on robust indicators in each of these three areas. Effective health promotion action on healthy eating, physical activity and tobacco control will make the most important contributions to reducing the burden of NCDs in the global population.

7. A central focus on equity both between and within nations, and a specific focus on addressing the needs of disadvantaged groups.

As an NGO with a specific global mandate for health promotion the IUHPE has a unique and important role and responsibility in providing advice and influencing outcomes. It has a network and specific working groups of leading experts and organizations, and a strong presence in all global regions.

The International Society for Physical Activity and Health

The International Society for Physical Activity and Health (ISPAH) is an international professional society of individual members who are interested in advancing the science and practice of physical activity and health. One of its important goals is to advocate for research funding and policies (legislative and non-legislative) that can improve opportunities and environments for physical activity throughout the world.

Physical activity promotes well-being, and physical and mental health, prevents disease, improves social connectedness and quality of life, provides economic benefits and contributes to environmental sustainability. In this area as well "there is no one single solution to increasing physical activity; an effective comprehensive approach will require multiple concurrent strategies to be implemented" (The Toronto Charter for Physical Activity: A Global Call to Action 2010). The Toronto Charter for Physical Activity is a comprehensive health promotion programme and a call for all countries, regions and communities to strive for greater political and social commitment to support health-enhancing physical

activity for all. It outlines the direct health benefits and co-benefits of investing in policies and programmes to increase the levels of physical activity.

Whole of school programmes; transport policies and systems that prioritise walking, cycling and public transport; structured and unstructured physical activity throughout the day; urban design regulations and infrastructure that provide for equitable and safe access for recreational physical activity, and recreational and transport-related walking and cycling across the life course; public education, including mass media to raise awareness and change social norms on physical activity; physical activity and NCD prevention integrated into primary health care systems; community-wide programs involving multiple settings and sectors and that mobilise and integrate community engagement and resources; and sports systems and programs that promote "sport for all" and encourage participation across the lifespan represent seven best investments to increase population levels of physical activity which, if applied at sufficient scale, will make a significant contribution to reducing the burden of non-communicable diseases and promote health (Global Advocacy for Physical Activity (GAPA), the Advocacy Council of the International Society for Physical Activity and Health (ISPAH) 2011).

Architecture Sans Frontières: International (http://www.asfint.org)

It was founded as a result of an increased interest in social and environmental issues in relation to the built environment.

Its aim is to promote in an independent way equitable architecture, town planning and construction methods, which are socially responsible and respect diverse human cultures while preserving historical heritage of people.

They focus their efforts on fair and sustainable development, social responsibility, ethical trade, social equity and inclusion, appropriate technologies, materials and labour, social production of habitat, transnational dialogue and community building, and recognise habitat as a fundamental human right and see housing as a process and not a product.

It collaborates with many international and local partners working for sustainable development, participatory processes, slum improvement and social responsibility.

As stated in the report of the Canadian Population Health Initiative about *Urban Physical Environments and Health Inequalities* (Canadian Population Health Initiative 2012), a healthier environment, achieved mainly by improving income security, housing and access to water for lower income people, not only curbs public health risks linked to substandard living conditions but also offers better conditions for children to learn and thrive and for adults to be productive citizens and workers.

WWF International recognises that most people essentially desire the same thing: a life where needs are met; to be safe and healthy; to be able to explore interests and realise potential; and to improve well-being.

It focuses on creating more just and equitable societies—providing food, water and energy for all—through the sustainable management of the Earth's natural capital. Solutions lie in such areas as reducing waste; using better seeds and better cultivation techniques; bringing degraded lands back into production; and changing diets—particularly by lowering meat consumption in high-income countries. The Living Planet Report 2012 documents the "state of the planet": the changing state of biodiversity, ecosystems and humanity's demand on natural resources, and explores the implications of these changes for biodiversity and humanity (www.panda.org/lpr).

Relationship with National and International Governmental Agencies

As stated earlier in this chapter, NGOs operate independently of government, but they also entertain close interactions with them both at the national and international levels.

Interaction, consultation and cooperation with NGOs are clearly encouraged by the WHO Constitution. In 1948, the first World Health Assembly (WHA) adopted a set of working principles governing admission of NGOs into official relations. The objectives are to establish with each of them a programme of evidence collection, consultation with a broad range of actors and analysis, to identify and develop propositions for more effective and useful interfaces and relationships between NGOs and WHO. Organized into national, regional and global networks, this has widened the range of interests that WHO has to interact with in its mandate to improve global health (WHO/Civil Society Initiative 2002c).

Global health initiatives such as NCD prevention and control and national or foreign policy development processes such as building capacity strategies through knowledge and know-how development are involving NGOs as major actors. Among multilateral donors and development partners the emphasis on enhancing relations with NGOs is also strong with programme support being channelled through international NGOs.

Health promotion NGOs share WHO's overarching principles and approaches to NCD prevention and control, i.e. human rights; the recognition that non-communicable diseases are a challenge to social and economic development; universal access and equity; a life-course approach; evidence-based strategies; and the empowerment of people and communities.

A number of informal dialogues with non-governmental organizations at the global and regional levels were organized in preparation of the UN High-level Meeting of the General Assembly on Non-Communicable Diseases to examine how in complementarity with other major organizations NGOs could play their part through a shared action plan and concerted response to address the economic, political, cultural and social determinants of NCDs and of health and sustainable development.

But these principles and approaches often differ when it comes to implementation as they too often relate to the biomedical approach and to the strengthening of health systems when it is well known that there is not one single system to be privileged as they all have a significant impact on health.

Conclusions

The past three decades have witnessed the consolidation and institutionalisation of health promotion. A diverse range of practitioners and independent voluntary associations of people acting together for a common purpose (NGOs) identify implicitly or explicitly with this field, contribute to its discourse and practice and advocate for the recognition of its role in the pursuit of the public's health (Potvin and Jones 2011). All have similar objectives to focus on positive health, and improve health and quality of life conditions and environments to enable people to lead an active, productive and meaningful life. They also have a central focus on equity both between and within nations, and on addressing the needs of disadvantaged groups.

They all value and explore participatory approaches founded on the sharing of knowledge among all stakeholders, the development of a collective vision, the empowerment of communities to take charge of their life and the transfer of best practices.

A collective global response to NCDs requires initiatives by coalitions of stakeholders including NGOs capable of exercising transnational influence, as well as the idea of a coordinating mechanism to provide leadership across all initiatives.

Shared values and objectives, regulatory systems through transversal governance methods, adaptation, genuine integration of all stakeholders' interests and effective collaboration amongst various actors are all prerequisites.

Producing ideas, methods and tools close to public decision-making; understanding and anticipating; and debating and enlightening are the imperatives the whole of the international community of health promotion professionals endeavours to implement in their own context.

References

Abel, T. (2007). Cultural capital in health promotion. In *Health and modernity, the role of theory in health promotion*. New York: Springer Science+Business Media, LLC, Chapter 5.

Campostrini, S., & McQueen, D. (2011a). *White paper on surveillance and health promotion, international union for health promotion and education*. France: St-Denis.

Campostrini, S., & McQueen, D. (2011b). *White paper on surveillance and health promotion, international union for health promotion and education*. France: St-Denis.

Canadian Population Health Initiative. (2012). Urban physical environments and health inequalities: A scoping review of interventions. https://secure.cihi.ca/free_products/UrbanPhysicalReport2012EN_web.pdf.

Global Advocacy for Physical Activity (GAPA) the Advocacy Council of the International Society for Physical Activity and Health (ISPAH). (2011). *NCD prevention: Investments that work for physical activity*. Retrieved February 2011, from www.globalpa.org.uk/investmentsthatwork.

Huber, M., Knottnerus, J. A., Green, L., van der Horst, H., Jadad, A. R., Kromhout, D., et al. (2011). How should we define health? *BMJ, 343*, d4163.

Kickbusch, I. (2007). Health governance: The health society. In *Health and modernity, the role of theory in health promotion*. New York: Springer Science+Business Media, LLC, Chapter 9

Kickbush, I. (2010). The food system: A prism of present and future challenges for health promotion and sustainable development. Health Promotion Switzerland. http://www.ilonakickbusch.com/kickbusch-wAssets/docs/White-Paper—The-Food-System.pdf.

Kickbush, I. (2010). Implementing health in all policies: Adelaide 2010. Department of Health, Government of South Australia.

Lin, V., Jones, C., Synnot, A., & Wismar, M. (2012). Synthesizing the evidence: How governance structures can trigger governance actions to support health in all policies. In D. V. McQueen, M. Wismar, V. Lin, C. M. Jones, & M. Davies (Eds.), *Intersectoral governance for health in all policies, structures, actions and experiences*, World Health Organization on behalf of the European Observatory on Health Systems and Policies, Chapter 2

Marmot, M. (2009). Presentation at the 7th WHO World Conference on Health Promotion, Sub-plenary Round 2, Convergent Strategies, Divergent Histories, Emergent Opportunities: Health Promotion, Social Determinants of Health and Primary Care, October 27.

McQueen, D. (2011). In IUHPE key messages on NCDs prevention and control. http://www.iuhpe.org/uploaded/Activities/Advocacy/IUHPE%20Key%20Messages%20_LONG_WEB.pdf.

McQueen, D. (2012). *The global programme on health promotion effectiveness: A bold concept with few resources*. Perspectives in Public Health published online, SAGE on behalf of the Royal Society for Public Health, Retrieved from http://rsh.sagepub.com/content/early/2012/04/10/1757913912442268.

NCD Alliance discussion paper: Recommendations to the UN secretary-general for effective partnerships. The Case for a Global Coordinating Platform for NCDs. http://ncdalliance.org.

Potvin, L., & Jones, C. (2011). Twenty-five years after the Ottawa charter: The critical role of health promotion for public health. *Canadian Journal of Public Health, 102*(4), 244–248.

Shilton, T., Sparks, M., Lamarre, M.-C., & Jackson, S. (2011). *BMJ, 343*, d5359. doi:10.1136/bmj.d53592011).

Speller, V. (2007). Collective and individual responsibilities for health, both physical and mental. Principles and Practice of Health Promotion. In: Public Health Textbook, Health Knowledge. Public Health Action Support Team. http://www.healthknowledge.org.uk/public-health-textbook/disease-causation-diagnostic/2h-principles-health-promotion/responsibilities-health-physical-mental.

Stiglitz, J. (2006). *Making globalization work*. New York: W.W. Norton & Company Inc.

Tackling Non-communicable Diseases to Enhance Sustainable Development. (2012). NCD alliance briefing paper

The Toronto Charter for Physical Activity: A Global Call to Action. (2010). *International Society for Physical Activity and Health*. Retrieved from www.globalpa.org.uk

Vakil Anna, C. (1997). *Confronting the classification problem: Toward a taxonomy of NGOs*. Windsor, ON, Canada: University of Windsor.

WHO. (1986). *Ottawa charter for health promotion*. Geneva: WHO.

WHO/Civil Society Initiative. (2002a). *WHO's interactions with Civil Society and Nongovernmetnal Organizations*. Geneva: WHO.

WHO/Civil Society Initiative. (2002b). *WHO's interactions with Civil Society and Nongovernmetnal Organizations*. Geneva: WHO.

WHO/Civil Society Initiative. (2002). *WHO's interactions with Civil Society and Nongovernmetnal Organizations*. Geneva: WHO http://www.who.int/civilsociety/documents/en/RevreportE.pdf.

Wikipedia (2012a) From Wikipedia, the free encyclopedia. http://en.wikipedia.org/wiki/Non-governmental_organization#Definition.

Wikipedia (2012b) From Wikipedia, the free encyclopedia. http://en.wikipedia.org/wiki/Non-governmental_organization#Definition.

Wikipedia (2012c) From Wikipedia, the free encyclopedia. http://en.wikipedia.org/wiki/Non-governmental_organization#Definition.

Willetts, P. (2012). *What is a non-governmental organization?*. UNESCO Encyclopaedia of Life Support Systems. London: City University. Retrieved July 18, 2012.

Health Literacy as a Lens for Understanding Non-communicable Diseases and Health Promotion

Sandra Vamos and Irving Rootman

Introduction

Health literacy is a relatively recently developed concept, which has the potential to increase our understanding of both non-communicable diseases (NCDs) and health promotion. This chapter begins with a discussion of the concept of health literacy. It is followed by its relevance for NCDs. The commonly used definitions of health literacy that exist are presented. The relevance and the role of health literacy in relation to chronic disease prevention and management in the global context follow. A discussion of existing evidence on the effectiveness of health literacy interventions in relation to chronic disease prevention and management is then presented. Examples of promising approaches from several countries that have been active in addressing health literacy are also provided. The chapter concludes by discussing the implications and emerging opportunities of these examples for other countries and the global community concerned about NCDs.

S. Vamos (✉)
Innovative Health Inc., 2506-1189 Melville Street, Vancouver, BC, Canada V6E 4T8
e-mail: sandravamos@gmail.com

I. Rootman
School of Public Health and School Policy, University of Victoria, 1428 W. 6th Avenue, Vancouver, BC, Canada V6H 4H4
e-mail: irootman@telus.net

The Concept of Health Literacy

Health literacy is an essential capacity for living a healthy life. While the concept of health literacy first appeared in the literature more than 35 years ago, interest in it has increased dramatically. Until recently, interest in health literacy was concentrated in the United States led by physicians. However, over the past decade interest in it has grown in other developed countries such as Canada, Australia and the United Kingdom as well as other European Union countries led by people with a background in the social sciences and health promotion (Paasche-Orlow 2009). Its importance for the promotion of health has also been recognized by international organizations such as the World Health Organization (WHO), the International Union for Health Promotion and Education (IUHPE) and the European Union (EU). For example, health literacy has been mentioned as an area of priority action in the European Commission's Health Strategy 2008–2013 (Commission of the European Communities 2007) where it is linked to the core value of citizen empowerment, and the priority actions for the promotion of health for different age groups.

As an important evolving field, health literacy appears to be repackaging a number of key concepts in health promotion and health education based on varying perspectives central to theory and practice in these fields (Nutbeam 2000). Much of the ongoing exercise has been triggered by a wish to move away from the original narrow medical concept of health literacy to a much broader concept, which is associated with skills contributing to individual and social empowerment. This transition of moving a health literacy focus outside of primarily health-care settings has potential to highlight health literacy as an asset and as a preventive public health perspective.

As suggested, this interest in the evolving concept of health literacy has developed from the following three main perspectives: (1) health care; (2) health promotion; and (3) education.

Health Care Perspective

The *health care* perspective, which developed in the United States, was stimulated by physician-researchers concerned about the impact of low literacy in relation to patient care. They developed some tools to measure what they considered to be health literacy and applied them to study the impact of "health literacy" on patient outcomes. This "health literacy as a risk factor model" exposed the relationship to low literacy, patient decision-making, prescription medication compliance and capacity to self-manage chronic disease (Nutbeam 2008). This stimulated interest of professional bodies such as the American Medical Association (AMA) and led to research on the effectiveness of various kinds of interventions in medical practice to address low health literacy as well as to policy and other initiatives in the United States. Over the years, many international experts would claim that our sphere of health has expanded beyond the "confines" of the health-care system and it is necessary for individuals to have the essential skills enabling them to become informed, engaged and active citizens able to make daily health decisions (Kickbusch et al. 2005). The view that health literacy is needed in sickness *and in health* began stimulating further discussion.

The Health Promotion Perspective

The *health promotion* perspective arose out of interest of key global leaders in the field of health promotion who saw health literacy as an outcome

of health education and health promotion and was subsequently picked up by researchers and practitioners in a number of countries throughout the world.

Health promotion involves a combination of approaches for promoting health including community development, organizational change, public policy implementation, communication and education (WHO 1986). These strategies focus on building individuals' and communities' capacities through a combination of educational, motivational and skill-enhancement techniques and environmental supports that may encourage/enhance behavioural and environmental change. By influencing both individuals' capacities and providing environmental supports, meaningful and sustained change in the health of individuals and communities (psychosocial and physical environments) can occur (Frankish 2011). Health literacy is seen as an outcome of effective health promotion by increasing capacities to access and use health information to make appropriate health decisions and maintain health.

The Education Perspective

The *education* perspective stems from health education and health-care researchers being concerned about the link between health and education around the globe. The term "health literacy" was first used in a 1974 paper entitled Health Education as Social Policy (Simonds 1974). Health literacy was described as health education meeting "minimal standards" for all school-grade levels while discussing health education as a policy issue affecting the education system, the health-care system and mass communication (Ratzan 2001).

Health is the first of the seven cardinal principles of education that posits the health of the individual as essential to the vitality of the nation and education as an essential component in one's ability to function successfully in society. The conceptualization of health literacy as an asset has its roots in educational research in literacy, concepts of adult education and health education and promotion (Nutbeam 2008). Improving health literacy in a population involves effective school health education and adult education (Nutbeam 2008; St Leger 2001). Furthermore, health literacy is an important factor enabling individuals to make daily decisions with essential life skills about health and well-being. It is also viewed as an asset to be built, as a lifelong process, and as an outcome to health education and promotion that supports greater empowerment in health decision-making across the lifespan. Health literacy helps strengthen the links between the fields of health and education (Kickbusch 2001).

There are evident relations between these three perspectives. Rather than thinking of a lack of health literacy simply as a risk factor for a poor disease-related health outcome (a kind of deficit model), it is possible to think of health literacy as an asset using a broad-ranging health promotion model. To conceptualize health literacy as an asset, it is viewed as a concept, a process, an outcome and a public health goal. Health literacy is a "key outcome from health education" for which health promotion could legitimately be held accountable; health literacy "significantly broadens the scope and content of health education and communication," both of which are critical operational strategies in health promotion (Nutbeam 2000, p. 264). Furthermore, Abel (2008) differentiates between the role of health literacy in medical settings versus health promotion contexts. In the former case, health literacy would be concerned with "… people's abilities to read and understand medical information, be it in written form or conveyed in personal encounters such as doctors visits"… (p. 169). Health promotion approaches do not focus on illness experiences, but rather the focus usually is much broader and emphasizes healthy general living conditions and people's chances to live healthy lives. In both settings, health literacy means understanding the conditions that determine health, knowing how to change them and adjusting practices accordingly (Abel 2008).

All three perspectives also share the term, "Three Noble Truths of Health Literacy". First, people (i.e. patients, public, practitioners or policymakers) are unlikely to act on or support health literacy practices or work unless they "know" about it, "care" about it and "believe"

in it. Second, those people who are "motivated" are more likely to take action on health literacy practices or work if they have the skills and "resources" for action and a "supportive" environment. Finally, people who take the desired action(s) on health literacy practices or work are more likely to maintain such action(s) if they receive "internal" or "external" reinforcement (Frankish 2011 adapted from Green and Kreuter 1999).

Definitions of Health Literacy

Partly as a result of these aforementioned different perspectives, different definitions of the concept have been developed. The European Health Literacy Project (HLS-EU) Consortium recently conducted a systematic literature review to identify definitions and conceptual frameworks for health literacy (Sorenson et al. 2012). The review resulted in 17 definitions and 12 conceptual models. For example, in the United States, the following definition, which reflects the *health care* and *education* perspectives, has been adopted widely: "The degree to which individuals have the capacity to obtain, process, and understand basic health information and services needed to make appropriate health decisions" (Institute of Medicine 2004). In Europe, the following definition, which first appeared in WHO glossary of health promotion terms, reflects the *health promotion* perspective: "the cognitive and social skills which determine the motivation and ability of individuals to gain access to, understand, and use information in ways which promote and maintain good health" (Nutbeam 1998).

More recently, other definitions have been put forward, some of which reflect attempts to merge the three perspectives. For example the definition proposed by the Canadian Expert Panel on Health Literacy is as follows: "the ability to access, understand, evaluate and communicate information as a way to promote, maintain and improve health in a variety of settings across the life-course" (Rootman and Gordon-El-Bihbety 2008, p. 11). This operational definition is a commonly cited definition of health literacy in Canadian research and practice.

Similarly, two other definitions merge the three perspectives and highlight the importance of skills by the several parties involved (consumers and various providers). Comparable broader views can be seen in the following two definitions:

> The ability to make sound health decision(s) in the context of everyday life—at home, in the community, at the workplace, the healthcare system, the market place and the political arena. It is a critical empowerment strategy to increase people's control over their health, their ability to seek out information and their ability to take responsibility (Kickbusch et al. 2005, p. 4).
>
> The wide range of skills, and competencies that people develop to seek out, comprehend, evaluate and use health information and concepts to make informed choices, reduce health risks ad increase quality of life (Zarcadoolas et al. 2006, p. 55).

Based on their analysis of these and other definitions, the authors of the review suggest their own "all inclusive" comprehensive definition, namely:

> Health literacy is linked to literacy and entails peoples' knowledge, motivation and competencies to access, understand, appraise, and apply health information in order to make judgments and take decisions in everyday life concerning healthcare, disease prevention and health promotion to maintain or improve quality of life during the life course (Sorenson et al. 2012).

While we applaud their efforts to develop a definition that captures the essence of the definitions from the literature that they considered, it is likely that the debate on the definition of health literacy will continue with a growing international consensus that none of the existing definitions fully address the capacity of health systems or health professionals to inhibit or enhance the skills and capabilities that individuals and communities require to be health literate (Rudd et al. 2012, Chapter 2). Furthermore, the variety of definitions that exist "enables the complex context of health literacy to be viewed and explored using different paradigms and within different contexts" (Begoray et al. 2012, Chapter 8). We agree with this viewpoint and rather than imposing our own favourite definition, we will simply indicate which definition is being used in the various examples that are presented.

Relevance of Health Literacy for Non-communicable Diseases

NCDs are the leading cause of deaths worldwide. Sixty-three percent of these deaths are due to mostly one of the four chronic diseases: cardiovascular diseases, cancers, respiratory diseases and diabetes (Bloom et al. 2011). Increasing chronic disease rates are associated with worse health outcomes and higher health-care costs. Low levels of health literacy are also related to poor health outcomes and higher health-care costs.

According to Rootman and Gordon-El-Bihbety (2008), people with limited health literacy may:

- Overuse hospitals and emergency rooms
- Have reduced access to services and information (e.g. free cancer-screening clinics, community health services)
- Be less likely to act on important public health alerts (influencing health outcomes)
- Make less use of preventive services (e.g. mammograms, pap tests)
- Be more likely to misunderstand instructions about prescription medication and make medication errors
- Be unable to manage chronic conditions (e.g. diabetes, high blood pressure, asthma)

Health literacy as currently measured has been found to be associated with NCDs (Martin et al. 2011; Canadian Council on Learning 2008). Individuals with limited health literacy are more likely to have chronic conditions and are less able to manage them effectively (Williams et al. 1998). Limited health literacy has also been found to have an adverse effect on the interaction between the patient, provider and health system in relation to NCD (Mancuso and Rincon 2006). On the other hand, improved health literacy has been found to be associated with better health outcomes and is a critical factor in managing NCDs (Williams et al. 1998; Rosenfeld et al. 2011; Schillinger et al. 2002; Johnston et al. 2006). Health literacy has also been found to be associated with knowledge of NCD (Gazmararian et al. 2003) and health literacy interventions have been found to reduce health disparities in NCD management (Paasche-Orlow et al. 2005).

Evidence on Effectiveness of Health Literacy Interventions

There have been several recent reviews of evaluations of health literacy interventions. These reviews have concluded that there have been a limited number of rigorous evaluations of health literacy interventions. In addition, they have suggested that interventions can tend to adopt one or more of the following strategies to address individual and/or systemic health literacy barriers:

- Improve knowledge and skills of individuals for decision-making (i.e. consumers, chronic disease prevention and management)
- Build the knowledge and skills of health providers
- Improve access to accurate, appropriate and relevant health information
- Improve usability of health-care services

The Canadian Public Health Association (2006) conducted a review of health literacy interventions in relation to chronic disease. It was found that most studies had been in the area of cancer screening interventions. The report also noted that another area of research had examined chronic disease management efforts in primary care settings, especially for diabetes.

The scope of health literacy continues to expand around the globe. Six extensive systematic literature reviews have been completed, two just recently, whereby possible findings may provide further insight into "what" and "how" interventions may improve health literacy. Table 11.1 summarizes such recent work (adapted from Mitic and Rootman 2012, unpublished). Although the research has not always produced conclusive results, we are able to take away some of the key points. These include the following:

- Effects of limited health literacy include increased preventable hospital visits, increased medication errors and mortality, and have a negative impact on self-management of chronic conditions.
- Interventions focusing on self-care and self-management reduce emergency room visits and hospitalizations and reduce disease severity.

- Few rigorous evaluations exist.
- Call for broader scope of inquiry (beyond doctor–patient) to include a range of settings and systems focusing on a community-based and empowerment approach.

It is clear that the scientific evidence on the effectiveness of health literacy interventions is limited, variable and mixed. Nevertheless, there is sufficient evidence to suggest that it is worthwhile to continue to work on health literacy as a promising approach that could be applied to NCDs. In addition, there are some encouraging examples of approaches that are being used in a number of countries around the world that might be adapted to other countries interested in using health literacy systematically as a means of addressing NCDs.

Examples of Promising Approaches from Different Countries

There are a number of health literacy initiatives throughout the world. Approaches vary by size and scale, and some initiatives focus directly on health literacy while others focus more broadly on building the literacy and/or specific skills that may support health literacy. We have selected several examples from countries that have been particularly active in using health literacy to address NCDs or have done something that is innovative and promising in relation to health literacy and NCDs. We have chosen one example from selected countries to highlight different approaches. Each is described in text boxes below. We have also listed some additional health literacy initiatives. These examples are not exhaustive.

The United States

- The United States has probably done more than any other country in relation to health literacy, perhaps more from a *health care* and *education* perspective than a *health promotion* perspective, although there are examples of the latter as well.

Table 11.1 Major systematic reviews of health literacy interventions, behaviours and outcomes

Author(s)	Method	Findings	Conclusion	Health literacy definition	Link to NCD
Pignon et al. (2005)[a]	Systematic review of research published between 1980 and 2003 on the effect of interventions on the health outcomes of persons with low health literacy. Included controlled and uncontrolled trials that measured literacy	Only five articles examined the interaction between literacy level and the effect of intervention. Mixed results	Drawing conclusions difficult because of limitations in study design, interventions tested and outcomes assessed. Further research required	Defined Low Literacy: "an inability to read, write, and use numbers effectively, is common and is associated with a wide range of adverse health outcomes"	Examined the effects of interventions for people with "low literacy" on health knowledge, health behaviours and use of health care resources, intermediate markers of disease status and morbidity or mortality
Hauser and Edwards (2006)[b]	Reviewed research on health literacy interventions published prior to 2007	Few rigorous evaluations exist. While the most widespread initiative used is simplifying reading material using clear language and pictures, there is no evidence that this improves health outcomes. Although multimedia presentations may improve knowledge in both the literate and the less literate, they do not appear to change health-related behaviours	Community development is a promising avenue that requires more exploration. Creation of innovative evaluation tools required	"the ability to access, understand, evaluate and communicate information as a way to promote, maintain and improve health in a variety of settings across the life-course"	Low literacy found to be associated with poor management of chronic disease and less use of preventive services as well as less knowledge about chronic disease. It also appears to be associated with higher rates of certain chronic diseases
King (2007)[c]	Review of published and grey literature related to health literacy interventions in Canada and internationally. Also conducted key informant interviews	Majority of health literacy interventions involve accessing and understanding, with few focused on appraising or communicating health information. Limited information found on the effectiveness of health literacy interventions. Some evidence to support the finding that a participatory educational and empowerment approach is effective	Barriers to evaluation of programs were time, money and lack of provider expertise. Further investigations suggested: • Health literacy interventions focused on appraising health information • Cultural issues • Health-care professional training • Sources of health information • Learner and patient perspectives	Used the Canadian Health Literacy definition to limit the scope of scan: "Health literacy is the degree to which people are able to access, understand, appraise and communicate information to engage with the demands of different health contexts in order to promote and maintain good health across the life-course." (Rootman and Gordon-El-Bihbety 2008)	Scan showed a participatory educational approach (using participatory educational methods for learners to identify, research and learn about health issues) appears to be effective in health promotion, disease prevention programs

Clement et al. (2009)[d]	Systematic review of randomized and quasi-randomized controlled trials that focused on complex interventions for people with limited literacy or numeracy. Searched eight databases from 1966 to 2007. Predominantly North American	Knowledge and self-efficacy were outcomes most likely to improve, but not necessarily related to health outcomes	While the review focused on two specific aspects of health literacy (reading ability and numeracy) many interventions included wider empowerment and/or community participation aspects. The implementation of literacy/ numeracy interventions might most usefully be embedded within this broader approach to health literacy	Literacy and numeracy skills are two key components of the review and within the wider concept of health literacy	The health literacy process generates knowledge and skills which enable a person to help navigate three domains of the health continuum: (1) being ill or as a patient in the health-care setting; (2) as a person at risk of disease in the disease prevention system; and (3) as a citizen in relation to the health promotion efforts in the community, the work place, the educational system, the political arena and the marketplace

(continued)

Table 11.1 (continued)

Author(s)	Method	Findings	Conclusion	Health literacy definition	Link to NCD

Sheridan et al. (2011)[c]	Conducted a systematic evidence review that evaluated the effectiveness of interventions designed to mitigate the effects of low health literacy through either single or multiple literacy-directed strategies	Found several discrete design features that improved participant comprehension in one or a few studies (e.g. presenting essential information by itself or first, presenting information so that the higher number is better, presenting numerical information in tables rather than text, adding icon arrays to numerical information, adding video to verbal narrative). Furthermore, we found a few studies that provided consistent, direct evidence that intensive mixed-strategy interventions focusing on self-management reduced emergency department visits and hospitalizations, and that intensive mixed-strategy interventions focusing on self- and disease management reduced disease severity	To continue to advance the field of health literacy research should:
			• Focus on confirming the effectiveness of discrete design features or mixed-strategy interventions that, to date, have shown success only in limited populations
			• Explore yet untested interventions. Such interventions might include interventions to
			  - Increase motivation to process information (e.g. fotonovelas); interventions that work around the problem of low health literacy (e.g. patient navigators); and interventions that change physician behaviour, practice structure or existing health policy
			  - Continue to explore the features that make health literacy interventions successful. Although a combination of intervention features has been shown to ensure the success of interventions, paring away ineffective features could save delivery time and be more cost-effective
			• Explore the best ways to disseminate and implement effective health literacy interventions. Such an effort might be aided by creating a central, accessible library of literacy-directed interventions
				Used a US definition: *Health literacy is* "the degree to which individuals can obtain, process, and understand the basic health information and services they need to make appropriate health decisions." (Institute of Medicine 2004)	Found a few studies that provided consistent evidence that intensive mixed-strategy interventions focusing on self-management reduced emergency room visits and hospitalizations. Intensive mixed-strategy interventions focusing on self-care and disease management reduced disease severity. Whenever possible, these latter interventions should be considered for use in clinical practice

| Sorensen et al. (2012)[f] | A systematic literature review was performed to identify definitions and conceptual frameworks of health literacy. A content analysis of the definitions and conceptual frameworks was carried out to identify the central dimensions of health literacy and develop an integrated model | The review resulted in 17 definitions of health literacy and 12 conceptual models. Based on the content analysis, an integrative conceptual model was developed containing 12 dimensions referring to the knowledge, motivation and competencies of accessing, understanding, appraising and applying health-related information within the health care, disease prevention and health promotion setting, respectively | A model is proposed integrating medical and public health views of health literacy. The model can serve as a basis for developing health literacy-enhancing interventions and provide a conceptual basis for the development and validation of measurement tools, capturing the different dimensions of health literacy within the health care, disease prevention and health promotion settings | Identified global definitions. Health literacy is a term first introduced in the 1970s | Health literacy is concerned with the capacities of people to meet the complex demands of health in a modern society. Health literate means placing individual, family and community health into context. This includes understanding which factors are influencing health, knowing how to address factors and taking responsibility for well-being |

Source: Adapted from Mitic and Rootman. (2012). *An inter-sectoral approach to improving health literacy for Canadians*. Vancouver, British Columbia: Public Health Association of British Columbia [unpublished]. http://www.phabc.org/modules.php?name=Contentpub&pa=showpage&pid=182

[a]Pignon, M., DeWalt, D., Sheridan, S., Berkman, N., & Lohr, K. (2005). Interventions to improve health outcomes for patients with low literacy: A systematic review. *Journal of General Internal Medicine*, 20(2), 185–192

[b]Hauser, J. & Edwards, P. (2006). *Literacy, health literacy and health: a literature review*. Ottawa, ON: Expert Panel on Health Literacy, Canadian Public Health Association

[c]King. J. (2007). *Environmental scan of interventions to improve health literacy*. National Collaborating Centre for Determinants of Health

[d]Clement, S., et al. (2009). Complex Interventions to improve the health of people with limited literacy. A systematic review. *Patient Education and Counceling*, 75, 340–351

[e]Sheridan, S., Halpern, D., Viera, A., et al. (2011). Interventions for individuals with low health literacy: A systematic review, *Journal of Health Communication*, 16, 30–54

[f]Sorensen, K., VAN DEN Broucke, S, Fullam, J., et al. (2012). Health literacy and public health: A systematic review and integration of definitions and models. *BioMed Central Public Health*. http://www.biomedcentral.com/1471-2458/12/80

Box 1 The US National Action Plan to Improve Health Literacy (2010)

The National Action Plan to Improve Health Literacy is a blueprint consisting of information about health literacy, a vision and seven strategic goals related to improving health literacy for the nation. Each of the seven goals offers possible actions and approaches using case studies and real-life strategies with town-hall Web links. The document is based on the principles that (1) everyone has the right to health information that helps them make informed decisions, and (2) health services are delivered in ways that are understandable and beneficial to health, longevity and quality of life.

Box 2 Canadian Expert Panel Report on Health Literacy: A Vision for a Health-Literate Canada (2008)

The Canadian Expert Panel Report on Health Literacy is considered as Canada's milestone report and a significant health literacy initiative itself. The document contains information about health literacy and calls for policies, programmes and research to improve health literacy and reduce health disparities in Canada. The Expert Panel's report shows that low health literacy is a serious and costly problem that will likely grow as the population ages and the incidence of chronic disease increases. The report summarizes promising Canadian-wide, provincial/territorial and local initiatives, which use different approaches and are directed at specific groups. Implications and recommendations are provided.

• Other promising examples from the United States include the following: AMA Task Force; AMA Curricula; Institute of Medicine (I.O.M.) Expert Committee on Health Literacy; Health Literacy Missouri Health Education Assessment Project (HEAP—School Health Project); Healthy People 2020 Objectives on Health Literacy; Research; Development of Measurement Tools (2003 National Adult Literacy Survey; 2006 Adult Literacy and Life Skills Survey); National Network of Libraries of Medicine (Health Literacy Listservs); Centers for Disease Control Healthy Literacy resources and training materials.

Canada

• Canada may be considered second to the United States in terms of work on health literacy, although more from a health promotion perspective.
• Other promising examples from Canada include the following: National Literacy and Health Program; Calgary Charter on Health Literacy; British Columbia Health Literacy Networks; A Plan to Improve Health Literacy

in Canada (draft); Prototype Health Literacy Collaborative; National Conferences on Literacy and Health; Canadian Council on Learning analyses of National Data on Health Literacy (including mapping); National Council on Health Literacy; BC Senior Citizen's Health Literacy Workshop Program; School Health Research Network.

Europe

Europe is involved in collaborative health literacy initiatives, many with a health promotion perspective. A cutting-edge project, centred in Maastricht University, is the development and pilot testing of the first international health literacy survey.

• Other promising examples from Europe include the following: IUHPE Priority Action Areas 2011–2015 (Health Literacy falls within Health Promotion Action Area); European Health Policy Forums Gastein, Health Literacy Europe Network.

Box 3 The European Health Literacy Survey (HLS-EU)

The HLS-EU is the first international survey to measure health literacy. It measures health literacy in various EU regions, and cultures creating datasets and an awareness of its societal and political impact. The importance of health literacy is understood whereby inadequate health literacy means less knowledge and use of preventive health services. It is carried out by many European countries and funded by the EU. The intended results of the project include providing input for practical political strategies on health literacy.

The United Kingdom

The United Kingdom is home to innovative initiatives, many of which focus on all three perspectives (health care, health promotion and education). "*Skilled for Life*" is an example of a well-recognized national program with the goal of helping the UK health sector develop a more skilled and flexible workforce. It is notable as it integrates health literacy into already existing programs.

Box 4 Skilled for Life

"*Skilled for Life*" is an adult skills program in the United Kingdom. The program integrates learning modules for developing skills particular to health, literacy and health literacy within other learning situations and pre-existing programs. It contains a large number of resources and courses that are available online. For example, it contains tools for staff in the health-care workforce to develop personal skills related to effective communications and health and delivery and patient safety. *Skilled for Life* has already developed and tested protocols, methods and produced learning resources for many vulnerable groups.

- Other promising examples from the United Kingdom include the following: UK Health Literacy Network; Department of Health—Health Inequalities Strategy (health literacy component of policy).

The Netherlands

- The Netherlands is currently involved in cross-cutting health literacy work across sectors, stemming from all three perspectives (health care, health promotion and education) with perhaps a greater focus on the latter two.

Box 5 National Health Council

An active health alliance comprising nearly 60 member organizations including pharmaceutical companies, insurance companies, hospitals, professional organizations, patient organizations and universities. Meetings entail the sharing of best practices and examples of work involve health literacy activities to train hospital staff, redesigning health education materials and advising on policy to service providers.

Australia

In Australia school-based and community-based health literacy initiatives appear to be prominent to encourage healthy decision-making, reflecting a health promotion and education perspective. Addressing lifestyle risk behaviours and the uptake of healthy decisions among target audiences in the Australian population are common approaches to chronic disease prevention. For example, innovative whole-school health programs (consistent with health promoting schools approach) versus "traditional" pedagogical health programs for K-12 students are suggested as a way that could promote healthy behavioural changes.

- Other promising examples from Australia include the following: Mental Health Literacy Initiatives; School-based Health Promotion Campaigns.

China

developing a regional action plan to promote health literacy. A set of recommendations was made to accelerate actions to achieve the MDG. For example, effective health literacy interventions can be scaled up with a focus on the core content areas of health literacy to combat NCDs, including the use of low-cost, simple but effective health education interventions.

Hong Kong

- Hong Kong is a city recognized for its participation in health-promoting schools (HPS), from both a health promotion and education perspective. The HPS concept arose through the influence of the *Ottawa Charter for Health Promotion* (WHO 1986) and is well known as a key setting for health promotion. The goal of the HPS initiative is to "facilitate higher levels of health literacy by helping individuals tackle the determinants of health better as they build the personal, cognitive and social skills for maintaining good health" (Lee 2009, p. 11). Many countries and global regions participate in HPS, including the Asia Pacific region (including Hong Kong), European Union (European Network of Health Promoting Schools), the United States, Canada, Australia and South Africa just to name a few.

Box 8 (continued)

outside agencies and organizations, etc.). The model takes an interdisciplinary approach to integrate health across the curriculum and empowers students to make decisions related to personal, family, community health and public health.

Singapore

- A promising example from Singapore is the National Health Literacy Plan, which is currently being implemented.

Israel

- Promising examples include the following: Refuah Shlema: Cultural liaisons in the community; Community intervention for diabetes control among the adult Arab population.

Thailand

- Promising examples include the following: Thai Health Literacy Scale; National Health Literacy Survey.

Taiwan

- A promising example is a national study of health literacy in all 12-year-old children in Taiwan.

Implications and Emerging Opportunities: Directions for Moving Forward in the Global Arena

Health literacy is congruent with scaling up prevention on NCDs and efforts in the field can contribute to improving health and well-being in populations around the world. We have seen an increase in interest, momentum and profile of global health literacy work. We have also seen a number of initiatives in various countries, regions and settings using different approaches to developing, implementing and evaluating health literacy action towards NCDs. Across the globe the recognition of the challenges related to the complexities of both the health literacy field and to the broad field of chronic diseases is widely accepted. This reality is the impetus leading to important discussions, emerging opportunities and recommended actions in the global arena.

Developed Versus Low–Middle-Income (Developing) Countries

While NCDs are commonly perceived as frequently afflicting those of affluence, there is an upward trend in the incidence of these diseases in low- and middle-income (developing) countries. According to the WHO, NCDs led to 36 million deaths in 2008, with approximately 90 % of these deaths occurring in low- and middle-income countries (Alwan et al. 2011). The WHO predicts that globally, deaths from NCDs are likely to increase by 17 % over the next 10 years, with the greatest increase projected in the African region (27 %) followed by the Eastern Mediterranean region (25 %) (WHO 2009). WHO prepared 193 NCD country profiles from the United Nations high-level meeting with global leaders on NCD prevention and control in New York in September 2011. In a one-page per country presentation format using graphs, the WHO report provides information on the prevalence, trends in metabolic risk factors (cholesterol, blood pressure, body mass index and blood sugar), and behavioural risk factors, alongside data on the country's capacity to tackle the diseases (Alwan et al. 2011). According to the report, the death rates due to NCDs are closely related to country income. In low-income countries the proportion of premature NCD deaths under 60 years was 41 %, three times the proportion in high-income countries. Furthermore, common preventable risk factors underlie most NCDs. The leading risk factors globally for mortality include (1) raised blood pressure (responsible for 13 % of deaths globally); (2) tobacco use (9 %); (3) raised blood glucose (6 %); (4) physical inactivity (6 %); and (5) overweight and obesity (5 %). These risk factors are a leading cause of death and disability regardless of economic development. According to the report, exposure to the four main behaviour risk factors is universal and trending upwards.

Health literacy is a lens and asset for practical application in all countries towards (1) better understanding and addressing NCDs, and (2) sustained action to help address the social determinants of health. Health literacy is a broad set of knowledge and skills related to healthy decision-making and empowerment, whether accessing and making the best use of the services or programs available, capacity to make informed lifestyle choices or taking an active role in the determinants of health (Kickbusch and Nutbeman 2000). This recognition leads us to tangible "proactive" actions related to daily activities contributing to and supporting chronic disease prevention, self-care and self-management.

Terminology and Process: Navigating the Public Health Map

The aforementioned UN high-level meeting not only helps show the shared universal complexities of NCDs but also can be used to reflect the notion that health literacy can be viewed as a bridging concept for *knowledge and practice*. If health literacy is to be a lens to better understand NCDs, it is first necessary to know what health literacy is. Next, once others know about it, they will need to care about it before using it as a lens. Individuals can be motivated through raising awareness regarding health literacy. Highlighting the universal and life-long relevance along with the practical importance as an asset in everyday life and in relation to NCDs is fundamental. It is also important to gain political traction highlighting benefits and discussing approaches to action.

However, with this exercise come caveats. Recalling that health literacy stems from three different perspectives (health care, health promotion,

education)—health literacy is a term that can describe a concept, process and a range of outcomes to health promotion and education approaches and activities under the broad public health umbrella. Similar to the health literacy concept, it is also important to note that terminology and relationships between terms and processes can also vary in the health promotion and health education fields. While definitions and concepts can be complex in nature, are emerging in scope and reflect cultural bias, clarifying meaning and relationship between terms is central to the development of practical action (Nutbeam 1998).

Whereas the sole purpose and focus of this chapter is not to conduct a comprehensive cross-cultural comparison of definitions, theories or international quality assurance mechanisms, different uses and housing of term(s) may drive interpretations and actions in a field. This is noted after taking global stock of the many innovative examples mentioned above from the field that have been particularly active in using health literacy in many ways and with many partners to address NCDs.

Highlighting the international interest on common approaches for health promotion and education, a recent meeting took place at the University of Ireland, Galway, in June 2008, jointly organized by the IUHPE, the Society for Public Health Education (SOPHE) and the US Centers for Disease Control (CDC), with participation by international leaders, to discuss the development of core competencies and common approaches to academic programs, accreditation and professional standards (Barry et al. 2009; McQueen 2009). According to a recent article entitled *Development and Utilization of Professional Standards in Health Education and Promotion: US and UK Experiences*, one of the most striking differences revealed is the different use of terminology around both the *roles* (i.e. health educator, health educator specialist, health promotion specialist, public health practitioner/specialist, health trainer, etc.) and the *systems* and *processes* (i.e. certification, accreditation, competencies). According to the authors: "We need to understand the different meanings that terminology has both in definition and in application in practice in different contexts." (Speller et al. 2009, p. 40).

While this particular meeting was not focused on health literacy or NCDs—*roles, systems* and *processes* do underpin the continuum of actions and supports for each in relation to health education and health promotion. *Consequently, targeting of the workforce and provision of learning opportunities that enhance the understanding and abilities of all partners to better support health literacy efforts are evident.* However, different governing bodies and approval processes can make it challenging to compare standards and procedures across the globe (Speller et al. 2009). This consensus conference is an example of a facilitated international discussion on key approaches for improved professionalization of health promotion and education practitioners. An important point concluded was to explore the adoption of educational improvements through local, regional and national strategies, which have international implications. Integrating health literacy concepts to support health education and promotion efforts within respective contexts builds a notable foundation for global professionalism and workforces to improve well-being (Vamos and Hayos 2011). Regardless of whether health education and health promotion are viewed as entities in and of themselves, or embedded under the public health umbrella, health literacy is a common skill set to support all practitioners amidst diverse terminology and process and to address NCD.

Future Directions

Many people have now realized that health literacy is more than providing brochures and health information to patients. It is a cross-cutting idea, which shows promise as a global approach to dealing with the broad array of causes, prevention and the management of NCDs. Health literacy goes beyond a narrow concept and traditional silos individual behaviours, health education and health promotion and addresses the environmental, political and social factors that determine health.

However, we remain at a time when the supports and sustainability of health and education systems are in question and people are encouraged to adopt more self-care and self-management. With this status quo, as examples, we might consider looking for the following indicators to demonstrate that health literacy is improving in relation to NCDs.

People with enhanced health literacy may:

Access

- Have access to services and information (e.g. free cancer-screening clinics, community health services)
  - % of people know where to go to access information about chronic disease prevention and/or to managing their chronic condition
- Make more use of preventive services (e.g. mammograms, pap tests)
  - % of people who received the care that they needed
- Avoid hospitals and emergency rooms
  - % of patient visits

Comprehend

- Be more likely to understand instructions about prescription medication and avoid medication errors
  - % of people who report no problems following prescription medication instructions
- Be more likely to act on important public health alerts related to NCD (influencing health outcomes)
  - % of people who are aware of the key messages delivered in the alert (knowledge)
  - % of people who are aware of the local public health programming, activities and initiatives that support or promote the messages (awareness)
  - % of people who believe in the message (beliefs, attitudes, perceptions)
  - % of people who have acted on the messages and/or alert provided (behaviours)

Evaluate

- Be more critical of the health-related information that they receive or obtain
  - % of people who ask questions about the information that they receive related to health
  - % of people who consider the sources of the information that they receive
  - % of people who asses the quality of the information that they receive

Communicate

- Be more able to manage chronic conditions (e.g. diabetes, high blood pressure, asthma)
  - % of people who can effectively communicate with their health-care provider about their chronic disease or illness
  - % of people who are very comfortable speaking to their health-care provider about concerns they may have about their condition and/or their medication
  - % of people who have a strong support system
  - % of people who believe that they have the information they need to make the daily lifestyle changes to adopt more self-care and self-management
  - % of people who plan accordingly and make the necessary daily personal adjustments to manage their condition

Where to from Here

We would like to conclude with a summary of possible and emerging opportunities related to future global health efforts on health literacy and NCDs. Health literacy is everyone's business. We recognize that countries and jurisdictions vary with respect to their existing use of a health literacy lens and their current degree of activity to focus such activity to understand and address NCD. The list below shows possible examples categorized using three key action areas (Mitic and Rootman 2012). These examples can be implemented by a range of partners committed to improving health literacy in different settings or sectors (i.e. health care, education, community, government, workplace). This is not an exhaustive list.

Possible emerging roles and opportunities include the following:

1. Knowledge Development (Research and Evaluation)
   (a) Continue to identify existing, emerging and promising health literacy practices
   (b) Develop initiatives targeting specific health issues, settings and population groups, giving particular attention to main population groups with lowest health literacy levels (i.e. children/youth, older

adults, immigrant populations, indigenous groups) and focus on chronic disease areas (i.e. cardiovascular disease, cancer, respiratory disease, diabetes, obesity in children)
   (c) Involve multiple sectors including the general public to help determine the health literacy needs
   (d) Include health literacy factors in the evaluation of public health interventions in areas such as chronic disease prevention and management
   (e) Build on existing evidence and experience
   (f) Rigorously evaluate health literacy efforts
   (g) Develop means for sharing knowledge, results and experience (vary channels and formats to disseminate findings that effectively reach and influence health professionals, public and policy-makers)

2. Raise Awareness and Capacity Building
   (a) Educate practitioners, policy-makers, decision-makers and health practitioners in the field about the need to communicate health literacy and its contribution to improvements in health outcomes and decreased costs
   (b) Conduct town-hall meetings, increase awareness within communities and general public and gather information on health literacy concerns, abilities in relation to NCDs and improving health
   (c) Adapt resources and tools (plain language, culturally and linguistically appropriate)
   (d) Leverage technology (social media, Web sites) and interactive ehealth tools to disseminate health information in a timely fashion in multiple formats to the public and to meet specific patient needs
   (e) Ensure that all health and safety information meets the needs and capacity of patients (i.e. aging population, multicultural groups)
   (f) Provide tools and resources that enable health professionals to expand their health information seeking skills
   (g) Build capacities of health and education providers and systems
   (h) Develop health education and health

literacy curricula for early childhood, K-12, postsecondary institutions, medical schools, adult learning

   (i) Integrate health literacy concepts into existing curricula and programmes

   (j) Require certification for all teachers who teach health education in schools

   (k) Provide professional development opportunities to integrate health literacy concepts for all health professions (i.e. continuing education requirements in health literacy)

   (l) Train more librarians and reference staff in health literacy skills and health information technologies

   (m) Focus both on improving skills and providing supports to people especially to those with lower skill levels to reduce health disparities

3. Build Infrastructure and Partnerships

   (a) Strengthen engagement and partnerships between health (hospitals), education (schools, academia), businesses, government (all levels) and community sectors (organizations, libraries) to integrate health literacy awareness issues, campaigns and interventions

   (b) Commit fiscal (funding) and human resources (positions) to support health literacy efforts in these partnerships

   (c) Develop and/or enhance national, state/provincial health literacy standards or benchmarks to guide efforts for all health professionals

   (d) Create patient-friendly environments that are easy to navigate (i.e. conducive to communication, assistance with forms, incorporate visuals)

When health literacy is addressed, health-literate individuals have increased health knowledge and skills to effectively prevent disease and make healthier lifestyle choices. Enhancing health literacy means that individuals are able to play a crucial role in chronic disease prevention, self-management and self-care. In order to self-manage chronic disease on a daily basis, individuals must be able to access health information, understand it (often for complex medical routines), plan and make lifestyle adjustments requiring informed decisions and communicate with health care providers and other supports. When health literacy is addressed professionals, organizations and systems informed and concerned about health literacy increase the effectiveness of supports, interactions, services and products that are part of this equation.

We have been witness to the growing attention and developments of health literacy in national agendas across the globe. Health literacy has recently been included in one of the four *IUHPE Future Priority Areas for 2011–2016* under *"Health Promotion Systems"* after the 20th World IUHPE Conference held in Geneva, Switzerland (IUHPE 2011). This has led to a newly formed IUHPE Network/Working Group on Health Literacy. This interest is an example of a global resource reflecting the investment, support and promotion for current and forthcoming health literacy activities. Health literacy works in synergy with the other identified IUHPE priority action areas such as *"Non-communicable Disease Prevention and Control"*. It is hoped that ongoing global efforts can continue to be evidenced within these linked fields for sustainable improvements leading to well-being for all.

References

Abel, T. (2008). Measuring health literacy: Moving towards a health-promotion perspective. *International Journal of Public Health, 53*, 169–170.

Alwan, A., Armstrong, T., Cowan, M., & Riley, L. (2011). *Non-communicable disease profiles 2011*. Geneva, Switzerland: WHO Press.

Barry, M. M., Allengrante, J. P., Lamarre, M. C., Auld, M. E., & Taub, A. (2009). The Galway consensus conference. International collaboration on the development of core competences for health promotion and health education. *Global Health Promotion, 16*(2), 5–11.

Begoray, D. L., Gillis, D., & Rowlands, G. (2012). Concluding thoughts on the future of health literacy. In D. L. Begoray, D. Gillis, & G. Rowlands (Eds.), *Health literacy in context: International perspectives*. Hauppauge, NY: Nova Sciences Publishers, Inc.

Bloom, D. E., Cafiero, E. T., Jané-Llopis, E., Abrahams-Gessel, S., Bloom, L. R., Fathima, S., et al. (2011). *The global economic burden of noncommunicable diseases*. Geneva: World Economic Forum. Retrieved March 22, 2012 from http://www3.weforum.org/docs/WEF_Harvard_HE_Global Economic BurdenNon Communicable Diseases_2011.pdf.

Canadian Council on Learning. (2008). *Health literacy in Canada: A healthy understanding*. Retrieved February 26, 2012 from http://www.ccl-cca.ca/pdfs/HealthLiteracy/HealthLiteracyReportFeb2008E.pdf.

Canadian Public Health Association. (2006). *Health literacy interventions*. Ottawa, ON: Canadian Public Health Association.

Clement, S., Ibrahim, S., Crichton, N., Wolf, M., & Rowlands, G. (2009). Complex interventions to improve the health of people with limited literacy: A systematic review. *Patient Education and Counseling, 75*(3), 340–351.

Commission of the European Communities. (2007). *Together for health: A strategic approach for the EU 2008–2013*. Retrieved March 20, 2012 from http://ec.europa.eu/health/ph_overview/Documents/strategy_wp_en.pdf.

Frankish, J. (2011). *Health literacy models and frameworks* (unpublished).

Gazmararian, J., Williams, M., Peel, J., & Baker, D. (2003). Health literacy and knowledge of chronic disease. *Patient Education and Counseling, 51*, 267–275.

Green, L. W., & Kreuter, M. W. (1999). *Health promotion planning: An educational and environmental approach* (2nd ed.). Palo Alto, CA: Mayfield Publishing Co.

Hauser, J., & Edwards, P. (2006). *Literacy, health literacy and health: A literature review*. Unpublished report prepared for the Expert Panel on Health Literacy. Ottawa, ON

Institute of Medicine. (2004). *Health literacy: A prescription to end confusion*. Washington, DC: National Academies Press.

International Union for Health Promotion and Education. (2011). *IUHPE Health promotion action areas for 2011–2016*. Geneva, Switzerland: IUHPE. Retrieved February 25, 2012 from http://www.iuhpe.org/uploaded/.../PriorityAreas_2011-2015_ENG.pdf.

Johnston, L., Ammary, N., Epstein, L., Johnson, R., & Rhee, K. (2006). A trans-disciplinary approach to improve health literacy and reduce disparities. *Health Promotion Practice, 3*, 331–335.

Kickbusch, I. (2001). Health literacy: Addressing the health and education divide. *Health Promotion International, 16*, 289–297.

Kickbusch, I., & Nutbeam, D. (1998). Health promotion glossary. *Health Promotion International, 13*, 349–364.

Kickbusch, I., & Nutbeman, D. (2000). Advancing health literacy: A global challenge for the 21st century. *Health Promotion International, 15*(3), 183–184.

Kickbusch, I., Wait, S., & Maag, D. (2005). *Navigating health: The role of health literacy*. Retrieved February 18, 2012 from http://www.emhf.org/resource_images/NavigatingHealth_FINAL.pdf.

King, J. (2007). *Environmental scan of interventions to improve health literacy*. Antigonish, NS: National Collaborating Centre for Determinants of Health.

Lee, A. (2009). Health-promoting schools: Evidence for a holistic approach to promoting health and improving health literacy. *Applied Health Economics and Health Policy, 7*(1), 11–17.

Mancuso, C. A., & Rincon, M. (2006). Impact of health literacy on longitudinal asthma outcomes. *Journal of General Internal Medicine, 21*, 813–817.

Martin, L., Schonlau, M., Haas, A., Derose, K., Rudd, R., Loucks, E., et al. (2011). Literacy skills and calculated 10-year risk of coronary heart disease. *Journal of General Internal Medicine, 26*(1), 45–50.

McQueen, D. (2009). The Galway consensus. *Global Health Promotion, 16*(2), 3–4.

Mitic, W., & Rootman, I. (2012). *An intersectoral approach to improving health literacy for Canadians: A discussion paper*. Victoria, BC: Public Health Association of British Columbia. Retrieved May 2, 2012 from http://www.phabc.org/modules.php?name=Contentpub&pa=showpage&pid=182.

Nutbeam, D. (1998). Health promotion glossary. *Health Promotion International, 13*(4), 349–364.

Nutbeam, D. (2000). Health literacy as a public health goal: A challenge for contemporary health education and communication strategies into the 21st century. *Health Promotion International, 15*, 259–267.

Nutbeam, D. (2008). The evolving concept of health literacy. *Social Science & Medicine, 67*(12), 2072–2078.

Paasche-Orlow, M. K. (2009). Bridging the international divide for health literacy research. *Patient Education and Counseling, 75*, 293–294.

Paasche-Orlow, M. K., Parker, R. M., Gazmararian, J. A., Nielsen-Bohlman, L. T., & Rudd, R. R. (2005). The prevalence of limited health literacy. *Journal of General Internal Medicine, 20*(2), 175–184.

Pignon, M., DeWalt, D., Sheridan, S., Berkman, N., & Lohr, K. (2005). Interventions to improve health outcomes for patients with low literacy: A systematic review. *Journal of General Internal Medicine, 20*(2), 185–192.

Ratzan, S. (2001). Health literacy: Communication for the public good. *Health Promotion International, 16*(2), 207–214.

Rootman, I., & Gordon-El-Bihbety, D. (2008). *A vision for a health literate Canada report of the expert panel on health literacy*. Retrieved February 15, 2012 from http://www.cpha.ca/uploads/portals/h-l/report_e.pdf.

Rosenfeld, L., Rudd, R., Emmons, K. M., Acevedo-García, D., Martin, L., & Buka, S. (2011). Beyond reading alone: The relationship between aural literacy and asthma management. *Patient Education and Counseling, 82*, 110–116.

Rudd, R. E., McCray, A. T., & Nutbeam, D. (2012). Health literacy and definitions of terms. In D. L. Begoray, D. Gillis, & G. Rowlands (Eds.), *Health literacy in context: International perspectives*. Hauppauge, NY, USA: Nova Sciences Publishers, Inc.. Chapter 2.

Schillinger, D., Grumach, K., Piette, J., Osmond, D., Daher, C., Palacios, J., et al. (2002). Association of health literacy with diabetes outcomes. *Journal of the American Medical Association, 288*, 475–482.

Sheridan, S. L., Halpern, D. J., Viera, A. J., Berkman, N. D., Donahue, K. E., & Crotty, K. (2011). Interventions for individuals with low health literacy: A systematic review. *Journal of Health Communication, 16*(3), 30–54.

Simonds, S. K. (1974). Health education as social policy. Health Education. *Monograph, 2*, 1–25.

Sorensen, K., Van den Broucke, S., Fullam, J., et al. (2012). Health literacy and public health: A systematic review and integration of definitions and models. *BioMed Central Public Health, 12*(80). Retrieved February 15, 2012 from http://www.biomedcentral.com/1471-2458/12/80.

Speller, V., Smith, B. J., & Lysoby, L. (2009). Development and utilization of professional standards in health education and promotion: US and UK experiences. *Global Health Promotion, 16*(2), 32–41.

St Leger, L. (2001). Schools, health literacy and public health: Possibilities and challenges. *Health Promotion International, 16*(2), 197–205.

State of Victoria, Department of Health. (2011). *Victorian public health and well-being plan 2011–2015.* Melbourne, VIC: Prevention and Population Health Branch, Victorian Government, Department of Health.

Vamos, S., & Hayos, J. (2011). Putting health education on the public health map in Canada: The role of higher education. *Journal of Health Education, 41*(5), 310–318.

WHO. (1986). *Ottawa charter for health promotion.* Ottawa, ON: World Health Organization, Health and Welfare Canada, Canadian Public Health Association.

WHO. (2009). *New network to combat non-communicable diseases.* Retrieved March 16, 2012 from http://www.who.int/mediacentre/news/releases/2009/noncommunicable_diseases_20090708/en/.

Williams, M. V., Baker, D. W., Parker, R. M., & Nurss, J. R. (1998). Relationship of functional health literacy to patients' knowledge of their chronic disease. A study of patients with hypertension and diabetes. *Archives of Internal Medicine, 158*(2), 166–172.

Zarcadoolas, C., Pleasant, A., & Greer, D. S. (2006). *Advancing health literacy: A framework for understanding and action.* San Francisco, CA: Wiley.

From Healthy Public Policy to Intersectoral Action and Health-in-All Policies

Vivian Lin and Bronwyn Carter

Introduction

Many of the determinants of non-communicable diseases (NCDs) lie outside the remit of the health-care system. The prevention of NCDs, therefore, necessitates action from all sectors to address the determinants of NCDs and incorporate a concern for the health and equity impacts into their policy development process. The 1986 Ottawa Charter (World Health Organization 1986) pointed to the importance of healthy public policy (HPP) as a key strategy for improving health. These strategies have been applied to public policy measures on specific NCD risk factors, such as tobacco. The clustering of NCD risk factors, however, underlies the general distribution of health inequities, including NCDs. More comprehensive intersectoral action (ISA), involving government, civil society and private sector partnership, is needed, and at multiple levels.

The 1997 World Health Organization (WHO) report on Intersectoral Action for Health (World Health Organization 1997) reinforced the impor-

V. Lin (✉)
School of Public Health, International Union for Health Promotion and Education, Plenty Rd, Bundoora, Melbourne, VIC 3086, Australia

La Trobe University, Melbourne, VIC 3086, Australia
e-mail: v.lin@latrobe.edu.au

B. Carter
School of Public Health, La Trobe University, Melbourne, VIC 3086, Australia

tance of collaboration working across sectors. The 2008 release of the report of the WHO Commission on Social Determinants of Health (World Health Organization 2008b) again drew attention to the need for action outside the health sector, if the health equity gap is to be closed. More recently, the Health-in-All Policies (HiAP) approach has been proposed as a governance innovation to address health equity and social determinants of health. Such an approach aims to create the enabling conditions for ISA as well as provide a framework for HPP on specific risk factors.

This chapter outlines the rationale for using the HiAP approach for NCDs, and reviews successes and failings related to HPP and ISA. The chapter considers suggestions about how HiAP can be applied to NCDs and concludes with lessons as governments begin to adopt HiAP.

Experiences to Date: HPP and ISA

Since the advent of the Ottawa Charter, there have been numerous examples of HPP enacted in relation to specific NCD risk factors, such as tobacco, diet, physical activity and alcohol. These policies aim to "make healthy choices easy choices".

Tobacco control is a well-established and particularly successful model for HPP. Exemplar elements of the HPP approach for tobacco include banning of cigarette sales to minors, banning of tobacco advertising, enlargement of tobacco warning labels and use of graphic warnings (World Health Organization 2005b). These policy measures

D.V. McQueen (ed.), *Global Handbook on Noncommunicable Diseases and Health Promotion*,
DOI 10.1007/978-1-4614-7594-1_12, © Springer Science+Business Media, LLC 2013

are specifically directed to reducing tobacco consumption, but there are also policies which have brought shared benefits (or co-benefits) to the health sector as well as other arenas of public policy. For instance, the increased tax on tobacco products raised both the price signal for smokers as well as government revenue, and the banning of smoking in workplaces and public spaces helped to prevent exposure to second-hand smoke as well as enhance productivity and amenities. In these examples, the health policy objectives are achieved through policy measures in other sectors, and bring benefits to these other sectors.

Similarly, HPP has been applied for some time to nutrition—such as labelling of ingredients (Department of Health and Ageing 2011; The Australian National Preventive Health Agency 2012; World Health Organization 2012a, c), and to alcohol—such as blood alcohol limits for drivers, banning of advertising and limiting hours of bars and pubs (The Australian National Preventive Health Agency 2012; World Health Organization 2012a, c). Increasing enactment of public policies with co-benefits has been seen in relation to physical activity—through improvements in public transportation (thus increasing opportunities for incidental physical activity and improving mobility) and creating green spaces (thus improving recreational opportunities as well as physical environment) (World Health Organization 2004a, 2009; Centre Disease Control n.d.).

Regulatory policies related to NCD risk factors are not sufficient, however, for prevention. Policy intent can only be achieved through a combination of legislative enforcement, community education, policies in micro settings and development of alternative products. For example, schools and communities can initiate policies and education to limit sun exposure for children (Collins et al. 2001), and non-government organizations (NGOs), such as The Heart Foundation, can endorse healthier foods or work with industry to develop healthier products, such as lean meats (Heart Foundation of Australia n.d.). The health insurance industry and the medical profession can offer incentives for lifestyle counselling and support. Employers can offer health-promoting workplace-based programs (Bellew 2008). ISA—partnerships between government agencies, civil society and private sector at local and national levels—are an integral part of NCD prevention efforts and complement HPP.

Healthy cities have been a particularly important development where local public policies and ISA are integrated in a setting which also encompasses a variety of micro-settings (such as workplaces, schools, neighbourhoods, hospitals, markets). While outcome evaluation has been limited, process evaluations point to decision-makers being more responsive to community needs, increased citizen participation, greater collaboration between organizations, more engagement with diverse communities and skill improvement for participants (Kegler et al. 2007, 2008, 2009).

HPP and ISA have not necessarily been easy to enact. Experiences suggest that the key ingredients for success for an integrated settings approach (such as healthy cities) are high-level support or champion, meaningful entry points and action-orientation, appropriate organizational locus for coordination and implementation, specific authority and resourcing and integration of activities into ongoing management decision-making (World Health Organization 2005a). At the same time, expected barriers can be lack of political and/or organizational support, lack of resources, insufficient understanding of concept and co-benefits, competing priorities and inadequate partnership development and management skills (Harpham et al. 2001; Berkeleya and Springett 2006; O'Neill and Simard 2006; World Health Organization 2008a, 2012a, b, c).

HPP and ISA have contributed to providing an enabling environment for individuals to exercise choice about how they manage potential risks to health. Without targeting specific communities with complementary strategies, an unanticipated consequence may be an increase in health inequalities (World Health Organization 2008a, b). In addressing risks and problems in the broader environment, these strategies can deliver whole of population benefits.

As in all social change efforts, HPP and ISA require strong skills in coalition and partnership work. While these have been recognised as health promotion workforce competencies in recent years (Australian Health Promotion Association 2009; Barry et al. 2009), they are not traditionally part of the education of the health care or public health workforce in general. Thus, some of the failings have been related to "health imperialism"— where other sectors are told what to do in the name of health while their core concerns are elsewhere—and non-sustainability of efforts. An important lesson from these earlier efforts in HPP and ISA is to focus on co-benefits for different sectors, creating win–win situations for partners, and consider what organizational mechanisms and processes are needed to continue initial efforts and maintain momentum for action.

The Health-in-All Policies Approach

The notion of HiAP came into international thinking in 2006 when the European Union adopted Council Conclusions on HiAP at its meeting in Brussels. Following a conference in Kuopio, Finland, there was explicit acknowledgement that population health status has positive repercussions for overall social and economic development as well as for health expenditures, that many policies with overlapping health objectives would benefit from intersectoral collaboration, and that broad action across policy sectors complements the more specific tasks carried out in the health sector. This Council Conclusions called for further development of the knowledge base and methodology for understanding how health determinants are affected by public policies at all levels, along with investigation and development of coordination mechanisms to ensure that health considerations are taken into account in decision-making. Member states were invited to undertake health impact assessment of major policy initiatives, paying specific attention to policy impacts on equity, and to take into account in formulating and implementing national policies the added value offered by cooperation between government sectors, social

partners, the private sector and NGOs (Council of the European Union 2006).

The EU health ministers further declared in Rome in 2007 their commitment to strengthening multisectoral approaches and processes at European, national, regional and local levels (European Union 2007). The importance of acting at multiple levels and on health determinants was recognised as relevant to "tobacco control, nutrition and physical activity, alcohol-related harm, drug dependence, mental health, occupational health and safety, health and environment, health and migration, healthy ageing, preventing accidents and injuries, and addressing issues related to sexual health" p. 6 (European Union 2007).

In 2010, The Adelaide Statement on Health in All Policies was adopted following a meeting jointly convened by the WHO and the South Australia Government, outlining the key principles and pathways that contribute to action for health across all sectors of government (World Health Organization and Government of South Australia 2010). The Statement argues for "joined-up government"—an approach to governance that recognises the interdependent nature of public policymaking, and adopts strategic plans that set out common goals, integrated responses and increased accountability for government departments. Partnership with civil society and the private sector is integral to this governance approach.

The HiAP approach is different from the HPP and ISA approaches. HPP tends to be more focused on policy measures that address specific health conditions or risk factors. It is focused on adopting particular policy instruments for specific policy outcomes, it may or may not require continuing engagement across sectors and it does not point to an approach to governance. ISA is similarly focused on particular issues, and points to partnership across government sectors. It is also inclusive of civil society and private sector organization at various levels. But it is not necessarily oriented toward policy.

By 2010, whole of government HiAP approaches have been reported from 16 countries and regions in the world: Australia, Brazil, Cuba, England, Finland, Iran, Malaysia, New Zealand,

Northern Ireland, Norway, Quebec, Scotland, Sri Lanka, Sweden, Thailand and Wales. In each case, the formal adopt of HiAP was preceded by emergence of ad hoc intersectoral initiatives to address health equity and informed by a government vision for health which was broader than healthcare delivery and recognised the role of social determinants. All initiatives addressed health effects of lifestyle/behavioural factors and/ or working and living conditions, although there was more attention on the broader environmental factors and individual lifestyle issues. Nearly all countries undertook a mixture of universal and targeted approaches in their attempt to both improve health for all, as well as address health equity and needs of vulnerable population groups.

Tools Used for Operationalising HiAP

A variety of tools and instruments have been used when implementing HiAP. Notably, these include governance structures (inter-ministerial and interdepartmental committees, cross-sector action teams, integrated budgets and accounting, partnership platforms, community consultations), shared activities (joint workforce development, cross-cutting information and evaluation systems) and analytical tools (health lens, health impact assessment, health equity impact assessment) (European Observatory on Health Systems and Policies 2006; Department of Health South Australia 2010; Shankardass et al. 2011).

Health impact assessment (HIA) has been used in a majority of HiAP initiatives to date (Shankardass et al. 2011). HIA has been shown to be an effective tool in supporting intersectoral decision and policymaking in Europe (European Observatory on Health Systems and Policies 2007) and is recognised as an important tool for the implementation of HiAP (European Union 2007).

In all instances of implementation of HiAP, a particular problem was identified and acted upon through one or more interventions. These entry points for HiAP indicate the specific sectors to be involved as well as demonstrate the role that the health sector plays. While entry points have always been important for ISA and HPP, an HiAP framework allows for multiple entry points to be addressed simultaneously.

South Australia uses a health lens analysis as a way of engaging with other agencies, with a basic 5-step process: (1) engage (for example, joint working group to agree on policy focus); (2) gather evidence (quantitative and qualitative research, critical appraisal); (3) generate advice (report and recommendations); (4) navigate policy decision-making (output approved by lead agency and Health Dept); and (5) evaluate (process and impact). These activities are overseen by a Chief Executives group, with the Department of Premier and Cabinet as the HiAP lead agency, and the state strategic plan forms the basis for joined-up government (Department of Health South Australia 2010) (Fig. 12.1).

The South Australia approach is comparable to the health promotion lens developed by the Pan American Health Organization, which attempts to incorporate an understanding of the social, cultural, political, environmental and economic conditions and structures that affect the lives, and health, of individuals and communities, as well as build on strengths and assets of communities and institutions (PAHO 2008). These principles are then built into all aspects of health program planning, delivery and evaluation, and assist with mainstreaming health promotion in the health system. HiAP is comparable in that the health lens is mainstreamed into other institutions.

Another increasingly common policy tool is HIA (Kemm et al. 2004). In Norway, HIA is used as a policy instrument to promote ISA while social and land use planning is used at the municipal level. Wales has adopted the use of health equity impact assessment as a rapid policy analysis tool which includes community participation. In Thailand, all projects with possible harmful effects are required to conduct HIA in their decision-making process, but HIA can also be undertaken proactively by any government organization at the policy and planning stage, or be requested by local community that may have concerns about impacts of specific policies. HIA is institutionalised in

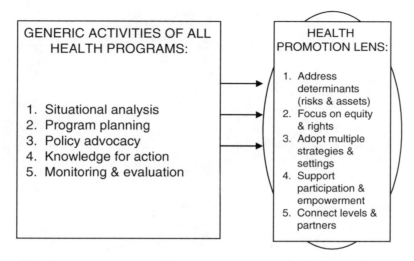

Fig. 12.1   The Health Promotion Lens. *Source*: Adapted from Pan American Health Organization (2008)

Thailand as the process is overseen by the National HIA Commission (Department of Health South Australia 2010).

Participants at the Adelaide meeting argue that HiAP works best when there is a clear mandate for joined-up government, systematic processes take account of interactions across sectors, mediation occurs across interests, engagement occurs with stakeholders outside of government, practical cross-sector initiatives build partnerships and trust and accountability, and transparency and participatory processes are present (World Health Organization and Government of South Australia 2010).

In order to improve effectiveness of action on social determinants of health, the WHO has developed an electronic platform to share tools and experiences. The website lists several tools and resources for governance and sector linkages containing material such as examples of policy for SDH and HiAP, resources for ISA and impact assessment, examples of programs implemented by local government and sectoral briefing papers and reports in relation to the education, housing, transport, social policy and environment sectors (Table 12.1).

Further resources available on the website include common ground and bridging differences in ISA, governance for mainstreaming (in relation to gender), public health legislation and promoting conditions for and facilitating participation.

Table 12.1   Action: SDH—tools and resources for action on SDH, by topic

Governance
Building governance
Implementing intersectoral action
Governance structures and instruments
Levels of government
Mainstreaming
Public health legislation
Sector linkages
Education
Housing
Transport
Social policy
Environment
Promoting participation
Participation conditions
Facilitating participation

Source: Adapted from World Health Organization 2010

Applying HiAP to NCD Prevention and Control

HPP and ISA have been long recognised as essential for controlling NCD risk factors—i.e. tobacco, alcohol, nutrition, physical activity and mental health. In the lead-up to the UN High Level Meeting on NCDs in New York in October 2011, international consultations and research also recognised the value of HiAP.

The first global ministerial conference on healthy lifestyles and NCD control committed to action on NCDs using the HiAP approach, identifying the potential for fiscal policies and regulations and other measures to reduce risk factors for NCDs (Moscow Declaration 2011). Focusing on the policy level, the potential HiAP interventions for the prevention of NCDs are apparent in the following areas: urban planning, taxation, pricing/subsidies, production and marketing of goods, health promotion financing and legislative mandates (United Nations 2011; World Bank 2011a, b).

HiAP can be applied to NCD prevention and control from three different entry points: risk factors or conditions, population groups (including life course and communities) and sectors. Entry points may be the starting point for single-policy measures but offer strategic points for ongoing dialogue and more extensive policy action.

Risk Factors/Conditions

Tobacco control provides one of the best known examples of HiAP applied to a key NCD risk factor. Multisectoral policy measures aimed at reducing tobacco use under the WHO Framework Convention on Tobacco Control (FCTC) typically require that legislative arms of government enact laws and bans; ministries of revenue implement tax increases on cigarettes; agricultural policies limit tobacco growth; and industry associations adhere to guidelines on advertising and promotion of cigarettes (see Table 12.2) (World Bank 2011a).

HiAP can be applied to other NCD risk factors, as seen in Table 12.2.

Finland's North Karelia project is an example of a comprehensive policy intervention, targeting several risk factors concomitantly. Using policy instruments such as those discussed above, interventions addressing environmental determinants and targeting diet, exercise and smoking achieved significant reduction in mortality due to chronic heart disease.

The New York City (NYC) restaurant project is an example of another local HiAP approach

Table 12.2 Examples of priority interventions to address risk factors for NCDs

Risk factor	Example intervention
Tobacco use	Accelerate implementation of the Framework Convention on Tobacco Control
	Raise taxes on tobacco
	Enforce bans on tobacco advertising, promotion and sponsorship
	Ban smoking in public places and protect people from tobacco smoke
	Offer help to quit tobacco use and warn about the dangers of tobacco use
Excessive dietary salt intake	Regulate salt concentration limits in processed and semi-processed foods
	Reduce dietary salt levels through voluntary action by food industry
	Promote low-sodium salt substitutes
	Implement information and education campaigns to warn about the harm from excessive salt intake
Harmful alcohol use	Increase taxes
	Ban advertising
	Restrict access
Unhealthy diets, physical inactivity, obesity	Introduce taxes for unhealthy food
	Provide subsidies for healthy food
	Promote labelling
	Administer marketing restrictions
Cardiovascular risk	Facilitate access to and promote combinations of drugs for individuals at high risk of NCDs
Environmental pollution	Subsidise and promote the use of cookstoves that use cleaner fuels
	Reduce emissions of harmful urban air pollutants from vehicles through better technology and greater use of mass transit
	Reduce exposure to agro-industrial chemicals and waste by ensuring clean water for irrigation and managing pesticide use for crops and vegetables

Sources: Expanded from *Toward a Healthy and Harmonious Life in China; Stemming the Rising Tide of Noncommunicable Diseases*. 2011. The World Bank. Adapted from "Priority action for the noncommunicable diseases" 2011. Lancet 377: 1438–47, cited by World Bank (2011a)

addressing risk factors. This project brought together the health and hospitality sectors, resulting in significant reductions in the use of *trans* fats as well as reduced smoking rates

(World Bank 2011b). Fit City NYC is another local HiAP project. This program provides free training sessions in active design guidelines for urban planners and architects, through involvement of multisector local council departments including building, transport, planning, parks, housing and schools, as well as interagency partnerships with academic institutions and architectural peak body representatives and private companies (Lee 2011).

Chile's alcohol policy reforms are an example of an HiAP approach. A collaborative project group involving international partners and an intersectoral committee including education, agriculture, transport and other sectors, drafted a National Alcohol Strategy, addressing alcohol from a societal perspective. Policy measures were introduced across sectors, including lower drink driving blood alcohol limits and increased penalties for drunk drivers as well as taxes on spirits (Peña 2012).

Table 12.3 Life course approach for NCD prevention and control

Stage of life	Policy opportunities
Foetal development and maternal environment	Subsidy for healthy food, targeted at low SES women
Infancy and early childhood	Subsidy for healthy food, targeted at low SES families
	Early childhood development programmes
Adolescence	Regulating food advertising
	School lunch programme
	Banning of alcohol and tobacco sales to minors
Adulthood	Health insurance incentives for keeping physically active
	Active transport
Aging and older people	Age-friendly cities
All stages	Safe communities
	Banning smoking in public spaces and workplaces

Source: Adapted from Hill et al. cited by World Bank (2011a)

Population Group/Life Course

An HiAP approach can also be applied to a life course approach to NCD prevention. Opportunities exist across the lifespan for lifestyle modification to reduce the risk of progression to NCDs. Reducing risk factors at the population level is possible within a conducive economic and legal environment, made possible by supportive government policy. Table 12.3 identifies policy opportunities addressing the need for access to healthy food for pregnant women and children; banning of promotion of tobacco and alcohol to adolescents; active lifestyles; older age-friendly environments; and safe communities and protection from exposure to passive smoking for all ages (World Bank 2011a).

Childhood obesity has become a major concern internationally. The childhood obesity prevention project EPODE is an example of a public–private partnership multi-stakeholder approach. The EPODE capacity building project which originated in France and subsequently has been developed in other countries based on the French experience aims to implement preventive

measures regarding diet and obesity at the local level, mobilising resources and securing additional funds through private–public partnerships as long as the prescribed rules are followed (World Health Organization 2009).

Built on the EPODE program, with the support of state and national governments, the South Australian OPAL programme uses a community-based approach coordinated through local government with the aim of reducing childhood overweight/obesity and increasing physical activity. For example, as part of the "Eat Well and Be Active Strategy", policy measures will be used to improve the built, social and natural environments as well as to ensure good governance, strong partnerships and workforce planning, which support healthy eating and physical activity (OPAL 2012).

The geographically based UK Health Action Zones (HAZ) are another example of a population group-based HiAP approach, with a particular emphasis on disadvantaged groups and partnership with local communities (Crawshaw et al. 2003). For example, one HAZ project working at the subregional level successfully put health on the agenda of other agencies at district

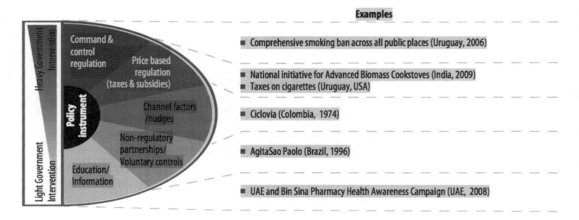

Fig. 12.2 A wide range of possible policy interventions to reduce NCDs. *Source*: "Effective Responses to Noncommunicable Diseases: Embracing Action Beyond the Health Sector", Health, Nutrition and Population Discussion Paper. 2011. Washington DC: World Bank, cited by World Bank (2011b). Reproduced with the permission of World Bank Publications

and strategic levels, through using HIA in developing a regional transport strategy. This HAZ project took a whole of systems approach, providing funding for cross-sector initiatives with a focus on addressing wider determinants of health and reducing health inequalities. Specific goals included promoting healthy employment opportunities and addressing the needs of older people as well as those undergoing cardiac rehabilitation (Springett 2005).

Sectors

Involvement of various sectors other than health is at the core of HiAP. A wide range of possible policy interventions are in use through existing intersectoral collaboration efforts, including with finance, agriculture, education, urban design and transport, together with civil society and the private sector (Fig. 12.2).

For example, various laws, guidelines and self-regulatory codes govern the advertising and promotion of food at country and international levels, but existing regulations do not consider food a special category from a public health viewpoint. Consumer protection laws have been used in cases against large food companies but there is scope for further development of the

HiAP approach in the food sector. More specifically in relation to marketing of food to children, minimal regulation is in place for non-traditional forms of marketing and the growing use of promotional activities in developing countries. Food advertising is not regulated in the majority of countries surveyed in the WHO global review of regulation of marketing of food to children, nor are specific restrictions in place on timing and content of television advertisements directed at children, in-school marketing and sale of food products, Internet marketing, sponsorship, product placement and sales promotions (World Health Organization 2004b).

The Republic of Slovenia adopted the HiAP approach, being the first government to review the health effects of agriculture policy at the national level. HIA was shown to be a useful tool in raising broader public health issues on the agricultural policy agenda (Lock et al. 2003). Policy opportunities in the agricultural sector with consequent health benefits were identified, such as financial support to increase production and yield (thereby preventing health problems associated with unemployment amongst farmers). Opportunities for joint work between health and agricultural sectors were identified to promote consumption and stimulate demand, through transferring production to fruits and vegetables and increasing demand through public procurement (Lock 2011).

The World Bank report on NCD prevention and control in China (World Bank 2011a) proposed that an HiAP approach be a key aspect of the national strategy, given that NCDs in China account for over 80 % of annual mortality and contribute 68.6 % of the total disease burden. More importantly, social and environmental determinants of chronic disease such as poverty and growing urbanisation contribute to the higher prevalence of NCDs and key risk factors among the poor in China, e.g. smoking prevalence among men aged 15–69 in China is among the highest in the world and is higher in less educated men in rural and western regions (World Bank 2011a). These risk factors and determinants of chronic disease in China would be addressed by comprehensive ISA involving a whole of government approach, rather than by the health sector targeting vulnerable groups and acting alone (Shankardass et al. 2011).

Table 12.4 identifies policy opportunities for the government in China, with sectors other than health as the entry point, addressing the need for access to healthy food, reduction of tobacco use and alcohol abuse, increased physical activity and improved access to coordinated care. A task-force identifying priorities and allocating funds for multisectoral action is suggested as a first step in adopting an HiAP approach, with a view to considering HiAP for adoption as national policy, as done by the European Union in 2006 (World Bank 2011a).

These recommendations for China are relevant to most countries, although priorities, specific measures and sequencing of policy action might vary.

Table 12.4 HiAP for NCD prevention and control in China

Sector	Policy opportunities
Finance	Subsidy for healthy food production
	Increasing prices for tobacco, alcohol, oils
	Removal of subsidy for harmful products, such as tobacco and sugar
Agriculture/food	Salt reduction in processed food
	Reduction of *trans* fat in food
	Crop substitution for tobacco
	Maintaining adequate land for agriculture and local food system development
Environment	Enforcement of environmental pollution standards
	Green spaces and physical activity facilities as part of housing development
Infrastructure, transportation	Better public transportation
	Road planning to facilitate cycling and walking
	Safe communities
Education	School breakfast/lunch programmes
	Sun protection measures
Social protection	Single-payer system
	Funding for care planning and coordination
Law enforcement	Penalties for violating smoke-free environment, excessive drinking, occupational and environmental pollution
Media	Ban inclusion of smoking and alcohol in TV and films
	Ban advertising of cigarettes and alcohol
Private sector	Workplace programmes

Source: Adapted from World Bank (2011a)

Lessons for Implementation of HiAP

HiAP experiences to date point to highly heterogeneous approaches for integrated management, but often linked either to development of primary health care or where intersectoral strengthening at local or regional level was itself a government goal. The specific structures used for joined-up government sectors include cabinet committees, steering committee, independent organizational unit, unit integrated into existing structure and network of committees (Shankardass et al. 2011).

From these early days of the implementation of the HiAP approach, emerging lessons relate to models for cross-sectoral interaction; governance structures; new roles for health departments; and mechanisms for NCD prevention

Table 12.5 Models for intersectoral interaction

Informative	Cooperative	Cooperation and coordination	Coordination	Coordination and integration	Integration
–	Brazil	England	Malaysia	Cuba	Iran
	New Zealand	Sri Lanka	N. Ireland	Finland	Norway
		Wales	Quebec	Thailand	
			Scotland		
			S. Australia		
			Sweden		

Source: Adapted from Shankardass et al. (2011)

and control. A variety of models for interaction between health and other sectors can be found, as seen in Table 12.5, occurring on a continuum ranging from simple information sharing to more intensive modes of integration (Shankardass et al. 2011).

A sustained approach to HiAP requires an ongoing structure and process for engagement. Governance structures are, therefore, critical for continued engagement across different sectors, if not different levels of government. Governance structures can be used to lead to a variety of decisions and actions that underpin the ultimate adoption of HiAP (McQueen et al. 2012). Case studies of intersectoral governance in European countries suggest that different structures are effective for different types of actions, as seen in Table 12.6.

The lessons from the European case studies essentially point to the following key success factors for HiAP (McQueen et al. 2012):

- Political will—presence of political support or interest
- Partnerships and constituents' interests—support from stakeholders outside government as well as across portfolios/departments
- Political importance of the specific health issues identified—expectation that a policy solution will be found
- Immediacy of the problem—time-limited response expected

- Leadership—may be political or bureaucratic
- Context—situational landscape as well as political landscape
- Resources—governance structures and actions require human and financial resources
- Implementation practicalities—solutions need to be feasible and workable

In order to work effectively across sectors, health departments/ministries will need to adopt new roles and capabilities. These include the following: understand the political agendas and administrative imperatives of other sectors; bring evidence base of policy options and strategies; assess comparative health consequences of policy options; create regular platforms for dialogue and problem-solving; work with other departments to achieve co-benefits; and evaluate effectiveness of intersectoral and integrated policymaking. Building the capacity of health departments and other sectors will also be necessary.

Creating a governance framework is a critical step. A cross-sectoral body, advised by non-government interests, is a first practical step to undertake analysis of the distribution of NCD risks and prioritise possible measures. Ideally, an NCD Commission could bring together key actors across government as well as outside government, to propose policy measures and oversee their implementation for prevention of NCDs, and ensuring health equity concerns are incorporated into NCD prevention policy and planning.

Table 12.6 Relationship between governance structures and governance actions

Intersectoral governance structures		Governance actions								
		Evidence support	Setting goals and targets	Coordination	Advocacy	Monitoring and evaluation	Policy guidance	Financial support	Providing legal mandate	Implementation and management
Government level	Ministerial linkages	–	✓	✓	–	✓	–	–	✓	–
	Cabinet Committees and Secretaries	–	✓	✓	✓	–	–	–	–	–
Parliament level	Parliamentary Committees	✓	–	–	✓	✓	✓	–	✓	–
Bureaucratic level/(civil service)	Interdepartmental committees and units	✓	–	✓	✓	✓	✓	–	–	✓
	Mega ministries and mergers	–	–	✓	–	–	–	–	–	✓
Managing funding arrangements	Joint budgeting	–	–	✓	–	–	✓	✓	–	✓
	Delegated financing	–	–	✓	✓	–	✓	✓	✓	✓
Engagement beyond government	Public engagement	✓	✓	–	✓	–	✓	–	–	–
	Stakeholder engagement	–	–	–	✓	–	✓	✓	✓	–
	Industry engagement	–	–	✓	–	–	–	✓	–	–

Source: Adapted from McQueen et al. (2012)

References

Australian Health Promotion Association. (2009). *Core competencies for health promotion practitioners.* Maroochydore, QLD: Australian Health Promotion Association.

Barry, M., Allegrante, J., Lamarre, M. -C., Auld, M. E., & Taub, A. (2009). The Galway consensus conference: International collaboration on the development of core competencies for health promotion and health education. *Global Health Promotion, 16*(2), 5–11.

Bellew, B. (2008). *Primary prevention of chronic disease in Australia through interventions in the workplace setting: An evidence check rapid review brokered by the Sax institute for the Chronic Disease Prevention Unit.* Melbourne, VIC: Victorian Government Department of Human Services.

Berkeleya, D., & Springett, J. (2006). From rhetoric to reality: Barriers faced by health for all initiatives. *Social Science & Medicine, 63*, 179–188.

Centre Disease Control. (n.d.). *US National activity plan.* From http://www.physicalactivityplan.org/theplan.php.

Collins, L., Stoneham, M. J., et al. (2001). Preventing skin cancer in Queensland: An evaluation of a community shade creation project. *Environmental Health, 1*(2), 87–94.

Council of the European Union. (2006). Council Conclusions on Health in All Policies (HiAP), 2767th Employment, Social Policy, Health and Consumer Affairs Council meeting, Brussels.

Crawshaw, P., Bunton, R., & Gillen, K. (2003). Health action zones and the problem of community. *Health & Social Care in the Community, 11*(1), 36–44.

Department of Health and Ageing. (2011). *Labelling logic. Review of food labelling law and policy.* Commonwealth of Australia: Department of Health and Ageing.

Department of Health South Australia. (2010). *Implementing health in all policies.* Adelaide, SA: Department of Health Government of South Australia.

European Observatory on Health Systems and Policies. (2006). *Health in all policies prospects and potentials.* Finland: Ministry of Social Affairs and Health Finland.

European Observatory on Health Systems and Policies. (2007). *The effectiveness of health impact assessment scope and limitations of supporting decision-making in Europe.* Copenhagen: World Health Organization.

European Union. (2007). Declaration on Health in All Policies. *Health in All Policies: achievement and challenges.* Rome.

Harpham, T., Burton, S., & Blue, I. (2001). Healthy city projects in developing countries: The first evaluation. *Health Promotion International, 16*(2), 111–125.

Heart Foundation of Australia. (n.d.). *Healthy eating.* From http://www.heartfoundation.org.au/healthy-eating/Pages/default.aspx.

Kegler, M. C., Ellenberg Painter, J., Twiss, J. M., Aronson, R., & Norton, B. L. (2009). Evaluation findings on community participation in the California Healthy Cities and Communities program. *Health Promotion International, 24*(4), 300–310.

Kegler, M. C., Escoffery, C., Alcantara, I., Ballard, D., & Glanz, K. (2008). A qualitative examination of home and neighborhood environments for obesity prevention in rural adults. *International Journal of Behavioral Nutrition and Physical Activity, 5*, 65.

Kegler, M. C., Norton, B. L., & Aronson, R. (2007). Skill improvement among coalition members in the California Healthy Cities and Communities Program. *Health Education Research, 22*(3), 450–457.

Kemm, J., Parry, J., & Palmer, S. (2004). *Health impact assessment: Concepts, theory, techniques and applications.* Oxford: Oxford University Press.

Lee, K. (2011). *Active design guidelines promoting physical activity and health in design.* Alberta: WHO Collaborating Center for NCD Policy University of Alberta School of Public Health.

Lock, K. (2011). *HIA of agriculture and nutrition policies in Slovenia.* From: http://www.docstoc.com/docs/77149661/HIA-of-agriculture-and-nutrition-polices-in-Slovenia.

Lock, K., Gabrijelcic-Blenkus, M., Martuzzi, M., Otorepec, P., Wallace, P., & Dora, C. (2003). Health impact assessment of agriculture and food policies: Lessons learnt from the Republic of Slovenia. *Bulletin of the World Health Organization, 81*(6), 391–398.

McQueen, D., Wismar, M., Lin, V., Jones, C. M., & Davies, M. (2012). *Intersectoral governance for health in all policies.* European Observatory on Health Systems and Policies. Copenhagen.

Moscow Declaration. (2011). *First Global Ministerial Conference on Healthy Lifestyles and Noncommunicable Disease Control.* Moscow.

O'Neill, M., & Simard, P. (2006). Choosing indicators to evaluate Healthy Cities projects: A political task? *Health Promotion International, 21*(2), 145–152.

OPAL. (2012). *Eat well be active strategy 2011–16.* From http://www.sahealth.sa.gov.au/wps/wcm/connect/public+content/sa+health+internet/healthy+living/healthy+eating/eat+well+be+active+strategy+2011-16.

Pan American Health Organization. (2008). *Mainstreaming health promotion in PAHO.* Revised Framework—Draft July. Washington, DC: Pan-American Health Organization.

Peña, S. (2012). *Health in all policies.* A global contribution to the WHO Global Conference on Health Promotion in Helsinki 2013.

Shankardass, K., Solar, O., Murphy, K., Freiler, A., Bobbili, S., & Bayoumi, A. (2011). *Getting started with health in all policies: A resource pack.* Report to the Ministry of Health and Long-Term Care. Ontario, Prepared by the Centre for Research on Inner City Health (CRICH) in the Keenan Research Centre of the Li Ka Shing Knowledge Institute of St. Michael's Hospital.

Springett, J. (2005). Geographically-based approaches to the integration of health promotion into health systems: A comparative study of two Health Action Zones in the UK. *Promotion and Education, Suppl 3*, 39–44.

The Australian National Preventive Health Agency. (2012). *ANPHA First Year Highlights Report 2011–*

2012. Retrieved July 27, 2012, from http://www. anpha.gov.au/internet/anpha/publishing.nsf/Content/ highlights-1st+year.

United Nations. (2011). *Resolution adopted by the General Assembly*. Political Declaration of the High-level Meeting of the General Assembly on the Prevention and Control of Non-communicable Diseases. New York

World Bank. (2011a). *Toward a healthy and harmonious life in China: Stemming the rising tide of non-communicable diseases*. Human Development Unit, East Asia and Pacific Region. Washington.

World Bank. (2011b). *The growing danger of non-communicable diseases, acting now to reverse course*.

World Health Organization. (1986). *The Ottawa charter for health promotion*. First International Conference on Health Promotion, Ottawa. From http://www.who. int/healthpromotion/conferences/previous/ottawa/en/ index.html.

World Health Organization. (1997). *Intersectoral action for health. A cornerstone for health-for-all in the twenty-first century*. Report of the International Conference. Halifax, Nova Scotia, Canada.

World Health Organization. (2004a). *Global strategy on diet, physical activity and health*. Geneva: World Health Organization.

World Health Organization. (2004b). *Marketing food to children: The global regulatory environment*. Geneva: World Health Organization.

World Health Organization. (2005a). *Settings-based initiatives to address environmental risks to children's health—What works?* (Annex 3). In Consultation report—Healthy Environments for Children Alliance,

Inter-regional Consultation, Improving Children's Environmental Health in Settings, Experiences and lessons for policies and action. Entebbe, Uganda.

World Health Organization. (2005b). *WHO framework convention on tobacco control*. From http://www.who. int/fctc/about/en/index.html.

World Health Organization. (2008a). *City leadership for health*. Geneva: World Health Organization.

World Health Organization. (2008b). *Closing the gap in a generation: Health equity through action on the social determinants of health*. Commission on Social Determinants of Health—final report. Geneva: World Health Organization.

World Health Organization. (2009). *Population-based prevention strategies for childhood obesity*. Geneva: World Health Organization.

World Health Organization. (2012). *Global strategy on diet, physical activity and health*. Retrieved July 27, 2012, from http://www.who.int/dietphysicalactivity/ en/index.html.

World Health Organization. (2012). *Healthy cities evaluation*. From http://www.who.int/healthy_settings/ types/cities/en/index.html.

World Health Organization. (2012). *Management of substance abuse. Global strategy to reduce harmful use of alcohol*. Retrieved July 27, 2012, from http://www.who. int/substance_abuse/activities/gsrhua/en/index.html.

World Health Organization and Government of South Australia. (2010). Statement on health in all policies: Moving towards a shared governance for health and well-being. Adelaide. *Health Promotion International, 25*(2), 258–260.

Section III

Approaches to NCDs

Population Health Intervention Research: A Fundamental Science for NCD Prevention

13

Louise Potvin

Studies indicate that most noncommunicable diseases (NCDs) are linked to various degrees to lifestyle and behavioral risk factors (McGinnis and Foege 1994; Mokdad et al. 2004). Logically, it follows that NDCs and associated mortality, morbidity, and other social costs can be prevented through decreasing the population prevalence of those risk factors (Smedley and Syme 2000). In this chapter, we argue that because of the complexity of the ecosystems that shape the population prevalence of NCD risk factors, there is still much uncertainty about which actions are required by whom to influence the population prevalence of risk factors.

Current etiological models, even the most complex ones, are limited to identifying potential causal pathways that go from ecosystemic conditions to population prevalence of risk factors to morbidity and mortality. For example, the systemic model of the obesity system developed for the British Foresight Report on obesity maps several dozens of variables and their feedback loops, into a very complex graphic representation (Government Office of Science 2007). Strength of this and other similar models is that they represent vital and necessary knowledge for identifying the risk factors and conditions that should be targeted

L. Potvin (✉)
Department of Social & Preventive Medicine
and Institut de recherche en santé publique,
University of Montreal, 7101 Parc Avenue, Room
3028, Montreal, QC, Canada H3N 1X70
e-mail: Louise.potvin@umontreal.ca

by public health programs and policy. They offer a variety of intervention points for public health and other actors in the prevention arena. Their major weakness however is that they provide very little clue on how to modify those conditions: on the type of public health programs and policy that should be implemented, by whom, where, and how, in order to affect those conditions and achieve foreseeable population health goals. Other types of studies and scientific efforts are required for that, studies that aim to develop a body of knowledge about the implementation and effectiveness of policy and programs aimed at changing the population distribution of risk factors and conditions involved in the etiology of NCDs.

The Moving Target of NCD Prevention: The Example of Tobacco

The spectacular reduction of tobacco consumption achieved in North America and in most Northern European countries during the last quarter of the twentieth century is often recognized as one of the major victories of public health. Indeed, starting in the late 1960s, and following the US Surgeon General's report on the adverse health consequences of tobacco smoking (US Department of Education, Health, and Welfare 1964), a wide variety of smoking cessation and tobacco use prevention efforts have been tried, implemented, disseminated, and scaled up. As of the end of 2012, the Cochrane Tobacco

D.V. McQueen (ed.), *Global Handbook on Noncommunicable Diseases and Health Promotion*,
DOI 10.1007/978-1-4614-7594-1_13, © Springer Science+Business Media, LLC 2013

Addiction Group (www.cochrane.tobacco.org) has published more than 70 review reports on tobacco prevention, smoking cessation, and government policy, synthesizing results from hundreds of interventions.

Since the 1970s, the use of tobacco has declined steadily in most western countries (Schaap et al. 2008). This decline was accompanied by a decrease in cardiovascular mortality for which smoking is one of the major risk factors (Unal et al. 2003). It is estimated that the 32 % reduction in smoking prevalence in the USA between 1980 and 2000 was responsible for 12 % of all the deaths from coronary heart diseases that were prevented in the USA during that same period (Ford et al. 2007). Overall, it is estimated that about 50 % of the reduction in coronary heart disease mortality during the last quarter of the twentieth century in developed countries can be attributed to the reduction of behavioral risk factors (Ford et al. 2007). Such data confirms some of the early promises of epidemiology that the identification of modifiable risk factors would lead to the reduction of their prevalence and ultimately to preventing diseases, suffering, and death.

However, a deeper examination of global trends in tobacco consumption shows that there is still much to accomplish for the prevention of tobacco-related mortality. After almost 50 years of efforts, tobacco is still killing on a massive scale globally (Ezzati and Lopez 2003; Jha 2009). In Western countries, where most of the prevention efforts have taken place and where significant reduction in tobacco consumption was achieved, the prevalence of smokers seems to stagnate somewhere between 15 and 25 %, (OECD 2009). More preoccupying is the fact that in all countries for which data is available, those who have stopped smoking are more likely to be from higher socioeconomic groups (Schaap et al. 2008). Consequently, the prevalence of smokers is now much higher among individuals in lower socioeconomic status groups (Barbeau et al. 2004), and more difficult to reach by standard cessation programs and tobacco reduction policy. In addition, the reduction of smoking in Western countries was accompanied by a displacement of the tobacco industry's marketing efforts which are now concentrated in regions of emerging economies, especially in

Eastern Europe and Asia (Gilmore and McKee 2004). Drawing lessons from the tobacco prevention policies and programs in Western countries, the tobacco industry adjusted its practices to develop new markets. "As the transnational tobacco companies successfully established new markets, they adapted aggressive marketing strategies used in high-income countries. Many of these strategies are illegal or severely restricted in high-income countries" (Lee et al. 2012, p. 117). Nowadays, 80 % of smokers reside in low- and middle-income countries and about 50 % of smoking-related deaths are occurring in low-income countries (Jha 2009). The tobacco epidemic has gone global (Proctor 2004) and has become a marker of social health inequalities (Frohlich 2008).

This example illustrates what becomes increasingly clear for epidemiologists and public health practitioners: the social conditions that shape population prevalence of risk factors (Rose 1992) are complex, multifaceted, and made of interrelated systems. Attempts to modify some of those conditions in populations through policy and programs may have impacts well beyond the conditions that were targeted by those interventions. Epidemiologists, and social epidemiologists in particular, have criticized etiological models of disease causation that propose a linear representation, from distal to proximal, of chains of causes (Krieger 1994, 2008). Instead, they propose models that take into account all aspects that influence human lives, from biology to the ways in which societies are organized (Dahlgren and Whitehead 1991; Mackenbach and Stronks 2004; World Health Organization 2008). For public health practitioners, these complex and multilevel models often translate into an ecological or an ecosystemic approach to chronic disease prevention (Richard et al. 2011; Institute of Medicine 2002) as a way of dealing with the complexity of the social world.

The Ecological Paradigm and the Context of Prevention Interventions

In the 2002 report on the *Future of the Public's Health in the 21st Century*, the Institute of Medicine (2002) strongly suggested the use of the ecological model for the planning and implementation of prevention. Ecological model recognizes that population prevalence of chronic diseases is rooted in the complex interplay of conditions that run across the many systems that form a society. To be effective prevention should encompass this complexity. There exist many variations and formulations of the ecological model for health (Richard et al. 2011). Typically these models represent individuals' behaviors and their determinants within their context and in interaction with the context as well (Trickett 2009). Ecological models conceive of individuals' behavioral risk factors as being influenced by the many systems and subsystems in which they belong and interact with other individuals throughout their life course. These systems vary in size, from household and family to workplace, to community, and to nation. In many representations, each system is embedded into a more inclusive, higher level system. Furthermore, since higher level systems are social settings, an ecological perspective on health also encompasses the so-called social determinants of health (WHO 2008). Therefore, ecological interventions to reduce the prevalence of risk factors in a population are generally comprehensive and multi-strategical (Institute of Medicine 2012). They seek to implement activities aimed at modifying environmental and social conditions in multiple relevant settings and these activities encompass a variety of strategies through which environments can be modified (Richard et al. 1996).

The actual WHO global strategy for addressing the tobacco epidemic, the Tobacco Free Initiative (WHO 2012a), is an example of the application of a comprehensive ecological model. At the core of this initiative, the MPOWER strategy proposes six types of activities that comprise most of the known effective interventions to reduce smoking prevalence. These are the following: (1) monitor tobacco use and prevention policies; (2) protect people from tobacco smoke; (3) offer help to quit tobacco use; (4) warn about the dangers of tobacco; (5) enforce bans on tobacco advertising, promotion, and sponsorship; and (6) raise taxes on tobacco (WHO 2012b).

One prominent feature of the ecological paradigm for prevention is the integration of a systemic perspective (Green et al. 1996; Stokols 1996; McLaren and Hawe 2005). Populations live in, and create, ecosystems composed of interrelated subsystems which include all the elements of the social and physical environments that support life. By definition, such systems are open systems, meaning that changes in any subsystem impact other subsystems through a series of feedback loops that characterize systems' functioning (Richard et al. 2011). Likewise, comprehensive population- and community-based prevention interventions are increasingly conceived as systems operating within those ecosystems (Hawe et al. 2009; Potvin and McQueen 2008; Trickett 2009), implying also reciprocal feedback loops between the interventions and the contexts in which they are implemented. In other words, population-based prevention interventions are not just a series of activities that are planned and implemented with resources that are totally situated outside of the setting of interest. These activities form systems of action that may or may not be resourced from external sources but are supported by delivery systems that engage with the community in which they are implemented (IOM 2012; Poland et al. 2008). To effectively change conditions that shape the prevalence of risk factors, prevention strategies must be culturally relevant and adapted to the characteristics of the settings (populations and communities) in which they are implemented (Trickett 2009) and they must be supported by some participatory mechanisms that engage with local populations (Viswanathan et al. 2004).

Context and the dense network of interactions among the various environments that compose one's context are increasingly recognized as fundamental elements, not only for understanding the population distribution of NCDs but also in the design and implementation of prevention efforts and in their evaluation (IOM 2012; Poland et al. 2008). Dealing with context in the implementation of prevention has become one of the major challenges not only in the design and implementation of NCD prevention but also in the constitution of a body of scientific knowledge to inform prevention (Potvin et al. 2005; Ruetten and Gelius 2011). Prevention interventions, in the form of policy or programs, can no longer be conceived as coming entirely from outside of the population concerned. Although there is some kind of externality in terms of resources, knowledge, and practices that are associated with NCD prevention, the manner in which such external elements are adapted and integrated in context is seen as constitutive of the effectiveness of such interventions (Poland et al. 2008; Trickett 2009).

This raises fundamental questions about the traditional neglect of issues related to external validity in health sciences and about the relevance and limitations of generalizing the results of population health intervention experimentations across settings (Green 2006; Green and Glasgow 2006). If adaptation and intervention–context interactions are essential elements for intervention effectiveness, then knowledge derived from experimentations in prevention can only be considered as the best plausible hypothesis for designing and implementing prevention in another setting. Indeed, beyond the mere recognition that implementation variations exist across sites not much is known about what produces local implementation variations of prevention policy and programs (Clavier et al. 2012a, b), and how to adapt those programs as a function of the various contexts, in order to maximize effectiveness. Aggregating empirical results from intervention experimentations across settings is unlikely to provide insights into how interventions interact with context and what makes those interactions effective. As a complement to epidemiology—a science that illuminates problems, their prevalence, and their causes and which provides invaluable knowledge about the causal pathways that lead to the population prevalence of NCDs—there is a need for developing a science of solutions that will provide valid scientific knowledge on the design, implementation, sustainability, diffusion, and scaling up of prevention efforts and their variations. This is exactly the goal of the nascent field of population health intervention research.

Beyond Evaluation: Population Health Intervention Research

There is a rich and productive field of research called evaluation that has been thriving for almost half a century. Rooted in the "Great society" objectives of the 1960s, early developments in the field of evaluation were linked to the ambitious program of using scientific means to transform society for the public's good (O'Connor 1995). The "experimenting society" as one of the pioneering figure of this field explained would be continuously studying attempts to improve social conditions and use the knowledge produced to inform further improvements (Campbell 1969, 1991). During the past decades, evaluation has developed as a scientific field, with its own journals, professional associations, and graduate training programs. The interventions evaluated cover a wide range of social, health, and economic issues at scales that vary from individual to global. Because it is also closely associated with judging the value of interventions and decision making, the field of program evaluation has often been discussed as a planning and management tool instead of a scientific endeavor.

In health research particularly, the term evaluation is not widely used to discuss the development of knowledge concerning interventions. In medicine and other health professions, clinical epidemiology has become the science through which knowledge about practice and clinical interventions is developed, synthesized, and disseminated into evidence-based practice (Sackett et al. 1985). There is now a general consensus about the distinction between epidemiology as a science that seeks to describe and understand the distribution and causes of diseases and clinical epidemiology, the study of clinical practices that relates to diagnosis and therapy in the context of patient care (Sackett 2002).

In the field of population and public health there is an analogous attempt to distinguish between research focusing on the causes of the population distribution of diseases and risk factors and research focusing on the interventions that are developed and implemented in attempts to modify these distributions through changes in social and physical environment. Population health intervention research (PHIR) is defined as the use of scientific methods to produce knowledge about interventions designed and implemented within or outside of the health sector with the intention to change the distribution of health and its determinants in a population (Hawe and Potvin 2009). Although there are many areas of overlap between PHIR and evaluation, the former appears as a specific subfield for population and public health and clearly identifies a specific object (population health intervention) for scientific enquiries. Hawe and Potvin (2009) further define population health interventions as coordinated actions, in the form of policy or programs intended to change the conditions that shape population health. Morabia and Costanza (2012) noted the overlap between the conceptual and methodological territory claimed by PHIR and the US-based tradition of community intervention research. The latter, a typical multidisciplinary field in which public health and community psychology researchers have been very active, is generally defined as the study of community-based interventions aimed at disease prevention and at the promotion of community well-being.

In population and public health, early attempts in the 1980s and 1990s to "experiment" with, and change, the social and community conditions that shape behavioral risk factors and ultimately, population health, were mainly undertaken by academic researchers to test scientific hypotheses. The Stanford Five City Project (Fortmann et al. 1995), the Minnesota Heart Health Project (Luepker et al. 1994), the Kaiser Family Foundation Community Health Promotion Grant Program (Wagner et al. 2000), and the tobacco prevention COMMIT trial (COMMIT Research Group 1995) are examples of such community trials designed and implemented by academic researchers. It became clear in the late studies such as the Kaiser Family Foundation and the COMMIT trial that in order to be effective community interventions need to be flexible and adaptations to contextual conditions are necessary. Relevant questions for such trials were no longer

whether community approaches to prevention work but instead what mix of activities is likely to be effective in which context (Fisher 1995), shifting the emphasis away from the intervention itself towards local capacity to implement and sustain interventions. This coincided with an increasing preoccupation with the sustainability of such initiatives once the research project is completed, making important distinctions between intervention delivery systems that are created through research projects and community service delivery systems that are the vehicle through which such projects can be continued and sustained (Altman 1995). Indeed, one important caveat associated with early community prevention trials was that even in the case of effective interventions, delivery systems created through research funding that were mainly serving research objectives were not necessarily transferred nor transferable to existing community structures.

In the same manner that clinical epidemiology is now an important contributor to the improvement of therapeutic practices in clinical settings, we suggest that population health intervention research will provide critical knowledge for evidence-based NCD prevention. Most robust research findings in clinical epidemiology come from studies that take place within regular care delivery systems with regular clinicians. In many cases research is integrated within care delivery systems and such integration has been shown to increase the relevance of research for practice, increase innovation in practice, and decrease the lag between scientific discovery and improvement in clinical practice. This proximity between research and delivery systems is even more critical for the nascent field of PHIR in which intervention context plays a dual role. First, as implied by the systemic ecological model, the effectiveness of population interventions is linked to the manner in which interventions adapt and are made relevant with regard to local conditions. Second, as community prevention trials have shown, delivery systems created for supporting community interventions driven and funded by research are not sustainable once research is over nor are they directly transferable to other communities.

The Role of Context in PHIR

As objects of scientific inquiries, population health interventions can, and should, be studied using a variety of questions. From an evidence-informed practice perspective, we suggest that with regard to a problematic issue in population health, and given that there is sufficient knowledge about the causal web of risk factors and social determinants at the root of the problem, several relevant questions need to be formulated to guide research on how to modify the distribution of those risk factors and social determinants in the population. Table 13.1 presents a typology of research questions that can potentially be addressed with regard to potential interventions.

The first type of question is concerned with the hypothetical exploration of what could work to modify the conditions that shape the distributions of given risk factors in the population. Providing valid answers to this type of questions implies a theoretical or an empirical exploration of potential solutions for a defined problem. Theoretical exploration entails the use of one or several social change theories in order to design an intervention that would translate relevant theoretical principles into actions. The empirical exploration of potential interventions by scientific means entails developing synthetic reviews of interventions that have been designed and studied to address an issue that is similar to the one at hand. This exploratory work results in aggregating the intervention effects across contexts in order to derive average effects that constitute the best effective hypothesis for any given context. Indeed, statistical inference works only in one direction, from the sample to the population. It is the role of the researcher to make the case that the particular context in which effective interventions are to be implemented belongs to the same "population" of contexts for which an intervention has demonstrated effects. Even when this is the case, cultural adaptations still need to be developed, and it is the task of the implementation system to operate and integrate those adaptations.

All the following questions are concerned with specific interventions. One weakness often mentioned when dealing with population health intervention research is the lack of relevant implementation details in most intervention descriptions (Egan et al. 2009). Furthermore, there is no generally agreed definition of what constitute such interventions, what they are made of, and what makes them effective. For Hawe, Shiell, and Riley (2004) for example, it is not so much the specific activities that form the important components of an intervention but rather it is the social mechanisms that these activities are triggering. The activities (or events) that form the observable, empirical elements of any given intervention are indeed context bound and result from interactions between interventionists' objectives and resources, the mechanisms that need to be triggered to operate the desired changes in risk factor prevalence, and the conditions in the local context (Hawe et al. 2009; Potvin et al. 2012).

Table 13.1 Typology of research questions in relation to population health interventions

Type of question	Methodological recommendations to provide valid answer
What could work?	Theoretical exploration of potential interventions given actual state of knowledge
	Synthetic review of existing studies on interventions that addressed same or similar issues
Could "it" work?	Trial of specific interventions in controlled conditions with adequate counterfactual
Does "it" work?	Observation of the chain of effects (proximate, intermediary, and distal) that follow an intervention implemented with contextual constraints
How does "it" work?	Observation of the interactions between context and intervention that produce (or not) the intended chain of effects
Is "it" sustainable/replicable/scalable?	Observation of an intervention's capacity to produce similar chains of effects through time and in other contexts

The second type of questions pertains to intervention's efficacy. It concerns an intervention's potential effects when it is implemented in ideal conditions. Following an experimental design, the intervention is randomly assigned to ecological units that come from the same population. Contextual conditions are controlled for in attempts to isolate the intervention as the main cause of observed changes. In a classic experiment, delivery systems that insure fidelity in program implementation are juxtaposed to or simply replace existing local systems. This was the case for the Catch Study (Perry et al. 1990) in which 96 primary schools in four states were randomly assigned in either of the three arms, two experimental and one control. In schools from the two experimental arms, intervention activities and classroom curriculums developed by researchers were implemented under the close supervision of researchers, leaving little room for local adaptation. In another type of experiment, the Kaiser Family Foundation Health Promotion Program has randomly assigned volunteer communities to receiving resources and training to develop activities to increase community activation in order to address issues that were identified locally (Wickizer et al. 1998). In this case, local conditions were not controlled for but their interactions with the intervening mechanisms resulted in variations in the activities implemented by local service delivery systems with the support of resources provided by the research.

The third, fourth, and fifth type of questions all concern the study of interventions implemented through local service delivery systems in response to local issues. In all those cases, intervention is designed mainly by professionals and the role of research is to accompany the intervention without attempting to control and impose intervention activities or mechanisms at play. In such cases, it is hypothesized that interventions are going to be responsive to contextual conditions and that their form will evolve with the changing contextual conditions (Potvin et al. 2001). Research is not testing specific preestablished intervention hypothesis but it deploys observational methods, with or without a control group, to analyze and understand the conditions that shape the intervention's activities as they unfold, as well as their effect on a variety of potential outcomes (Potvin and Bisset 2008). Most of the evidence regarding the effect of tobacco prevention interventions at the population level was derived from observational data analyzed by researchers who were following interventions implemented by regular service delivery systems (Hopkins et al. 2001).

There is still a healthy debate in the public health literature about the superiority of the randomized controlled cluster trial to derive evidence about whether an intervention is producing a desired effect (Fuller and Potvin 2012; Macintyre 2011). It is not the intention of this chapter to enter into this debate. What needs to be recognized from the perspective of population health intervention research is the variety of questions that can legitimately be addressed to build a knowledge base about population health interventions. Many of these questions require the use of observational methods. In fact, whenever one is trying to open the black box of complex interventions and to understand how these interventions are producing effects, and how these effects can be reproduced through time (sustainability) and across settings (diffusion and scalability), one does not have much choice but to use observational methods that can also be implemented as complementary to randomized trial (Corrigan et al. 2006).

PHIR and Implementation Systems

Population-based NCD prevention requires implementation systems that can support complex, systemic interventions that are continuously adapted to local conditions. True to ecological approach, and recognizing that the health sector alone does not control the levers by which most social determinants can be modified (Institute of Medicine 2002; WHO 2010), such systems are usually composed of numerous stakeholders with a variety of roles the health system alone is not able to fulfill. As exemplified in Fig. 13.1, activities, services, and policies are the result of interactions and sharing of resources between those

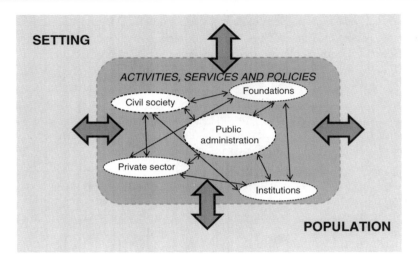

Fig. 13.1 Implementation system for population health interventions

stakeholders. The dotted lines representing the contours of the various structures indicate the permeability and numerous exchanges between context, the various stakeholders, and the systems created to support interventions (Potvin and McQueen 2008). The double arrows between the setting and the intervention system indicate that they coevolve, changes in local conditions inducing changes in the intervention and effective interventions producing changes in settings (Potvin et al. 2001).

As illustrated in Fig. 13.2, research on population health interventions developed and implemented by service implementation systems requires that a research infrastructure be coupled with the intervention system. This research apparatus may vary in size and complexity but ideally in addition to population health research capacity there should be some liaison capacity that facilitates both the translation of practice problems into researchable scientific questions and the communication of research results into actionable conclusions (Clavier et al. 2012a, b). Critically, as illustrated in Fig. 13.2, this coupling of research with implementation system provides the latter with a communication channel with the research sector which facilitates access to scientific knowledge. It also facilitates reflexivity of practice as a means to reveal how intervention is shaped by contextual conditions

in interactions with practitioners and other partners' motivations and theoretical underpinnings (McQueen 2007). Organized reflexivity (Potvin and Bisset 2008; Potvin et al. 2010) is a type of evaluation practice that aims to illuminate conditions that allow an intervention to be produced and reproduced, and to situate its components and results, in context.

Another implication of Fig. 13.2 is that all components of the intervention and their interactions with the implementation system are potentially relevant for research. A comprehensive knowledge base on population health interventions would provide scientific knowledge about whether an intervention works but also how effects are produced, for whom, and in which conditions. Potvin, Haddad, and Frohlich (2001) list five families of questions that go beyond the usual dichotomy between outcome and process evaluation. The questions pertain to relevance and ways to ensure that an intervention addresses an issue that is real for the concerned populations; coherence between the intervention's objectives and actions and their adaptation to local culture; the intervention's achievements or how actions are produced, including conditions of scaling up, dissemination, and sustainability; the intervention's effects and impact; and the intervention's responsiveness to local conditions through its evolution.

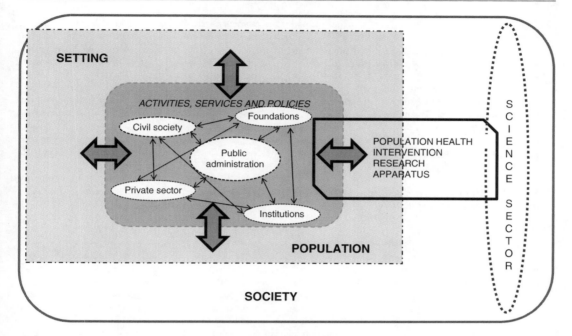

Fig. 13.2 Relationship between PHIR apparatus and implementation system

Conclusion

Attempts to change the distribution of risk factors and the social determinants of NCDs require complex population health interventions that mobilize actors from many sectors who implement a variety of activities that potentially affect many systems that shape these distributions. Because of their complexity and their necessary adaptation to local conditions, there are large areas of uncertainty with regard to how these interventions interact with implementation context. For many of these comprehensive intervention strategies the possibility of harmful and undesirable effects is still present. Prevention interventions are thus still largely based on trials and errors informed by previously evaluated trials.

Most of the actual research in prevention aims at identifying risk factors and their specific pathways and contributions to NCDs. In this chapter we have argued that progress in evidence-based prevention will be linked to the development of a science of population health intervention. Such a science would aim at developing scientific knowledge bases for such interventions and that could be used to

develop theoretical propositions about the planning, implementation, diffusion/sustainability/scaling up, and evaluation of such interventions. Furthermore, to be relevant and contribute to NCD prevention, a large proportion of studies should be conducted about practices, programs, and policies planned and implemented by public health service delivery systems in order to identify which interventions work, how they work, for whom, and under which conditions. Not only would the development of such research infrastructure allows the development of badly needed knowledge, but it also increases service delivery implementation systems' reflexivity. This in turn should theoretically increase the effectiveness of prevention.

References

Altman, D. G. (1995). Sustaining interventions in community systems: On the relationship between researchers and communities. *Health Psychology, 14*, 526–536.

Barbeau, E. M., Krieger, N., & Soobader, M. J. (2004). Working class matters: Socioeconomic disadvantage, race/ethnicity, gender, and smoking in NHIS 2000. *American Journal of Public Health, 94*(2), 269–278.

Campbell, D. T. (1969). Reforms as experiments. *American Psychologist, 24*(4), 409–429.

Campbell, D. T. (1991). Methods for the experimenting society. *American Journal of Evaluation, 12*, 223–260.

Clavier, C., Gendron, S., Lamontagne, L., & Potvin, L. (2012a). Understanding similarities in the local implementation of a healthy environment programme: Insights from the policy studies. *Social Science & Medicine, 75*, 171–178.

Clavier, C., Sénéchal, Y., Vibert, S., & Potvin, L. (2012b). A theory-based model of translation practices in public health participatory research. *Sociology of Health & Illness, 34*, 791–805.

COMMIT Research Group. (1995). Community intervention trial for smoking cessation: II. Changes in adult cigarette smoking prevalence. *American Journal of Public Health, 85*, 193–200.

Corrigan, M., Cupples, M. E., Smith, S. M., Byrne, M., Leathem, C. S., Clerkin, P., et al. (2006). The contribution of qualitative research to designing a complex intervention for secondary prevention of coronary heart disease in two different health care systems. *BMC Health Services Research*. doi:10.1186/1472-6963-6-90.

Dahlgren, G., & Whitehead, M. (1991). *Policies and strategies to promote social equity in health*. Stockholm: Institute of Futures Studies.

Egan, M., Bambra, C., Petticrew, M., & Whitehead, M. (2009). Reviewing evidence on complex social interventions: Appraising implementation in systematic reviews of health effects of organizational-level workplace interventions. *Journal of Epidemiology and Community Health, 63*, 4–11.

Ezzati, M., & Lopez, A. D. (2003). Estimates of global mortality attributable to smoking in 2000. *The Lancet, 362*, 847–852.

Fisher, E. B. (1995). Editorial: The results of the COMMIT Trial. *American Journal of Public Health, 85*, 159–160.

Ford, E. S., Ajani, U. A., Croft, J. B., Critchley, J. A., Labarthe, D. R., Kottke, T. E., et al. (2007). Explaining the decrease in U.S. deaths from coronary heart disease, 1980–2000. *The New England Journal of Medicine, 356*, 2388–2398.

Fortmann, S. P., Flora, J. A., Winkleby, M. A., Schooler, C., Barr Taylor, C., & Farquhar, J. W. (1995). Community intervention trials: Reflections on the Stanford five-city project. *American Journal of Epidemiology, 142*, 576–596.

Frohlich, K. (2008). Is tobacco use a disease? *CMAJ, 179*, 880–882.

Fuller, D., & Potvin, L. (2012). Context by treatment interactions as the primary object of study in cluster randomized controlled trials of population health interventions. *International Journal of Public Health, 57*, 633–636.

Gilmore, A. B., & McKee, M. (2004). Moving East: How the transnational tobacco industry gained entry to the emerging markets of the former Soviet Union—Part 1: Establishing cigarette imports. *Tobacco Control, 13*, 143–150.

Government Office of Science. (2007). *Foresight. Tacling obesities: Future choices—Project report*. London, UK: UK Governmennt's Foresight Programme. Accessed October 2012, from http://www.bis.gov.uk/assets/foresight/docs/obesity/17.pdf

Green, L. W. (2006). Public health asks of systems science: To advance our evidence-based practice, can you help us get more practice-based evidence? *American Journal of Public Health, 96*, 406–409.

Green, L. W., & Glasgow, R. E. (2006). Evaluating the relevance, generalization, and applicability of research. *Evaluation and the Health Profession, 29*, 126–153.

Green, L. W., Richard, L., & Potvin, L. (1996). Ecological foundations of health promotion. *American Journal of Health Promotion, 10*(4), 270–281.

Hawe, P., & Potvin, L. (2009). What is population health intervention research? *Canadian Journal of Public Health, 100*(1), I8–I14.

Hawe, P., Shiell, A., & Riley, T. (2004). Complex interventions: How "out of control" can a randomised controlled trial be? *British Medical Journal, 328*, 1561–1563.

Hawe, P., Shiell, A., & Riley, T. (2009). Theorising interventions as events in systems. *American Journal of Community Psychology, 43*, 267–276.

Hopkins, D. P., Briss, P. A., Ricard, C. J., Husten, C. G., Carande-Kulis, V. G., Fielding, J. E., et al. (2001). Reviews of evidence regarding intervention to reduce tobacco used and exposure to environmental tobacco smoke. *American Journal of Preventive Medicine, 20*(2S), 16–66.

Institute of Medicine. (2002). *The future of the public's health in the 21st century*. Washington, DC: The National Academies Press.

Institute of Medicine. (2012). *An integrated framework for assessing the value of community-based prevention*. Washington, DC: The National Academies Press.

Jha, P. (2009). Avoidable global cancer deaths and total deaths from smoking. *Nature Reviews. Cancer, 9*, 655–664.

Krieger, N. (1994). Epidemiology and the web of causation: Has anyone seen the spider? *Social Science & Medicine, 39*, 887–903.

Krieger, N. (2008). Proximal, distal and the politics of causation: What's level got to do with it? *American Journal of Public Health, 98*, 221–230.

Lee, S., Ling, P. M., & Glantz, S. A. (2012). The vector of tobaaco epidemic: Tobbacco industry practices in low and middle-income countries. *Cancer Causes & Control, 23*, 117–129.

Luepker, R. V., Murray, D. M., Jacobs, D. R., Mittlemark, M. B., Bracht, N., Carlaw, R., et al. (1994). Community education for cardiovascular disease prevention: Risk factor changes in the Minnesota Heart Health Program. *American Journal of Public Health, 84*, 1383–1393.

Macintyre, S. (2011). Good intentions and received wisdom are not good enough: The need for controlled trials in public health. *Journal of Epidemiology and Community Health, 65*(7), 564–567.

Mackenbach, J. P., & Stronks, K. (2004). The development of a strategy for tackling health inequalities in the Netherlands. *International Journal for Equity in Health, 3*, 11. doi:10.1186/1475-9276-3-11.

McGinnis, J. M., & Foege, W. H. (1994). Actual causes of death in the United States. *JAMA: The Journal of the American Medical Association, 270*, 2207–2212.

McLaren, L., & Hawe, P. (2005). Ecological perspectives in health research. *Journal of Epidemiology and Community Health, 59*(1), 6–14.

McQueen, D. V. (2007). Critical issues in theory for health promotion. In D. V. McQueen, I. Kickbusch, L. Potvin, J. M. Pelikan, L. Balbo, & T. Abel (Eds.), *Health & modernity. The role of theory in health promotion* (pp. 21–42). New York, NY: Springer.

Mokdad, A. H., Marks, J. S., Stroup, D. F., & Gerberding, J. L. (2004). Actual causes of death in the United States, 2000. *JAMA: The Journal of the American Medical Association, 291*(10), 1238–1245.

Morabia, A., & Costanza, M. C. (2012). Population health intervention research (PHIR): Should we fear the "P"? *Preventive Medicine, 54*, 291–292.

O'Connor, A. (1995). Evaluating comprehensive community initiatives: A view from history. In I. J. P. Connell, A. C. Kubisch, L. B. Schorr, & C. H. Weiss (Eds.), *New approaches to evaluating community intiatives. Concepts, methods, and contexts* (pp. 23–63). New York, NY: The Aspen Institute.

OECD. (2009). Tobacco consumption among adults. In *Health at a glance 2009: OECD indicators*. Paris: OECD Publishing. Downloaded in May 2013, from: http://www.oecd.org/health/health-systems/44117530.pdf

Perry, C. L., Stone, E. J., Parcel, G. S., Ellison, R. C., Nader, P. R., Webber, L. S., et al. (1990). School-based cardiovascular health promotion: The child and adolescent trial for cardiovascular health (CATCH). *Journal of School Health, 60*(8), 406–413.

Poland, B., Frohlich, K. L., & Cargo, M. (2008). Context as a fundamental dimension of health promotion program evaluation. In L. Potvin & D. V. McQueen (Eds.), *Health promotion evaluation practice in the America: Research and values* (pp. 300–317). New York, NY: Springer.

Potvin, L., Bilodeau, A., & Gendron, S. (2012). Trois conceptions de la nature des programmes: Implications pour l'évaluation de programmes complexes en santé publique. *The Canadian Journal of Program Evaluation, 26*, 91–104.

Potvin, l., Gendron, S., Bilodeau, A., & Chabot, P. (2005). Integrating social science theory into public health practice. *American Journal of Public Health, 95*, 591–595.

Potvin, L., & Bisset, S. L. (2008). There is more to methodology than method. In L. Potvin & D. V. McQueen (Eds.), *Health promotion evaluation practices in the Americas: Values and research* (pp. 63–80). New York, NY: Springer.

Potvin, L., Bisset, S. L., & Walz, L. (2010). Participatory action research: Theoretical perspectives on the challenges of research action. In I. Bourgeault, L. Dingwall, & R. De Vries (Eds.), *The Sage handbook of qualitative methods in health research* (pp. 433–453). London, UK: Sage.

Potvin, L., Haddad, S., & Frohlich, K. L. (2001). Beyond process and outcome evaluation: A comprehensive approach for evaluating health promotion program. In I. Rootman, B. Hyndman, M. Goodstadt, D. V. McQueen, L. Potvin, J. Sprengett, & E. Ziglio (Eds.), *Health promotion evaluation: Principles and perspectives* (European Series, Vol. 92, pp. 45–62). Copenhague: WHO Regional Publications.

Potvin, L., & McQueen, D. V. (2008). Practical dilemmas for health promotion evaluation. In L. Potvin & D. V. McQueen (Eds.), *Health promotion evaluation practices in the Americas: Values and research* (pp. 25–45). New York, NY: Springer.

Proctor, R. N. (2004). The global smoking epidemic: A history and status report. *Clinical Lung Cancer, 5*, 371–376.

Richard, L., Gauvin, L., & Raine, K. (2011). Ecological models revisited: Their uses and evolution in health promotion over two decades. *Annual Review of Public Health, 32*(32), 307–326.

Richard, L., Potvin, L., Kishchuk, N., Prlic, H., & Green, L. W. (1996). Assessment of the integration of the ecological approach in health promotion programs. *American Journal of Health Promotion, 10*(4), 318–328.

Rose, G. (1992). *The strategy of preventive medicine*. Oxford, UK: Oxford University Press.

Ruetten, A., & Gelius, P. (2011). The interplay of structure and agency in health promotion: Integrating a concept of structural change and the policy dimension into a multi-level model and applying it to health promotion principles and practice. *Social Science & Medicine, 73*, 953–959.

Sackett, D. L. (2002). Clinical epidemiology: What, who, and wither. *Journal of Clinical Epidemiology, 55*, 1161–1166.

Sackett, D. L., Haynes, R. B., & Tugwell, P. (1985). *Cinical epidmiology; a basic science for clinical medicine* (1st ed.). Boston, MA: Little Brown.

Schaap, M. M., Kunst, A. E., Leinsalu, M., Regidor, E., Ekholm, O., Dzurova, D., et al. (2008). Effect of nationwide tobacco control policies on smoking cessation in high and low educated groups in 18 European countries. *Tobacco Control, 17*, 248–255.

Smedley, B. D., & Syme, S. L. (2000). *Promoting health: Intervention strategies from social and behavioral research*. Washington, DC: National Academy Press.

Stokols, D. (1996). Translating social ecological theory into guidelines for community health promotion. *American Journal of Health Promotion, 10*(4), 282–298.

Trickett, E. J. (2009). Community psychology: individuals and interventions in community context. *Annual Review of Psychology, 60*, 395–419.

Unal, B., Critchley, J. A., & Capewell, S. (2003). Impact of smoking reduction on coronary heart disease mortality trends during 1981–2000 in England and Wales. *Tobacco Induced Diseases, 1*(3), 185–196.

US Department of Health, Education and Welfare. (1964). *Smoking and health. Report of the Advisory Committee to the Surgeon General of the Public Health Service.* Washington, DC: US Government Printing Office. Obtained in October 2012, from http://profiles.nlm. nih.gov/ps/access/NNBBMQ.pdf

Viswanathan, M., Ammerman, A., Eng, E., Garlehner, G., Lohr, K. N., Girffith, D. et al. (2004). *Community based participatory research: Assessing the evidence.* Evidence report/ Technology Assessment No 99. AHRQ Publication 04-E022-2. Rockville, MD: Agency for Healthcare Research and Quality.

Wagner, E. H., Wickizer, T. M., Cheadle, A., Psaty, B. M., Koepsell, T. D., Diehr, P., et al. (2000). The Kaiser Family Foundation community health promotion grant program: Findings from an outcome evaluation. *Health Services Research, 35*, 561–589.

WHO. (2008). *Closing the gap in a generation: Health equity through action on the social determinants of health.* Geneva: World Health Organization.

WHO. (2012a). *The tobacco free initiative.* Downloaded in August 2012, from www.who.int/tobacco/en/

WHO. (2012b). *MPOWER brochures and other resources.* Downloaded in August 2012, from www.who.int/ tobacco/mpower/publications/en/index.html

WHO and the Government of Southern Australia. (2010). *Adelaide statement on health in all policies: Moving towards a shared governance for health and well-being.* Downloaded in September 2012, from www.who.int/ social_determinants/hiap_statement_who_sa_final.pdf

Wickizer, T. M., Wagner, E., Cheadle, A., Pearson, D., Beery, W., Maeser, J., et al. (1998). Implementation of the Henry J. Kaiser Family Foundation's Community Health Promotion Grant Program: a process evaluation. *The Milbank Quarterly, 76*(1), 121–147.

Planning and Management of Cross-Sectoral Programs: Strategies to Address NCDs

14

Ligia de Salazar

Introduction

It had been clearly demonstrated that the causal conditions of non-communicable chronic diseases are interdependent: poverty, inequities in opportunities and exposure to risks, access to health services, as well as unbalance in power relations, which not only influence but also enhance the increase of prevalence of these diseases, especially in developing countries (Duncan et al. 1993). Reducing socioeconomic and health inequalities has therefore been on the agenda of policy-makers in a number of countries and international organizations (Vega and Irwin 2004). Nevertheless, the underlying mechanisms that determine health inequalities are not fully understood, which makes it hard for policy-makers to create well-targeted public policy and programs that include intersectoral actions.

There is a robust empirical evidence illustrating the existence of health inequalities and association between socioeconomic position and health inequalities. Roses (2007) and Sundmacher et al. (2011) have indicated that where there exists poverty concentration, with low infrastructure and low cohesion levels, the

health worsens, as well as other aspects of the well-being. Likewise, the need to articulate plans of development with plans for improvement of the health conditions has been highlighted; not doing so could result expensive and perpetuate the poverty (World Diabetes Foundation 2010).

Intersectoriality has been defined as a "public health practice with potential to allow local public health units to address the social determinants of health and reduce health inequities" (National Collaborating Centre for Determinants of Health 2012). It refers to actions undertaken by sectors possibly outside the health sector, but not necessarily in collaboration with it. One of the limitations to develop intersectoral actions is the availability and quality of information and evidences, regarding the mechanisms that facilitate the harmonious articulation between sectors, the know-how.

Additionally, the programs are formulated from optics of sectoral planning and implementation, although this type of actions requests an intersectoral management, supported and fortified with systems of information, surveillance, and evaluation, in order to contribute to decision-making processes with the participation of diverse sectors, as response to the targeted situation. In conclusion, the burden, magnitude, and unequal distribution and consequences of non-communicable diseases, NCDs, have been widely documented (OMS 2008; Gobierno de Chile 2011; Ministerio de la Salud de Brasil 2011; De Salazar 2011a); however this is not the case for the processes to build and sustain intersectoral work.

L. de Salazar (✉)
FUNDESALUD, Calle 58 Norte # 5BN-75,
Apto 12-04, Torre 5, Condominio Parques
de la Flora, Cali, Colombia
e-mail: ligiadesalazar@gmail.com

D.V. McQueen (ed.), *Global Handbook on Noncommunicable Diseases and Health Promotion*,
DOI 10.1007/978-1-4614-7594-1_14, © Springer Science+Business Media, LLC 2013

This chapter focuses on issues related to the above limitations, which considers the nature, organizational culture, functioning processes, and resources of associated sectors, to build alliances and intersectoral management that facilitate and strengthen cross-intersectoral interventions.

The Problem

Why Interventions Addressing Non-communicable Chronic Diseases Have Not Produced the Expected Results, Especially in Developing Countries?

A variety of factors can be highlighted as contributors to the above situation. In this chapter we refer to the most common and critical, according to the experience of the author in Latin American countries, as well as global literature review. Below are listed the main findings of the bibliographic search to face NCDs, with the goal of putting the science and the knowledge at the service of the intersectoral program management.

Weak Public Policies and Health Systems to Defend Health Rights and Health Equity

Even though the SDH should be considered in any comprehensive response to face NCDs, given that these (SDH) influence and are influenced by contextual factors within a determined political and social organization, in the practice, this is not the case, and the majority of interventions restrict their focus to preventive measures related with the risk factors of these diseases, without taking into account the context that produces and reproduces the inequitable distribution of these diseases, as well as the consequences. In the few occasions in which the SDHs are taken into account, only specific SDHs are accounted, not a group of them, as it had been recommended (Ward et al. 2011).

With population and territories as subject of change, the response to the NCDs has to have a population reach, in which the individuals are considered within a group, part of a society, and a territory. Some authors (Daniels et al. 2000) have insisted in that the health sector could do a lot to remediate the consequences in health of the social and economic disparities (Casas-Zamora and Gwatkin 2002). In the last three decades as per Mahmoud (Larned 2010), the involved organizations in global health have expanded, but their objectives are narrow and the goals are for short term, focusing in specific diseases and communities, more than in the strengthening of the systems as a whole.

The prior has led to the fragmentation and inequity in the financing of health programs and lack of continuity in the care. Therefore it requires public policies and reforms to the health systems so that they contribute to rectify these limitations, as well as expand their acting on the social determinants of population's health, under health as a right and social justice principles. It is noteworthy that in the published studies by four countries in Latin America, big part of the proposals has focused in the access to the health services, under the component of health service reorientation (Fig. 14.1).

Complexity of NCD Interventions Has Not Been Considered in the Practice

Lack of understanding of the complex and multifactorial nature of NCD interventions is the second problem; as a result of it, the theoretical foundations for the design and planning of interventions are weak. From the focus of the sciences of complexity, these interventions are multifactorial involving the participation of several sectors and levels of action; therefore the answer is also complex as well (Cocho 2005; García-Vigil 2010). It requires structural changes during long periods of time, and innovative management approaches to sustain the process of change.

Complexity has been defined as a scientific theory, which recognizes that some systems show behavioral phenomenon, which cannot be explained through conventional analysis; and therefore, a complex system cannot be reduced to the quantity of components that integrate it, because the specificity of what does make it work as such would be lost (Hawe et al. 2004).

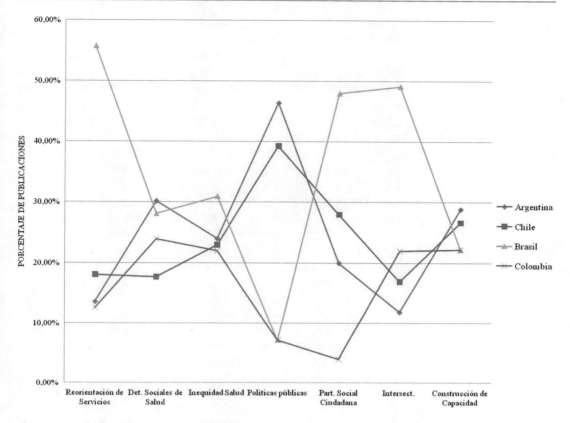

Fig. 14.1 Publications for country and health component 2007–2012 (four countries). *Source*: De Salazar, L. (2012). Abordaje de la equidad en intervenciones en Promoción de la Salud en los países de la UNASUR. Tipo, alcance e impacto de intervenciones sobre los determinantes sociales de la salud y equidad en salud. Cali, Colombia: CEDETES—Ministerio de Salud y Protección Social

In this regard, Craig and colleagues (2008) affirm that although there is no clear limit between the simple and complex interventions, and the number of components and the effects may vary, it is recognized that few interventions can be considered really simple. The complexity has two connotations: the first, referred to a property of the intervention and the second, as a property of the system where the intervention is implemented (Shiell et al. cited by De Salazar 2009); both dimensions have to be subject to investigation and practice.

Complexity theory explains in certain way the emphasis that some authors (McMichael 1999) give to environment as context for human health, materialized in the "ecosystem approaches" to health and sustainability (Parkes et al. 2003), including proposals for a "socio-ecologic systems perspective," as well as the convergence of research, policy, and practice, seeking to relink social and ecological understandings of health (Kay et al. 1999; Forget and Lebel 2001; Waltner-Toews 2004, 2009).

Lack or Insufficient Evidences and Competences to Address Complex Interventions

The ignorance of both the complexity of the NCD problem and the interventions to respond to them and contexts where they are produced is perhaps one of the main causes of the poor reached results. It is therefore necessary to look for strategies that in a sustained manner will help identify the roots of the problem and the factors that influence the effectiveness of the responses, considering that the success is valued by not only the non-presence of an event of interest but also the preparation and resilience to respond to new ones.

The results of a systematic review, assessing the impact and effectiveness of intersectoral action on the social determinants of health and health equity done by the National Collaborating Centre for Determinants of Health (2012), found that "the studies focused their interventions on populations experiencing social and/or economic disadvantage; few described assessing and comparing the impacts of interventions in marginalized groups with the impacts of such interventions in other groups within the population. The majority of studies did not specifically analyze the health equity implications of the interventions in terms of multiple factors of disadvantage. It is possible that some initiatives would improve the health of marginalized populations without changing the gap between marginalized and privileged groups. While the interventions reviewed here focused on marginalized communities, the majority were downstream and midstream interventions. For example, none of the included studies that focused on racialized communities addressed the issue of institutionalized racism. Previous work has noted the challenge of addressing upstream determinants of health."

The extension of the research agenda, as well as the strengthening of structures to achieve it, is an imperative. In this regard Krieger et al. (2010) affirm that it is required to identify the political, economic, cultural, and ecologic priorities of the society in its historical context, which requires evidences, knowledge, and action. The articulation of lessons learned from practice, as well as information and surveillance systems to the program management, could contribute to give response to the prior limitations. In order for the impact of the research results to transcend the scientific publishing, the evidences and information have to be communicated to several audiences, taking into account the rationality that underlies the decisions-taking processes.

Lack of Capacity Building Strategies to Face NCDs

An additional drawback is the absent or the weak competencies as well as institutional and human capacities, to respond to the increasing trends of NCDs, and risk factors, addressing equity issues through determinants of health. As pointed by Gortmaker et al. (2011), risk factors such as the obesity epidemic have been escalating for four decades; yet sustained prevention efforts have barely begun. On his behalf Krieger suggests that it is required to clarify the theoretical structure that compromises the analysis, intellectually and epistemologically, on how the societies produce and reproduce the social inequities, the political dominance, the work relations, the ways of life, and the ecological context, and how the societies shape and are shaped by its context. Data from Table 14.1 shows that the capacity building component is one of the less developed, or has not been the priority theme of publication.

Reductionist Approaches and Protocols Fragmented and Disarticulated: Practice Influenced by Threaten and Changing Contexts

Alleyne et al. (2010) make allusion to the global discussions around the action strategies to face the NCDs, where the countries have assumed compromises to put in practice the action plan of the global strategy and adopt coherent approaches with the development of intersectorial policies. This explicitly implies articulating the interventions to give response to the NCDs, within the strategies of poverty reduction and in the relevant social and economic policies.

There is a lack of integrated and proactive approaches across the fields of health promotion, public health, and primary health care, working in the same territory and scenarios; this fact affects the quality of health care, as well as the optimal use of the often limited resources. The integration of actions within *existing systems*, into both health and non-health sectors, can greatly increase the influence and sustainability of policies and programs.

Table 14.1 Publications for country and health component 2007–2012 (four countries)

Variables / PAÍS	Reorientación de Servicios		Det. Sociales de Salud		Inequidad Salud		Políticas Públicas		Part. Social Ciudadana		Intersectorialidad		Construcción de Capacidad		Total Dctos. por países	Total % por países
	Cantidad	%	Cantidad	%	Cantidad	%	Cantidad	%	Cantidad	%	Cantidad	%	Cantidad	%		
Argentina	27	13.57	29	30.21	24	24.00	13	46.43	5	20.00	14	11.86	13	28.89	125	20.46
Chile	36	18.09	17	17.71	23	23.00	11	39.29	7	28.00	20	16.95	12	26.67	126	20.62
Brazil	111	55.78	27	28.13	31	31.00	2	7.14	12	48.00	58	49.15	10	22.22	251	41.08
Colombia	25	12.56	23	23.96	22	22.00	2	7.14	1	4.00	26	22.03	10	22.22	109	17.84
Total	199	100.00	96	100.00	100	100.00	28	100.00	25	100.00	118	100.00	45	100.00	611	100.00
% por variable	32.57 %		15.71 %		16.37 %		4.58 %		4.09 %		19.31 %		7.36 %			

Source: De Salazar, L. (2012). Abordaje de la equidad en intervenciones en Promoción de la Salud en los países de la UNASUR. Tipo, alcance e impacto de intervenciones sobre los determinantes sociales de la salud y equidad en salud. Cali, Colombia: CEDETES—Ministerio de Salud y Protección Social

The verticality and sectoral planning and management of programs impose barriers for the implementation of more comprehensive and integrated approaches, and also the neoliberal policies present in most countries, focused on the law market, more than to guarantee the right to health of the population. Furthermore, most efforts are isolated and not institutionalized, because countries often lack relevant policies, legislation, as well as tools to measure the level of vulnerability and health consequences of the negative influence of SDH on health equity.

Alliances to Undertake Intersectoral Actions to Face NCD Epidemic and to Create Healthy Populations and Scenarios

Intersectoral action has been widely recognized as an important and key factor to reduce the inequities in health to improve the health conditions in the population. Despite this recognition, there is limited information and protocols of approach that clarify the interrelations and mechanisms that facilitate the harmonious relations between sectors.

Developing countries work under limited institutional and territorial infrastructures and with poor mechanisms for intersectoral management. Many of the problems to implement effective responses relate to structural and functional incoherence between health systems and the necessary conditions to guarantee the success of intersectoral work. To respond to this situation countries and institutions continue to focus on irrelevant actions such as creating new interventions, changing the name of previous ones, and "strengthening" them by adding new scope of actions; yet, these interventions continue to operate within same rigid structures and vertical logic.

The response as pointed by Alleyne et al. (2010) and Butterfoss and Kegler (2009) WHO, recommend the establishment of alliances between the public and private sector, as well as among countries, in order to work for a common objective, overcoming the organizational limitations. To make them work Butterfoss and Kegler (2009) highlight that for the alliances to work and to be sustainable, its infrastructure has to be monitored and evaluated in addition to functions and processes; the programs designed to reach its mission, goals, and objectives; as well as the changes in the health state, organizations, systems, and participating sectors. The prior information has to be shared to decision makers and policies formulators; and even most importantly, it should be produced with their participation, in order to contribute to increase its use.

Impacts and effectiveness evaluations of health equity alliances and intersectoral action to undertake upstream interventions should include both empirical outcome measures as well as processes. It is important to describe not only outcome trends but also the processes that produce them. Thus, intersectoral management, activities, tools, roles, and responsibilities undertaken should be considered in any evaluation, in order to build evidence on intersectoral action on health equity and the social determinants of health, according to specific context.

Weak or Absent Articulation of Information, Monitoring, and Surveillance Systems, for Knowledge and Evidence Production

Going from Data to Information and Evidences for Planning, Evaluating, and Following Up NCD Interventions

There is not enough relevant and strong evidence on the reach and impact to work intersectorially (Pagliccia et al. 2010), to convince decision takers and policy formulators on the need and importance to invest in initiative of this type (Vega and Irwin 2004). The recent literature points out that many of the main themes of study in relation with NCDs have to do with technical aspects related with data procurement, processing, and analysis of data around the distribution and frequency of NCDs and risk factors in the populations. Therefore, the processes of planning, managing, and use of information, directed to generate actions that can accomplish significant changes, have not received the attention deserved (De Salazar 2007, 2012). Also, few efforts have been done in developing countries to confront the applicability of effectiveness and impact evidences of intersectorial actions, which are produced in countries with different sociopolitical conditions.

The concept of evidence that has prevailed until now is based on the discipline, unknowing the systematic and contextual character of the social processes of change; these last mentioned are reactive, more than proactive, when it comes to decision making. Hence, we deal with the dilemma of modifying the concept of evidence to make it more coherent with this type of processes of change, or expand the criteria and indicators to value the success and impact of the intervention, using innovative methodological indicators and approaches.

The evidence in this case would be judged by not only changes in the frequency of events of interest but also complying with rules related with the methodological rigor of scientific studies, such as selection bias, blinding, and sample size, among others. Additional criteria should be included, related with the appropriateness of problem definition; quality of intervention design (logic framework); quality of the implementation of intervention—according to context changes and demands, not necessarily to adherence to a defined protocol; as well as logical and robust arguments to attribute observed outcomes to the intervention (time frame to reach the results; trend measures).

The Response

What Strategies and Tools Have Contributed to the Successful Planning and Implementation of Effective Interventions?

Several initiatives worldwide have been recommended to develop comprehensive approaches aimed at the prevention and control of chronic NCDs and their associated risk factors. Although the recommendations have been produced in diverse context, there are some common aspects: integral responses that compromise diverse actors and spheres of action; combination of initiatives at short, mid, and long term; product of sustained efforts on behalf of the promoting agents of these;

application of strategies to reduce the vulnerability of specific population groups; protocols that include complementary actions, acting simultaneously in different fronts of the causal chain, in order to accomplish greater impacts at a lesser social and economic cost; construction of local capacity and development of resilience with a preventive and proactive orientation (ISDR 2007, 2008); and systems of information, monitoring, and evaluation, linked to the managing and governance of these initiatives (De Salazar 2007, 2011b).

Developing countries face many limitations to implement the above recommendations, the most frequent obstacles being those related with the design and implementation of NCD surveillance and information systems; the lack of appropriate methodological approaches to evaluate the impact and effectiveness of NCDs of complex interventions; and the existence of political and health systems of which structure and regulation not only hinder but also impede the accomplishment of certain conditions needed to guarantee the success of these interventions, such as the intersectorial work, which requires new approaches for the management and governance of these initiatives.

In order to move forward, it is important to better position issues related to program and policy planning, intersectoral management, and impact evaluation in the public sphere and agenda. We need to bring sustainable processes for the development of skills, organizational structures, social networks, resources, capacity building, and responsibilities to create health and well-being. We should also reflect on how we can better contribute to regional development and focus not solely on what we can do but also on what we are supposed to do.

In this proposal we take into account the accumulated body of knowledge about these topics, as well as the gaps and limitations that until now have favored or impeded the performance of these interventions. Policies, programs, protocols, and technological developments will be analyzed.

To develop and implement a comprehensive and integrated approach to respond to NCD challenges, several recommendations have been identified: wider scope of interventions—clearly addressing equity and SDH; population approaches, which also include the territory where this population lives as intervention target; sustainable processes aiming to create favorable conditions to produce health and well-being: creation of sustainable healthy settings and territories; health systems focused on health care, not only on health service provision; comprehensive integrated protocols—heath care oriented; monitoring and evaluation research—linked to decision-taking processes and practice; and intersectoral management and governance.

It is required to identify guidelines and mechanisms that support the construction of approach, integrals to the NCDs; for it, it is necessary to articulate and integrate visions, positions, strategies, and resources. Following are some guidelines and strategies to put in practice these recommendations, with the goal to put the science and the knowledge at the service of the intersectorial management of NCD-focused programs.

Population-Based Approaches for Interventions, Which Include the Territory Where People Live

Approaches to NCD prevention and control should be population based and incorporate complementary interventions that apply to the population as a whole and not exclusively to those at risk. Population-based interventions require the coordination of institutions and communities through sustainable and cost-effective intersectoral efforts. This places intersectoral management and governance as a key issue for the success of comprehensive and integrated interventions.

Population-based approaches for reducing health inequities also include the territory where the population or subgroups of this population live. The main reason to include the territory as subject of action is exactly there, as it is where policies, laws, budget, and social and cultural networks take place. On the other hand, it is important to identify needs and demands of specific groups of the population, who have specific characteristics and problems due to the

differential effect of SDH on their health and ability to respond to them. Being context specific, while providing common principles and definitions, has been recommended by Health Impact Assessment WHO Center for Health Development (2012).

In countries where the politics, health systems, legislation, and organizational structure are weak or contradictory to the guidelines and actions to reduce the inequities in health acting on the SDH, but at the same time, they have decentralized structures that facilitate the implementation of processes of change, it is the case of the municipalities, where the mechanisms of managing or governance around has to or can be strengthened: intersectoral action, financings, alliances, organizational structure, resources, and construction of capacity to intervene in decisions that affect health and life quality of the populations. In this case the advances and changes have to be visible in a permanent way doing advocacy in higher levels, using massive media and social movements.

The first guideline to give response to the prior recommendation would be to fortify the investigation on the influence to the social determinants of health SDofH on the population's health, and on the impact and effectiveness of interventions. The comparison and differences between the different subgroups of the population in relation with the two prior variables help to improve the impact of interventions. According to evidence all interventions should address essential components to reach an effective response its operation adapts to the characteristic of the specific groups and contexts; in other words, we could standardize the components but not the ways to implement them.

In this sense the NCDs are a mean and a goal to improve population's health, supported in a package of strategies and technologies that contribute to fortify the response of institutions and the society, acting in coordinated and synchronized manner on the main causes of these diseases, represented in structural factors around the equity in health and social determinants, behavior risk factors, and existence of protective environments/territories.

Wider Scope of NCD Interventions, Clearly and Intentionally Addressing Equity and SDH

The demand for more comprehensive and holistic interventions to give effective responses to the NCDs requires an integral vision of the social determination of life, not only of health; this vision has philosophical, political, social, economic, and technical implications. The practice from this perspective is more political and social; the interventions in health have to be articulated to development plans; the reach of the action to prevent and control NCDs transcends actions on the risk factors, to incursion in the creation of healthy environment and territories; the health care becomes a rock of the action, not only the provision of health services.

On another side, the use of evidences for planning and management of health policies and programs should envision health as a political process supported not only in scientific information but also in practical experiences and, even more important, in specific circumstances that combine political as well as technical and social issues.

The above circumstances cannot always be controlled; however, a wider comprehension of the process of decision making will facilitate this objective. On the other hand the processes of change, in order to be sustainable, require a consensus in relation with the fundamental orientation—strategic and axiological frame—based on the legal frame (IUHPE 2011; De Salazar et al. 2011). In relation with this point Lang and Rayner (2012) affirm that "the connection between evidence, policy, and practice, is often hesitant, not helped by the fact that public health can often be a matter of political action—a willingness to risk societal change to create a better fit between human bodies and the conditions in which they live. Modern public health had almost forgotten the primacy of the human–environmental interface; the interface of human and ecosystems health now deserves to be central for policy making."

Action within and between sectors, at the local, regional, provincial, national, and global levels, is needed to influence the social and economic landscape that enables the health and well-being of the population. The prior includes actions at various levels and of different complexity, which are complementary and have to be performed concomitantly through upstream, midstream, and downstream actions. The first as per the National Collaborating Centre for Determinants of Health (2012) are those that "include reform of fundamental social and economic structures and involve mechanisms for the redistribution of wealth, power, opportunities, and decision-making capacities"; midstream on the other hand are those which "seek to reduce risky behaviors or exposures to hazards by influencing health behaviors or psychosocial factors and/or by improving working and living conditions; they generally occur at the community or organizational level; finally, the downstream interventions occur at the micro and/or individual level and mitigate the inequitable impacts of upstream and midstream determinants through efforts to increase equitable access to health care services."

IUHPE (2011) also sent key messages to tackle NCDs, recommending the adoption of a comprehensive health promotion approach and the coordination of actions that impact on the determinants that underpin the NCD epidemic across populations.

It is important to take into account these differences of complexity for the design of interventions, as it was stated by the National Collaborating Centre for Determinants of Health (2012). The difference of complexity influences the decisions, governance, managing, and financing of NCD programs, responding to a different rationality and ways to operate these concepts. Therefore, contributor factors such as participation mechanisms, alliances, type of evidences and information to stakeholders, and advocacy, among others, need appropriate methodological approaches and context-specific tools.

According to Lang and Rayner (2012) point of view, a complex ecological thinking is required, considering ecological public health as a field of action and a process for continuing knowledge building, "which it articulates modern thinking about complexity and system dynamics, addressing questions of non-linearity, variations in scale, feedback, and other emergent qualities of nature, biology, and human behavior. This means more than just evidence, and includes the open pursuit of social values, highlighting the role of interest groups, and debate across society not just within restricted scientific circles."

Comprehensive and Integrated Approaches, Health Care Oriented: Health Systems Oriented to Health Care, Not Only to Health Service Provision

To achieve the above recommendations to face NCDs, a change in approaches and structures is needed. We need to move from risk behavior to vulnerable contexts. This implies a deeper understanding of issues related to equity, the differential influence of social determinants of health, and the role of different players to cope with changing environments. Changes in methodological approaches, which contribute to a more effective planning and evaluation process, as well as for producing and using information and knowledge to institutionalize practices; local capacity building; community—civil and social—participation to empower people to participate in decision making, around public policies and resource allocation.

Many initiatives worldwide have attempted to incorporate a comprehensive approach to the prevention and control of chronic NCDs and their associated risk factors (Agency for Healthcare Research and Quality 2003). One of the recommended approaches is the denominated "social quality theory," which refers to the people's capacity to participate in the social and economic life and in the development of their communities, under conditions that fortify its potential and well-being (Beck cited by Ward et al. 2011).

The use of the social quality theory approach, according to Beck 1998, helps in understanding the problems and the planning and implementation to prevent and control these diseases. It encompasses a set of conditional factors: socioeconomic security (linked to social justice), social cohesion (linked to solidarity), social inclusion (linked to equity value), and social empowerment (linked to human dignity). The author calls the attention on the intimate linkages

between systems and individuals, and thus provides an understanding of both within the same theoretical framework (Beck cited by Ward et al. 2011).

Another fundamental strategy has been the strengthening and articulation of three essential public health functions: health policies, program planning, and management; intersectoral practice; as well as health impact and effectiveness evaluation. It requires the development of a theoretical and operational framework that will help understand the factors associated with NCD interventions, and to produce relevant information geared towards action, that is, to move from data to information and to public health practice. While the articulation of these public health functions is greatly needed, the advances so far have been little.

Several mechanisms, approaches, and procedures have been suggested, but despite the efforts made, we are very far from the expected target. A clear example is the increasing intention to strengthened information and surveillance systems, in order to produce relevant and valid information about health inequities and the influence of social determinants, using the results of monitoring and evaluation research as inputs.

Monitoring, Surveillance, and Evaluation Research: Linked to Decision-Making Processes and Practice

The contribution of the surveillance and information systems to develop evidences on impact and effectiveness of interventions oriented to the prevention and control of NCDs is unquestionable. We begin by considering that the evidences in public health are something more than data and information; they become a motor and anchorage of sustained processes of development in order to improve the population's health and life quality.

The concepts and criteria to judge impact and effectiveness. The reflection and consensus on concepts and criteria to judge the impact and effectiveness of intersectorial interventions, of which complexity has already been the theme of analysis, have to be done in the context of processes of decision making, central objective of the knowledge and evidences produced to improve the practice. In this type of interventions we need to take into account that the truth is not absolute or static, but contextual, relative, and dynamic. On the other side, we need to keep in mind that not only the knowledge is produced by the investigators and academics, but also there is a lot to learn from those that constantly are facing unknown realities in the scientific literature.

The criteria to value the impact and effectiveness of interventions to give response to the NCDs have to take into account not only outcome measure, in relation with changes of frequency of the events of interest, but also information about the quality of the design and implementation of the interventions, as well as the processes and mechanisms that make the intervention works (De Salazar 2010; De Salazar and Gómez 2011). Gortmaker et al. (2011) point out other variables of the process of implementation of these interventions such as the articulation of clinical, preventive, and health promotion programs, and surveillance and continuous monitoring and evaluation of progress and effectiveness.

Methodological approaches. The complexity of evaluating the impact of intersectoral actions on the social determinants of health to improve health equity calls for more rigorous approaches to evaluate intersectoral action along a continuum, taking into account intersectoral processes, tools, and strategies used to support such processes, and the implementation and health equity impacts of interventions. Richter (2010) suggests that the investigation in social determinants of health—SDH—requires a change of orientation and adopting stronger explanatory focuses using innovative and useful tools.

The National Collaborating Centre for Determinants of Health (2012) made recommendations to assess the impact of intersectoral actions. One approach to narrowing health inequities considers the gap between those who are worst off in society and those who are best off. Additionally, interventions can focus on reducing social inequities throughout the whole population and creating better opportunities for health across the socioeconomic continuum. For the evaluation the author suggests a comparison of the targeted and reference group, to identify whether any observed improvement affects differently the marginalized and more privileged groups.

The Centre for Health Development, 2012, calls the attention about the type of decision that will be taken with the evaluation results. "If economic interests dominate decision-making, it will be important to consider appropriate robust and validated methods to monetize the costs and benefits of better health outcomes and equity. This is specifically not easy in the case of health determinants and outcomes because of the complex and often distal causal pathways between policies, programs and projects, and health outcomes" (WHO Center for Health Development 2012).

Mixed approaches. Evaluations of the health equity impacts of intersectoral actions include both empirical outcome measures and processes. It is important to describe not only outcomes but also the processes that produce the observed results. Information, knowledge, and evidences from long-term, large, controlled quantitative studies, complemented with well-designed qualitative studies, involving the opinions of stakeholders, to better understand the impact of intersectoral actions, and the influence of contextual factors, are necessary. The mixed approaches have a higher probability to identify significant changes on the events of interest, and also support the identification of valid and relevant association between interventions and outcomes. Richter (2010) suggests, "it is very obvious that the status quo in research on social determinants of health, needs a change to a stronger accentuation of explanatory approaches."

Given that the relationships between sectors and how these relationships contributed to outcomes are often not clearly understood and therefore not reported, it is difficult to attribute the changes to the interventions. Successes and failures of the programs and policies may have been the result not necessarily of the intervention, but of other contextual factors. The published studies generally provided few details about the process, context, successes, and challenges of the intersectoral interventions and how these were related to the observed outcomes.

One of the promising methodologies for advocacy and involvement of stakeholders in the evaluation is the systematization of interventions; it supports the understanding and acting on contradictory processes where different interests and actors often coincide and collide at the same time.

Systematization has been defined as a qualitative methodological approach, which assumes a dialectic conception of the world, reality as a totality, reality as a historical process, and reality in permanent movement, and recognizes that we are part of that reality that we want to know; that we are characters that participate in the construction of the history; and that the theory and the practice, the objective and the subjective, are contradictory poles which coexist in that reality. In the systematization underlies a plural notion of character (Jara cited by Galeano et al. 2012), which therefore recognizes that all the men and women, independently of the social place occupied and of its moment of the vital cycle, are in capacity of generating scientific knowledge (Galeano et al. 2012). This way in the systematization, the epistemological preoccupation is not centered in expressing if an experience is or was effective—if it fulfilled or not with the objectives set—but instead in pointing the reasons that mediated for such experience to occur in a determined manner, to understand and learn from the occurred, and to provide information to those interested in this intervention.

The systematization results are used to make public health advocacy. In this regard, Tim Lang and Geof Rayner (2012) said, "advocacy requires a political savvy not reflected in the mantras of evidence based policy. But if public health is understood more in terms of managerial actions than of visions and movements, the risk is that the possibility of the field being about altering circumstances to enable health fades."

Also this kind of research provides information that supports the capacity building process, as Bunch et al. 2011 said, "it helps to construct a system that involves organizing, ranking and linking a series of facts and elements that are apparently scattered in order to better understand and interpret community and social practices in local contexts." The combination of short-, medium-, and long-term initiatives demands permanent efforts in order to reduce vulnerability and build resilience as a preventive and proactive strategy.

Long-Term Capacity Building Processes: The Contribution of the Healthy Settings Strategy

The mandatory question is the following: Should we wait for there to be a structural change to be able to act, or should we initiate a process of change of which the goal would exactly be to promote operative policies and structures that make possible the practice of the right to health and the equity in services and opportunities for the population? In our opinion the second alternative is not only more logic but also more ethical. However, this alternative sets as requirement a change of direction, where the purpose in this case is to not only resolve a problem or a health condition but also use this situation to promote and invigorate processes of change that permeate the policy and structures as well as the systems and institutions responsible to sustain them.

In that sense intersectoral action can be thought of as both a strategy and a process to promote shared goals in a range of areas, including policy, research, management, governance, funding, and practice. In this way knowledge is created from practice focusing in the process for social change, not only on final outcomes. Action within and between sectors, at the local, regional, provincial, national, and global levels, is needed to influence the social and economic landscape that enables the health and well-being of the population (National Collaborating Centre for Determinants of Health 2012).

The approach of the inequities in health demands long-term actions, which implies a planning, organization, financing, and, above all, a long-range process of construction of capacity, especially when the political and social systems are adverse to this new political and social perspective in public health. Strategies are created not only to give response to a determined problem but also to be prepared to face new challenges. New sociopolitical situations create new threatening situations and therefore the abilities and capacities of the individuals have to be fortified, as well as of the groups and institutions, using sustained processes of change. In this proposal the problem or the situation to change becomes objective or strategy to invigorate and articulate efforts of the sectors and actors of the development, to build and maintain the health of the collective. Usually we plan and evaluate according to the solution of a determined problem, but we do not do the same with the process and even less the long-range ones.

Planning and Management of Intersectoral Programs to Prevent and Reduce Health Inequities and NCDs

Different strategies and actions for planning and management of intersectoral programs to prevent and reduce health inequities and NCDs are proposed here considering the strengths and limitations of most of the developing countries. First we start with a health concept which is envisioned as a product of a sociopolitical process aimed to address the determinants of health; second, tools, mechanisms, and strategies to build and sustain this process are subject of analysis: *NCDs as Entry Points to develop resilience and local development; alliances, context-specific, and process-oriented approaches; impact and effectiveness evaluation of NCD interventions; and the contribution of NCD surveillance and information systems. In this last point it is considered that the evidences in public health are something more than data and information; they become motor and anchorage of sustained processes of development to improve the health and quality of life of populations.*

Intersectorial management has attracted a lot of attention in recent years. Much has been said about the need to act and to work intersectorially; yet little has been done on understanding how to do it. In order to be successful, intersectoral management requires an adjustment of systems, structures, organizations, and technology at various levels and contexts. Intersectoral programs in the context of societal normative factors which determine the social structures, policies, and relationships within a society is not a simple issue: social justice, solidarity, equal values, and human dignity are involved.

Before we undertake intersectoral work we must think about the implications of the collaborative or the articulated work. Stokes and Brower (2005) point that this implies answering ourselves questions about the origins of the respective sectors and the tensions between them that define their distinctiveness. According to this author, intersectoral and intergovernmental management has become more explicit as our knowledge of networks and governance increases.

The problem of the information availability was also highlighted by Stokes and Brower (2005), when affirming that there are challenges to make available the information for those that need it, which is an easier task when the actors are no part of the table of negotiation, or the nets, or even more, when they ignore what is going in the partners net. An additional concern is the relation between the governability of the state and the potential unbalance of the power relations between the partners; therefore the access to information has to do with both the management and accountability of not only decision makers but citizens also.

Approaches to governance and management that are more appropriate to complex situations and interventions must be explored. Lebel et al. (2006) have demonstrated that "governance for resilience in regional social–ecological systems is effective if: it is participatory (building trust, shared understanding, and promoting engagement by stakeholders); involves polycentric and multilayered institutions (that allow adaptive responses at appropriate scales); and in which accountable authorities focus attention on equity and adaptive capacity of vulnerable groups and society."

In this proposal we take into account the accumulated body of knowledge on the subject, as well as the gaps and limitations that have, until now, favored or impeded the performance of these interventions. This is how the policies, programs, approach protocols, and technological developments will be target of intervention. Also the appropriateness of tools to measure the level of vulnerability and health consequences in specific groups of the population, as the negative influence of the social determinants and inequities in health.

Health as a Product of a Sociopolitical Process Aimed to Address the Determinants of Health

The perspective of health as the product of a capacity building process has not received the attention it deserves, despite its contribution to creating knowledge and competences and capacity to cope with complex and adaptive systems (De Salazar 2011c). The process itself could act as a strategy and a powerful tool to bridge not only capacity building and resilience but also health and sustainable development. In this sense Waltner-Toews and Wall (1997) point the necessity that the individuals, communities, and ecosystems—territories—should be part. The scope and role played by the different systems and actors are not static, and, on the contrary, are dynamic and adaptive to the context; thus, it needs to be adjusted continuously to the new demands and challenges; so independent of external influences, the process continues its progress to produce the expected results. This adaptation is what some authors will denominate "social resilience" (Kay et al. 1999; Regier and Kay 2002; Sendzimir et al. 2004), relating resilience and complexity within the focus of ecohealth–ecosystems. Lang and Rayner 2012, referring to this aspect, state, "the connection between evidence, policy, and practice is often hesitant, not helped by the fact that public health can often be a matter of political action—a willingness to risk societal change to create a better fit between human bodies and the conditions in which they live."

To build and sustain this process of capacity and resilience construction, the application of strategies, mechanisms, and technical tools is required, which will be treated below.

Tools, Mechanisms, and Strategies for Initiation and Implementation

This section presents strategies and tools to create, implement, and sustain intersectoral initiatives aimed at the prevention and control of NCDs. It considers the nature, organizational culture, functioning, and resources of populations and territories to construct alliances that allow and facilitate the putting into practice the intersectoral actions.

NCDs as Entry Points to Develop Resilience and Local Development

The perspective of capacity building and resilience as critical aspects of processes of change is a strategy to deal with complex adaptive systems. The process itself could act as a bridge between health and sustainable development.

The creation and improvement of intersectoral management tools require a better understanding of what are the most appropriate and effective entry points for strategies to act as catalyst of changes: alliances, adoption of innovative information, monitoring and surveillance systems linked to the management of these initiatives, as well as the development of innovative indicators of success and relevant evaluation approaches that account for the complexity nature of most of the NCD interventions are needed.

NCDs could convert themselves as entry points to generate new organizational ways of planning, of relations and empowerment of resources and efforts around policies and programs to build and maintain the population's health. In this sense the NCDs are a mean and a goal to accomplish a same purpose, the population's health, supported in a package of strategies and technologies that contribute to strengthen the response of institutions and the society in its ensemble, acting in coordinated and synchronized manner on the main causes of these diseases, represented in structural factors around the equity in health and social determinants, behavior risk factors, and existence of protective environments/territories.

In countries where the politics, health systems, legislation, and organizational structure are weak or contradictory in relation with the reduction of inequities and intersectoral work, it is recommended to initiate the process with local scenarios. Bailey (2010) and Fawcett and others (2010) point that having common objectives between the allies helps in creating a unified sense to the mission and supporting the collective compromise to improve the population's health. In this same sense they recommend the creation of intersectoral initiatives and partnerships into existing programs.

The intervention should respond to common values according to the nature of the problem of interest, as well as the nature of the intervention to respond to it. Although each intervention has specificities, there are common aspects to all the projects (WHO Center for Health Development 2012), one of them being the "cross-sectoral management, where interests, activities and resources of the different fronts converge in order to contribute to the building and implementation of proposals to face the NCDs from the approach of the SDH and the equity, in an integral and integrated manner overcoming the traditional sectoral and individualists approaches."

The healthy settings could fortify and be fortified participating in an agenda of development, with agreed actions, oriented to build and maintain processes of change and social projection. In this regard Pahl-Wostl et al. (2007) and Steyaert and Jiggins (2007) pointed out, "social learning focused on the development of shared meanings, new institutions, and capacity at the level of the social entity as a result of participation and collaboration, and learning generated by feedback between project outcomes and the problem context."

Alliances: Context-Specific and Process-Oriented Approaches

The intersectoral approach is supported in the nature of the institutions, its organizational culture, functioning, and partners' own resources so that from there, alliances can be built that allow and facilitate the implementation of intersectoral actions in pro of the improvement of health conditions and well-being in populations.

In this sense, throughout the strategy values will be built and fortified, strongly associated with the approach of SDH and equity, which are common to various health problematic, such as socioeconomic security, access/use of opportunities and resources, social cohesion, and social groups that share social values and regulations. The prior aspects are shaped and they shape the institutional nature, governability, organizational structure, and use of local resources, fortifying the local capacity to participate in decision taking. These are key aspects for the initiation and sustainability

of alliances, as well as their articulation with higher levels, through strategies of communication, social movements, and advocacy.

A recent systematic review conducted by the National Collaborating Centre for determinants of health (2012) to assess the impact and effectiveness of intersectoral action showed the following results: " the strongest effects were observed with more downstream interventions for population health outcomes such as intersectoral collaborations to improve immunization rates and oral health among vulnerable populations. Midstream intersectoral interventions have shown moderate to no impact on the social determinants of health and health equity. The association between upstream interventions and health outcomes is less conclusive."

An experience about intersectoral action is the denominated "watershed management approach" which could be an excellent approach to accomplish the expectative of the intersectoral management and guarantee sustainable development (Bunch et al. 2011). This approach takes into account both the human health and the spatial units where it is produced, combining health with the natural resources; an example is the strategy of healthy settings. However Parkes and Horwitz (2009) alert on the risk that the initiatives that are based only in the spatial conception create a disjuncture between the objects of management and biophysical processes. The author calls the attention on the fact that although healthy settings have an explicit "ecological" and systemic orientation (Green et al. 1996; Poland et al. 2000; Dooris 2005), such approaches often overlook the specific ecosystems within which their healthy cities, schools, workplaces, or hospitals are embedded.

In the practice, the intervention is articulated and integrates programs and functions of the associate institutions, in order to increase the sustainability and cost-effectiveness of these. This articulation facilitates the governability as well as the monitoring and evaluation of the initiative to fortify it. The systems of information, surveillance, monitoring, and evaluation, and processes of the formulation of policies, are an important part of the proposal.

Identifying and engaging key stakeholders including communities, affected people, private sector, and the media, among others, will be facilitated after a clear definition and consensus about their roles and responsibilities. The reach and role played by the different actors in complex and adaptive systems are not static; on the contrary, they are in permanent change in order to respond to new demands and challenges. To this adaptation is what some authors denominate "resilience" (Kay et al. 1999; Regier and Kay 2002; Sendzimir et al. 2004), relating resilience and complexity within the approach of eco-health–ecosystems. Walters-Toews and Wall (1997) see in the health perspective as process of permanent construction, the opportunity to fortify the resilience complex adaptive systems.

Many actions have been subject to research and intervention, but there is still a lot to do, especially around systems of information and surveillance; as well as evaluation of the viability, sustainability, and differential impact and consequences of NCD interventions. A key research issue is related with the process of change and technologies that are effective, viable, and sustainable according to diverse contexts. Methodological approaches to support aspects related with governance, alliances, budgeting and financing, priority setting, and collaborative and intersectoral work.

Impact and Effectiveness Evaluation: Contribution of NCD Surveillance and Information Systems

There is limited experience on intersectoral management; given that we function from planning optics and implementation of sectoral programs, there are no appropriate indicators that give account of the performance, impact, and results of these interventions; it is therefore required to design and implement strategies for the management of intersectoral programs, where surveillance, monitoring, impact evaluation, and advocacy are articulated around the process of decision making agreed upon for the accomplishment of the program goal.

The complexity of evaluating intersectoral actions on the social determinants of health demands relevant and valid methodological approaches that address both the outcomes as well as the building process. Context-specific, complex, and process-oriented approaches for intersectoral action require similarly appropriate mechanisms for assessing their impact and effectiveness (National Collaborating Centre for Determinants of Health 2012).

An evaluation model combining different methodological approaches has been applied and tested in different Latin American countries (De Salazar 2010; De Salazar and Gómez 2011). It makes use of available information and surveillance results to identify trends of changes, while at the same time contributes to institutional and local capacity building to address local issues, converting surveillance on a capacity building and empowerment tool. It supports the establishment of community monitoring and surveillance systems, the recovery of local practices, and the construction of local capacity to produce and use information for action. The application of this model has resulted in increased awareness about the problem and effective ways to address it and contribute to local development.

The evaluation model uses secondary data from surveillance and information systems, complemented with information from qualitative research to identify and understand issues related with the quality of the intervention design and implementation, as well as the contextual factors that could have influenced the intervention achievement and outcomes. The model is available at www.fundacionfundesalud.org.

If surveillance and information systems provide updated and valid data, they could be used to develop long-term studies, to be strengthened with well-designed qualitative studies involving the intended beneficiaries, to better understand the processes and effects of intersectoral action on health equity. The prior aspects should be considered at the light of the needs and demands of information to give account and do advocacy so that participant networks will be continuously informed on the advances, performance, and critical aspects to fortify the initiatives.

Many challenges remain and need to be resolved in order to produce knowledge, evidences, and appropriate tools coherent with the conditions and specific characteristics of the countries and localities. The challenges include the following: criteria to appropriately define the problem, identifying the grade of vulnerability, inequities, and differential consequences in the health of collectives and specific groups of the population; criteria to formulate relevant and answerable questions; methodological approaches that adjust to the nature of the complex interventions and to the necessities of information of decision makers; and internal and external validity of the results, taking into account the accomplishment of parameters on which the analytic studies are based on. It is highly recommended to establish alliances between international, national, and local institutions and governments and organized communities to plan and develop research agendas and actions that fortify the processes of change and, even more, that help making advocacy in front of different instances for the creation, adoption, and adaptation of proposals, which have demonstrated impact and effectiveness. The most important is to start now and follow up the process of change.

References

Agency for Healthcare Research and Quality (AHRQ). (2003). *National healthcare disparities report.* Rockville, MD: Agency for Healthcare Research and Quality (AHRQ), US Department of Health and Human Services. Resource document. AHRQ. Accessed July 15, 2012, from http://archive.ahrq.gov/qual/nhdr03/nhdr2003.pdf.

Alleyne, G., Stuckler, D., & Alwan, A. (2010). The hope and the promise of the UN Resolution on non-communicable diseases. *Globalization and Health, 6,* 15.

Bailey, S. (2010). Focusing on solid partnerships across multiple sectors for population health improvement. *Preventing Chronic Disease, 7*(6), A115.

Bunch, M., Morrison, K., Parkes, M., & Venema, H. (2011). Promoting health and well-being by managing for social–ecological resilience: The potential of integrating ecohealth and water resources management approaches. *Ecology and Society, 16*(1), 6.

Butterfoss, F., & Kegler, M. (2009). Toward a comprehensive understanding of community coalitions: Moving from practice to theory. In R. J. DiClemente et al. (Eds.), *Emerging theories in health promotion practice and research* (pp. 157–193). San Francisco, CA: Jossey-Bass.

Casas-Zamora, J., & Gwatkin, D. (2002). *Las muchas dimensiones de la equidad en la salud.* Resource document. Revista Panamericana de Salud Pública. Resource document. Scielo. Accessed June 30, 2012, from http://www.scielosp.org/scielo.php?script=sci_arttext&pid=S1020-49892002000500001&lng=en.

Cocho, G. (2005). Sociedades complejas: Enfermedades complejas. In B. Ruelas, R. Mansilla, et al. (Eds.), *Las ciencias de la complejidad y la innovación médica* (pp. 111–132). México: UNAM/SSA/Plaza y Valdez.

Craig, P., Dieppe, P., Macintyre, S., Mitchie, S., Nazareth, I., & Petticrew, M. (2008). Developing and evaluating complex interventions: The new Medical Research Council guidance. *BMJ, 337*(7676), a1655.

Daniels, N., Kennedy, B., & Kawachi, I. (2000). Justice is good for our health. In J. Cohen & J. Rogers (Eds.), *Is inequality bad for our health?* Boston, MA: Beacon.

De Salazar, L. (2007). *Haciendo funcionar los sistemas de vigilancia en América Latina. Una mirada política y gerencial para incrementar viabilidad, sostenibilidad e impacto de la vigilancia de factores de riesgo asociados con Enfermedades Crónicas No Transmisibles, ECNT.* Cali, Colombia: Programa Editorial Universidad del Valle.

De Salazar, L. (2009). *Evidencias de efectividad en salud pública y promoción de la salud. Reflexiones sobre la práctica en América Latina y propuestas de cambio.* Cali, Colombia: Programa Editorial Universidad del Valle.

De Salazar, L. (2010). *Evaluación Programa Comunitario de Promoción de la Salud Cardiovascular Implementado por Promotores de Salud.* Cali, Colombia: OPS—NHLBI.

De Salazar, L. (2011a). *¿Funcionan y son efectivas las intervenciones para prevenir y controlar las Enfermedades Crónicas? ¿Qué dice la evaluación?* Cali, Colombia: Programa Editorial Universidad del Valle.

De Salazar, L. (2011b). Articulación de sistemas de vigilancia en salud pública a la evaluación de efectividad de programas. *Colombia Médica, 42*(3), 342–351.

De Salazar, L. (2011c). *Reflexiones y posiciones alrededor de la evaluación de intervenciones complejas. Salud pública y promoción de la salud.* Cali, Colombia: Programa Editorial Universidad del Valle.

De Salazar, L. (2012). *Abordaje de la equidad en intervenciones en Promoción de la Salud en los países de la UNASUR. Tipo, alcance e impacto de intervenciones sobre los determinantes sociales de la salud y equidad en salud.* Cali, Colombia: CEDETES— Ministerio de Salud y Protección Social.

De Salazar, L., & Gómez, S. (2011). *Abordaje de las Enfermedades Crónicas. Lecciones de la práctica.* Cali, Colombia: Programa Editorial Universidad del Valle.

De Salazar, L., Vélez, J., & Rojas, M. (2011). Evidencias en salud pública, algo más que datos e información— motor del cambio social. Análisis de la situación de salud y de los determinantes sociales para el diseño de la política municipal de salud pública de Cali. *Global Health Promotion, 18*(1), 139–142.

Dooris, M. (2005). Healthy settings: Challenges to generating evidence of effectiveness. *Health Promotion International, 21*(1), 55–65.

Duncan, B., Schmidt, M., Achutti, A., Polanczyk, C., Benia, L., & Maia, A. (1993). Socioeconomic distribution of noncommunicable disease risk factors in urban Brazil: The case of Porto Alegre. *Bulletin of the Pan American Health Organization, 27*(4), 337–349.

Fawcett, S., Schultz, J., Watson-Thompson, J., Fox, M., & Bremby, R. (2010). Building multisectoral partnerships for population health and health equity. *Preventing Chronic Disease, 7*(6), 1–7.

Forget, G., & Lebel, J. (2001). An ecosystem approach to human health. *International Journal of Occupational and Environmental Health, 7*(2 Suppl), S3–S38.

Galeano, C., Magaña, A., & Gómez, S. (2012). *Guía para la Sistematización de Intervenciones en Salud Pública y Promoción de la Salud*. Cali, Colombia: CEDETES, Universidad del Valle—Ministerio de Salud y Protección Social.

García-Vigil, J. L. (2010). Las enfermedades crónicas y neoplásicas desde las ciencias de la complejidad y la atención primaria. *Revista Médica Instituto Mexicano de Seguro Social, 48*(1), 7–12.

Gobierno de Chile. (2011). *Metas 2011–2020 Elige vivir sano. Estrategia Nacional de Salud para el cumplimiento de los Objetivos Sanitarios de la Década 2011–2020*. Resource document. Ministerio de Salud. Accessed June 30, 2012, from http://www.minsal.gob.cl/portal/url/item/c4034eddbc96ca6de0400101640159b8.pdf.

Gortmaker, S., Swinburn, B., Levy, D., Carter, R., Mabry, P., Finegood, D., et al. (2011). Changing the future of obesity: Science, policy, and action. *The Lancet, 378*(9793), 838–847.

Green, L., Richard, L., & Potvin, L. (1996). Ecological foundations of health promotion. *American Journal of Health Promotion, 10*(4), 270–281.

Hawe, P., Shiell, A., & Riley, T. (2004). Complex interventions: How "out of control" can a randomised controlled trial be? *British Medical Journal, 328*(7455), 1561–1563.

International Strategy for Disaster Reduction (ISDR). (2007). *Words into action: A guide for implementing the Hyogo framework for action 2005–2015: Building the resilience of nations and communities to disasters*. Geneva, Switzerland: United Nations, ISDR.

International Strategy for Disaster Reduction (ISDR). (2008). *Towards national resilience: Good practices of national platforms for disaster risk reduction*. Geneva, Switzerland: United Nations Secretariat of the International Strategy for Disaster Reduction (UN/ISDR).

International Union for Health Promotion and Education (IUHPE). (2011). *Advocating for health promotion approaches t o non-communicable diseases prevention*. Key messages from The International Union For Health Promotion And Education In the lead up to the United Nations High Level Meeting on NCDs New York, September 2011. Resource document. IUHPE. Accessed June 20, 2012, from http://www.iuhpe.org/uploaded/Activities/Advocacy/IUHPE%20Key%20Messages%20_LONG_WEB.pdf.

Kay, J., Boyle, M., Regier, H., & Francis, G. (1999). An ecosystem approach for sustainability: Addressing the challenge of complexity. *Futures, 31*(7), 721–742.

Krieger, N., Alegría, M., Almeida-Filho, N., Barbosa da Silva, J., Barreto, M., Beckfield, J., et al. (2010). Who, and what, causes health inequities? Reflections on emerging debates from an exploratory Latin American/North American workshop. *Journal of Epidemiology and Community Health, 64*(9), 747.

Lang, T., & Rayner, G. (2012). Ecological public health: The 21st century's big idea? An essay. *BMJ*. doi:10.1136/bmj.e5466.

Larned, M. (2010). The big question: What is the most pressing health crisis and how can it be solved? *World Policy Journal, 27*(2), 3–6.

Lebel, L., Anderies, J., Campbell, B., Folke, C., Hatfield-Dodds, S., Hughes, T., et al. (2006). Governance and the capacity to manage resilience in regional social–ecological systems. *Ecology and Society, 11*(1), 19.

McMichael, A. J. (1999). Prisoners of the proximate: Loosening the constraints on epidemiology in an age of change. *American Journal of Epidemiology, 149*(10), 887–897.

Ministerio de la Salud de Brasil. (2011). Plan de Acciones estratégicas para el enfrentamiento de las enfermedades no transmisibles (ENT) en Brasil 2011–2022. Secretaría de Vigilancia en Salud. Departamento de Análisis de Situación de Salud. Brasilia: Ministerio de la Salud.

National Collaborating Centre for Determinants of Health. (2012). *Assessing the impact and effectiveness of intersectoral action on the social determinants of health and health equity: An expedited systematic review*. Antigonish, NS: National Collaborating Centre for Determinants of Health, St. Francis Xavier University.

Organización Mundial de la Salud (OMS). (2008). Prevención y control de las enfermedades no transmisibles: aplicación de la estrategia mundial. Informe de la Secretaría. 61ª Asamblea Mundial de la Salud. Resource document WHO. Accessed June 20, 2012, from http://apps.who.int/gb/ebwha/pdf_files/A61/A61_8-sp.pdf.

Pagliccia, N., Spiegel, J., Alegret, M., Bonet, M., Martinez, B., & Yassi, A. (2010). Network analysis as a tool to assess the intersectoral management of health determinants at the local level: A report from an exploratory study of two Cuban municipalities. *Social Science & Medicine, 71*(2), 394–399.

Pahl-Wostl, C., Craps, M., Dewulf, A., Mostert, E., Tabara, D., & Taillieu, T. (2007). Social learning and water resources management. *Ecology and Society, 12*(2), 5.

Parkes, M., & Horwitz, P. (2009). Water, ecology and health: Ecosystems as settings for promoting health and sustainability. *Health Promotion International, 24*(1), 94–102.

Parkes, M., Panelli, R., & Weinstein, P. (2003). Converging paradigms for environmental health theory and practice. *Environmental Health Perspectives, 111*(5), 669–675.

Poland, B., Green, L., & Rootman, I. (Eds.). (2000). *Settings for health promotion: Linking theory and practice*. London, UK: Sage Publications.

Regier, H., & Kay, J. (2002). Phase shifts and flip-flops in complex systems. In T. Munn (Ed.), *Encyclopedia of global environmental change* (Social dimensions of global environmental change, Vol. 5, pp. 422–429). Chichester, UK: Wiley.

Richter, M. (2010). It does take two to tango! On the need for theory in research on the social determinants of health. *International Journal of Public Health, 55*(5), 457–458.

Roses, M. (2007). *Consideraciones sobre cohesión social y protección social en Salud*. IX Conferencia Iberoamericana de Ministros de Salud, Iquique, Chile. Resource document. Organización Panamericana de la Salud. Accessed March 15, 2012, from http://www.paho.org/Spanish/D/Roses_MOHIquique.pdf.

Sendzimir, J., Balogh, P., Vari, A., & Lantos, T. (2004). The Tisza river basin: Slow change leads to sudden crisis. In S. Light (Ed.), *The role of biodiversity conservation in the transition to rural sustainability* (Science & technology policy, Vol. 41, pp. 261–290). Amsterdam, The Netherlands: Ios Press.

Steyaert, P., & Jiggins, J. (2007). Governance of complex environmental situations through social learning: A synthesis of slim's lessons for research, policy and practice. *Environmental Science and Policy, 10*, 575–586.

Stokes, B. F., & Brower, R. S. (2005). Intergovernmental and intersectoral management: Weaving networking, contracting out and management roles in to third party government. *Public Performance & Management Review, 29*(1), 7–17.

Sundmacher, L., Scheller-Kreinsen, D., & Busse, R. (2011). The wider determinants of inequalities in health: A decomposition analysis. *International Journal for Equity in Health, 10*(30), 1–13.

Vega, J., & Irwin, A. (2004). Tackling health inequalities: New approaches in public policy. *Bulletin of the World Health Organization, 82*(7), 482.

Waltner-Toews, D. (2004). *Ecosystem sustainability and health: A practical approach*. Cambridge, UK: Cambridge University Press.

Waltner-Toews, D. (2009). Food, global environmental change and health: Ecohealth to the rescue? *McGill Journal of Medicine, 12*(1), 85–89.

Waltner-Toews, D., & Wall, E. (1997). Emergent perplexity: In search of post-normal questions for community and agroecosystem health. *Social Science & Medicine, 45*(11), 1741–1749.

Ward, P., Meyer, S., Verity, F., Gill, T., & Luong, T. (2011). Complex problems require complex solutions: The utility of social quality theory for addressing the social determinants of health. *BMC Public Health, 5*(11), 630.

WHO Center for Health Development. (2012). *Expert consultation. Impact assessment as a tool for Multisectoral Action for Health. Summary and Recomendations*. June 20–22. Kobe, Japan. Resource document. World Health Organization. Accessed June 15, 2012, from http://www.who.int/kobe_centre/iamsa_consultation_final_summary_report.pdf.

World Diabetes Foundation. (2010). *Cumbre de Diabetes de América Latina*. Salvador, Bahia, Brasil. 30 June–2 July.

The Public Policy Approach: Governments, Institutions, Welfare States and Social Justice

15

Evelyne de Leeuw

Introduction

In this chapter it will be argued that, more than ever, action to control non-communicable disease should be grounded in a networked, theory-driven, evidence informed and community-based public policy agenda. We will illustrate this conclusion with observations on the nature of political theory, the evidence required, and practical indices of what communities can do to engage in the process to control the social determinants of their health. This is the core remit of the Ottawa Charter (World Health Organization, Canadian Public Health Association & Health Canada 1986) which sees as its main strategies to reorient health services, create supportive environments, and develop personal skills and community action towards building healthy public policy.

To arrive at these conclusions three narrative strands need to be braided. First, the roots of modern industrial welfare states are briefly explored, and it is demonstrated that altruistic concerns for the well-being of all people were not necessarily on the minds of the architects of these systems. Considering the current rhetoric around health equity, social determinants of health, and action on NCDs these roots posit real challenges.

Second, it will be argued—commensurate with a number of colleagues predominantly from the fields of social epidemiology and social health sciences—that action on, and policy for, NCDs and health equity cannot, and should not, be a party political issue. Using the work by John Rawls on social justice it is contended that the left and the right of the political spectrum can find common ground on equitable (public) (health) policy, and that subsequently it is not the substance of any policy that is contentious, but rather the issue of coalescing (power) interests in parliamentary and social deliberation.

Third, a description is presented how the power of reductionist and technocratic argument has hijacked the policy process. This will be illustrated with—the undeniable triumph of—the smallpox eradication campaign. Although the record shows that the success of the campaign depended on a long-term fluctuating complex of global politics, resourcing, technological advances and social discourse, proponents of current global disease eradication programmes argue for relatively naïve, linear and reductionist approaches. Although the argument is not that such programmes are bound to comprehensively fail, with confidence it is maintained that simplism does not enable ample and durable policy solutions that are broadly implementable for the benefit of all. More than anything else, the non-communicable disease epidemic requires a thoughtful and rigorous, value-driven, policy response.

E. de Leeuw (✉)
Faculty of Health, Deakin University, Pigdon's Road, Waurn Ponds, Geelong, VIC 3220, Australia
e-mail: Evelyne.deleeuw@deakin.edu.au

D.V. McQueen (ed.), *Global Handbook on Noncommunicable Diseases and Health Promotion*,
DOI 10.1007/978-1-4614-7594-1_15, © Springer Science+Business Media, LLC 2013

Welfare State Architecture

It is widely accepted that when Iron Chancellor Otto von Bismarck introduced the first state health insurance system in the modern world in 1883, it was by no means his intent to develop a welfare state with full community health protection in the fledgling German nation. Rather, his programmes of social legislation (which eventually also included accident insurance, disability compensation and old age pension) were purely politically motivated.

On the one hand these programmes were designed to pre-empt any repeat of the revolutionary spirit that had swept through Europe in the middle of the nineteenth century, including sentiments that were in the 1880s revitalised by the works of Friedrich Engels and Karl Marx, and the emergence of social democrats in the German parliament. Bismarck referred to his movement as "applied Christianity" or "State Socialism" (which would in his view be balancing the more radical and undesirable "Workers' Socialism"). On the other hand there were productivity considerations: with the establishment of the package of social legislation (particularly the health, accident and disability components) the workers' masses would be provided with a minimal level of existence security. These first welfare state efforts indeed served both purposes, with almost as a contingency effect the broad accessibility of health care systems for those in work, and subsequently healthcare provision to the masses.

One might see parallels with developments across the Channel: when the 1848 turmoil swept through Europe, Britain saw the passing of the Public Health Act for England and Wales initiated by Sir Edwin Chadwick. Chadwick, an authoritarian Benthamite, has a connection with Von Bismarck; he has been described in a more recent biography as "Prussian" in perspective (Brundage 1988) for his arrogance and single-mindedness. Interestingly, Chadwick is celebrated now as one of the architects of systemic and infrastructural public health interventions, but at the time was facing stiff opposition from a medical establishment that argued that deprivation, not the disease caused by it, was the cause of British misery. Politically convenient, when the Parliament after decades of deliberation passed its legislation (Roberts 2009) it preferred a technocratic engineering solution, and not the "social engineering" approach advocated by some doctors—this would have upset the entire class system (Hamlin 1998). Hall (1998) even argues that Chadwick's solution was primarily successful *because* it meant the maintenance of class status quo. Of course, McKeown's observation (1976) should be acknowledged that the sanitary and welfare innovations initiated by Chadwick and his fellow "hygienists" have dramatically improved population health statistics over time, and that medical interventions have had a more limited and often more focused (on specific diseases, or specific proximal determinants of health conditions) effect. But Chadwick's argument toward establishing universal and comprehensive public health for all can only retrospectively, in a world where health scholarship talks of determinants of health and inequities in health, be seen as a population-wide health reform.

In spite of such retrospective criticism, the work of the Hygienists is generally heralded as marking a revolutionary turning point in the development of modern health, and by some—also because of Chadwick's work on the Poor Law—as critical in the establishment of the modern welfare state.

Another pivotal Anglo-Saxon personality in that development was Sir William Beveridge.

Chadwick and Beveridge (and Bismarck could be added) are often mentioned as being advocates of a similar type of welfare state. Both have been described as authoritarian, liberal, and convinced of the appropriateness of their own analysis. However, Beveridge even more than Chadwick, was exceptionally fortunate in his capacity to exploit his times and contexts. Beveridge ... "like Chadwick (...) had the knack of offending just those people whose acquiescence was essential to the realization of his hopes" (Fraser 1979).

Originally a member of the Fabian Society (a British group of socialists advocating incremental social change) he eventually became a member of the Liberal party. His Beveridge Report, published in 1942 and widely seen as the foundation of modern Western welfare states, was never supposed to have happened: war-time Cabinet thought they could silence the media-savvy and outspoken Beveridge by appointing him to chair a commission to do a (for all intents and purposes back-room) review of welfare state issues. The incredibly well-planned launch of the report came at an auspicious moment: just after Britain's first victory at El Alamein, when the general mood turned to a hope for much better times. The timing and language of the Report struck a chord.

Beveridge was an avid advocate of social reform to address the five "Giant Evils" of Want, Disease, Ignorance, Squalor and Idleness, and proposed a general insurance scheme that would allow all citizens to access base-line income, education, and health care. The report thus was the critical foundation stone for the National Health Service in Britain, and similar schemes elsewhere in the world. It should be noted, though, that the Beveridge health systems in the comparative health systems research literature are considered conceptually radically different from the Bismarck systems (Bonoli 1997; Arts and Gelissen 2002). "Beveridge" systems make for universal coverage, whereas "Bismarck" systems only cover certain populations for certain risks (until recently, in many modern welfare states applying the Bismarck system, this has been extended to almost the entire population for nearly all risks excluding elective surgery. This is nevertheless not the primary ideological remit of the system). Sometimes Bismarck systems are classified as "occupational" schemes, as defined occupational groups are members of defined schemes with defined benefits (Ferrera 1993): and still, in Germany, health insurance arrangements follow, and are administered by, occupational classes and their representations (Geissler 2011). Interestingly, contemporary welfare perspectives on the concept of "occupation" do no longer exclusively see this in the context of paid work: "Occupation, that is, purposeful activity, is a central aspect of the human experience" (Wilcock 1993). "Mothering" for some women and "playing" for children are thus occupational designations as legitimate as those assigned to blue and white collar workers— this occupational perspective would open up new vistas for a welfare state policy that values a wider occupational conceptualization...

Beveridge framed his great intent thus: "The proposals in the report are concerned not with increasing the wealth of the British people, but with so distributing whatever wealth is available to them in total, as to deal first with first things, with essential physical needs" (Beveridge 1942, p. 171). Almost counter-intuitively to this ambition, though, with the introduction of the National Health Service also a pattern of use became apparent, first described by Hart (1971) as the "inverse care law": *the availability of good medical care tends to vary inversely with the need for the population served.*

Long before the landmark Black report (describing the social gradient in health inequities for the first time in epidemiologically sound ways), Titmuss (1968) observed that "… the higher income groups know how to make better use of the service; they tend to receive more specialist attention; occupy more of the beds in better equipped and staffed hospitals; receive more elective surgery have better maternal care, and are more likely to get psychiatric help and psychotherapy than low-income groups—particularly the unskilled."

But the mechanism creating and sustaining inequity is more perverse than just "knowing" by the higher income groups how make use of existing services better than others, and extends the inverse *care* law into a general inverse *services* law. The leading social epidemiologists of our time (Syme, Wilkinson, Marmot, Kawachi, Berman) have time and again affirmed that those welfare states with the greatest redistributive income policies (resulting in a Gini-coefficient close to zero, cf. Gini 1912; a zero value approaches complete income equality, the maximum value of one indicates complete income inequality) also have the most equitable health status. Such income policies and resulting population health measures would indeed suggest that social-democratic egalitarianism effectively enables all groups in society to access any service required. This would then refute the inverse services law. Recent research from Sweden, usually presented as residing at the vanguard of such countries, demonstrates that income level per capita relative to population mean does not fully explain overall health status: persons earning an amount of × Swedish Kroner are significantly healthier than persons whose income is exactly the same × Swedish Kroner, but derived from welfare or other support payments (Sabel et al. 2007). Data were controlled for any other imaginable variable, and the inescapable conundrum becomes: how is the very nature of a welfare payment unhealthier than earned income?

However, low Gini coefficients do not always indicate high health status (or the reverse). The riddle becomes even more fascinating when we look at recent data from Costa Rica (Rosero-Bixby and Dow 2009). This Central American nation is another shining example often proffered as generating higher health outcomes. But factually, the Gini coefficient for Costa Rica is located substantially under the global median (that is, more than half of the world's nations have greater income equality than Costa Rica) according to UN data (UNDP 2008), whereas per capita GDP is about one-tenth of that in the USA. Yet, life expectancy of Costa Ricans is among the highest in the world, and when we would look at life expectancy at age 80, *the* highest in the world. As if this fact in itself is not yet staggering enough, Costa Rica is perhaps the only country in the world that does not display a social gradient in mortality (Rosero-Bixby et al. 2005; Wilkinson and Pickett 2007). Either this is an extraordinary fluke, or the Costa Ricans must be on to something!

As of yet, the evidence and arguments for what is going on in Costa Rica is relatively scant. Some argue that such excellent health data can be attributed to good governance and social justice parameters in the public sector, and general policies addressing social inequity (Navarro et al. 2006), although Navarro and his colleagues demonstrate that with such policies population health indicators improve, without saying anything about reductions in the gap between the most well-off and the marginalised. Wilkinson and Pickett (2007) suggest that integrated packages dealing with the underlying causes of inequity and social exclusion would be the recipe. Rosero-Bixby et al. (2005) argue for follow-up research validating their hypothesis that Costa Rica is so successful because (a) it has a targeted (Bismarck) health insurance system in addition to (b) a pro-portion of 78.8 % of the total health budget spent on public health measures (compared to 44.6 % in the United States).

As social and health inequities, as well as social exclusion and situations of (ethnic, gender, or class) privilege by their very nature pertain to sections of the population, the only way forward must be the development of specific policies for specific issues and specific people. Welfare state policies have been incredibly successful; they have established, in many cases, the conditions for equal access for all, and have increased average health levels of national populations substantially. But welfare state policies have been less effective at providing specific services to marginalised, indigent, and socially excluded groups in society: they have been ineffective addressing issues of health inequity. Many welfare state politicians struggle with this reality. Policies that would be allocating specific resources and opportunities to particular groups seem to run counter to what many welfare state politicians believe is legitimate in the "universal" system they have designed.

A Welfare State and Lifecourse Perspective

In the above there may have been a suggestion that there is a degree of uniformity in welfare state design, with two types of "delivery systems," the Bismarck and Beveridge models. In fact, however, there has been a lively if not fierce debate around welfare state typologies. Clare Bambra (2007) has summarised different typologies, and how they pertain to public health research. An aggregate typology could consist of four types, a liberal (with as a dominant example the USA), conservative (Germany), social-democratic (Sweden) and Familistic/Confucian (Italy/Taiwan). Considering the welfare state creed dictating "womb to tomb" or "cradle to grave" support mechanisms, mapping types of welfare states against stages in the lifecourse seems a particularly effective way of demonstrating how intersectoral policies in modern nation-states impact on service provisions impacting on health (Table 15.1).

Table 15.1 Welfare state types and selected parameters of lifecourse policy impact

Parameter	Model			
	Liberal	Conservative	Social-democratic	Familistic
Dominant example	USA	Federal Republic Germany	Sweden	Italy (Confucian: Taiwan)
Funding principle	Basic safety-net	Subsidiarity	Collective tax based	Basic insurance
Degree of interventionism	Low	Medium (through state and corporatist actors)	High (state only)	Low
Society is composed of…	Individuals	Families	Individuals	Families
Stages in the lifecourse				
Infant Mortality Rate (typical—deaths per 1,000 live births)[a]	Medium (~6.75) Wide distribution	Low (~4.23) Narrow distribution	Low (~3.42) Narrow distribution	Medium (~6.65) Medium distribution
Parental leave[b]	Absent	Limited (<3 months); employer co-payment; mostly maternity	Extensive (~1 year); state paid; equal maternity/paternity	Absent or limited (<3 months); state/employer co-payment; maternity only
Schooling[c]	Through cost recovery payments	Primary/secondary: access for all. Tertiary: subsidiarity	Access for all	Primary/secondary: access for all. Tertiary: subsidiarity
Entry in the labour market	Early	Late	Early	Late
Job mobility	High	Low	Low	Low
Social inequality	High	Medium	Low	High
Social inequality over time	Instable	Stable	Stable	Instable
Retirement (pre-GFC)[d]	Self-funded: no age limit	Insurance-funded (state/corporatist): ~65	State funded: ~67 or capacity determined	Insurance-funded (state/corporatist): ~57
Third and Fourth Age care	Self-funded	State funded with income limits	State funded with income limits	Self-funded
Disability support[e]	Absent	Through employer and state-based agencies	State determined; supplementary services	Through family, supplemented by employer and state-based agencies

[a]Based on Bambra, C. (2011) Work, Worklessness, and the Political Economy of Health. Oxford University Press, Oxford. Table 2.2

[b]Based on The Danish National Centre for Social Research: www.sfi.dk/Default.aspx?ID=3172

[c]Based on Organization for Economic Co-operation and Development: stats.oecd.org/Index.aspx?DatasetCode=RGRADSTY

[d]Based on Organization for Economic Co-operation and Development: www.oecd.org/…/0,3343,en_2649_34747_39371887_1_1_1,00.html

[e]Based on Fisher, K.R., R. Gleeson, R. Edwards, C. Purcal, T. Sitek, B. Dinning, C. Laragy, L. d'Aegher & D. Thompson (2010) Occasional Paper no. 29: Effectiveness of individual funding approaches for disability support. Australian Government Department of families, Housing, Community Services and Indigenous Affairs, Canberra

Where this chapter is about the public policy approach to prevention and management of non-communicable disease it would be too much of a diversion to discuss the political and value systems that have created and continue to perpetuate these different ways of looking at the role of the state (if any) in social support mechanisms. There are strong philosophical and belief foundations for most of the institutional choices different states make, and these would determine the possibility and feasibility of particular policy options. For instance, in Germany there is a strong belief in the necessity of intergenerational justice, laid down in a welfare state principle from the 1950s, the "Generationenvertrag" (the Generations Compact, following the Social Compact identified by De Tocqueville 1835, 1840) which has received recent attention to be enshrined in the German Constitution.

Such principles, values, cultural beliefs and their resultant development of both civil society and public sector organization as well as the range of implicit and explicit rules are commonly known as "institutional arrangements." Table 15.1 looks at the lifecourse from such an institutional perspective (Kohli 2007). The differences identified between the four types of welfare states have been embedded—sometimes purposely, often implicitly—in the institutional arrangements dictating the ways societies deal with health and other social matters. Public policy is both the resultant and one of the foundations of these institutions, and Bambra and Beckfield (2011) have recently started a compelling argument that a rigorous international comparative research effort needs to be mounted to establish links between institutional arrangements and population health.

There is, of course particularly in nations with only a few political parties dominating the democratic and political discourse, a tendency to paint pictures of the policy system in stark contrasts: social democrats (including "Labour" parties) and Democrats would opt for an extensive welfare state, Big Government and all public services accessible to all, whereas liberal conservatives and Republicans would opt for leaner and (sometimes) meaner government. Policy options that would lead to greater population health equality

would intuitively seem to stem more easily from "left" approaches to government, but Wilkinson and Pickett (2010) for national governments, and de Leeuw (2009) for urban health programmes have argued that (health) equity really is without political colour.

A Rawlsian Conundrum

We thus arrive at a point where it seems important to discuss what role and *meanings* "public policy" and "public health" have acquired in the course of the evolution of welfare states. More in particular, it seems important to consider the meaning of the word "public" in each. The general connotation associated with "public" would be "government" or "population"; in many European languages a translation of "public health" involves a certain designation of "the people," e.g., *folke*sundhed (Danish) or *volks*gezondheid (Dutch), whereas the public in "public policy" would translate as *regering* (Danish) or *overheid* (Dutch): government. These linguistic issues reveal a tension when it comes to public health policy: is this the public's health policy, or public sector health policy? We believe it is this very same tension that is at the heart of reducing inequities in health, or rather, develop policies that enable "the science and art of preventing disease, prolonging life, and promoting mental and physical health and efficiency through the organized community efforts for the sanitation of the environment, the control of communicable infections, the education of the individual in personal hygiene, the organization of medical and nursing services for the early diagnosis and preventive treatment of disease and the development of social machinery to ensure to every individual a standard of living adequate for the maintenance of health, so organizing these benefits as to enable every citizen to realize his birthright of health and longevity" (the first, and still authoritative, definition of public health cf Winslow 1920).

This isn't simply a game of words. The tension, at a philosophical level, relates to John Rawls' theory of social justice (Rawls 1971), or, as Laswell would frame it for politics: the question who gets what (1936)? Rawls' Principle of Equal Liberty postulates that "…each person is to have an equal right to the most extensive basic liberties compatible with similar liberties for all." This principle is then balanced by the Difference Principle, stating that "…social and economic inequalities should be arranged so that they are both (a) to the greatest benefit of the least advantaged persons, and (b) attached to offices and positions open to all under conditions of equality of opportunity." This is, unfortunately, not the place to discuss in detail the conceptual merits and challenges of Rawls' theory of justice to the health (care) domain, nor compare Rawls with more recent, and possibly more adroit, philosophical approaches to health equity such as Sen's capability approach (see Ruger 2006). But what needs to be emphasised here is that Rawls' two principles have earlier quite successfully bridged the political tensions that we have outlined above. In Britain, Tony Blair's Third Way politics (sometimes lumped together with contemporaries like the US Clinton—1993–2001—and German Schroeder—1998–2005—governments)   was explicitly inspired by the duality of these principles, although—through exegesis—some British communitarianist political philosophers have found Rawls' views too individualistic and liberal (Hale 2004). In The Netherlands and Belgium, traditionally   coalition-driven   parliamentary democracies with a plethora of political parties, Rawls' views enabled so-called Purple Coalitions (between the red of Labour and blue of Liberals), in The Netherlands, 1994–2002 between Liberal Democrats (D66), Labour (PvdA), and Liberals (VVD—in the European context, liberals are considered right-of-centre), and in Belgium, 1999–2007 between Flemish and Walloon Social Democrats and Liberal parties (supplemented initially by the Flemish and Walloon Green Parties).

Lehning (2002) has described in detail how Rawls bridged the political divide in The Netherlands on five historical issues: income redistribution, the liberalism-communitarianism debate, the question whether to send troops to Kosovo, the nature of the multicultural nation state, and rights versus obligations in era of rapid technological and social change. Rawls' Theory of Social Justice became, in a very practical way, the philosophical tool in The Netherlands to build government coalitions.

The success of such coalition building may work better in multi-party political systems. In bipartisan systems where government is formed by one party versus another, such Rawlsian bridging would lead to governments of national unity, in which opportunities to advance specific issues on party political platforms would vanish. Furthermore, coalition governments in multi-party systems will still face parliamentary opposition, and although "Rawls" may appear to be the "great political leveler," bridging ideological and moral divides, politically (that is, around issues of power and control over resources, cf. de Leeuw 1993) the game always continues.

Nevertheless, the bottom-line of the above argument is clear: the discourse on roles and responsibilities between individual, community and systems level interventions and policies for health is not naturally owned by the "left" or the "right": the public's health can very well be public sector health, and equity in health can be achieved by reconciling preconceived ideological differences.

Returning for a moment to the welfare state typologies presented above (Table 15.1) several "outlying" states can be identified that do not measure up to the typical lifecourse health consequences suggested by our classification. We already mentioned Costa Rica, and within the familistic/Confucian type Singapore comes to the fore. Although this small nation-state by many standards could be designated a liberal welfare state, its health measures are not commensurate with the type. DeVol (2011) describes how the country explicitly invests in its people. With its people the only abundant resource available, high education levels, and investments in public health care and health promotion would sustain the viability of the country. Ham (2001) also describes how the country in its post-colonial era freed itself from British institutional shackles and found its own "Third Way" in health policy development. The drive to invest in people capacities, combined with novel health insurance and health savings approaches means that Singapore with a comparatively minimal GDP percentage spent on health (about 3 %) still ranks sixth in health system performance (WHO 2000). Clearly, institutional arrangements set the stage for new approaches to equitable health policy development.

The Limitations of the Stages Heuristic: Smallpox Eradication

Another issue on the role of public policy in public health needs to be explored: could "the Century of the Welfare State" have happened *because* of (and not *in spite* of) the complexity of the social issues faced by industrial and post-industrial nations in the twentieth century?

The development of a dominant medical-industrial complex could be seen as one of the great accomplishments of the industrial and welfare state era. Health care, since medicine started its professionalisation drive in the mid-nineteenth century, has seen an enormous expansion with many great victories, including highly effective public health measures such as vaccination. One of the results of these apparent technological triumphs has been the strong belief in the effectiveness and universal applicability of reductionist approaches, not just to health care and public health, but consequently to the development and implementation of health policy.

And who wouldn't be proud of the great, unequivocal technological triumph of humankind over one of its worst scourges, smallpox? Dr. Walt Orenstein, the deputy director for Immunization Programs of the Bill & Melinda Gates Foundation, definitely voiced that pride in 2010 when he said on The Takeaway[1]: "Now, in perpetuity, we not (sic! EdL) have any deaths from small pox (…) It was an amazing accomplishment (…) By knowing your disease, following it, tracking it, you can begin to adjust your strategy." And thus the Foundation has allocated substantial resources, in fact more than any government ever did in WHO's smallpox eradication programme (cf. Barrett 2006), toward a number of global disease control, containment and eradication (polio, guinea worm and malaria) programmes.

The Gates Foundation's role and views on not just disease eradication but more generally global health issues are important, albeit biased, drivers of a certain type of health policy. Sabatier and colleagues (2007) have criticised this type of policy and its development as drawing on a — faulty — stages heuristic. In policy science, the proponents of the stages heuristic claim that policy development in its essence is composed of a simple, linear series of steps or stages that each need to be passed. Such stages might include problem formulation, inventory of solutions, selection of best policy option, allocation of resources, policy adoption, implementation and (ideally) evaluation. Superficially, and certainly in the visible and formal policy processes we can see almost daily in the media, these are indeed the steps in the process. But there is mounting evidence that the reality of policy making is much more complex, messy, iterative, and often simply wicked and symbolic. Anyone with more than a passing interest in politics would know that often problems are connected to solutions (rather than the other way around), selected policy alternatives are demonstrably ineffective, or that implementation has in fact started before policies are adopted.

The stages heuristic, therefore, is wishful thinking, and the reliance on technocratic power and prowess an effective veil of ignorance (with a Rawlsian pun intended!). Fortunately there are potent conceptual and theoretical alternatives to the stages heuristic in policy development.

To illustrate these we return to the saga of smallpox eradication. Aaron Wildavsky (1977) famously postulated his "Paradox of Time": past successes lead to future failures (p.106). It must be assumed that this Paradox only has validity because we fail to appreciate the complexity of the evidence. The accounts that Birn (2011) and Barrett (2006) provide suggest that a programmatic conclusion such as Orenstein's ("intervene → monitor → adapt → resource → intervene → monitor → adapt," etc.) is a gross

---

[1] The Takeaway is a unique partnership of global news leaders. It is a co-production of PRI (Public Radio International) and WNYC Radio in collaboration with the BBC World Service, The New York Times and WGBH Boston.

oversimplification of what actually happened, both in terms of international diplomacy and advances in medical and social technology. Birn starts off with the "McKeown Argument" (that biomedical disease control occurs after systems change already leads to declines in mortality and morbidity): when the global community, through its elected body (the World Health Organization, on initial proposal by the Soviet Union), decided to embark on the smallpox eradication programme, the disease was already in retreat in most countries. Several of these, notably in Europe and the Americas, had had inoculation and vaccination programmes for sometimes nearly a century. It was not exclusively the biomedical model of health that had achieved disease control victories in those countries, but rather the establishment of effective health and social awareness and infrastructures that facilitated monitoring, control and containment (i.e., strong "institutional arrangements," following the above argument). The very nature of the smallpox pathogen and its exclusive human-to-human transmission enabled such awareness and infrastructure; the biomedical intervention was simply the technological tool to give the pathogen its last push into history.

Perhaps the best way of explaining the evidence of complexity of smallpox eradication in a policy context comes from the classical Greek analysis of the field of knowledge. Flyvbjerg (2001) discusses Aristotle's "The Nicomachean Ethics" to demonstrate the contemporary value of techne, phronesis and episteme, together contributing to Sophia (wisdom): "whereas episteme concerns theoretical know why and techne denotes technical know how, phronesis emphasizes practical knowledge and practical ethics" (p.56). Sound policy development for health thus explores and appreciates all three types of knowledge, and in its considerations explicitly connects them.

There is another reason why (public) (health) policy development and implementation must transcend the mere reductionist and technical approach. Thus far this chapter has emphasised the importance of political discourse in policy formulation, but possibly more importantly, good policy must also be implemented. Fortunately,

there is a solid scholarly basis in the social and political sciences to guide that endeavour. As is so often the case in social science, different perspectives on the implementation issue (and its research and evaluation) vie for prominence. Adil Najam's 5C model (based on a systematic review of sustainability policies in the Global South) is attractive for its graphic simplicity: in a pentagon he describes how content, context, commitment, capacity, and clients & coalitions all interconnect (Najam 1995). At the other end of the conceptual spectrum, in terms of abstraction, we find Hill & Hupe's multi-level governance approach (Hill and Hupe 2006): they maintain that implicit and explicit institutional arrangements at the individual, organizational and systems level allow for interactions between constitutive (setting rules), directive (steering rules) and operational (practical rules) governance for better policy development and implementation coordination. Somewhere in the middle Mazmanian and Sabatier (1989) can be located.

Their approach is more useful than either Najam's and Hill and Hupe's, as it provides insight in some of the factors that emerged above in the description of the smallpox eradication programme.

Policy implementation (and by inference, the policy development discourse that it is part of) is dependent on three categories of variables: the nature and extent of the problem addressed by the problem (variables A in Fig. 15.1), the ability of the agency that leads the implementation efforts to plan and resource implementation (B), and factors outside the immediate control of the policy-making and implementing agency that are required in support of implementation efforts (C). The accounts of the decade long efforts in smallpox eradication suggest that the (A) factors were well-understood, or could be developed incrementally and iteratively (for instance, the design of the bifurcated vaccination needle, which was then made available by the Wyeth corporation, and subsequent WHO research that demonstrated that stainless steel needles could be sterilised and re-used, thus minimising some of the logistics required).

But factors (B) and (C) were poorly or simply not at all understood, haphazardly addressed or at

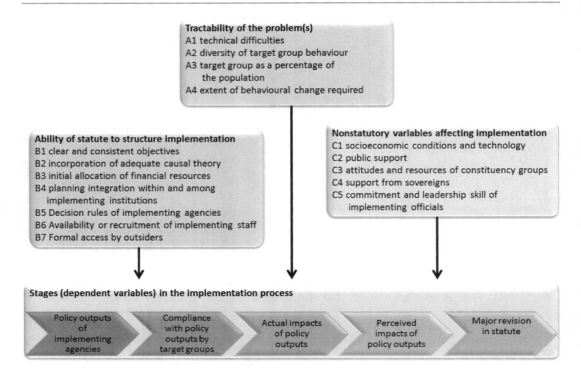

Fig. 15.1 Variables involved in the implementation process (adapted from Fig. 2.1 in Mazmanian, D.A. & P.A. Sabatier (1989) Implementation and public policy—with a new postscript. University Press of America, Lanham/New York/London)

the mercy of wildly fluctuating public opinion. Indeed, as both Birn (2011) and Barrett (2006) intimate, it was nothing less than a miracle that the campaign succeeded at all, particularly where sustainable resourcing was stagnant and left often to the initiative of the small team at WHO under the leadership of Donald Henderson. One might say that in the twenty-first century global health efforts through public–private partnerships and corporate charitative involvement has transcended the naïve public welfare state resourcing models of the twentieth century and has embraced far more astute public relations and social media approaches. But diffident resource commitments continue, the Global Fund has reduced its allocations to global efforts, and communities most affected by global health scourges still have not found a voice in corporate public relations (Townsend et al. 2012).

This touches upon a final observation before we move on to our policy views particular to NCDs. The smallpox eradication campaign has been lauded as the one great collaborative effort between the two superpowers during the Cold War. The Soviet Union was the first to propose the campaign in the World Health Assembly, and eventually was involved in large-scale vaccine supplies. The USA never fully resourced the campaign to its formal commitments, but made its massive organizational and logistics know-how available. Birn suggests that the myth of collaboration should be rewritten into a tale of complementary strengths. An analysis that yet has to be carried out, though, is how this complementarity played out in the global geopolitical Realpolitik. Smallpox, it appears, was eradicated first and most effectively in the spheres of influence of the two blocs. It may not be a surprise that the last cases of the disease were identified in the Horn of Africa, in areas that had not been colonised by any of the allies of the two blocs and traditionally were regarded as without strategic assets (Somalia and Ethiopia, and a disputed swathe of Kenya). If anything, our hypothesis suggests that disease control in a globalised era radically transcends the technical issues part of the set of variables for policy implementation.

NCDs: The Public's Policy More Than Ever

In this chapter a few observations are formulated. The traditional architecture of the welfare state was not designed for the attainment of high health equity. A more incisive set of (public) (health) policies can and must be designed to deal with population health, and in particular with health equity. Such policies are not aligned with traditional political belief systems, and work by John Rawls suggests that party political divides can be bridged. Other post-colonial institutional arrangements (e.g., Singapore) also deliver approaches toward health equity through novel public policy. The chapter also demonstrated that the dynamics of policy making and implementation far transcend the orthodox stages heuristic, and that an emphasis on technological and reductionist approaches wouldn't necessarily lead to better policy and better health.

The pathogenic pathways of noncommunicable diseases, including the social determinants that exacerbate their causes and provide opportunities for health promotion, are not just a fraction more complex than the infectious disease field. They are vastly more complex and wicked, and require a rigorous public policy approach strongly grounded in institutional arrangements that facilitate health equity through action on social determinants of health. The arguments advanced in this chapter would suggest that better, more (phronesis, episteme and techne) evidence-based, comprehensively community driven and theory-based health policy development is the only way to deal with NCDs. Most of all, though, it appears that the adoption of an agenda for health promotion policy (whether they are called whole-of-government, Healthy Public Policy, or Health in All Policies) based on values embedded in, among others, the Ottawa Charter and Jakarta Declaration can be our only alternative.

References

Arts, W. A., & Gelissen, J. (2002). Three worlds of welfare capitalism or more? A state-of-the-art report. *Journal of European Social Policy, 12*(2), 137–158.

Bambra, C. (2007). Going beyond the three worlds: regime theory and public health research. *Journal of Epidemiology and Community Health, 61*, 1098–1102.

Bambra, C., & Beckfield, J. (2011). *Institutional arrangements as candidate explanations for the US mortality disadvantage*. Background paper for the NAS/IOM panel on Understanding International Health Differences in High-Income Countries. The National Academies/Institute of Medicine, Washington (scholar.harvard.edu/jbeckfield/files/bambra_and_beckfield_2012.pdf) last Accessed August 21, 2012.

Barrett, S. (2006). The smallpox eradication game. *Public Choice, 130*, 179–207.

Beveridge, W. (1942). *Social insurance and allied services. Report by Sir William Beveridge*. New York, NY: The MacMillan Co.

Birn, A. E. (2011). Small(pox) success? Erradicação da varíola: medida do sucesso? *Ciência & Saúde Coletiva, 16*(2), 591–597.

Bonoli, G. (1997). Classifying welfare states: A two-dimension approach. *Journal of Social Policy, 26*(3), 351–372.

Brundage, A. (1988). *England's "Prussian" minister: Edwin Chadwick and the politics of government growth 1832 1854*. University Park: University of Pennsylvania Press.

de Leeuw, E. (1993). Health policy, epidemiology and power: the interest web. *Health Promotion International, 8*(1), 49–52.

de Leeuw, E. (2009). Evidence for healthy cities: reflections on practice, method and theory. *Health Promotion International, 24*(S1), i19–i36.

De Tocqueville, A. (1835, 1840). *Democracy in America*. London: Penguin Classics. 2003 edition and translation.

DeVol, R. (2011). *The eight Best innovation ideas from around the world*. The Atlantic, http://www.theatlantic.com/business/archive/2011/11/the-8-best-innovation-ideas-from-around-the-world/248695/ (last Accessed August 21, 2012)

Ferrera, M. (1993). *Modelli di solidarietà*. Bologna: Il Mulino.

Flyvbjerg, B. (2001). *Making social science matter: Why social inquiry fails and how it can succeed again*. Cambridge, UK: Cambridge University Press.

Fraser, D. (1979). Review of William Beveridge: A biography by Jose Harris. *The Historical Journal, 22*(4), 1031–1032.

Geissler, J. (2011). Health policy in Germany: Consumer groups in a corporatist polity. Ch. 9. In H. Löfgren, E. DeLeeuw, & M. Leahy (Eds.), *Democratising health: Consumer groups in the policy process*. Cheltenham: Edward Elgar Publishing.

Gini, C. (1912). *Variabilità e mutabilità*. Tipografia di P: Cuppini, Bologna

Hale, S. (2004). The communitarian "philosophy" of New Labour. In S. Hale, W. Leggett, & L. Martell (Eds.), *The third Way and beyond. Criticisms, futures, alternatives* (pp. 87–107). Manchester: Manchester University Press.

Hall, P. (1998). *Cities in civilization*. Oxford: Blackwell.

Ham, C. (2001). Values and health policy: The case of Singapore. *Journal of Health Politics, Policy and Law, 26*(4), 739–745.

Hamlin, C. (1998). *Public health and social justice in the age of Chadwick: Britain 1800–1854*. Cambridge: Cambridge University Press.

Hill, M., & Hupe, P. (2006). Analysing policy processes as multiple governance: Accountability in social policy. *Policy & Politics, 34*(3), 557–573.

Kohli, M. (2007). The institutionalization of the life-course: Looking back to look ahead. *Research in Human Development, 4*(3–4), 253–271.

Lehning, P. B. (2002). Rawls in The Netherlands. *European Journal of Political Theory, 1*(2), 199–214.

Mazmanian, D. A., & Sabatier, P. A. (1989). *Implementation and public policy. With a new postscript*. Lan-ham, MD: University Press of America.

McKeown, T. (1976). *The role of medicine—Dream, mirage or nemesis*. London: Nuffield.

Najam, A. (1995). *Learning from the literature on policy implementation: A synthesis perspective*. Laxenburg, Austria: International Institute for Applied Systems Analysis.

Navarro, V., Muntaner, C., Borrell, C., Benach, J., Quiroga, Á., Rodríguez-Sanz, M., et al. (2006). Politics and health outcomes. *The Lancet, 368*, 1033–1037.

Rawls, J. (1971). *A theory of justice*. Cambridge: The Belknap Press of Harvard University Press

Roberts, M. J. D. (2009). The Politics of Professionalisation: MPs, Medical men, and the 1858 Medical Act. *Medical History, 53*, 37–56.

Rosero-Bixby, L., & Dow, W. H. (2009). Surprising SES gradients in mortality, health, and biomarkers in a Latin American population of adults. *Journals of Gerontology Series B—Psychological Sciences and Social Sciences, 64*(1), 105–117.

Rosero-Bixby, L., Dow, W. H., & Laclé, A. (2005). Insurance and other socioeconomic determinants of elderly longevity in a Costa Rican panel. *Journal of Biosocial Science, 37*(6), 705–720.

Ruger, J. P. (2006). Ethics of the social determinants of health. *The Lancet, 364*(9439), 1092–1097.

Sabatier, P. A. (2007). The need for better theories. In P. A. Sabatier (Ed.), *Theories of the policy process* (2nd ed., pp. 3–17). Boulder, CO: Westview.

Sabel, C. E., Dorling, D., & Hiscock, R. (2007). Sources of income, wealth and the length of life: An individual level study of mortality. *Critical Public Health, 17*(4), 293–310.

Titmuss, R. M. (1968). *Essays on the welfare state*. London: Allen and Unwin.

Townsend B., Martin E., Löfgren H., de Leeuw E. (2012). Global Health Governance: Framework Convention on Tobacco Control (FCTC), the Doha Declaration, and Democratisation. *Administrative Sciences, 2*(2), 186–202.

UNDP. (2008). *Human development report 2007/2008: Fighting climate change: Human solidarity in a divided world*. New York: United Nations Development Program.

WHO (2000). *Health systems: improving performance*. World Health Report. WHO, Geneva

Wilcock, A. (1993). A theory of the human need for occupation. *Journal of Occupational Science: Australia, 1*(1), 17–24.

Wildavsky, A. (1977). Doing better and feeling worse: The political pathology of health policy. *Daedalus, 106*(1), 105–123.

Wilkinson, R. G., & Pickett, K. E. (2007). The problems of relative deprivation: Why some societies do better than others. *Social Science & Medicine, 65*(9), 1965–1978.

Wilkinson, R., & Pickett, K. (2010). *The spirit level. Why greater equality makes societies stronger*. London: Bloomsbury Press.

Winslow, C. E.-A. (1920). The untilled fields of public health. *Science, 51*(3106), 23–33.

World Health Organization, Canadian Public Health Association & Health Canada. (1986). The Ottawa charter for health promotion. *Health Promotion, 1*(4), 1–5.

Accelerating Action on NCDs: Understanding and Applying a Social Determinants of Health Framework for Change

16

Erma Manoncourt

Non-communicable Diseases (NCDs) in Low and Middle-Income Countries: Is the Social Determinants of Health (SDH) Framework a "Magic Wand?"

Informed by regional initiatives on the prevention and control on NCDs throughout the world, coupled with the latest scientific evidence, the High-Level Meeting on Non-Communicable Diseases noted in its concluding declaration that an estimated 36 million of the 57 million global deaths were due to four prominent NCDs (i.e., heart diseases, cancers, diabetes, chronic respiratory diseases); and nearly 80 % of these deaths occurred in developing countries, plus increasing incidence indicated that they would also be their most common causes of death by 2030 (Giles 2010, UN General Assembly 2011). Michael Marmot and others have made a strong case that tackling NCDs is not merely a health problem, but also a development concern that reflects the roles that inequity and social justice play in this phenomena. For low-income countries, tackling NCDs represents an additional burden that complicates other efforts being implemented to address infectious diseases; and the combination of this dual disease burden are interlinked to pov-

erty and slow development to the extent that many may not reach the Millennium Development Goal (MDG) targets by 2015. Analyzing the rise of NCDs in all middle- and low-income country regions, Nikolic et al. (2011) also point out that these countries are experiencing high NCD prevalence at earlier stages of economic development but their treatment and service delivery efforts are compounded by short timeframes and lower capacity to respond. The World Economic Reports of 2009 and 2010 reinforced this perspective when identifying NCDs as a global threat with negative economic ramifications, especially for poor countries. While the increased prevalence of NCDs is problematic throughout the world, its increased incidence in low and middle-income countries creates a double burden that (1) competes with national efforts to address other competing development and humanitarian priorities such as combating communicable diseases, addressing maternal and perinatal conditions and tackling nutritional deficiencies; and (2) has the potential to undermine social and economic gains that have been made over the past two decades.

Of course, the common risk factors for NCDs are well-documented—tobacco use, unhealthy diet and poor nutrition, physical inactivity, and inappropriate alcohol use. Evidence shows that these factors tend to cluster among disadvantaged groups and communities who often live in poor environments with the least access to health services and information. Current research also indicates that beyond addressing the complex set of

E. Manoncourt, Ph.D. (✉)
International Union of Health Promotion
and Education, 15 Rue Daval, Paris 75011, France
e-mail: emanoncourt@gmail.com

D.V. McQueen (ed.), *Global Handbook on Noncommunicable Diseases and Health Promotion*,
DOI 10.1007/978-1-4614-7594-1_16, © Springer Science+Business Media, LLC 2013

risk factors that are associated with NCDs, there is an urgent need to tackle the underlying conditions and fundamental root causes of these risks and gross health inequalities within and among countries. For example, the Brazilian experience presents evidence that proactive measures to reduce health disparities accompanied by socioeconomic progress can result in measurable improvements in the health of children and mothers in a relatively short interval (Barros et al. 2010). While it is agreed globally that the concept of "social determinants of health" focus on the economic and social conditions that govern people's lives and affect their health and well-being, in practice they may be identified differently by various organizations, among countries or within local communities, depending on the unique challenges faced by each. Internationally, the final report of Commission on Social Determinants of Health (CDSH), supported by the World Health Organization (WHO), identified several underlying causes that contribute to ill health risks and inequities and raised the alarm for immediate, renewed action. The fundamental causes specified were: "early child development; women and gender equity; unemployment; unsafe workplaces; urban slums; globalization; and lack of access to health systems" (WHO 2010). Given its equity-focused agenda in low and middle-income countries, the United Nations Children's Fund (UNICEF) has further identified a complex range of political, social, and economic factors that contribute to inequities faced by families and their children. These include but are not limited to:

- Gender discrimination
- Ethnic, linguistic, minority, and religious discrimination
- Discrimination due to disability status
- Structural poverty
- Natural or manmade disasters
- Geographic isolation
- Cultural and social norms
- Weak governance

Taking into account different cultural and political contexts, social factors as determinants of health are not isolates; but rather interact with each other to produce health consequences and impact on other development priorities. Income,

early childhood, food, housing, and security do not exist in a vacuum. The quality of SDH is shaped by political, economic and social forces that differ by nation, region, and municipality (Raphael 2008). In a complementary manner, the Voluntary Health Association of India (VHAI) has signaled the importance of recognizing the health system, itself, as a social determinant of health, which is influenced by and influences other social determinants such as gender, employment and income, geographic location, ethnicity, and provided evidence of the relationship to the use of basic maternal and child health services (Mukhopadhyay 2009/2010). Therefore, applying a SDH framework to NCDs necessitates putting equity considerations at the center of all policy and prevention efforts, which is based on five lessons learned from the field:

- Health inequities exist in all countries, only the extent and degree may vary
- Attention to equality is an ethical imperative that is essential for stability
- Investments in primary health care yield positive health outcomes
- Focus on underserved and missed populations or groups is important to tackling health inequities
- Studying differential health outcomes helps identify inequities and disparities that are experienced by different population groups and communities

Nikolic et al. (2011) argue that despite the magnitude of the NCD challenge, as well as overall economic and social costs, in both middle and low-income countries, there is considerable space for action. They stress the importance of targeting NCD risk factors to promote healthier lifestyles through focused prevention efforts and facilitating strategic adaptation measures to mitigate the impact of NCDs on economies, health systems, households and individuals rather than simply emphasizing heavy investments in treatment. Their perspective sets the groundwork for applying a SDH framework to help clarify the full range of factors—both medical and nonmedical—around which prevention activities can be focused and sustainable responses can be developed.

A strategic and concerted focus on the Social Determinants of Health, applied to NCD prevention efforts, will also involve developing a range of programs and interventions that span the life course and improve the conditions of daily life of individuals, families, and communities (Bégin 2009; Potvin et al. 2010). These activities would range from early child development and education, employment and working conditions, income and access to resources, training, people and places, transport, climate change, and sustainability. In addition, applying SDH on NCD also involves developing social capital by empowering individuals and communities to participate and take greater control over their lives and strengthening social cohesion and equity as a contribution to social normative change. Similarly, a WHO analysis of local government action on SDH in six European countries (Denmark, England, Latvia, the Netherlands, Spain, and Sweden) identified six key implementation factors—each warrants consideration and could inform NCD prevention activities: the level of inter-sectoral cooperation, policy coherence, the strength and communication of the evidence base, capacity, managing the political context and knowledge transfer (Grady and Goldblatt 2012).

In 2000, the WHO Global Strategy for the Prevention and Control of Non-Communicable Diseases acknowledged the necessity for comprehensive approaches to respond to the global NCD epidemic. This led to the implementation of population-based interventions such as antismoking campaigns, physical activity and cancer screening programs, reduced marketing and higher taxation of unhealthy foods to make positive differences in reducing NCD risks. In a complementary manner, there has also been a focus on primary prevention programs and development of cost-effective health care service delivery systems that target high-risk individuals or those already suffering from NCDs. This has led to increased attention being placed on a package of essential NCD interventions, which have a high impact or are cost-effective, affordable, and feasible. As a result, evidence from high-income countries showing reductions in CVD mortality, cancer deaths, and morbidity associated with diabetes, chronic respiratory diseases and other NCDs have shown the value of primary health-care interventions for early detection, prevention and management. This has also contributed to the rise of individual behavior change programs for the self-care and management of chronic disease since lifestyle issues are often conceived as individual responsibility. However, SDH helps policy-makers and practitioners to realize the importance of tackling "the causes of the causes" and minimize "blaming the victim" approaches (Lins et al. 2010) Clearly, population-wide and individual behavior strategies are necessary, but are insufficient without additional attention to addressing SDH related to chronic disease prevalence, if the ultimate aim of decreased NCD morbidity and mortality is to be attained.

Taking into account rising NCD levels in low and middle-income countries coupled with the realization that many of these countries are often characterized by limited resources that must also address communicable disease challenges and by health systems that tend to be more oriented towards acute rather than chronic care, it is clear that current approaches to address NCD prevention need rethinking. To bolster inadequate health system capacity to respond to CHDs, there is an imperative to include interventions that address the wider social determinants of health as an essential complement to reinforce selective, cost-effective health-care interventions and population–wide prevention strategies—a threefold approach towards NCD reduction.

Social Determinants to Address NCDs in Low and Middle-Income Countries: Is Poverty Reduction Fundamental to Accelerated Action?

Middle-income and low-income countries often face similar challenges and vulnerabilities. There remains an unfinished development agenda in middle-income countries (MICs) and heightened vulnerability among their poorer neighbors. An analysis of progress on the MDGs reveals that one of their greatest social challenges is reducing poverty and social disparities, which are key root causes for health inequities and ongoing development threats, as reflected by the increasing gap between the "have's" and "have not's". Currently, it is estimated that almost three-quarters of approximately 1.3 billion people existing below the $1.25 a day poverty line currently live in middle-income countries, compared to only a quarter living in the poorest states ,mostly in Africa (Sumner 2010). The current poverty scenario is further complicated by the fact that at least five major global threats can undermine accelerated progress towards equitable development: the food and financial crises, rapid urbanization, climate change and ecosystem degradation, escalating humanitarian crises and rising fiscal austerity.

As with other priority health issues, prevailing social and economic conditions influence people's exposure and vulnerability to NCDs, as well as related health-care outcomes and consequences (WHO 2010). Poor socioeconomic conditions can be closely linked with NCDs, and as noted by the WHO, the rapid rise in the magnitude of these health problems is therefore predicted to impede poverty reduction initiatives in low-income countries and communities (WHO 2010). Even in high-income countries, there is strong evidence on the links between poverty and lower life expectancy, and strong associations between a host of social determinants, especially education and income levels, and NCD prevalence. A similar pattern is found in low and middle-income countries: the poor are worst off and have higher vulnerability and risk for NCDs (e.g., diabetes, heart disease, obesity, asthma) in all countries, regardless of the level of development.

While acknowledging positive efforts had been made to control major diseases and strengthen health systems, Marmot (2005) also highlighted the necessity of taking into account the important role of social justice and the negative effects of poverty on health outcomes. As he stated "To reduce inequalities in health across the world, there is a need for a third major thrust that is complementary to the development of health systems and relief of poverty, to take action on the social determinants of health." By focusing on social, economic, and political factors that impact on health and well-being, a SDH framework helps to (1) highlight the cyclic relationship between poverty and NCDs[1] and (2) reframe and transform national development agendas by taking into account the interdependency between NCDs and the health-related dimensions of other competing development priorities, such as education, social protection.

As such, a SDH framework to NCD prevention requires a heightened attention to inequities and disparities among and within countries. Since inequities, like social determinants, are often interdependent, poor families and their children face, during their life cycle, a series of difficulties in accessing adequate goods and services for the full development of their capabilities, and this lack of access perpetuates the poverty cycle for the next generations (Bull and Mittlemark 2010). A study carried out in Port Alegre, Brazil (Published in 2008), investigated the relationship between cardiovascular disease and socioeconomic conditions. Ecological analysis of the association between early mortality and CVD was carried out in the population of 45–64 year olds and socioeconomic conditions in 74 districts. The CVD mortality was found to be 3.3 times higher in poorer districts than in districts with better socioeconomic conditions: districts with better socioeconomic conditions had 123 deaths/100,000 population and districts with poorer socioeconomic conditions had 402 deaths/100,000 population (PAHO/WHO 2011a). Other families and their children are vulnerable but not reached by NCD prevention efforts because of social exclusion or discrimination related to class, gender, race, ethnicity or religion. These forms of inequities create distinct vulnerabilities resulting in lack of opportunity, loss of rights and various forms of social exclusion. For example, gender may determine different levels of access to nutrition and education, while ethnicity may result in deprivations in education and employment opportunities.

---

[1] The outcome document at the High-Level Meeting on NCDs in 2011 noted that NCDs and risk factors worsen poverty and poverty contributes to rising rates of NCDs.

The combination of different inequity factors such as gender, poverty and discrimination based on minority status can have an accumulated negative, life-long impact. For example, studies have shown that children from rural, socially excluded groups, compared to urban peers, enter adulthood without the same preparation or access to opportunities that could increase their earning potential and exit from poverty. This contributes to an intergenerational cycle of poverty that underpins the NCD risk factors.

While there is no uniform approach or consensus to defining, identifying or measuring poverty which is most often determined by income thresholds, it is clear that its nature and dynamics are multifaceted and often intergenerational. At any age, poverty is closely related to poor health, nutrition, hunger and other factors that make it difficult to realize one's full attention (UNICEF 2010a, b). However, from a SDH perspective, an understanding of child poverty provides a more sensitive lens to measure the poverty interplay with NCDs because childhood is a window of opportunity for development, and poverty experienced by children, even over short periods, can have a life-long negative and irreversible effects.

Based on a child rights framework, colleagues at the Townsend Centre for International Poverty Research conceptualized the phenomenon of childhood poverty as a compilation of eight deprivations rather than a monetary definition alone (Gordon 2008). While children living in poverty experience a lack of household income to purchase basic needs, they are also exposed to other areas of deprivation which are non-monetary in nature:

– Lack of access to formal education
– Lack of access to food
– Lack of access to clean water
– Lack of access to health care services
– Lack of access to sanitation facilities
– Lack of access to adequate shelter
– Lack of access to adequate information

Childhood poverty is most detrimental during the formative years. The UNESCO 2010 Education for All Report noted that early childhood can create the foundations for a life of expanded opportunity—or it can lock children into a future of deprivation and marginalization and yet every year millions of children start school handicapped with the experience of malnutrition, ill health and poverty in their early years. Poverty links have been found with childhood obesity because of poor and insufficient diets—of course, obesity is one of the risk factors for such chronic diseases as Type 2 diabetes. Moore et al. (2008) have also documented that childhood poverty had direct correlations with chronic diseases such as anemia and asthma. These findings are further compounded by the reality that in relative terms poor children in living in low and middle-income countries are more even more vulnerable than those living in developed countries. Measuring and studying the trends of childhood poverty in a country is useful in identifying and understanding the patterns of disparity and provide the foundation for developing multi-dimensional strategies to eradicate poverty and injustice, two key social determinants that also impact on NCDs. Addressing poverty and childhood poverty in particular, should be an imperative for NCD prevention.

Applying a SDH Framework to Accelerate Action on NCDs: What Does It Really Mean?

The Commission on SDH (WHO 2008) highlighted three key actions that should guide the application of a SDH approach:

– Improve daily living conditions
– Tackle the equitable distribution of power, money and resources
– Measure and understand the problem (health inequity) and assess the results of action

In practice, applying a SDH framework in NCD in programming is rights-based and puts "equity" as a foundational principle for action. Inherently, it also implies putting attention on reaching the most marginalized and most disadvantaged who are the least likely to have access to necessary services or benefit from current development policies and health programs. A change of focus is required if acceleration is to be effective as noted in Fig. 16.1.

SDH Focus	Supporting Strategies
SDH for NCD prevention is a national and local priority	▪ Promote the inclusion of SDH in Poverty Reduction Strategies (PRS) and National Development Plans and related policy and budget instruments ▪ Promote the participation of children, young people and women in analysing SDH and working on disaster risk reduction (DRR) strategies

Fig. 16.1 SDH focus with supporting strategies

Strategically framing NCD prevention within a SDH framework provides an opportunity to broaden policy formulation that incorporates both health and non-medical/social considerations which contribute to NCD prevalence and address disparities in a more targeted manner. At the same time, emphasizing the SDH-NCD link provides another channel through which the public can be engaged in taking individual and collective actions that reinforce health service delivery and broader environmental interventions and ultimately lead to a more comprehensive response to combating NCDs.

In contrast to the medical model of health, the SDH perspective supports a model of health that is perceived to be largely socially determined and posits that addressing socioeconomic and environmental factors can lead to positive health consequences. As such, SDH provides an analytical and programmatic framework for NCD prevention programs and interventions and as such, positions local governments as key actors in NCD prevention because they have the primary responsibility for planning and/or delivering many of the services that are crucial to addressing critical social determinants of health and NCD risks, such as: education, transport, housing and urban planning. In fact, participants at the Pan American Forum for Action on Non-Communicable Diseases (PAFNCD) held in Brasilia in May 2012 agreed that in addressing NCDs more effectively, collective action will yield greater impact on disease prevention, and reliance only on individual behavior change initiatives is no longer sufficient for sustainable development (PAHO/WHO 2012). The Pan American Forum conclusions reinforce the position of participants at the Entebbe Conference in 2010 who strongly advocated for the integrating

a SDH approach with NCDs given its recognition that individual behaviors are not always an individual choice and health behavior is also determined by a complex array of social, political and economic conditions that dictate the distribution of resources, power and health (Lins et al. 2010).

More specifically, the SDH perspective also helps foster a comprehensive approach to NCD prevention by identifying and framing the non-medical—i.e., social, economic, political, and environmental—factors that influence the distribution of health and illness linked to NCDs in a population. For example, the Toronto Charter of Physical Activity promotes comprehensive or "whole of community" initiatives that target people where they live, work and enjoy leisure time, and results have demonstrated significant increases in physical activity thereby reducing health risks linked to NCDs. Seven key actions, considered as investments, that could make a difference in tackling physical inactivity, as an important NCD risk factor, were found to be most effective: (1) prioritizing physical activity in schools via "whole of school, concept"; (2) putting in place transport policies and systems that prioritize walking, cycling and public transport; (3) formulating urban design regulations and infrastructure that provide equitable and safe access for recreational physical activity and transport-related walking and cycling across the life cycle; (4) integrating NCD prevention and physical activity within the primary health care system; (5) increasing public education, including mass media, to raise awareness and change social norms on physical activity; (6) implement community-wide programs across multiple settings and sectors while mobilizing and integrating community engagement and resources; and (7) providing sports systems and promotions that promote "sport for all" and encourage participation by all ages, from the very young to the aged.

Consistent with a SDH framework, implementation of the Charter also led to the systematic establishment partnerships and collaborative action across society was also emphasized within the comprehensive approach—the regulatory framework and infrastructure of the public sector, business planning expertise and workplace interventions by the private sector and civil society monitoring of actions and results, complemented by research and evidence provided by academic institutions. Additionally, lessons learned from the Toronto Charter show that the focus should be on providing brief, practical advice; linking community–based action to complement individual behavior change; and providing public education to increase knowledge, shift community norms and values as a means of motivating the population, both individually and collectively.

Maintaining a balance between NCDs and other development priorities—How can a SDH framework make a difference in setting program focus and policy direction in low and middle-income countries?

Given its "health-related" orientation, the SDH framework accepts and builds on the synergistic interplay between of NCDs and other development priorities, such as female literacy, girls' education, poverty reduction. How SDHs are defined operationally and for program planning and design is defined by each country's particular needs and priorities. The goal is not a perfect "definition" of SDH but rather a systematic analysis of the underlying or root causes of major risk factors that contribute to NCDs and their manifestation in varying country contexts as a foundation for design NCD prevention programs. These causes (poverty, social and cultural norms, etc.) are also implicated in communicable diseases and other development problems. Health promotion, as a discipline, provides tools and insights that are useful in developing NCD prevention strategies.

As Amuyunzu-Nyamongo (2010) pointed out, the determinants of NCDs, similar to other health problems, are influenced by a much wider range of individual, social and socio-economic factors than the health sector alone. In considering the projected rise in morbidity and mortality of cardio-vascular disease and other chronic diseases in sub-Saharan Africa from 28 to 60 % and from 35 to 65 %, respectively she further noted that addressing a single risk factor or condition is unlikely to achieve broad-based, population level change. Therefore, applying a Social Determinants Framework to NCD prevention requires a health-related rather than health-directed approach and leads to refocusing policy and reformulating programs to address four intersecting inequalities:

- Economic inequalities: wealthier quintiles have increased power and influence to those with higher incomes and put excluded groups at the receiving end of an unfair distribution of assets and opportunities
- Spatial inequalities: structures and patterns of economic growth which result in excluded groups living in places that make them harder to reach and/or easier to ignore as well as in geo-environmental precarious situations making them more prone to suffering the consequences of natural and man-made disasters
- Cultural inequalities: forms of discrimination and devaluation that perpetuate social exclusion by treating excluded groups as inferior
- Political inequalities: concentration of economic power and influence among a limited dominant group and the denial of voice and influence in the decision-making that affect the lives of excluded groups and their communities

Sir Richard Jolly aptly explained this interaction as follows:

While each one of these inequalities reflects an injustice, it is their mutually reinforcing interaction that explains the persistence of social exclusion over time and its resistance to "business as usual" approaches. Caste, race, ethnicity, language and religion are among the most common markers of exclusion. And as elsewhere in society, gender cuts across all these so that women and girls from marginalized groups generally fare worse than men and boys. (Kabeer 2010)

Prioritizing NCD Interventions in Humanitarian Action: Is SDH Still Relevant in Emergency Situations?

Unrest, armed conflict, disasters and disaster risks exacerbate already existing vulnerabilities and inequalities of those affected, disproportionately affect poor countries, erode development gains and set back progress in achieving the MDGs, as well as overshadow concerns about NCDs. As is often in times of peace, poor and marginalized families are at greater risk in situations of armed conflict, natural disasters and other emergencies. However, an emphasis on immediate response for life-saving measures and safety in these situations often means attention to NCDs may be considered to be of secondary importance. For families and children, who are victimized already by drought, famine or other results of war, NCDs can become a "silent killer" which is overlooked in the glare of fighting and natural catastrophes. However, the integration of a SDH framework into Early Recovery (ER) and Disaster Risk Reduction (DRR) interventions is paramount, since it facilitates a clearer synergy between immediate, emergency response and longer-term development initiatives and health interventions. In fact, opportunities for NCD interventions should be integrated with communicable disease management systems even during emergency situations taking into account on-the-ground realities and available resources since many of the same underlying causes for unrest and insecurity also contribute to increased risks to NCDs, especially among the poor and most disadvantaged. By placing more attention on the causes rather than only the diseases themselves, NCD prevention activities can target the core problems (Fig. 16.2).

Two major activities are crucial to applying a SDH framework to DRR and early recovery efforts. First, there is a need to partnering with NGOs and local communities to identify social determinants that are relevant in their situation and then using this information to develop Disaster Risk Reduction activities that include the active participation of children and women (groups who are often the most at-risk in any disaster). This will contribute significantly to develop individual and community resilience and preparedness. Secondly, developing the workforce and institutional capacities of government agencies and civil society organizations engaged in emergency response to use a SDH framework in preparedness planning, is essential. This planning would also necessitate taking into account the contingency management of NCDs in case of emergencies, disasters or highly unstable situations as well as understanding how these situations could further acerbate social determinants underpinning the NCDs.

Governments, civil society, and international cooperating partners are increasingly developing

---

management

In the context of emergencies, a SDH approach would seek answers to the following questions: :

- What emergency situations or disasters pose the biggest risk and to what extent do they correlate to NCD patterns/trends, where do they occur, and who is most vulnerable and/or most affected?
- What are the underlying and root causes of the NCD vulnerabilities which are leading certain groups to suffer from emergencies or disaster risks? Why do these problems occur and how can they be prevented or ameliorated?
- Who or which individuals and/or institutions have a role in managing NCDs during an emergency or reducing disaster risks?
- What individual and/or institutional capacities are needed to address the disaster risks faced by individuals suffering from NCDs, both for those who are being denied their rights through disaster vulnerability, and those who have the duty to address these problems?

Fig. 16.2 Using SDH to inform DRR interventions linked to NCD management

DRR policies, networks, bodies and capacities. Much of the leadership behind the support for disaster risk reduction increasingly has come from NGOs and from the South. National platforms to advance disaster risk reduction have been established in an estimated 56 countries. Civil society and NGO disaster risk reduction networks[2] have been created and regional bodies, such as the Asian Disaster Preparedness Centre (ADPC), have been mandated to develop the capacity of governments and civil society. After responding to immediate needs of affected communities after a crisis or disaster, focus should be to ensure a smooth transition from immediate relief and early recovery, the latter being an opportune period to begin integrating SDH framework for NCDs. Examples of specific action are listed in Fig. 16.3.

Potential Multi-sectoral Strategies and Horizontal Partnerships/Collaboration: Who Else Should Be Involved in NCD Prevention Beyond the Health Sector?

The High-Level meetings on NCDs and SDH, respectively, have provided momentum and widened international discussions on complex, interrelated factors linked to national development agendas throughout the world. These insights, coupled with on-the-ground programs, have provided insights for accelerated action. But conferences come and go; therefore to maintain attention and pressure to act on the SDH dimensions of NCDs, there is an ongoing need to maintain this topic on the public agenda and in political discourse, especially in low and middle-income countries. This is an opportune time to engage with media channels (both print and electronic) as partners not just conduits of information. By keeping journalists and social media professionals regularly informed on the latest scientific evidence and its implications for national development priorities, an ongoing dialogue can be maintained.

In addressing obesity as a health and development concern, Jordan's experience shows that effective, adequately funded and long-term media advertising and public education campaigns can be instrumental in addressing NCDs (Al Hourani et al. 2011).

Rasanathan and Krech (2011) have posited that the prevention of NCDs requires collaboration between different sectors (including finance, trade, agriculture, housing, education, community planning, etc.) to address conditions that give rise to them and to implement policies that support people to minimize their exposure to risks. Health professionals, alone, are insufficient to address the social determinants that underpin NCDs—this requires linking to political and policy decision-makers, educators, social workers and other professionals who intervene in the lives of families and communities.

Iran's experience in road safety prevention provides a relevant example of the type of multisectoral and interdisciplinary work that is supported by a SDH perspective (Esmaeili et al. 2011). Highly committed to minimizing the consequences of negative social determinants of health and health inequalities, the Government formulated a SDH strategic plan and established a SDH Secretariat within its Ministry of Health and Medical Education. The Secretariat liaises and has worked with a wide range of researchers and professionals from other sectors to set a robust action agenda in 15 areas—all either directly or indirectly related to NCDs: (1) Traffic Accidents; (2) Early Child Development; (3) Mental and spiritual health; (4) Equitable health care delivery; (5) Unemployment and job security; (6) Nutrition and food security; (7) Healthy lifestyle; (8) Education, awareness and literacy; (9) Housing; (10) Environment; (11) Social support; (12) Marginalized, deprived and desert areas, (13) Economic security; (14) Equitable distribution of resources; and (15) Vulnerable groups such as households headed by women. One of the priority areas in the current Secretariat's SDH plan of action is traffic injuries, as these are a major burden of disease and a major source of health inequity in the country.

Considering the multi-dimensional nature of road traffic injuries, the initiative involved the

---

[2] The Global Network of Civil Society Organizations for Disaster Reduction is an international network of 300 civil society organizations in 90 countries.

SDH Focus	Supporting Strategies
Foster NCD prevention as an integral component of Emergency Preparedness	▪ Support the capacity development of national and sub-national partners to take into account and incorporate socioeconomic and cultural dimensions of NCDs in emergency preparedness planning and response including early recovery approaches. Formulate and implement mitigation and prevention strategies that take into account the particular vulnerabilities of persons suffering from NCDs as a fundamental input in preparedness planning (i.e. prioritize information dissemination on relevant household and community actions for self-care during disasters or in emergency situations, take care in building temporary shelter (where and how), if needed, that is conducive to persons suffering from chronic respiratory diseases, or make available alternative fuel cooking sources to reduce smoke that could also affect them); ▪ Ensure periodic training of health and social workers, including community agents, in emergency preparedness and response actions that linked to NCDs; ▪ Engage in contingency planning for WASH, Nutrition, Health, Education and Child Protection responses, especially in high NCD prevalence zones; ▪ Promote the development community and school emergency preparedness plans and policies for refugees and/or displaced people that factor in NCD issues and concerns; ▪ Adapt health and nutrition information systems, to incorporate information on SDH and NCDs, to facilitate rapid, evidence-based decision making.
Identification of differential risks according to vulnerable groups	▪ Include a robust assessment of disaster risk and SDH as linked to NCDs while promote sub-national assessments of NCD vulnerability and response capacity in high risk contexts as needed; ▪ Promote and strengthen national systems to assess and monitor SDHs and NCD risks, including people-centred early warning systems; ▪ Working with multi-sectoral partners, establish an evidence and research base on SDH-linked disaster risks with a focus on differential vulnerabilities and capacities of children and women.
Increased safety and resiliency for the most vulnerable groups, especially those suffering from NCDs	▪ Promote DRR knowledge and awareness at household and community level through behavior and social change communication; ▪ Strengthen social protection systems and policy strategies to mitigate against the impact of emergencies or disasters on persons suffering from NCDs; ▪ Promote health and nutrition strategies, that take into account NCD needs, as a means of increasing individual safety and community resilience; ▪ Promote an integrated programming approach that links national development and policy processes to community resilience strategies for NCD prevention, treatment, and self-care in specific high risk or unstable environments.

Fig. 16.3 Integrating SDH-focus actions on NCDs in disaster preparedness

health, insurance, police, and education sectors. It was implemented by applying a systematic community based approach to engage local action, enforcement of law and legislation, engineering, environment modification, education, emergency care and evaluation. For example, on a policy level, 10 % of the mandatory third party premium of all kinds of motor vehicles is used to finance the compensation for free medical care for accident victims and a 10-year strategic plan, which includes roles and responsibilities of different sectors has been developed by the Road Safety Commission and approved by parliament for implementation. These efforts were further complemented and reinforced by an innovative approach that included engaging primary, elementary and secondary school students as social change agents[3] and community awareness-raising through mass media. Preliminary results show a strengthened policy-community interface and a 17.9 % decrease in the number of traffic errors within 1 year of the beginning of this initiative.

Bogota, Colombia has established one of the world's most extensive bike path systems (Ciclo-Ruta). Between 2000 and 2007 the number of bicycle users increased from 22,700 to 83,500 and the number of deaths related to bikes decreased by 33 % (PAHO/WHO 2011b).

Role of Local Communities and Civil Society Pin Accelerating the Reduction of NCDs: To What Extent Are Community Voices and Opinions Factored into the SDH Application?

If we are to transform ourselves, we have to make every effort to step from the outside to the inside view, to begin to see the world through the eyes of the people we claim to be trying to help and not through the refracting lens of our own. A real change in our relationship with people will depend on our serious and consistent attempts to learn from them; our use of every contact to explore the people's own resources and capacities that will be the main source of innovation in public health and medical care; our sensitivity and response to and support of their control and decision-making powers to whatever extent they may want it (Steuart 1977).

Tackling NCDs requires interventions that take place in local communities and in the settings where people live, work, and play (Shilton 2011) and therefore community engagement is an

important element of social change that is needed to address NCDs. Working with communities and reaching the most marginalized in low and middle-income countries is easier said than done and often requires new, innovative ways of working. The International Union of Health Promotion and Education (IUHPE) recognizes that NGOs are an important resource and partner to governments given the influence they can wield in local communities and their ability to outreach in the most marginalized and poorest communities. Their ongoing role as change agents make them, especially those who work with marginalized groups or serve in poor communities, an effective "interpreter" of community norms, health perceptions, and local thinking that are related to different determinants of chronic diseases. As a first-line resource, they bring the ability to transform national NCD policies into community friendly action and understanding, which is relevant to NCD prevention.

A recent initiative in Senegal, "The Grandmother Project," provides strong evidence on how placing value and focus on the positive aspects of indigenous culture can bring about change from within local communities (Musoko et al. 2011). Based on the premise that culture is a key determinant, project results have proven that the inclusion of elders, as particularly grandmothers, in program implementation; strengthening intergenerational communication; and use of communication/education approaches based on dialogue and critical thinking are important to increasing community engagement to address social determinants that impact on adolescent girls' health and well-being. The project provides evidence on how strategies that reflect cultural norms and build on community positive traditions can bring about change in a relatively short period of time, but is sustainable.

The Voluntary Health Association of India (Mukhopadhyay 2011) has made a strong case for the social determinants approach through community mobilization, based on its experience implementing a project designed to foster holistic change by "uplifting the socio-economic and health status of vulnerable communities," especially in remote areas of the country. Therefore interventions have been conceived within the larger

---

[3] Students serve as police officers for the family and the community and are given the responsibility to issue traffic tickets (with the cooperation of traffic police).

context of development. In response to community felt needs, health interventions were used mainly as an entry point to establish rapport and foster community engagement. Therefore, besides health promotion and disease prevention activities, an even stronger emphasis has been placed on community development (i.e., formation of self-help groups, capacity building, income generation, and education), community organization (women's groups, farmers groups, etc.), mobilization of village committees (i.e., forming social action groups, linking with the local political structure "panchayat," education). Lessons learned suggested that the four key drivers are needed to apply a community-oriented SDH approach:

- Planning with the local community at onset
- Identifying and building on the community's strengths and allowing them to control the process
- Responding to various socioeconomic determinants to bring about a change in the health and general condition of the population
- Creative partnering within communities and their external environments

In Guarulhos, Sao Paulo, Brazil, 51 participatory health forums were held to identify and incorporate the requests of the population into the preparation of local health policies and plans, through 1,300 representatives from Local Health Councils. Participatory budgeting was one of the tools used to directly channel the community's wishes into local initiatives, including the measuring of the effects of policies, plans, projects and programs on the health and equity of the population (PAHO/WHO 2011a).

These actions collectively then contribute to building community resiliency and competence to make informed choices about various sustainable and equitable development options

Current Avenues and Future Opportunities to Accelerate Collective Action in Reducing NCDs: What Else Can Be Done?

Developing programmatic tools to apply SDH is underway in a variety of countries and lessons learned are still being documented and shared, as was evidenced at the 2011 Rio Conference on Social Determinants of Health (Nayyar 2011). In addition to the landmark work of the Commission and WHO leadership in supporting SDH implementation, other UN agencies that do not have a health-specific mandate have also been engaged in similar efforts and provide other opportunities for joint action, especially as it relates to low and middle-income countries, Having wider missions to tackle inequities and social justice within a development context, their work can provide additional insights in operationalizing SDH. For example, UNICEF's seminal report entitled "Narrowing the Gaps to Meet the Goals" challenged a common assumption that to focus on the very poorest children would be costly and time-consuming; and instead found that extending services to the most marginalized through an equity-based approach can deliver concrete, sustainable results (UNICEF 2010a). This premise is consistent with a SDH approach in development programming. Based on the UNICEF experience in addressing child poverty as an underlying determinant for health and other development disparities, five practical policy parameters found: (1) investing more in the most deprived, (2) using cost-effective interventions, (3) overcoming bottlenecks, (4) partnering with communities, and (5) making the most of available resources (working from an assets orientation). In terms of implementation, a seven step programming framework has been developed, which is also relevant to health promotion practice and NCD prevention (Fig. 16.4).

In a parallel and complementary manner, the United Nations Development Program (UNDP) has proposed a framework for accelerated efforts to meet the Millennium Development Goals (2010). It includes a systematic strategy to determine bottlenecks and possible high-impact solutions, which then result in developing a concrete plan of action with coordinated roles for governments and their development partners (UN and other international agencies, private sector, NGOs and other civil society organizations, etc.) for achieving the country's MDG priorities (Fig. 16.5).

Professional associations such as The International Union for Health Promotion and Education (IUHPE) have also taken up the

Step 1: Analyze deprivations (monetary and non-monetary) of children and their causes
Step 2: Select evidence-based, high impact intervention packages to prevent or mitigate these
deprivations
Step 3: Analyze system wide bottlenecks in supply & demand and obstacles to effective coverage
Step 4: Analyze barriers in the enabling environment such as social norms, legislation/policies,
budgets, governance/partnerships
Step 5: Implement and apply evidence based strategies to remove equity bottlenecks and barriers in
development programs and their strategies
Step 6: Incorporate equity focused intervention packages and strategies in National Development
Plans, Sector Wide Approaches (SWAps), Social Contracts and other strategic policy and
planning documents etc.
Step 7: Leverage national policies, budgets and partnerships (at all levels), including media, civil
society and private sector, and parliamentarians etc.

Fig. 16.4 Action steps to narrow inequities/gaps

Step 1: Identify the relevant MDG target that is off-track or unlikely to be met,
          and made evidence-based determinations on key interventions needed
Step 2: Identify and prioritize causal factors for the lack of success, for each
intervention
Step 3: Review and rank solutions according to their impact and feasibility[4]
Step 4: Develop a MDG Action Plan, including a monitoring and evaluation
component

Fig. 16.5 Steps to accelerate MDG

Commission's challenge. In a forthcoming position statement, IUHPE is advocating for five areas for accelerated action in SDH; each has direct implications for NCD prevention efforts:

- *Developing evidence of effective action on the social determinants of health equities.*

    This includes documenting and strengthening the evidence of what and how SDH impacts on NCDs, and under what conditions.

- *Disseminating resources, best practices and tools to support action health equity.*

    By nurturing communities of practice, policy dialogue and knowledge exchange on lessons learned can be facilitated and guidance packages developed.

- *Building workforce capacity.*

    This would entails incorporating a human rights and equity perspective in both policy and program design. It promotes expanding beyond a focus on health workers alone to other disciplines such as social workers, gender professionals and moving beyond government to civil society and NGOs partnerships.

- *Engaging in dialogue on governance.*

    This supports strengthening the interface between government and communities and recognizes their shared responsibility in tackling the underlying causes of NCD risks in a coordinated, fashion. This dialogue sets the foundation for a smoother interface between policy and practice.

- *Greater investment in health promotion.*

    NCD prevention efforts must expand beyond information and persuasive messages to actual dialogue and interaction with families and local communities. Health promotion, as a discipline, promotes skill sets that support community engagement and empowerment and when applied effectively can accelerate the achievement of desired results.

These efforts, coupled with innovative country initiatives and practitioner engagement, provide renewed impetus to health promotion strategies that can contribute to NCD prevention in low and middle-income countries. As the body of knowledge on the interface between SDH and NCD is strengthened, collaborative action between governments and communities is solidified, and engagement of non-health sectors tackling underlying causes is widened, the reduction of mortality and morbidity due to chronic diseases is attainable. At the same time, the transformational effect of a SDH approach in tackling the root causes of health inequities and disparities associated with NCDs can lead to longer term, sustainable development and therefore serves as critical function in helping these countries achieve the MDGs and their own national development priorities.

References

Al Hourani, H., Naffa, S., & Fardous, T. (2011). *National commitment to action on SDH in Jordon: Addressing Obesity*. Background Paper No. 18, World Health Organization for the World Conference on Social Determinants of Health in Rio de Janeiro, Brazil.

Amuyunzu-Nyamongo, M. (2010). Need for a multi-factorial, multi-sectorial and multi-disciplinary approach to NCD prevention and control in Africa. *Global Health Promotion, 17*(2 Suppl), 31–2.

Barros, F., Victora., C, Scherpbier, R., & Davidson, G. (2010). Socioeconomic inequities in the health and nutrition of children in low/middle income countries. *Revista de Saúde Pública, 44*(1), 1–16.

Bégin, M. (2009). Equité et déterminants sociaux de la santé: de l'urgence d'agir. *Global Health Promotion, 19*(3), 73–75.

Bull, T., & Mittlemark, M. (Eds). (2010). *Living Conditions and Determinants of Social Position Amongst Women of Child-bearing Age in Very Poor Ruralities: Qualitative Exploratory Studies in India, Ghana and Haiti*, IUHPE Research Report Series (Vol. V, No. 1).

Esmaeili, A., Haddadi, M., Manesh., A, Sirous, S., & Mesdaghinia, A. (2011). *School pupil police officer (Hamyare officer)—a national initiative based on social participation to improve road safety*. Background Paper No. 17, World Health Organization for the World Conference on Social Determinants of Health in Rio de Janeiro, Brazil.

Giles, W. H. (2010). Centers for Disease Control and Prevention, Division of Adult and Community Health. *Global Health Promotion 17*(Suppl 2), 3–5.

Gordon, D. (2008). *Measuring child poverty and deprivation, university of Bristol, Townsend Centre for international poverty research*. UNICEF Global Study on Child Poverty and Deprivations Workshop, Policy Analysis Techniques Related to Child Poverty and Disparities, University of Southampton, 18–28 August.

Grady, E., & Goldblatt, P. (Eds.). (2012). *Addressing the social determinants of health: the urban dimension and the role of local government*. Geneva, Switzerland: WHO.

Kabeer, N. (2010). Can the MDGs provide a pathway to social justice? The challenge of intersecting inequalities Sussex and New York: IDS & UN MDG Achievement Fund, p. 8.

Lins, N. E., Jones, C. M., & Nilson, J. R. (2010). Commentary—New frontiers for the sustainable prevention and control of non-communicable diseases (NCDs): A View from Sub-Saharan Africa. *Global Health Promotion 17*(Suppl 2), 27–30.

Marmot, M. (2005). Social determinants of health inequalities. *The Lancet, 365*, 1099–1104.

Moore, K. A., Redd, Z., Burkhauser, K., & Collins, A. (2009). *Children in poverty: Trends, consequences and policy options*. Child Trends Research Bulletin, Washington, DC, USA.

Mukhopadhyay, A. (2011). *Effective social determinants of health approach in India through social mobilization*. Background Paper No. 9, World Health Organization for the World Conference on Social Determinants of Health, in Rio de Janeiro, Brazil.

Mukhopadhyay, A. (Ed.) (2009/2010). Health for the millions: A social determinants approach. *Innovations in Practice, 35*(4 & 5), 1–15.

Musoko, A., Scoppa, C., & Manoncourt, E. (2011). *Dialogue Communautaire et Culture: Appuyer les filles pour un avenir meilleur*. Lessons Learned Document from The Grandmother Project, World Vision, Unpublished Paper, Rome, Italy.

Nayyar, K. R. (2011). *India's country experience in addressing social exclusion in maternal and child health*. Background Paper No. 8, World Health Organization for the World Conference on Social Determinants of Health in Rio de Janeiro, Brazil.

Nikolic, I. A., Anderson E., Stanciole, A. E., & Mikhail, Z. (2011). Chronic Emergency: Why NCDs Matter? Health, Nutrition, and Population, Human Development Network, The World Bank.

PAHO/WHO. (2011a). *Trends and Achievements in Promoting Health and Equity in the Americas: Developments from 2003 to 2011*. WHO: Washington, DC.

PAHO/WHO. (2011b). *Non-communicable diseases: Building a healthier future*. WHO: Washington, DC.

PAHO/WHO. (2012). *Pan American Forum for Action on Noncommunicable Diseases (PAFNCD)*. Brasilia, Brazil.

Potvin, L., Moquet, M., & Jones, C. (2010). *Réduire les inéqalités sociales en santé*. INEPS. Santé en Action: Paris, France.

Raphael, D. (2008). Getting Serious about SDH: New directions for public health workers. *Promotion and Education, 15*(3), 15–20.

Rasanathan, K., & Krech, R. (2011). Action on social determinants of health is essential to tackle non-communicable diseases. *Bulletin of the World Health Organization, 89*, 775–776. doi:10.2471/BLT.11.094243.

Shilton, T. (2011). *Advocating for health promotion approaches to non-communicable disease prevention*. IUHPE Key Messages in the Lead up to the United Nations High Level Meeting on NCDs, position statement, Paris, France.

Steuart, G. (1977). *The world is not round: Innovation and the medical wheel*. Speech given at APHA Conference in Washington, DC.

Sumner, A. (2010). *Global poverty and the new bottom billion: what if three-quarters of the world's poor live in middle income countries?* Institute of Development Studies, September.

UN General Assembly. (2011). *Outcome document*. High-Level Meeting on the Prevention and Control of Noncommunicable Diseases in New York, USA.

UNESCO, (2010). *EFA Global Monitoring Report, Reaching the Marginalized*. Oxford University Press: London.

UNICEF. (2010a). *Progress for children: achieving the MDGs with equity and narrowing the gaps to meet the goals*. New York, USA.

UNICEF. (2010b). *Child poverty and disparities in Egypt: Building the social infrastructure for Egypt's future*, Cairo, Egypt.

WHO. (2008). "Closing the gap in a generation: health equity through action on the social determinants of health," *Final Report of the Commission on Social Determinants of Health*, Geneva, Switzerland.

WHO. (2010). *Equity, social determinants and public health programmes*. WHO: Geneva, Switzerland.

Books

Closing the Gap in a Generation Health Equity through Action on the Social Determinants of Health. International Conference, 6–7 November 2008, London Global Health Promotion Supplement 1–2009.

(2010) Community Health Promotion Strategies to address non-communicable diseases in Africa. *Global Health Promotion, 17*(Suppl II).

Cardiovascular Health, Risk, and Disease: Primordial and Remedial Strategies

Darwin R. Labarthe

Introduction

Cardiovascular health, risk, and disease serve well as an example of chronic diseases of global health concern for discussion of health promotion and its role in improving population health. Several considerations support this view (Labarthe & Dunbar, 2012). Cardiovascular disease occurs in every region of the world. Its two leading components, ischemic heart disease and cerebrovascular disease (CVD), or stroke, are estimated globally to rank first and second in number of deaths each year, first and third as causes of disability, and first and fourth as contributors to years of healthy life lost. Cardiovascular disease shares several determinants with the other major chronic diseases (cancer, chronic respiratory diseases, and diabetes). Cardiovascular conditions therefore share with other major chronic diseases the appropriateness of broad health promotion strategies.

A spectrum of cardiovascular health states together constitutes an important object of health promotion (US Department of Health and Human Services, 2003). The expression "cardiovascular health, risk, and disease" emphasizes this perspective, which is explicitly more comprehensive than "cardiovascular disease" alone. This spectrum represents a progression from health to disease. It represents a wide range of potential opportunities for intervention, from the broadest approaches of population-wide health promotion to the most disease-specific and individualized clinical practices.

The goals of health promotion as it addresses cardiovascular health, risk, and disease are derived directly from this cardiovascular health spectrum (Healthy people, 2010). True it is that policies, programs, and practices aimed at cardiovascular health promotion are most clearly applicable prior to manifest expression of cardiovascular disease. However, the goals of cardiovascular health promotion and disease prevention reach across the full spectrum of outcomes—from maintaining health to reversing risk to ameliorating the consequences of overt disease.

Several major determinants of cardiovascular health, risk, and disease provide focus and rationale for health promotion efforts. A vast body of evidence has been developed over decades of research and experience regarding these determinants. Firm knowledge of their causal roles, their amenability to modification, and the impact of effective interventions provide a solid scientific foundation for cardiovascular health promotion (Labarthe, 2011).

D.R. Labarthe, MD, MPH, PhD (✉)
Department of Preventive Medicine,
Northwestern University Feinberg School
of Medicine, 680 N. Lakeshore Drive, Suite 1400,
Chicago, IL 60611, USA
e-mail: darwin.labarthe@northwestern.edu

D.V. McQueen (ed.), *Global Handbook on Noncommunicable Diseases and Health Promotion*,
DOI 10.1007/978-1-4614-7594-1_17, © Springer Science+Business Media, LLC 2013

Strategies of health promotion and disease prevention in the cardiovascular area are broadly of two kinds: primordial and remedial (Labarthe & Dunbar, 2012). They differ in their immediate goals as well as the points where they apply in the progression from health to disease. Primordial strategies are truest to the usual meaning of health promotion. They are intended to establish or sustain conditions of life so as to strengthen positive health assets, thereby averting development of risk in the first place. Remedial strategies, by contrast, are intended either to address already acquired risk or to remedy or limit the consequences of manifest disease.

Only through taking effective action can these strategies have practical impact. Past and present pleas, plans, and policies for action in cardiovascular health promotion attest to efforts to date and what they have contributed to improvements in population-level cardiovascular health (Labarthe, 2011). In every region of the world, greater investment in known effective interventions could achieve much greater impact than has been evident to date (Labarthe & Dunbar, 2012).

How the global challenges of cardiovascular health, risk, and disease might be addressed more effectively leads to the following question: What new directions toward this end might be anticipated in policy, practice, and research?

The Cardiovascular Health Spectrum

The major cardiovascular conditions, from a global health perspective, are the atherosclerotic and hypertensive diseases. These occur chiefly as either ischemic heart disease (IHD; also "coronary heart disease," CHD; also "heart attack") or CVD (also "stroke"). For each of these two conditions, a schematic figure illustrates the course of the typical individual case, as the status progresses from subclinical, or unapparent, disease to fatal outcome. Related circumstances progress as well, from latent to acute to post-event phases, as do time frames, from decades to seconds, in the development and outcome of the individual case (Figs. 17.1, 17.2) (Labarthe, 2011).

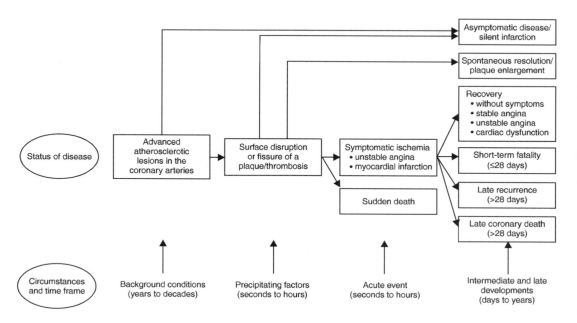

Fig. 17.1 Time course of the typical coronary event. Reprinted with permission from the author, Labarthe (2011)

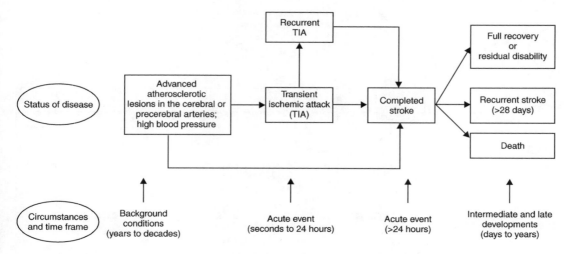

Fig. 17.2 Time course of the typical cerebrovascular event. Reprinted with permission from the author, Labarthe (2011)

Depicted in these figures are the late consequences of processes denoted as "background conditions" present over "years to decades." The figures largely represent the domain of clinical intervention and preventive cardiology. Epidemiologic indicators of IHD and CVD are predominantly numbers and rates of death from the far right, or downstream, end of the spectrum. Even these data are absent, incomplete, or unreliable in many parts of the world, especially in low-income countries. However, this fragmentary information is at present the best available basis for estimating the burden of disease and suggesting of trends, favorable or unfavorable, in the course of these conditions (Gaziano, Reddy, Paccaud, Horton, & Chaturvedi, 2006).

Across a whole population, from childhood to late adulthood, a spectrum of cardiovascular states is implied, from low risk to increased risk to presence of cardiovascular disease. This latter state may be represented by either an acute event (heart attack or stroke) or persistent chronic cardiovascular disease among those who survive. It is useful for a comprehensive approach to population health to recognize each of these states because distinct approaches to health promotion or disease prevention are applicable in each case (US Department of Health and Human Services, 2003).

More elaborate schemes to represent the cardiovascular health spectrum draw on evidence from high-income countries. There, population health data are far more extensive, including surveillance, through continuous probability sampling of the national population. Data of this kind, coupled with knowledge from decades of epidemiologic research and intervention experience, afford a more comprehensive picture of the fundamental process of cardiovascular health, risk, and disease. Figure 17.3, for example, presents a public health action framework for cardiovascular health promotion and disease prevention developed for the United States (US Department of Health and Human Services, 2003). Though this framework is an abstraction based largely on Western experience, it is believed to be valid in principle for cardiovascular health, risk, and disease anywhere in the world.

What does this framework contribute to understanding the role of cardiovascular health promotion? The upper three panels pertain to the cardiovascular health spectrum, first in terms of "the present reality" (middle panel), then a contrasting "vision of the future" (upper panel), and in between an array of "intervention approaches" considered instrumental in moving from the challenges of the present to a more salutary future.

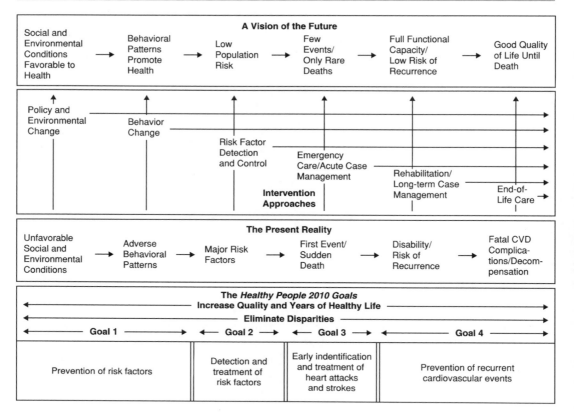

Fig. 17.3 A public health action framework to prevent heart disease and stroke. Adapted from the US Department of Health and Human Services (2003)

"The present reality" begins from the broadest conditions of society, as it illustrates the progression from unfavorable conditions through adverse population-level behavioral patterns to development of major risk factors, cardiovascular events, and their aftermath, with ultimate cardiovascular death. In "a vision of the future," rival realities are presented. This future is seen as attainable through the intervention approaches that correspond to each pair of alternatives—between the future and the status quo. Policy and environmental change, for example, is the path from unfavorable to favorable social and environmental conditions (vertical arrow). Notably, this approach may have consequences for other phases of the cardiovascular spectrum as well (horizontal arrow).

The main contributions of health promotion are at the level of social and environmental conditions, where the most far-reaching determinants of health are addressed. Effective action here can have consequences not only for cardiovascular

health but also for prevention of the other major chronic diseases as well. Attention to the lower panels of the framework will further underscore the unique contributions of health promotion, in relation to four distinct goals of heart disease and stroke prevention.

Goals of Cardiovascular Health Promotion and Disease Prevention

The *Public Health Action Plan* with its framework, above, was created as a guide to cardiovascular health promotion and disease prevention strategies for the United States, through 2020 and beyond (US Department of Health and Human Services, 2003). Goals for cardiovascular health could be cited from a variety of sources—national, regional, or global (Labarthe, 2011). This framework incorporates the goal for heart disease and stroke prevention published by the

US Department of Health and Human Services in the year 2000 to serve for the decade, to 2010; it was subsequently retained for the decade to 2020 as well (Healthy people, 2010; US Department of Health and Human Services, 2000):

> To improve cardiovascular health and quality of life through prevention, detection and treatment of risk factors, early identification and treatment of heart attacks and strokes, and prevention of recurrent cardiovascular events.

For purposes of the *Action Plan* and framework, the distinction between prevention of risk factors on the one hand and their detection and treatment on the other was critical. This would permit specific alignment between intervention approaches and their targets, especially distinguishing the main focus of health promotion—prevention of risk factors—from other intervention approaches.

From this perspective, strategies of prevention can be understood as having four distinct but complementary goals, shown in the bottom panel of Fig. 17.3. The overarching goals of Healthy People 2010 were to increase quality and years of healthy life and to eliminate health disparities (US Department of Health and Human Services, 2000). Any of the intervention approaches would be expected to contribute toward achievement of those goals. But for each of the four goals of cardiovascular health promotion and disease prevention, a distinct subset of approaches applies. For example, the goal of prevention of risk factors can only be attained through policy and environmental change and population-wide behavior change—tools of health promotion.

Documents abound that present goals for improving cardiovascular health, either explicitly or, among more recent examples, implicitly within the rubric of chronic diseases, or NCDs (Labarthe, 2011). The scope of these goal statements sometimes spans the full spectrum addressed in the *Action Plan* but is often restricted to one or another of these four goals. Three examples serve to illustrate commonalities and differences among statements of this kind:

- The World Health Organization (WHO) 2004 *Global Strategy on Diet, Physical Activity, and Health* called for development of comprehensive regional and national strategies to address all aspects of nutrition and physical activity. Elements of the strategies should include a life course perspective, a priority of reaching low-income populations, sensitivity to variations in prevailing patterns of diet and activity, and inclusion of evaluation, monitoring, and surveillance. Rapid reductions in the incidence of NCDs were to be expected following implementation of effective interventions. This strategy focuses on population-wide behavior change that would serve the goal of prevention of risk factors as well as further downstream benefits.

- The World Bank project, *Disease Control Priorities in Developing Countries*, was updated in 2006 after first being published in 1993 (Gaziano et al., 2006; Pearson et al., 1993). A broad range of conditions of major public health concern in developing countries is addressed in both editions. Most relevant here is the conclusion that "Population-wide efforts now to reduce risk factors through multiple economic and educational policies and programs will reap savings later in medical and other direct costs as well as indirectly in terms of improved quality of life and economic productivity" (Gaziano et al., 2006). Here the focus was the goal of reducing risks already established in the populations of developing countries.

- The Impact Goal for 2020 adopted by the American Heart Association (AHA)—the leading voluntary health agency in the United States in the cardiovascular arena—is as follows: "By 2020, to improve cardiovascular health of all Americans by 20 %, while reducing deaths from cardiovascular diseases and stroke by 20 %" (Lloyd-Jones et al., 2010). This shift in AHA's focus from cardiovascular death and disability to cardiovascular health has been called "a quiet revolution," for its potential impact in preserving and promoting cardiovascular health (Labarthe, 2012). It has entailed, for example, definition of cardiovascular health and specification of metrics by which to evaluate it at both individual and population levels (Fig. 17.4). For each metric, quantitative criteria are specified, separately for ages below 20 and 20 years and older.

"By 2020, to improve the cardiovascular health of all Americans by 20%, while reducing deaths from cardiovascular diseases and stroke by 20%."

Cardiovascular health metrics

Tobacco
Diet
Physical activity
Body mass index
Blood pressure
Blood cholesterol
Blood glucose

Fig. 17.4 The American Heart Association 2020 impact goal and the defining cardiovascular health metrics

Three levels, "ideal," "intermediate," and "poor," of cardiovascular health are distinguished, among persons free of clinically recognized cardiovascular disease. This 2020 goal implies population change from poor to intermediate and from intermediate to ideal cardiovascular health—and, potentially, to promote and preserve ideal cardiovascular health from the beginning. All of these activities relate to Goals 1 and 2 of the *Action Plan* (US Department of Health and Human Services, 2003).

Major Determinants of Cardiovascular Health, Risk, and Disease

What determines individual and population levels of cardiovascular health, risk, and disease? Until recently, "traditional" or "conventional" risk factors alone were cited in the discussion of cardiovascular disease prevention. Each of several factors, well documented through decades of epidemiologic research, could be described in terms of both its contribution to cardiovascular risk and the underlying determinants of the specific risk factor itself.

This approach is reflected in Table 17.1, which lists the main headings under which the most prominent determinants are reviewed in corresponding chapters in a recent text, *Epidemiology and Prevention of Cardiovascular Diseases: A Global Challenge* (Labarthe, 2011). The concept

Table 17.1 Determinants of cardiovascular health, risk, and disease

Dietary imbalance
Physical inactivity
Obesity
Adverse blood lipid profile
High blood pressure
Diabetes
Smoking and other tobacco exposure
Other personal factors
Social environment
Physical environment
Heredity and family history

Note 1: Social determinants of health represent the broadest conditions of life in which the foregoing factors are themselves determined
Note 2: The social–ecological framework represents the multilevel relationships among all determinants of health

behind this list is that patterns of diet and physical activity are fundamental behavioral factors; obesity is a consequence of dietary imbalance and physical inactivity; adverse blood lipid profile, high blood pressure, and diabetes are in turn consequences of dietary and activity patterns through and beyond obesity as an intermediary; tobacco use and exposure act separately from these; and other factors (including genetic and other hereditary influences) operate largely to foster or exacerbate these foregoing factors. This representation is incomplete, as noted, and requires addition of the concepts of social determinants of health and the social–ecological framework better to reflect the substantial influence of social and environmental conditions

(Committee on Assuring the Health of the Public in the 21st Century, 2003; World Health Organization, 2006).

Elevated prominence of "cardiovascular health" has another effect on a current view of determinants. The AHA metrics (Fig. 17.4) are now characterized as "health behaviors" and "health factors," no longer "risk behaviors" and "risk factors" as before (Lloyd-Jones et al., 2010). In parallel, a concept of "positive cardio-vascular health" is emerging in which positive psychological assets may operate independently from recognized adverse characteristics to pro-mote health, reduce disease incidence, and accel-erate recovery from acute events (Boehm & Kubzansky, 2012). Together, these developments add further to the recognized importance of health promotion, and prevention of cardiovascu-lar risk in the first place, as major strategic oppor-tunities in cardiovascular health.

Strategies of Cardiovascular Health Promotion and Disease Prevention

The goals for cardiovascular health promotion and disease prevention derived from the Healthy People process and depicted in Fig. 17.3 suggest two broad strategies of intervention. One addresses prevention of risk factors and, by implication, promotion of health in order to achieve this goal (Goal 1). The other addresses already acquired risk or manifest disease, through detection and treatment of risk factors, early identification and treatment of heart attacks and strokes, and prevention of recurrent cardiovascu-lar events (Goals 2–4) (US Department of Health and Human Services, 2000, 2003).

The first strategy can readily be seen as "pri-mordial," in the sense of this term as introduced by Strasser (1978). This approach was proposed as a means of "preserving entire risk-factor-free societies from the penetration of risk factor epidemics." The second strategy, by contrast, is "remedial." It works to reduce risk, increase survival of acute events when they do occur, and improve function and prognosis for those who survive.

Table 17.2 Dimensions of health promotion and disease prevention

Strategy
- Primordial/remedial (population-wide/high risk; primary/secondary/tertiary)
- Health promotion/disease prevention

Approach
- Policy and environmental change/behavior change/risk factor detection and control/emergency care and acute case management/rehabilitation and long-term case management/end-of-life care
- Lifestyle change/pharmacotherapy
- Single/multifactor intervention

Setting
- Community/worksite/school/health care facility/religious organization

This second strategy conforms closely to the dual "high-risk" and "mass" or "population-wide" strategies articulated by Rose (1981). It also sub-sumes the approaches long associated with pre-ventive cardiology: "primary," "secondary," and "tertiary" prevention. The first of these is to reduce the risk to avert an initial cardiovascular event; the second would seek to avert recurrent events; the third would improve function through rehabilitation following a prior acute event. (It should be noted that Goal 3, addressing the acute event, is not clearly identified with any of these terms.) Some ambiguity in usage (e.g., "primary prevention of hypertension" vs. "primary preven-tion of CHD"), as well as unnecessary complex-ity, favors the simpler distinction between primordial and remedial strategies.

Other dimensions of cardiovascular health promotion and disease prevention are also described, such as those listed in Table 17.2 (Labarthe, 2011). First, the primordial and reme-dial strategies are seen to correspond with the distinction between health promotion and disease prevention. Second, approaches can be described in various terms, such as those in Fig. 17.3; life-style or behavioral change versus pharmacother-apy; or single- versus multifactor intervention. Third, multiple settings for implementing inter-ventions may be identified. Still, other descrip-tors could be added. Those shown here are intended to point to a wide range of intervention opportunities at the practical level, where action happens. The broad distinction between primordial and remedial strategies, and health promotion and disease prevention, appears useful as an overarching concept in planning for public health action (Labarthe & Dunbar, 2012).

Taking Action: Pleas, Plans, and Policies

These strategic concepts, like the guidelines and recommendations often promulgated by authoritative bodies, can contribute to improving population health only with effective action to implement them. As strategies have been articulated in the cardiovascular arena, calls to action have accompanied them.

Pleas for implementation of accepted strategies have been published for more than a half-century, perhaps first in a notice to doctors and patients regarding preventive measures they could undertake (White et al., 1959). By the early 1980s, these calls rose to the level of WHO recommendations to Member States regarding prevention of CHD (World Health Organization Expert Committee, 1982). Beginning in 1992, the International Heart Health Society has periodically issued Declarations exhorting governments, nongovernment organizations, and multiple sectors of society to take action based on the knowledge of potentially effective policy initiatives. These were compiled in 2005 as a "platform document" to foster action for cardiovascular health throughout the world (International Heart Health Society, 2005).

The Institute of Medicine, in a 2010 report on cardiovascular health promotion in developing countries, stated: "The accelerating rates of unrecognized and inadequately addressed CVD [cardiovascular diseases] and related chronic diseases in both men and women in low and middle income countries are cause for immediate action" (Institute of Medicine, 2010). Most recently, the United Nations' High-Level Meeting of the General Assembly on the Prevention and Control of Non-communicable Diseases proposed 23

new commitments to efforts in NCD prevention and called on WHO to present options for meaningful action, by the end of 2012; a report on progress achieved, in 2013; and a comprehensive assessment of progress in 2014 (United Nations General Assembly, 2011).

Calls to action call for plans of action designed to apply chosen strategies and approaches. Examples of action plans found from the Americas, Europe, and South Asia are described elsewhere in some detail, including a case study of the (US) *Public Health Action Plan to Prevent Heart Disease and Stroke*, the source of Fig. 17.3 (Labarthe, 2011; US Department of Health and Human Services, 2003).

A well-known classic action plan for cardiovascular health promotion and disease prevention is the North Karelia Project in Eastern Finland, which began in 1972. The aim was to reduce blood pressure and cholesterol levels and achieve smoking cessation population-wide through a comprehensive program of policy change, population-wide behavior change, and change in the health care system. The exceptionally high rate of coronary mortality that stimulated the project was reduced substantially, to an even greater degree than predicted from the actual risk factor reductions that were achieved (Vartiainen et al., 1994).

Beyond the demonstrated impact on population health in North Karelia, this project established a model for policy development that has been replicated in many other countries, principally in central and eastern Europe. The concept was to take action within a subregion of a country, demonstrate its feasibility and impact, and elevate the effective policies to the national level, as was accomplished in Finland. This has been the model for the Country-wide Integrated Noncommunicable Diseases Intervention (CINDI) Program of WHO, which illustrates the successful merging of cardiovascular with other chronic disease initiatives (Grabowsky, Farquhar, Sunnarborg, & Bales, 1997).

Recent (though late) recognition of the contribution of cardiovascular conditions to the global burden of disease, especially in low- and middle-income countries, has stimulated wide discussion of the opportunities and challenges confronting effective health promotion efforts for these conditions, whether or not including the other NCDs. A more concerted approach to policy development is now in progress, in part as an outgrowth of events since 2000, reviewed in some detail in 2012 (Labarthe, 2012).

The United Nations Millennium Development Declaration, adopted in September 2000, presented a set of Millennium Development Goals (MDGs) that addressed global health issues—but only in relation to HIV/AIDS, malaria, and "other diseases" (United Nations General Assembly, 2000). The lack of any reference to cardiovascular and other chronic conditions produced an outcry of global proportions. Several prominent publications addressed this issue, collectively presenting arguments in support of global efforts in cardiovascular health promotion and disease prevention and in NCD prevention and control.

Two outcomes of special significance were publication of a 2010 report from the Institute of Medicine, cited above, *Promoting Cardiovascular Health in the Developing World: A Critical Challenge to Achieve Global Health*, and the convening in September 2011 of the United Nations General Assembly (UNGA) to focus on NCD prevention (Institute of Medicine, 2010; United Nations General Assembly 2011).

The Institute of Medicine report is noteworthy, in part, because it proposed integration of cardiovascular health promotion into global health activities at two levels. First, its 12 recommendations referred in all but 2 cases to NCDs together, not cardiovascular disease alone—despite its clearly explicit focus on cardiovascular health. Second, it called attention to models of organization and implementation in the arena of HIV/AIDS and the potential value for cardiovascular health promotion of emulating or joining in those efforts. This argument bears most directly on risk factor detection and treatment and on long-term case management, in terms of Fig. 17.3 above, but it may have relevance to earlier stage health promotion as well (Institute of Medicine, 2010).

In addition, the Institute of Medicine report recommended a new approach to implementation, in which the Global Alliance for Chronic Diseases would conduct (Institute of Medicine, 2010):

> … case studies of the CVD financing needs of five to seven countries representing different geographic regions, stages of the CVD epidemic, and stages of development. Several scenarios for different prevention and treatment efforts, training and capacity building efforts, and demographic trends should be evaluated. These initial case studies should establish an analytical framework with the goal of expanding beyond the initial pilot countries.

This proposal suggests a nodal center, at the national level, in each region of the world where models of policy development, implementation, and evaluation could catalyze work throughout the region.

The UNGA Meeting and its Declaration, noted above, have given a new level of prominence to cardiovascular and other chronic diseases, with a highly demanding charge to WHO as an outcome. The Declaration calls for reduction of risk factors and creation of health-promoting environments; strengthening of national policies and health systems; international cooperation including collaborative partnerships; research and development; monitoring and evaluation; and follow-up (United Nations General Assembly, 2011).

Meanwhile, WHO activities continue, to implement its *Global Strategy for the Prevention and Control of Noncommunicable Diseases*. A global status report in 2011 pointed to major forces behind the global expanse of the NCDs, stating that (World Health Organization, 2011):

> … the epidemic of these diseases is being driven by powerful forces now touching every region of the world: demographic ageing, rapid unplanned urbanization, and the globalization of unhealthy lifestyles. While many chronic conditions develop slowly, changes in lifestyles and behaviours are occurring with a stunning speed and sweep.

The principal interventions considered by WHO to be cost-effective and ready for immediate implementation are the following "best buys," at the population level:

Protecting people from tobacco smoke and banning smoking in public places

Warning about the dangers of tobacco use

Enforcing bans on tobacco advertising, promotion, and sponsorship

Raising taxes on tobacco

Restricting access to retailed alcohol

Enforcing bans on alcohol advertising

Raising taxes on alcohol

Reducing salt intake and salt content of food

Replacing trans fat in food with polyunsaturated fat

Promoting public awareness about diet and physical activity, including through mass media
And at the individual, health care level:

> Counseling and multidrug therapy ("a regimen of aspirin, statin, and blood pressure-lowering agents in people at high cardiovascular risk"), including glycemic control for diabetes for people ≥ 30 years old with a 10-year risk of fatal or nonfatal cardiovascular events ≥ 30 %; [and] Aspirin therapy for acute myocardial infarction.

Each of these interventions is expected to have substantial impact in cardiovascular health promotion and disease prevention. Together they offer an agenda for action that is hoped to be sufficient to offset and overcome the adverse social and environmental conditions that foster continued growth of this epidemic.

Finally, through the practical experience of programs at community, regional, or national levels, as well as decades of epidemiologic and other research, a number of points in support of cardiovascular health promotion and disease prevention have become established and can be summarized as follows (Labarthe, 2011):

- Experience with multifactor primary prevention has accrued from a large number of studies in the United States and much of the world. What can be learned from this body of work is the cornerstone of the case for prevention. Widespread interest in community approaches suggests increasing readiness over the past decade to take further action. Lessons of experience indicate foremost a need to implement the most promising and comprehensive interventions, in multiple populations, on a large enough scale and with sufficient duration to permit rigorous evaluation. This would offer the greatest opportunity to identify intervention approaches with potential for widespread dissemination and adaptation to local needs and resources.

- The fact of global occurrence of CVD on an epidemic level calls for application of current knowledge on a corresponding scale. The burden of risk is global in extent, and every region of the world is experiencing CVD on an epidemic scale. Distributions of particular risk factors vary among populations as do, therefore, their relative and respective population-attributable fractions for CHD and stroke. But the same factors are accountable everywhere.

- At a macroeconomic level, CVD and other chronic diseases demand a level of attention and urgency of action that have been seriously underappreciated until quite recently. The economic and social impact of lost productivity, especially—but not exclusively—in low- and middle-income countries would seem to compel action, the cost of continued inaction being unacceptable from the perspective of public health accountability. On the basis of cost-effectiveness analysis, substantial progress could be made by implementing presently affordable preventive measures.

- Modeling contributes importantly to explanation, description, and prediction of past, present, and future occurrence of CVD and other chronic diseases. Extending beyond the sometimes quite limited observations available, modeling offers insights that can influence decision making about health policy in positive ways. For example, reduction of population-wide risk factors has contributed to approximately half of the gain in CHD mortality in high-income countries in recent decades. This strategy is projected to make continuing major contributions in low- and middle-income countries in the future. Wider interest in modeling can also stimulate strengthening of data sources for future analyses.

- The visions expressed in several published statements from responsible organizations represent judgments that go beyond systematic review of evidence on a specific intervention. They reflect not only a sense of what such evidence says, but what it means in terms of societal interests and values. That such belief in the potential for CVD prevention is expressed strongly by many authoritative sources contributes significantly to the case for prevention.

- That counterarguments that continue to be raised regarding the case for CVD prevention should not be surprising, given competing interests, priorities, or interpretations of the evidence. Weighed against the elements of the argument in favor of CVD prevention, however, they are not persuasive to many in positions of accountability for the public's health.

New Directions

Past efforts are not without their successes but have been far from sufficient to meet the global challenge. In contrast, current directions and future possibilities are worthy of consideration. Salient themes in this review include the increased prominence of NCDs, including cardiovascular disease, in the global health arena; the fundamental importance of primordial as well as remedial strategies of prevention; and a shift toward positive concepts of cardiovascular health, beginning with recognition of the progression from cardiovascular health to risk to disease—both in the individual life course and in population health.

Briefly, these themes might be considered to suggest the following implications for policy, practice, and research:

- Policy: Balance is needed between investments in immediate- and long-term impacts. To concentrate only on remedial strategies is to consign future generations to a life course like those occurring today, with no improvement in prognosis. Without primordial prevention, the chronic disease burdens of nations will only grow, as the forces cited by WHO continue unabated.
- Practice: The major determinants of cardiovascular health, risk, and disease—and their

underlying influences—are amenable to modification and control to different degrees. It is imaginable that practical measures designed to improve patterns of diet and physical activity can be effective within definable populations, even while the deeper underlying forces continue to operate. Demonstration of successes in selected target populations may serve to mobilize greater political will and investment in a new phase of increasing momentum behind health promotion.

- Research: Evaluation of policies and practices in the sphere of cardiovascular health promotion and NCD prevention should include specific metrics such as those adopted for cardiovascular health, possibly expanded to encompass relevant measures for other NCDs, and broader indicators of positive population health assets. Fuller appreciation of the impact of interventions could result, again mobilizing new interest and investment.

If the Global Alliance for Chronic Diseases were to take up the recommendation of the 2010 Institute of Medicine report on cardiovascular health promotion, a model national policy framework and action plan within each global region could result (Global Alliance for Chronic Disease, 2011; Institute of Medicine 2010). A plan based on the foregoing suggestions could become a catalyst for each region and offer considerable promise of much-needed progress.

References

Boehm, J. K., & Kubzansky, L. D. (2012). The heart's content: The association between positive psychological well-being and cardiovascular health. *Psychol Bull.* doi:10.1037/a0027448.

Committee on Assuring the Health of the Public in the 21st Century. (2003). *The future of the public's health in the 21st century. Board on Health Promotion and Disease Prevention, Institute of Medicine.* Washington: The National Academies Press.

Gaziano, T. A., Reddy, K. S., Paccaud, F., Horton, S., & Chaturvedi, V. (2006). Cardiovascular disease. In D. T. Jamison, J. G. Breman, A. R. Measham, G. Alleyne, M. Claeson, D. B. Evans, et al. (Eds.), *Disease control priorities in developing countries* (2nd ed., pp. 645–662). Washington, DC: International Bank for Reconstruction and Development/World Bank.

Global Alliance for Chronic Disease. (2011) Fact sheet on global alliance for chronic diseases. Retrieved October 22, 2011 from www.ga-cd.org/who.php.

Grabowsky, T. A., Farquhar, J. W., Sunnarborg, K. R., & Bales, V. S. (1997). *Worldwide efforts to improve heart health: A follow-up to the catalonia declaration: Selected program descriptions*. Atlanta, GA: US Department of Health and Human Services, Centers for Disease Control and Prevention, National Center for Chronic Disease Prevention and Health Promotion.

Healthy people 2020: Improving the health of Americans. (2010). Retrieved March 20, 2011 from http://healthy-people.gov/2020/about/topicsobjectives2020.

Institute of Medicine. (2010). *Promoting cardiovascular health in the developing world: A critical challenge to achieve global health*. Washington, DC: National Academies Press.

International Heart Health Society. (2005) International action on cardiovascular disease: A platform for success based on International Cardiovascular Disease Declarations. Retrieved January 21, 2008 from www.internationalhearthealth.org.

Labarthe, D. R. (2011). *Epidemiology and prevention of cardiovascular diseases: A global challenge*. Sudbury, MA: Jones & Bartlett.

Labarthe, D. R. (2012). From cardiovascular disease to cardiovascular health: A quiet revolution? *Circulation. Cardiovascular Quality and Outcomes, 5*, e86–e92.

Labarthe, D. R., & Dunbar, S. B. (2012). Global cardiovascular health promotion and disease prevention: 2011 and beyond. *Circulation, 125*, 2667–2676.

Lloyd-Jones, D. M., Hong, Y., Labarthe, D., Mozaffarian, D., Appel, L. J., Van Horn, L., et al. (2010). Defining and setting national goals for cardiovascular health promotion and disease reduction: the American Heart Association's strategic impact goal through 2020 and beyond. *Circulation, 121*, 586–613.

Pearson, T. A., Jamison, D. T., & Trejo-Gutierrez, J. (1993). Cardiovascular disease. In D. T. Jamison, W. H. Mosley, A. R. Measham, & J. L. Bobadilla (Eds.), *Disease control priorities in developing countries* (pp. 577–594). Oxford, UK: Oxford University Press.

Rose, G. (1981). Strategy of prevention: lessons from cardiovascular disease. *British Medical Journal, 282*, 1847–1851.

Strasser, T. (1978). Reflections on cardiovascular diseases. *Interdisciplinary Science Reviews, 3*, 225–230.

United Nations General Assembly. (2000) Resolution adopted by the General Assembly: United Nations Millennium Declaration. New York, NY: United Nations; 18 September, 2000. A/RES/55/2.

United Nations General Assembly. (2011) Political declaration of the high-level meeting of the General Assembly on the Prevention and Control of Non-Communicable Diseases. New York, NY: United Nations; 16 September 2011. A/66/L.1.

US Department of Health and Human Services. (2000). *Healthy people 2010: With understanding and improving health and objectives for improving health* (2nd ed.). Washington, DC: US Government Printing Office.

US Department of Health and Human Services. (2003) A public health action plan to prevent heart disease and stroke. Atlanta, GA: US Department of Health and Human Services, Centers for Disease Control and Prevention.

Vartiainen, E., Puska, P., Jousilahti, P., Korhonen, H. J., Tuomilehto, J., & Nissinen, A. (1994). Twenty-year trends in coronary risk factors in North Karelia and in other areas of Finland. *International Journal of Epidemiology, 23*, 495–504.

White, P. D., Wright, I. S., Sprague, H. B., Katz, L. N., Stamler, J., Levine, S. L., et al. (1959). *A statement on Arteriosclerosis: Main cause of "heart attacks" and "strokes"*. New York, NY: National Health Education Committee Inc.

World Health Organization. (2006) Commission on social determinants of health. Geneva (Switzerland): World Health Organization. WHO/EPI/EQH/01/2006.

World Health Organization. (2011) Global status report on noncommunicable diseases 2010: Description of the global burden of NCDs, their risk factors and determinants. Geneva, Switzerland: World Health Organization; April 2011.

World Health Organization Expert Committee. (1982) Prevention of coronary heart disease (Technical Report Series 679). Geneva, Switzerland: World Health Organization.

Advocacy Strategies to Address NCDs: Actions to Increase the Profile of Physical Activity

18

Trevor Shilton, Adrian Bauman, and Fiona Bull

The Scientific Case for Greater Advocacy on Physical Activity

The World Health Organization identified physical activity in 2009 as the fourth leading contributor to risk of death from NCDs (World Health Organization, 2009). A more recent meta-analysis estimated that physical activity accounts for over five million deaths annually, very similar to the population health threat posed by tobacco smoking (Lee et al., 2012). The health evidence for the protective and health promoting effects of physical activity in adults and children, and across the age span, is compelling. Physical activity protects against death and disability from the major non-communicable diseases (NCDs),

T. Shilton (✉)
Cardiovascular Health Programs,
National Heart Foundation, Western Australia
Division, 334 Rokeby Road, Subiaco, Australia
e-mail: Trevor.Shilton@heartfoundation.org.au

A. Bauman
Prevention Research Collaboration,
School of Public Health, Sydney University,
Level 2 Medical Foundation Building k25, Sydney,
NSW 2006, Australia
e-mail: adrian.bauman@sydney.edu.au

F. Bull
Centre for Built Environment and Health,
The University of Western Australia,
M707, 35 Stirling Highway, Perth, WA, Australia
e-mail: fiona.bull@uwa.edu.au

as well as a range of other conditions, especially among older adults (Lee et al., 2012; Haskell et al., 2007). In relation to mental health physical activity is effective in preventing and treating depression and anxiety (Warburton et al., 2006).

In the context of an ageing community, physical activity has benefits in delaying dementia and improving cognitive function in the elderly (Colcombe & Kramer, 2003; Heyn et al., 2004; Physical Activity Guidelines Advisory Committee, 2008). Physical activity also prevents falls and promotes independent living in seniors (Sherrington et al., 2008). For children physical activity promotes healthy growth and development, fitness and healthy weight as well as providing benefits for cognitive development and academic performance (Roberts et al., 2009; Singh et al., 2012).

The extensive evidence on the health benefits of physical activity has led to many national Governments developing their own position statements and national guidelines on the recommended levels of physical activity. It is notable that these are mostly seen in developed countries where there has been more recognition of physical activity over recent years. In 2010 the World Health Organization launched their official evidence based recommendations for physical activity in adults and children (World Health Organization, 2010). These global guidelines are an important reference for many low and middle income (LMIC) countries that can now refer to these as an agreed consensus on the scientific evidence.

D.V. McQueen (ed.), *Global Handbook on Noncommunicable Diseases and Health Promotion*,
DOI 10.1007/978-1-4614-7594-1_18, © Springer Science+Business Media, LLC 2013

Table 18.1 Outline of physical activity advocacy milestones

Date	Physical activity milestones
1996	US Surgeon General's report "Physical Activity and Health"
1997	1st meeting of the International Physical Activity Questionnaire (IPAQ) ; hosted by WHO, leading to testing of IPAQ 2002–2003, and subsequent IPAQ dissemination for surveillance
2000–2010	Formation of Regional Physical Activity Networks
2002	CDC Community Guide published
2004	Launch of Global Strategy on Diet, Physical Activity And Health by WHO (World Health Assembly)
2004–2012	AGITA MUNDO established following the successful launch of the Global Strategy and providing a global network of researchers, practitioners, and policy makers from around the world; World Health Day on Physical Activity commenced as a day for celebration and advocacy for action on physical activity
2004	Establishment of the Journal of Physical Activity and Health
1999–2012	National and international physical activity training courses undertaken in the USA, Australia, and later in Latin America and elsewhere to build capacity in the workforce
2006	1st International Congress on Physical Activity and Public Health (ICPAPH) held in Atlanta, GA; celebration of the 10 year anniversary of the USSG report, and subsequent (2009) formation of ISPAH, an International Society for Physical Activity and Health
2007	Launch of GAPA as the Global Advocacy for Physical Activity as an advocacy group; comprised leading researchers and public health officials
2008	2nd International Congress on Physical Activity and Public Health (ICPAPH), Amsterdam, The Netherlands
2009	International Society for Physical Activity and Health (ISPAH) established
2010	3rd International Congress on Physical Activity and Public Health (ICPAPH), Toronto, Canada; Launch of the *Toronto Charter for Physical Activity: A Global Call for Action*
2010	Release of Burden of Disease Report by WHO identifying physical inactivity as the fourth leading risk factor for the prevention of NCDs
2010	Launch of the WHO's first official set of Guidelines on Physical Activity and Health
2010	Global launch of Exercise Is Medicine—an initiative led by the American College of Sports Medicine
2011	Release of *Noncommunicable Disease Prevention: Investments that Work for Physical Activity* by GAPA as part of advocacy activities linked to the UN High Level meeting on NCD Prevention 2011
2011	United Nations High level meeting on Noncommunicable Diseases; the political declaration fully recognized physical inactivity as one of four common risk factor and central to efforts aimed at the prevention of NCD
2012	GAPA, in collaboration with the regional physical activity networks and AGITA MUNDO, releases two key position statements on the need for a global target and indicator on physical inactivity as part of the Global NCD framework underdevelopment by WHO
2012	WHO General Assembly endorses the proposed set of five global targets and indicators which includes: global target to reduce NCDs by 25 % by 2025 and the target to reduce physical inactivity by 10 % by 2025

Table 18.1 outlines a recent history of physical activity advocacy milestones, starting with key documents and evidence syntheses, and subsequently identifying developments in surveillance tools, guidelines, networks, and the advocacy-specific activities

It is evident that the evidence on health benefits of physical activity is strong enough to warrant forthright Government action. Yet, despite progress outlined in Table 18.1, the overall response from Governments throughout the world has been limited, both in the absence of sustained investment and the scale of actions implemented.

This has led to physical inactivity being described as the "*Cinderella of NCD risk factors*" which they defined as "poverty of policy attention and resourcing proportionate to its importance" (Bull & Bauman, 2011). The lack of prioritization and policy response to addressing physical inactivity is even more surprising given that the potential benefits extend beyond the health sector and can potentially positively address other social and environmental issues such as global warming, traffic congestion, and social cohesion. To address the lack of priority given to physical activity, it is clear that increased advocacy is required.

Advocacy Needs of Physical Activity

Simply put, advocacy is a process for bringing about change. Most definitions describe an organized approach to promoting an issue and processes for mobilizing others to take action on the issue. The World Health Organization defines advocacy for health as a "combination of individual and social actions designed to gain political commitment, policy support, social acceptance and system support for a particular health goal or program" (WHO, 1995). Of importance in this definition is its orientation around systems and policy change. A supportive policy framework and regulatory environment is an essential building block for action aimed at increasing population levels of physical activity. Advocacy has at its heart the desire to change policies and systems to enable sustained change. Physical activity advocacy needs to focus on "upstream" actions aimed at achieving political commitment and advancing policies and system changes to advance physical activity. Its primary focus is not individual behavior change (Shilton, 2008).

Advocacy actions can be aimed directly at political leaders to bring about policy change or they may be indirectly applied to mobilize support for change through other stakeholders such as the media and professionals (Shilton, 2006). Table 18.2 describes five avenues for advocacy action and provides examples of methods that may be applied to advance advocacy in each area. These five areas of advocacy action are not discreet. Policy influence is often achieved through a combination of means such as encouraging coalitions of professionals, mobilizing citizen action, empowering those who lack a voice, or achieving coverage in the press.

Systematic Approaches to Physical Activity Advocacy: The Case of GAPA (Global Advocacy for Physical Activity)

Shilton (2008) described a systematic approach to creating and making the case for increased focus on physical activity. Drawing on experience from effective advocacy in other areas of public health Shilton outlines advocacy imperatives. These are illustrated in Fig. 18.1. These include making the case for physical activity as an urgent prevention priority, identifying the policy-relevance of action, mobilizing an advocacy strategy, partnerships with stakeholders, and having an overarching communications strategy to increase the profile of physical activity (Shilton, 2008).

The persistent imbalance between high levels of evidence and relatively low levels of policy commitment to physical activity has given rise to a better-mobilized advocacy movement for physical activity across the world. Global Advocacy for Physical Activity (GAPA) was incorporated as the Advocacy Council of the International Society for Physical Activity and Health (ISPAH) in 2010. Since this time GAPA has played a leading role in mobilizing evidence, policy

Table 18.2 Five avenues for advocacy action

	Avenues for advocacy				
	Political advocacy	Media advocacy	Professional mobilization	Community mobilization	Advocacy from within an organization
Example methods	o Influencing policy makers o Submissions o Ministerial visits o Representations	o Public relations o Media events o Press releases and conferences o Proactive and reactive media o Paid media	o Information mobilization o Web sites o Newsletters o Journals o Conferences o E-networks o Training	o Public agitation o Mass media o Mass events o Programs o Social networking o Letters to the editor o Letter writing o Rallys o Petitions	o E-news o Email o Intranet o Representation o Expert visitors o Presentations o Lunches and o Morning teas

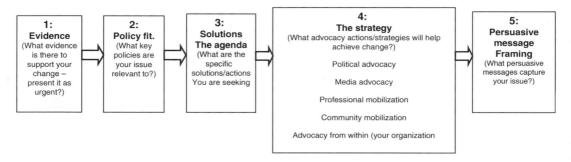

Fig. 18.1 Five imperatives for effective advocacy. Modified from Shilton (2008)

frameworks, and professional information regarding physical activity. Further to this, and reflecting the systematic advocacy framework above, GAPA has mobilized global action around five priorities for physical activity advocacy. GAPA has identified these priorities as their "core advocacy functions" and has formed a systematic program of global physical activity advocacy actions around them. A summary of these areas of action and the GAPA framework for advocacy is shown in Table 18.3.

The International Society for Physical Activity and Health (ISPAH), and its advocacy council Global Advocacy for Physical Activity (GAPA) has played a leading role in developing international consensus documents that aim to mobilize policies, action plans, and interventions for physical activity.

The Toronto Charter for Physical Activity: A Global Call for Action

A specific action of GAPA was the development of a clear position statement on the evidence and need to act directed at national governments. The *Toronto Charter for Physical Activity: A Global Call to Action* represents such a concise statement and was written as a global call for action on physical activity (GAPA, 2010). Developed over 2 years with extensive global consultation in multiple languages the Toronto Charter was launched at the 3rd International Congress on Physical Activity and Public Health (ICPAPH)

held in Toronto in May 2010. The Toronto Charter presents the case for why physical activity is a powerful investment for people, health and the economy and outlines a set of guiding principles for a population level action as well as a four-point framework for action. The framework calls for countries to take action to:

- Implement national policies and action plans;
- Introduce policies that support physical activity;
- Reorient services and funding to prioritize physical activity;
- Develop partnerships for action across all relevant sectors.

To support the use and dissemination across a variety of national and cultural contexts, the Toronto Charter has been translated into 21 languages, the majority of which were undertaken by volunteer advocates in each country following a standardized protocol. These are available at the GAPA Web site www.globalpa.org.uk/charter/translation.php. The GAPA Web site also provides a hub for mobilizing advocacy support, and at May 2013 the Toronto Charter had been endorsed by 939 individuals and 259 organizations from 161 countries on the site.

The Toronto Charter for Physical Activity was couched in the language of health promotion. It acknowledges the need for comprehensive (policy, environment, and system) approaches—ecological approaches to increasing physical activity. The focus of the Toronto Charter on the need for national policies and plans is consistent with the World Health Organization's Ottawa

Table 18.3   Global advocacy for physical activity (GAPA): Five core areas of Advocacy work

1. Disseminate physical activity information and evidence:

   GAPA has developed several important instruments for information mobilization including a Web site (www.globalpa.org.uk), e-newsletter, and members communiqués. In 2012 the flagship *Global Physical Activity Network* (GlobalPANet) was launched. GlobalPAnet aims to build knowledge and capacity in the global physical activity workforce through rapid and frequent dissemination of relevant scientific and policy material (www.globalpanet.com). The Web site fortnightly e-News circulates physical activity information from around the globe

2. Advocate for the development, dissemination, and implementation of national physical activity policies, action plans, and guidelines:

   Supporting the development of national policy is a central focus of the WHO Global NCD Action Plan 2008–2013 and a core element recommended in the 2004 Global Strategy for Diet, PA and Health. GAPA has advocated for national policy through presentations and engagement in consultation with efforts in individual countries (Examples include Thailand, Scotland, Canada, and the USA). In addition, GAPA has led an European based project in collaboration with the European physical activity network (HEPA Europe) to develop a Policy Audit Tool (PAT) and conduct a demonstration project in seven countries in 2009–2012. The experience from this project will support global dissemination of the PAT tool as a tool for assessing current and future policy level actions aimed at physical activity in specific countries. PAT is available at www.euro.who.int/hepapat

3. Advocacy for physical activity—within the NCD agenda and other related agendas at all levels and across all relevant sectors:

   This work aims to identify and communicate clear actions aimed at increasing physical activity. Initiatives in this area included the development of The Toronto charter for physical activity and the seven investments document. Both were developed with international consultation and are available at www.globalpa.org.uk
   The Toronto Charter sets out a four point framework for national actions and the seven investments provides details of the seven settings in which there is a sufficient evidence base for national actions to commence or be scaled up

4. Advocate for capacity building and the development of workforce training initiatives:

   Developing a knowledgeable and skilled workforce is necessary to underpin the development of national action on physical activity and is required at all levels within a country (state, regional, and local levels). Members of GAPA have been involved in contributing to various international training courses on physical activity since 2002 and more recently, GAPA has initiated training courses in advocacy in collaboration with the IUHPE. These courses were run for the first time in 2012

5. Advocate for establishing and strengthening regional networks and global collaboration amongst these:

   GAPA has played a key role in supporting communications between the regional physical activity networks and mobilizing them to form a common voice on issues related to physical activity in the global NCD agenda. During 2011–2012 this concerted advocacy ensured the position of physical activity within the UN High Level Meeting and regional consultation forums and in the period following the UN meeting as part of the discussions and consultation opportunities related to the Global NCD Monitoring Framework. This work is exemplified by the joint position statements released during 2011–2012 (available from www.globalpa.org.uk)

Charter (WHO, 1986) and its focus on the need for partnership and intersectoral action is consistent with subsequent WHO health promotion documents (WHO, 1997, 2011) (Fig. 18.2).

Noncommunicable Disease Prevention: Investments That Work for Physical Activity

A second example of GAPA's advocacy work is the development of another position statement in the lead up the United Nations High Level Meeting on Noncommunicable Disease Prevention and Control in September 2011 (United Nations, 2011a). The document,

Noncommunicable Disease Prevention: Investments that Work for Physical Activity, was written as a complement to the Toronto Charter (GAPA, 2011). The ISPAH Advocacy Council, GAPA was acutely aware that if advocacy to elevate the policy priority for physical activity was to be successful, politicians and policy makers would require evidence and guidance on where to invest. "Investments that Work" was written to provide specific guidance by identifying seven

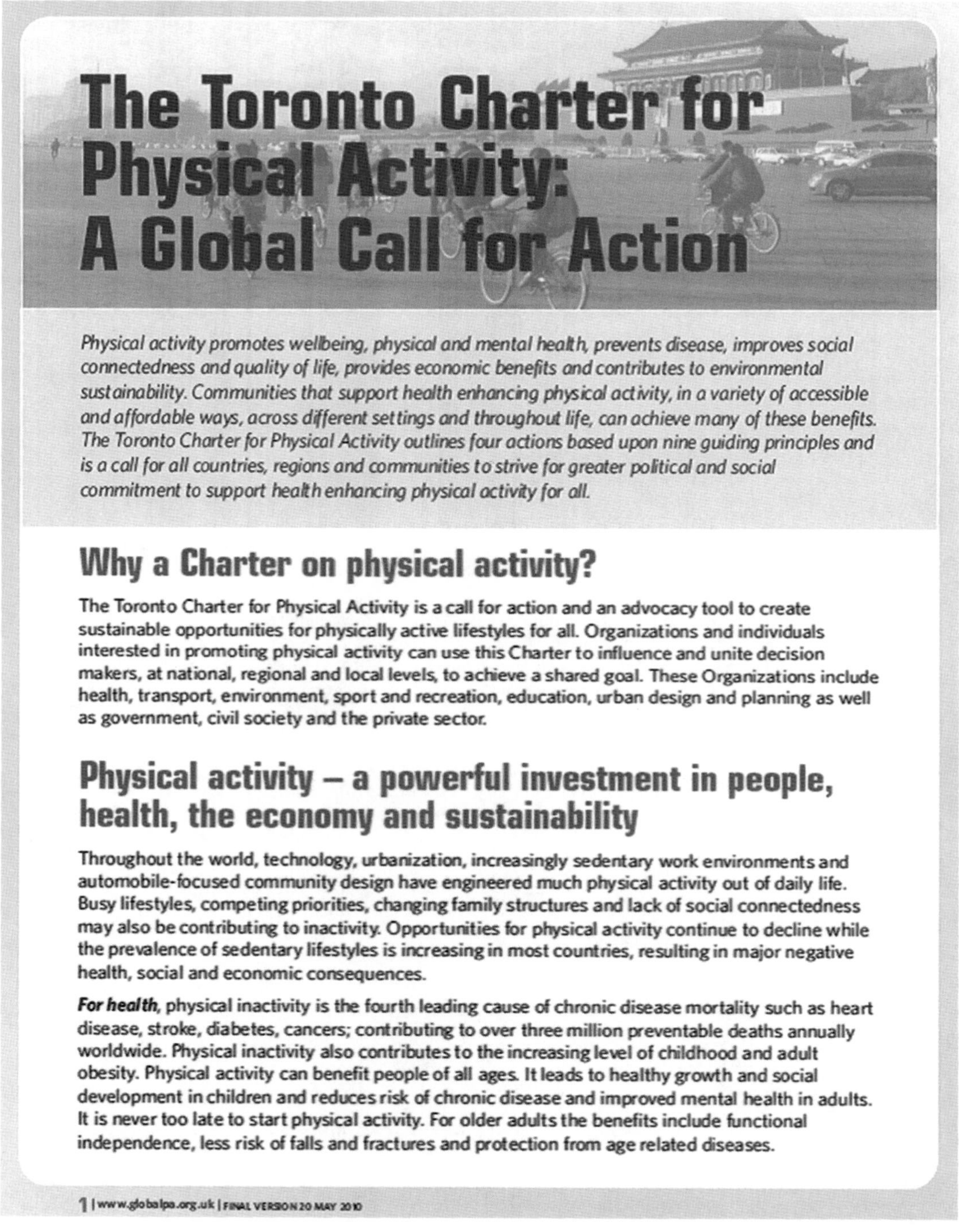

The Toronto Charter for Physical Activity: A Global Call for Action

Physical activity promotes wellbeing, physical and mental health, prevents disease, improves social connectedness and quality of life, provides economic benefits and contributes to environmental sustainability. Communities that support health enhancing physical activity, in a variety of accessible and affordable ways, across different settings and throughout life, can achieve many of these benefits. The Toronto Charter for Physical Activity outlines four actions based upon nine guiding principles and is a call for all countries, regions and communities to strive for greater political and social commitment to support health enhancing physical activity for all.

Why a Charter on physical activity?

The Toronto Charter for Physical Activity is a call for action and an advocacy tool to create sustainable opportunities for physically active lifestyles for all. Organizations and individuals interested in promoting physical activity can use this Charter to influence and unite decision makers, at national, regional and local levels, to achieve a shared goal. These Organizations include health, transport, environment, sport and recreation, education, urban design and planning as well as government, civil society and the private sector.

Physical activity – a powerful investment in people, health, the economy and sustainability

Throughout the world, technology, urbanization, increasingly sedentary work environments and automobile-focused community design have engineered much physical activity out of daily life. Busy lifestyles, competing priorities, changing family structures and lack of social connectedness may also be contributing to inactivity. Opportunities for physical activity continue to decline while the prevalence of sedentary lifestyles is increasing in most countries, resulting in major negative health, social and economic consequences.

For health, physical inactivity is the fourth leading cause of chronic disease mortality such as heart disease, stroke, diabetes, cancers; contributing to over three million preventable deaths annually worldwide. Physical inactivity also contributes to the increasing level of childhood and adult obesity. Physical activity can benefit people of all ages. It leads to healthy growth and social development in children and reduces risk of chronic disease and improved mental health in adults. It is never too late to start physical activity. For older adults the benefits include functional independence, less risk of falls and fractures and protection from age related diseases.

1 | www.globalpa.org.uk | FINAL VERSION 20 MAY 2010

Fig. 18.2 Toronto charter

areas where sufficient evidence exists to support investment, and which, if applied at sufficient scale would make the largest contribution to increasing physical activity. The seven areas identified are: whole of schools approaches; transport systems; urban design policy; primary

NON COMMUNICABLE DISEASE PREVENTION:

Investments that Work for Physical Activity

A complementary document to
The Toronto Charter for Physical Activity: A Global Call to Action

Physical inactivity is the fourth leading cause of deaths due to non communicable disease (NCDs) worldwide - heart disease, stroke, diabetes and cancers - and each year contributes to over three million preventable deaths.[1] Physical inactivity is related (directly and indirectly) to the other leading risk factors for NCDs such as high blood pressure, high cholesterol and high glucose levels; and, to the recent striking increases in childhood and adult obesity, not only in developed countries but also in many developing countries. Substantial scientific evidence supports the importance of physical inactivity as a risk factor for NCD *independent* of poor diet, smoking and alcohol misuse.

Physical activity has comprehensive health benefits across the lifespan: It promotes healthy growth and development in children and young people, helps to prevent unhealthy mid-life weight gain, and is important for healthy ageing, improving and maintaining quality of life and independence in older adults.

The most recent global estimates indicate that 60% of the world population are exposed to health risks due to inactivity.[2] Increasing population-wide participation in physical activity is a major health priority in most high and middle income countries and is a rapidly-emerging priority in lower income countries experiencing rapid social and economic transitions.

The **Toronto Charter for Physical Activity** (May 2010) outlines the direct health benefits and co benefits of investing in policies and programs to increase levels of physical activity.[3] Already translated into 11 languages, the Toronto Charter makes a strong case for increased action and greater investment on physical activity as part of a comprehensive approach to NCD prevention. The Charter was developed with extensive world-wide stakeholder consultation and calls for action in four key areas consistent with the WHO Global Strategy for Diet and Physical Activity: 1) national policy; 2) policies and regulations; 3) programs and environments; and 4) partnerships.

There is strong evidence to guide the implementation of effective approaches to increase physical activity.[4,5,6] Reversing downward trends in physical activity will require countries to commit to a combination of strategies aimed at the individual, social-cultural, environmental and policy determinants of inactivity. Physical activity is influenced by policies and practices in education, transportation, parks and recreation, media, and business, so multiple sectors of society need to be involved in the solutions. There is the clear need to inform, motivate and support individuals and communities to be active in ways that are safe, accessible and enjoyable. ***There is no one single solution to increasing physical activity, an effective comprehensive approach will require multiple concurrent strategies to be implemented.*** To support countries ready to respond, there are seven "best investments" for physical activity, which are supported by good evidence of effectiveness and that will have worldwide applicability.

Whole-of-community approaches where people live, work and recreate have the opportunity to mobilize large numbers of people.

1 | www.globalpa.org.uk | FEBRUARY 2011

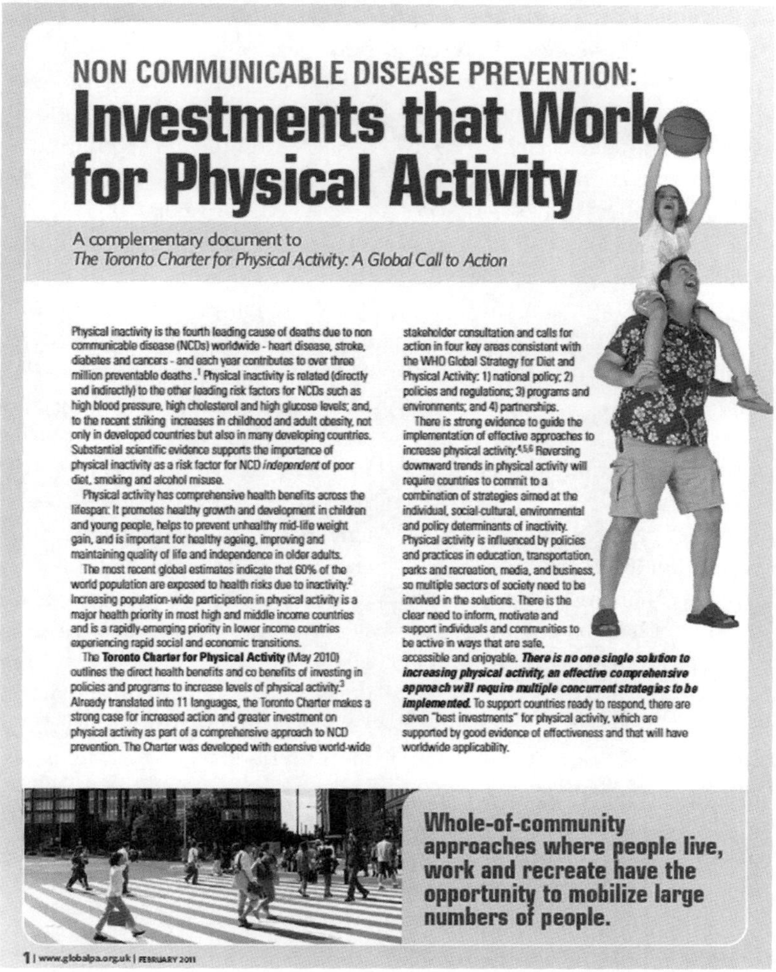

Fig. 18.3 Investments

health care; public education strategies; sports for all, and comprehensive community-wide programs. The latter area reflected the ideal approach is a combination of all elements in a coordinated way adapted to the contexts of specific countries and communities (Fig. 18.3 and Table 18.4).

Through the work of GAPA, the "physical activity movement" has endeavored to "fast track" political acceptance of the importance of physical inactivity through well-directed advocacy actions. The Toronto Charter and supporting documents communicate clearly and simply the body of science and present a powerful rationale for why physical activity should be prioritized among the solutions to the global NCD crisis.

Table 18.4 7 Investments that work for physical activity

1. *Whole-of-school* programs
2. *Transport policies* and systems that prioritise walking, cycling and public transport
3. *Urban design* regulations and infrastructure that provides for equitable and safe access for recreational physical activity, and recreational and transport-related walking and cycling across the life course
4. Physical activity and NCD prevention integrated into *primary health care* systems
5. *Public education*, including mass media to raise awareness and change social norms on physical activity
6. *Community-wide programs* involving multiple settings and sectors & that mobilize and integrate community engagement and resources
7. Sports systems and programs that promote "*sport for all*" and encourage participation across the life span

GAPA has called on nations to "act now on physical activity for better health, wellbeing and prevention of NCDs". To disseminate this message at key political meetings and specifically regional and global consultations conducted by WHO as part of the United Nations High Level Meeting, GAPA produced its smallest advocacy tool, namely, a "postcard" sized resource that summarizes the key strengths and progress that the physical activity movement can now claim. These key points include the following:

1. There is enough evidence on the benefits of physical activity to act now.
2. There are global physical activity Guidelines based on international scientific evidence and consensus.
3. Physical activity can be measured and monitored at the population level.
4. Physical inactivity is an increasing problem in high, low, and middle-income countries, particularly in countries experiencing rapid urbanization.
5. There are solutions—across different settings and these require cross-sector partnerships.

(Extracted from the GAPA advocacy postcard available at www.globalpa.org.uk).

One particular observation in recent years has been the continuing and central role of data from population surveillance and monitoring systems on physical activity. This has never been more evident than in the advocacy work surrounding the development of the Global NCD Monitoring Framework and the selection of a set of global indicators and targets. WHO was charged with developing a framework to monitor progress on the implementation of prevention activities in 2012–2013. Physical activity advocates were acutely aware that securing a global target on physical activity would be a key requirement for future policy success and would underpin country level response to the UN Political Declaration. Notably, the Secretary General of WHO Dr Margaret Chan stated "what gets measured gets done" (United Nations, 2011b). It was very clear that those issues which had agreed indicators and target within the Global Monitoring Framework would be very likely to receive stronger focus by both WHO and Member States in their National NCD actions plans and priorities.

Global and Regional physical activity networks responded to the opportunity presented by the UN High Level Meeting to act as a coordinated and clear voice on physical activity. Led by GAPA, they responded by rapidly mobilizing advocacy and specifically developing two Position Statements on the need for a global indicator and target on physical inactivity. Working together, GAPA, the Physical Activity Network of the Americas (RAFA–PANA), AGITA MUNDO, Health Enhancing Physical Activity (HEPA) European Network, the Asia Pacific Physical Activity Network (APPAN), and the African Physical Activity Network (AFPAN) agreed to a consensus statement that outlined the supporting evidence and case for inclusion of physical inactivity. The two position statements widely distributed to key government and non-government stakeholders to inform and influence the debate in the lead up and during the UN High Level Meeting. The position statements addressed the criteria set out for inclusion by the WHO and presented a solid argument and supporting evidence that:

- There is strong epidemiological evidence for physical inactivity as a leading contributor to death and disease burden.
- Physical activity is established as a core element of NCD prevention and coherent with major strategies.
- There is evidence of effective and feasible physical activity public health interventions, particularly in low resource contexts.
- The selected target is measureable, data collection instruments are available and already in use providing baseline data and the target is achievable allowing necessary time for progress.

Challenges for Physical Activity Advocacy

There is a clear and powerful need for all countries to increase the level and scale of their actions to reduce the levels of physical inactivity across all ages and there is emerging consensus regarding effective and efficient interventions where investments will make the biggest difference. The policy and advocacy initiatives outlined in this chapter represent good progress. However, further advocacy challenges remain and these are discussed briefly below.

In a rapidly changing world there are numerous socio-demographic changes that have profoundly impacted nations, cities and their inhabitants. Changes such as urbanization, mechanization, and greater reliance on the motorcar have resulted in declines in physical activity and increases in sedentary behavior. All countries have felt the impacts, while some changes have disproportionately impacted low and middle-income countries (LMIC).

There is a need for better identification and communication of interventions that are effective in increasing population levels of physical activity in LMIC. In high-income countries a challenge is to identify those interventions that best reach the lowest income groups. In addition, these interventions need to demonstrate that they can be scaled up from local to national level, and are applicable in other nations. In LMIC rapid urbanization has resulted in populations being displaced from the land. This often leads to poorer access to a healthy food supply and reliance on motorized transportation. Increasing dominance of the motorcar has resulted in declines in walking and cycling for transport. In addition vast tracts of urban space are being devoted to roads, often severing local communities from services and leading to increased road crashes and exposure to atmospheric pollutants. Rapid urbanization is often accompanied by chaotic urban planning, where citizens may be remotely located from employment, education, recreation, and public open space.

More studies are needed to illustrate the cost-effectiveness of physical activity interventions and demonstrate that these can be implemented at a cost that is low relative to public health benefit and savings in health-care costs.

There is a need to identify effective interventions that increase physical activity among older adults. In an ageing community keeping seniors active and healthy is vital for public health.

Physical activity is beneficial in the prevention of chronic diseases and also in bone health, injury and falls prevention, mental health, the maintenance of cognitive function and prevention of cognitive decline (Physical Activity Guidelines Advisory Committee, 2008).

In high-income countries a challenge is to identify those interventions that best reach the lowest income groups. In addition, these interventions need to demonstrate that they can be scaled up form local to national level, and are applicable in other nations.

The rise and diversification of electronic media has resulted in an increase in sitting for recreation, and a consequent decrease in energy expenditure. Television, computers, the Internet, DVDs, and games now are the most pervasive recreation for most children and a majority of adults in many societies—giving rise to increased risk of NCDs, obesity, and psychosocial problems. This is coupled with the increase of labor saving devices and technology in the workplace, resulting in work environments becoming dominated by the "sit-down job," with many previously manual tasks being replaced by computers or machines.

Rapid urbanization, chaotic urban planning, increasing motorized transportation, the rise and diversification of electronic media, and the crowded curriculum in our schools have resulted in declines in energy expenditure and have put pressure on available time for physical activity. These changes have adversely affected population physical activity and present advocacy opportunities—adding further weight to the arguments for policy intervention and cross-community approaches to physical activity. They bring into play a breadth of new stakeholders and potential partners, as well as synergies for physical activity with prominent community issues such as clean air, traffic congestion, community safety, and social capital. These issues add complexity to the physical activity movement, but they also offer opportunities for fruitful partnership, and joined up approaches that deliver co-benefits across causes.

A supportive policy framework and regulatory environment is an essential building block for public health action aimed at increasing population

Table 18.5 Text box [or panel]: Lessons to be learned from tobacco control advocacy for physical activity

Tobacco control is an outstanding example where over a period of 40 years or more there has been significant legislative reform and political action designed to protect citizens from harm or restrict the tobacco industry's ability to promote its deadly product. Many of these public health gains are attributable to tobacco-focused advocacy, targeting the general population, decision makers and professionals, through a series of mass media campaigns, informal advocacy, and targeted community mobilization

The results were important public health progress in tobacco control. This includes the first WHO-led global health treaty, the Framework Convention on Tobacco Control (FCTC). The international tobacco control movement has a well-developed and articulated consensus around effective strategies for tobacco control. These include increasing price, increasing taxation, smoke free policy, advertising bans, point of sale restrictions, health warnings, and cessation support

Yach et al. in 2005 described lessons that physical activity and nutrition advocates could take from the success in controlling tobacco. These included:

  Building a workforce of dedicated, persistent, media-savvy, and politically astute leaders and agitators

  Developing broad-based, well-networked coalitions for concerted advocacy

  Building global consensus around a comprehensive intervention package—agreed 10 point plan

  Addressing the issue of individual versus environmental action early, often and well [and recognizing the importance of both in tobacco control]

  Acknowledging that evidence of harm is necessary but not sufficient for policy change

  Ensuring that interventions known to be effective are fully implemented and reach all population segments

  Recognizing the importance of persistence, and that change can take decades of effort!

Adapted from Yach et al. (2005)

levels of physical activity. Advocacy has at its heart the desire to change policies and systems to enable sustained change. Successful policy led actions have been seen in other areas of public health, notable in tobacco control as illustrated in Table 18.5.

Certainly, relative to a decade ago physical activity can claim, on the basis of these criteria, to be a "rapidly emerging" discipline. As a sign of physical activity beginning to rise to policy prominence the United Nations, in its Political Declaration from the September 2011 High Level Meeting on Noncommunicable Disease Prevention and Control, refers to physical activity as one of the four "common" risk factors, along with unhealthy diet, tobacco use, and harmful use of alcohol (United Nations, 2011a).

Conclusion

Physical inactivity is a major contributor to death and disability. It is the fourth leading contributor to the burden of disease from NCDs. The health evidence for the protective benefits and health promoting effects of physical activity in adults and children is compelling. There is no doubt that, relative to the public health impact of physical

activity, physical activity suffers a lack of political support, funding, and policy priority. This is why a concerted global approach to physical activity advocacy has emerged, as outlined in this chapter. As long as the imbalance between physical activity evidence and policy action persists, a strong focus on advocacy is warranted. The lack of priority afforded to physical activity is even more surprising given its demonstrable contribution to ameliorating more "pervasive" social and environmental problems such as global warming, traffic congestion, and declining social cohesion. Supportive public policy combined with effective interventions and programs have a unique opportunity to increase public health and provide impressive co-benefits across a range of other social and environmental agendas. Successful demonstration of these wider co-benefits is required to add much-needed impetus to national and global physical activity actions.

References

Bull, F. C., & Bauman, A. E. (2011). Physical inactivity – The 'Cinderella' risk factor for NCD prevention. *Journal of Health Communication, 16*(sup 2), 13–26.

Colcombe, S., & Kramer, A. F. (2003). Fitness effects on the cognitive function of older adults: A meta-analytic study. *Psychology Science, 14*, 125–30.

Global Advocacy for Physical Activity: Advocacy Council of International Society for Physical Activity and Health. (2010). *The Toronto charter for physical activity: A global call to action.* Toronto, Canada: International Society for Physical Activity and Health.

Global Advocacy for Physical Activity: Advocacy Council of International Society for Physical Activity and Health. (2011). *Non communicable disease prevention: Seven investments that work.* Toronto, Canada: International Society for Physical Activity and Health.

Haskell, W., Lee, I., Pate, R., Powell, K., Blair, S., Franklin, B., et al. (2007). Physical activity and public health: Updated recommendation for adults from the American College of Sports Medicine and the American Heart Association. *Circulation, 116,* 1081–1093.

Heyn, P. H., Abreu, B. C., & Ottenbacher, K. J. (2004). The effects of exercise training on elderly persons with cognitive impairment and dementia: a meta-analysis. *Archives of Physical Medicine and Rehabilitation, 85,* 1694–1704.

Lee, I.-M., Shiroma, E. J., Lobelo, F., Puska, P., Blair, S. N., Katzmarzyk, P. T., et al. (2012). Effect of physical inactivity on major non-communicable diseases worldwide: an analysis of burden of disease and life expectancy. *Lancet, 380*(9838), 219–229. doi:DOI: 10.1016/S0140-6736(12)61031-9.

Physical Activity Guidelines Advisory Committee. (2008). Physical Activity Guidelines Advisory Committee report, 2008. Washington, D.C.

Roberts, C. K., Freed, B., & McCarthy, W. J. (2009). Low aerobic fitness and obesity are associated with lower standardized test scores in children. *The Journal of Pediatrics, 156*(5), 711–718.

Sherrington, C., Whitney, J. C., Lord, S. R., Herbert, R. D., Cumming, R. G., & Close, J. C. T. (2008). Effective exercise for the prevention of falls: A systematic review and meta analysis. *Journal of the American Geriatrics Society, 56*(12), 2234–2243.

Shilton, T. R. (2006). Advocacy for physical activity – from evidence to influence. *Promotion and Education, 13*(2), 119–126.

Shilton, T. R. (2008). Creating and making the case: Global advocacy for physical activity. *5*(5), 765–776.

Singh, A., Uijtdewilligen, L., Twisk, J., van Mechelen, W., & Chinapaw, M. (2012). Physical activity and performance at school: A systematic review of the literature including a methodological quality assessment. *Archives of Pediatric and Adolescent Medicine, 166*(1), 49–55.

United Nations. (2011a). *Political declaration of the high-level meeting on the prevention and control of non-communicable diseases.* New York: United Nations.

United Nations (2011b). Department of public information, news and media division. Sixty-sixth general assembly plenary 3rd, 4th & 5th meetings (AM, PM & night). Press statement 19th September 2011. Retrieved 22 April, 2013, from http://www.un.org/News/Press/docs//2011/ga11138.doc.htm.

Warburton, D. E., Nicol, C. W., & Bredin, S. S. (2006). Health benefits of physical activity: The evidence. *Canadian Medical Association Journal, 174,* 801–809.

World Health Organization. (1986). *Ottawa Charter for Health Promotion.* Geneva: World Health Organization.

World Health Organization (1995). *Report of the Inter-Agency Meeting on Advocacy Strategies for Health and Development: Development Communication in Action.* Geneva, Switzerland: World Health Organization.

World Health Organization. (1997). *The Jakarta Declaration on Health Promotion in the 21st Century.* Geneva: World Health Organization.

World Health Organization. (2010). *Global guidelines on physical activity for health.* Geneva: World Health Organization.

World Health Organization. (2009). *Global health risks: mortality and burden of disease attributable to selected major risks.* Geneva: World Health Organization.

World Health Organization. (2011). *Global status report on non communicable disease 2010.* Geneva: World Health Organization.

Yach, D., McKee, M., Lopez, A. D., & Novotny, T. (2005). Improving diet and physical activity: 12 lessons from controlling tobacco smoking. *British Medical Journal, 330,* 898–900.

Advocacy Strategies to Address NCDs: Tobacco Control

Michael Sparks

Good health is a major resource for social, economic and personal development and an important dimension of quality of life. Political, economic, social, cultural, environmental, behavioral and biological factors can all favor health or be harmful to it. Health promotion action aims at making these conditions favorable through advocacy for health.

Ottawa Charter (WHO 1986).

Overview

This chapter discusses the role that health promotion advocacy has taken in addressing non-communicable diseases (NCDs) through efforts to support tobacco control. The link between tobacco control and NCDs will be established. Health promotion advocacy will be explained in the context of the Ottawa Charter and evolving contemporary health promotion practice. This will be followed by a discussion of the contribution of tobacco control advocacy efforts to addressing NCDs on a global level, particularly through advocacy for full implementation of the World Health Organization Framework Convention on Tobacco Control (FCTC). Some brief case studies are presented to illustrate the practice of health promotion advocacy for tobacco control, and the chapter concludes with a discussion of successes and challenges for health promotion advocacy for tobacco control.

M. Sparks (✉)
Faculty of Health, University of Canberra
ACT 2601, Australia
e-mail: msparks@homemail.com.au

Tobacco Control and Non-communicable Diseases

The impact of NCDs on world health has been well established in previous chapters of this volume. It has been noted that NCDs including diabetes, cancer, respiratory diseases and cardiovascular diseases account for about 60 % of all deaths worldwide. Nearly 80 % of NCD-related deaths occur in low- and middle-income countries (WHO 2011; Glantz and Gonzalez 2012). The global burden of NCDs is growing and is projected to increase to 44 million people per year in 2020, up from 36 million in 2008.

In response to the growing burden of NCDs the United Nations held a high-level meeting with more than 30 heads of state in September 2011. That meeting adopted the Political Declaration of the United Nations High Level Meeting of the General Assembly on the Prevention and Control of Non-communicable Diseases, demonstrating ongoing global political will to address NCDs (Glantz and Gonzalez 2012; UN 2011). The Political Declaration recognised "that most prominent NCDs are linked to common risk factors" (UN 2011). The emphasis of the UN Political Declaration is on addressing the four major common risk factors (tobacco use, nutrition, alcohol use and physical activity) in order to make progress on the four most prominent NCDs (cardiovascular disease, cancer, chronic respiratory disease and diabetes) (UN 2011).

Among those common risk factors, tobacco use is the single most preventable cause of world mortality and is accordingly listed first among preventable risk factors for NCDs (WHO 2006, 2011). Tobacco use kills more than tuberculosis, HIV/AIDS and malaria combined—over five million people per year (WHO 2006; Lein and DeLand 2011). Tobacco use has been identified as a risk factor for six of the eight leading causes of death worldwide (WHO 2008a) and it costs the world hundreds of billions of dollars each year through tobacco-related disease health-care costs and reduction in productivity (Mackay et al. 2006). Tobacco use has been causally associated with heart disease, lung disease and cancer (Glantz and Gonzalez 2012). The impact of effective tobacco control measures on NCD has been found to be both profound and relatively quick. Reductions in tobacco use have been found to lead to a rapid decrease in NCDs and health-care costs within 12 months (Lightwood and Glantz 1997; Fichtenberg and Glantz 2000; Glantz and Gonzalez 2012).

The link between tobacco use and NCDs is clear. What is new is the integration of tobacco control efforts under a broader umbrella of global NCD reduction strategies. Intergovernmental organizations, particularly the World Health Organization and the United Nations, have been instrumental in supporting and advancing the push for greater tobacco control. The development of the FCTC within the WHO system acknowledged the great negative impact of tobacco use on global health and proposed a structure for systematically addressing a complex web of supply and demand factors. The inclusion of tobacco control with other common risk factors in the WHO 2008–2013 Action Plan for the Global Strategy for the Prevention and Control of Non-communicable Diseases assisted in getting United Nations attention and action such as the resolutions of the General Assembly on the prevention and control of NCDs in September 2011 (WHO 2008b; UN 2011).

The UN Political Declaration urges continued effort on the WHO FCTC, the WHO 2008–2013 Action Plan for the Global Strategy for the Prevention and Control of Non-communicable Diseases, the Global Strategy on Diet, Physical Activity and Health and the Global Strategy to Reduce the Harmful Use of Alcohol (UN 2011). The Declaration called for whole-of-government and whole-of-society efforts; the reduction of risk factors and the creation of health-promoting environments; the strengthening of national policies and health systems; and increased international cooperation including collaborative partnerships. The Declaration called for increased investment of Member States in research and development and in monitoring and evaluation of these multi-sectoral, multi-stakeholder efforts (UN 2011).

Advocacy and the Ottawa Charter

The principles of contemporary health promotion were set out in the Ottawa Charter in 1986 and have been further developed and refined by subsequent global conferences, and associations of health promotion professionals and health promotion researchers (Sparks 2012). Advocacy is one of the three key actions included in the World Health Organization's Ottawa Charter for Health Promotion (WHO 1986). Advocacy is a central element in an integrated health promotion approach to addressing a range of health and social issues, including tobacco control (WHO 2006).

But what is advocacy? The World Health Organization defines advocacy as "simply the process of influencing people to create change. Its lifeblood is good strategic communications—educating people about a need and mobilising them to meet it" (WHO 2006). Weiss (1999) takes the view that advocacy is a way of setting agendas and that advocacy includes consultations, information and lobbying; surveillance; and policymaking and decision-making. Wallack et al. (1993) write, "advocacy is a catch-all word for the set of skills used to create a shift in public opinion and mobilise the necessary resources and forces to support an issue, policy or constituency". Chapman and Wakefield (2001) argue that advocacy "should be assessed as a strategy or a means and not as an end in itself". They further add that public health advocacy is increasingly underpinned with theory, principles and practice guidelines, but note the majority of public health advocates are not working within a research or a scholarly setting and, therefore, work more on an instinctive framework than a theoretically grounded one (Chapman and Wakefield 2001).

From this sample of definitions there is some commonality that can be synthesised: Advocacy is a process of influencing change that utilises a number of methods to achieve its aims. Advocacy methods utilised to influence change in tobacco control are many and varied and include, but are not limited to:

- Media campaigns (radio, print, television, video)
- E-advocacy using twitter, social media, blogging, email and other electronic means
- Production and dissemination of evidence/persuasive information
- Information exchange/clearinghouse functions
- Surveillance (disease incidence, knowledge, attitudes, behaviour)
- Watchdog functions (litigation, compliance with law/policy, reports of industry activity)
- Modelling best practice (legislation, process)
- Opinion polling
- Generating and participating in debate
- Developing champions
- Community awareness
- Community mobilisation (for any of these activities)
- Non-violent resistance including protests, boycotts, culture-jamming, etc
- Training and capacity building for communities, organizations, governments
- Traditional political lobbying
- Letter writing (politicians, media sites, employers, etc.)
- Partnership development and support of like-minded organizations/alliances
- Coordination functions (national/regional/global)

While this list is long and includes many activities that extend beyond those some think of as traditional advocacy efforts, each type of activity can be seen to support advocacy efforts in tobacco control in an integrated understanding of advocacy. Such an understanding is underpinned by the concept that any activity may be considered a method of advocacy that helps to convey the anti-tobacco message or to assist advocates in advancing tobacco control issues (Wallack et al. 1993; Weiss 1999).

Though all tobacco control advocates will not necessarily participate in all of the aforementioned advocacy activities, any combination of them may be found in the advocacy efforts taking place at government, research, NGO or community levels. The case studies included in this chapter provide some insight into the range of activities undertaken in the name of tobacco control advocacy. Applying multiple strategies to advocate, enable and mediate for tobacco control is consistent with the health promotion principles articulated in the Ottawa Charter (WHO 1986). Using the Ottawa Charter action areas as a framework for holistic thinking about tobacco control advocacy, this breadth of activities is necessary to build healthy public policy, reorient health services, build capacity at the individual and community level and create supportive environments for health (WHO 1986). In a contemporary health promotion approach, a broad range of methods can be seen to support advocacy for tobacco control.

It should be clearly understood that the focus of this chapter is on advocacy for tobacco control. Advocacy for tobacco use is also actively engaged by major tobacco manufacturers through advertising, sponsorship, product placement, giveaways and attempts to influence policymakers. This type of pro-tobacco advocacy has been critically analysed elsewhere and is not further explored here, though it is always a form of counter-advocacy to tobacco control efforts.

Tobacco Control, Advocacy and the Framework Convention on Tobacco Control

Tobacco control has been a public health objective since the connection was made between smoking and lung cancer in the 1950s (Wynder and Graham 1950; Doll and Hill 1950, 1954). In the six decades that the link between smoking and cancer has been known, further causal connections have been established between tobacco use and other forms of cancer, cardiovascular disease and respiratory diseases (Wynder 1988; Stratton et al. 2001).

Advocacy for tobacco control began in earnest in developed countries following the establishment of the epidemiological connection between tobacco use and cancers. In Great Britain in 1962 the Royal College of Physicians released its report *Smoking and Health* which clearly established links between tobacco use, particularly cigarette smoking, and lung cancer (RCP 1962). In addition, the report was innovative in that it also called on government to respond with:

- More education of the public, especially school children, regarding the hazards of smoking
- More effective restrictions on the sale of tobacco to minors
- Restriction of tobacco advertising
- Wider restrictions on smoking in public places
- An increase in taxes on tobacco products
- Informing purchasers of the tar and nicotine content of the products
- Investigating the value of anti-smoking clinics to help people quit (RCP 1962)

The essence of these recommendations can still be seen at the core of contemporary tobacco control advocacy and is reflected and expanded in the articles of the World Health Organization's FCTC (WHO 2005). The release of the report is also important because it marks the first recorded use of media advocacy for tobacco control. The Royal College of Physicians engaged a public relations consultant to coordinate the launch of the report and held their first ever press conference to highlight the importance of the report, its findings and its recommendations (Arnott 2012). In taking this remarkable step forward the Royal College of Physicians may well be regarded as the first in a long line of tobacco control advocates.

Two years later, in early 1964, the Surgeon General of the United States released the first report of the Surgeon General's Advisory Committee on Smoking and Health. This report analysed all of the biomedical literature since Doll's early work and clearly established causal links between tobacco use and cancer. The Surgeon General's report is recognised as the first major action to implement tobacco control in the United States (CDC 2006). The report was seen as critical in gaining the attention of American citizens, private organizations, public agencies and elective officials and encouraging tobacco control advocacy.

Over the next three decades national and provincial governments enacted tobacco control measures with varying degrees of success with warning labels, banning of advertising in broadcast media and reporting and surveillance on tobacco-related diseases and the effectiveness of tobacco control. Resistance to tobacco control in the form of pressure from transnational tobacco companies resulted in less-than-optimum results even in the countries with the most advanced tobacco control measures (CDC 2006; Chapman and Wakefield 2001; Arnott 2012).

Non-government organizations (NGOs) and coalitions arose in many parts of the world to take on, and in many cases lead, the cause of tobacco control advocacy. Action on Smoking and Health (ASH) was created in the UK in 1971 and has become a leading force in tobacco control advocacy with ASH organizations now existing in Wales, Scotland, Australia, New Zealand and the United States (RCP 2012). In 1974 a number of existing health agencies including the Cancer Society, the Heart Foundation and the TB and Respiratory Disease Association formed the Canadian Council on Smoking and Health to take the lead on tobacco control advocacy in that country (Collishaw 2009). Voluntary Organization In The Interest Of Consumer Education (VOICE) was formed in New Delhi in 1993 and quickly become active in tobacco control advocacy when it sued British American Tobacco's Indian subsidiary over its tobacco advertising (Khanna and Misra 2000). At a regional level, the European Union created the European Bureau for Action on Smoking Prevention (BASP) in 1988 and it supported the development of other networks including the European Network on Young People and Tobacco (ENYAPAT) and a European Smoke-Free

Cities Network. The European Network for Smoking Prevention, an NGO network, was established in 1997 (Fleitmann 2000).

Case Study One: If at First You Do Not Succeed: Smoke-Free Mexico City

The first attempt by Mexico City legislators to pass smoke-free legislation was in early 2003 with proposals to restrict smoking in public places and workplaces. Due to pressure from restaurant and bar owner associations, the original proposal was weakened from 50 % of public places being reserved for non-smokers down to 30 %. Counter-advocacy arguments used at the time included questions of constitutionality, economic loss, implementation difficulty and that the proposal was out of step with the "smoking culture" of Mexico City. While the law was passed, regulations were never issued and the 2003 law was never practically enforced.

In early 2007 Mexico City legislators started work to amend the law to make all enclosed public places and workplaces there 100 % smoke free. Informed by evidence of the dangers of second-hand smoke, rising medical costs and tobacco-related disease mortality, the legislators again faced opposition from the hospitality industry as well as from smoker's rights groups. This time, however, there was strong political leadership and technical and financial support from national and international tobacco control NGOs. Mexico City Health Minister Manuel Mondragon led the push, persuading fellow assembly members that 100 % smoke free was easier to enforce than having both smoking and non-smoking areas in public places. This was further supported by evidence from the National Institute of Public Health in Mexico on the effects of second-hand smoke and the benefits of 100 % smoke-free environments. Media advocacy was used to emphasise the advantages of going 100 % smoke free. In early 2008 the Legislative Assembly of Mexico City approved the 100 % smoke-free law with an exemption for hotels to allocate up to 25 % of their rooms for smoking.

Mexico City's efforts to become a smoke-free city are of note in that they were undertaken at a municipal level during a time of much less certain national tobacco control activity. On the same day (26 February 2008) that Mexico City became the first jurisdiction in Mexico to go 100 % smoke free, the Mexican National Congress passed a weak federal tobacco control law that allowed for designated smoking areas. This led to confusion, legal challenges to the city legislation and counter-advocacy from the tobacco industry that stressed a position of harmonious coexistence. Once again, a coalition of tobacco control organizations used media advocacy to increase the awareness of the benefits of 100 % smoke-free environments and compliance increased in Mexico City bars and restaurants. Notably, approval ratings for the legislative approach also increased 16 % following the media campaign. This was considered a great success for tobacco control in Mexico City until 2009 when a new City Health Minister came into office—one who has not enforced the law and does not issue sanctions for non-compliance. This highlights the need for ongoing vigilance in monitoring the implementation and enforcement of legislation or policy change once it has been achieved.

(Adapted from Crosbie et al. 2011)

International advocacy networks also arose in response to the development of the FCTC and created links between previous national and regional structures. These new international advocacy networks also created stronger links between policy researchers and public health researchers and in doing so created a stronger and more credible voice for tobacco control advocacy on a global level (Farquharson 2003). GLOBALink was created in the late 1980s as a network to facilitate communication among tobacco control advocates and researchers worldwide (Mamudu and Glantz 2009). The International Non Governmental Coalition against Tobacco (INGCAT) was formed in 1995 by the International Union against Cancer, the International Union against Tuberculosis and Lung Disease and the World Heart Federation. The Framework Convention Alliance (FCA), a global NGO tobacco control group, was formed in 1998 to advance the development and acceptance of a framework convention (WHO 2009). The journal Tobacco Control was launched by the British Medical Journal in 1992 to provide a dedicated source of academic evidence to support global efforts to control tobacco.

The concept of a global legal instrument for advancing tobacco control arose in 1979 as a result of a report of the WHO Expert Committee on Smoking Control. This report called for the application of Article 19 of the World Health Organization Constitution and suggested that the World Health Assembly consider using its treaty-making powers to control the tobacco epidemic (WHO 1979, 2009). This idea was further explored a decade later in an article on the feasibility of an international legal framework for tobacco and alcohol control written by a Professor of International Law at the University of Vladivostok, V. S. Mihajlov (WHO 2009).

Professor Allyn Taylor wrote an article in 1992 proposing that WHO utilises its neglected constitutional authority to promote the development and implementation of international law to advance global public health (Roemer et al. 2005). In 1994, Professor Ruth Roemer of the University of California at Los Angeles School of Public Health, working with Professor Taylor, proposed the specific idea of a framework convention on tobacco control and campaigned to gain support for it from the World Health Organization and the global tobacco control community (Roemer et al. 2005; WHO 2009). Roemer and Taylor worked together over the next 2 years to develop a background paper with

options for the development of a framework convention.

In 1996 the WHO Executive Board adopted the resolution to develop what would become the FCTC and later that year the World Health Assembly adopted the resolution as well (Roemer et al. 2005). Not much concrete action took place within WHO until Gro Harlem Brundtland was elected Director General of WHO in 1998, announcing that tobacco control was to be one of her two priorities in office. Brundtland made resources available for tobacco control, established the Tobacco Free Initiative and began negotiations for the WHO FCTC (WHO 2009). The new Director General funded a media and social marketing campaign to highlight the need for comprehensive tobacco control and she ensured that resources and personnel were made available for tobacco control in all regions. The leadership shown by Dr. Brundtland was a significant fillip for the FCTC and its subsequent success (WHO 2009).

A working group was set up to develop the FCTC in 1999 and text for the Convention was drafted in 1999 and 2000. Member States negotiated the specific language of the document over the next 3 years. In May 2003 the FCTC was adopted by the World Health Assembly and it was opened for signatures on 16 June 2003. Following formal ratification by 40 Member States, the FCTC came into force 90 days later on 27 February 2005. As of August 2012 there are 176 parties to (Member States who have ratified) the convention (WHO 2009, 2012).

The development of the FCTC, like all good tobacco control advocacy processes, involved multiple stakeholders working together to WHO expert committees, academics, member states, NGOs and passionate individuals. They used evidence, persuasion and charisma to build support for this groundbreaking treaty while resisting internal opposition to the treaty as well as significant pressure from multinational tobacco companies to weaken or derail the FCTC. The already extant tools for effective tobacco control advocacy came together in a new way to deliver the world's first public health treaty, the most successful treaty in the history of the United Nations system (WHO 2009).

Table 19.1 Key provisions of the FCTC (WHO 2005)

Measures relating to the reduction of demand for tobacco
- Price and tax measure
- Non-price measures
- Protection from exposure to tobacco smoke
- Regulation of the contents of tobacco products
- Regulation of tobacco product disclosures
- Packaging and labelling of tobacco products
- Education, communication, training and public awareness
- Tobacco advertising, promotion and sponsorship
- Demand reduction measures concerning tobacco dependence and cessation

Measures relating to the reduction of supply of tobacco
- Illicit trade in tobacco products
- Sales to and by minors
- Provision of support for economically viable alternatives

Protection of the environment
- Protection of the environment and the health of persons

Question related to liability
- Liability

Scientific and technical cooperation and communication of information
- Research, surveillance and exchange of information
- Reporting and exchange of information
- Cooperation in scientific, technical and legal fields and provision of related expertise

The FCTC requires signatories or Parties to the Convention, to take action across a range of tobacco control measures as indicated in Table 19.1.

The range and breadth of coverage of the articles of the FCTC are such that signatories can only succeed in a timely way if they take an integrated approach to national tobacco control. To assist in reaching these complex goals the Tobacco Free Initiative of WHO has produced resources on a range of measures that can be taken in all countries under the banner of "MPOWER". The six components of the MPOWER program are as follows:

*M*onitor tobacco use and prevention policies
*P*rotect people from tobacco smoke
*O*ffer help to quit tobacco use
*W*arn about the dangers of tobacco
*E*nforce bans on tobacco advertising, promotion and sponsorship
*R*aise taxes on tobacco (WHO 2012)

WHO has produced and brought together documents and resources produced by its regional offices, tobacco control NGOs, academic institutions and government agencies to address specific issues related to the articles of the FCTC and how they can best be implemented within Member States. Impressively these resources are available in all six official languages of the WHO (English, French, Russian, Spanish, Arabic and Chinese). With multiple resources under each of the letters of the MPOWER mnemonic freely available on the Internet, policymakers and advocates alike can find useful information, guidance and examples of successful implementation of each of the articles of the FCTC.

With such a broad range of objectives in the articles of the FCTC (see Table 19.1), advocacy to advance the adoption and full implementation of the FCTC requires a sophisticated set of methods that will allow tobacco control advocates to monitor the degree of implementation across that range of articles and to ensure that they are working as effectively as possible with other advocates. Advocacy in this context is not limited to attempting to persuade lawmakers that they should enact specific provisions of the FCTC. Advocacy for full implementation of the FCTC in any given country requires analysis of the provisions that have already been enacted, the degree to which they are enforced and a strategy to implement any articles of the FCTC that have not yet been addressed . The specifics of the FCTC are not entirely prescriptive and give countries latitude in the application of some of its articles. In some cases the measures taken by a government are not seen as going far enough to satisfy tobacco control advocates.

Advocacy is most likely to be successful when seemingly diverse chronic disease-related interest groups band together to circulate common messages and call for unified action. By combining their voices to deliver the powerful message that comprehensive and integrated action can stop the global epidemic of chronic disease, advocates can make a real difference. There is power in numbers (WHO 2006).

The articles of the FCTC provide a clear tobacco control agenda for advocates in each signatory state. The existence of a set number of objectives gives greater clarity to advocates and enables them to organize advocacy efforts around articles of the FCTC that have not been sufficiently implemented in their countries. The FCTC has provided a framework for action as well as an impetus for national and regional collaboration. Because tobacco control in many nations is not entirely within the control of national governments, the need for tobacco control advocacy and action at the local level still exists. For example, in countries with a federal government system, states or provinces may have responsibility for legislation on issues such as tobacco taxes, smoke-free legislation and funding of cessation and other tobacco control programs (WHO 2008c; ACS CAN 2012).

Local tobacco control advocates can use the FCTC to separate the locally controlled tobacco control issues from the provincially or the nationally controlled issues and create a local action plan that supports provincial and national efforts. Reporting on local, provincial and state implementation of tobacco control measures can contribute to the development of a national tobacco control profile and can help advocates gauge how well their efforts compare to those in other jurisdictions (WHO 2008c). Regional structures can use reports of national achievements to analyse the need for specific forms of support or training within countries of the region (Fleitmann 2000; El Awa 2010; SEATCA 2012).

Case Study Two: Integrated Action at the Regional Level: The Southeast Asia Tobacco Control Alliance

In 2001 the Southeast Asia Tobacco Control Alliance (SEATCA) was formed as a multi-sectoral alliance to support tobacco control in ASEAN nations. SEATCA has a core group composed of representatives from government, the World Health Organization and leading tobacco control NGOs from across the region. The alliance works to identify the tobacco control priorities of nations in the region and support progressive policy development, strengthen national tobacco control working groups, generate more local evidence for advancing tobacco control policy and increase the number and capacity of tobacco control workers. SEATCA does this work through:

- Generating policy-driven evidence-based research
- Promoting active participation and knowledge sharing
- Multi-lateral discussions
- Capacity building and media advocacy
- Customised technical assistance

SEATCA advocates for a region-wide focus on issues by building meaningful partnerships, mobilising local NGOs and using regional workshops to build and maintain momentum for tobacco control. With support from philanthropic, government and academic institutions SEATCA develops and conducts policy-relevant research in the region and builds regional research capacity through mentoring local and regional researchers and connecting regional research with other international research projects. SEATCA also works with the World Health Organization's Western Pacific Regional Office (WPRO) to provide technical assistance to regional Member States and to compile a regional database on tobacco control.

Southeast Asian countries served by SEATCA range from those where tobacco control is sophisticated and advanced, to countries where tobacco control is still in a developmental phase. SEATCA successfully supports all of these countries by forming a sophisticated network that provides advocacy fellowships to train media advocates, builds local capacity and mentors other tobacco control advocates. SEATCA also provides a Regional Media Officer's Network to strengthen knowledge, sharing and communication among media officers.

(continued)

Case Study Two: (continued)

They also provide a news-monitoring system to specifically support activities that respond to tobacco industry tactics.

By providing support for clear communication across the region, including the identification of priorities and capacity gaps, SEATCA is aware of where its support is of greatest need but is also aware of where its wealth of human assets can most effectively be utilised. SEATCA provides a sophisticated structure that advances tobacco control advocacy through:

• Supporting research that provides evidence to inform good practice and strengthen advocacy.

• Mentoring and providing communication and networking tools for advocates and media officers ensure consistency of message, increase national and international media coverage and exponentially expand the tobacco control advocacy effort across the region.

• Establishing and maintaining a resource centre that provides online resources and a database to keep members up to date on research, policy development and best practice for tobacco control. This resource also serves as a virtual interactive online platform where members can make requests for assistance.

The strength of the SEATCA model is in its inclusiveness and its focus on sharing resources, mentoring and building capacity for tobacco control through well-integrated activity in the region. While the research, policy-development and technical support efforts of the Alliance extend beyond the traditional definition of advocacy alone, all of the efforts of the SEATCA can be seen to support the message that effective tobacco control saves lives. Comprehensive coverage of all the needs of tobacco control workers, not just one subset of workers in isolation, demonstrates best practice in support for tobacco control through an effective alliance.

The approach taken by SEATCA is entirely consistent with the principles of health promotion laid down in the Ottawa Charter, which states: "Health promotion strategies and programmes should be adapted to the local needs and possibilities of individual countries and regions to take into account differing social, cultural and economic systems" (WHO 1986).

(Adapted from SEATCA 2012)

Advocacy for tobacco control, within the context of the FCTC, can focus on any of the aspects of tobacco control covered by the articles of the Convention (see Table 19.1). This can mean advocacy at the community level, at local, provincial or national government level and with a broad range of sectors and stakeholders. Critical to achieving this range of tobacco control measures in a country is the development of a national coordination mechanism as called for in Article 5 of the FCTC (WHO 2005). Advocates in numerous countries have indicated the benefits of such a centralised function to ensure that strategies are well coordinated, integrated and appropriately reported (FCA 2007; WHO 2008c; Bureau of Health Promotion 2011; RCP 2012). The existence of such a national coordination mechanism can provide a solid foundation for local and provincial contributions to national plans and strategies as well as providing leadership, training, funding and consistent reporting frameworks for non-governmental advocates.

Such a coordination mechanism provides scope for nationally determined priorities to be implemented in a way that takes into account the contextual factors relevant to tobacco control within the country. Given that the majority of Members States of the United Nations are signatories to the FCTC and the fact that the level of implementation of the FCTC provisions varies greatly across these nations, the capacity to adapt to national contextual factors allows countries to report the current status of tobacco control in a realistic light. Just as contextual issues will affect the capacity of any UN Member State to enact all of the articles of the FCTC, so will these same contextual issues shape the need for coordinated advocacy.

Implementation reports from multiple countries within a region can further highlight contextual issues relevant to tobacco control such as traditional gender roles and tobacco use, the impact of tobacco on poverty, influence of the tobacco industry or regional support mechanism and technical assistance for tobacco control (Fleitmann 2000; FCA 2007; El Awa 2010; SEATCA 2012). In countries with weak commitment to tobacco control or countries that are not signatory to the FCTC, the coordination function for tobacco control advocacy may rest with an NGO or a civil society organization (Reddy 2005).

Some authors who discuss the role of advocacy for tobacco control emphasise the importance of advocacy efforts originating or predominantly being supported by civil society organizations in what is sometimes referred to as a "bottom-up" direction (Reddy 2005; Open Society Institute 2007; Lin 2010). This is aligned with traditional health promotion ideals and reflects the importance of the principle of empowerment in health promotion (Wallerstein 1992; Kirk et al. 2009). Advocacy activities at the community level include awareness-raising, political empowerment, contribution to research and developing evidence, and developing the capacity to perform watchdog tasks to ensure that legislation and policies are being enforced and to keep an eye on the local activities of the tobacco industry (Reddy 2005).

Advocacy for health promotion has achieved its greatest successes where there exist civil society movements, an enabling policy environment, sufficient government funding, health promotion capacity and social and cultural norms that support tobacco control. This has been most notable in developed nations where tobacco control has been on the public health radar for decades (Lin 2010).

It has been noted that tobacco control in Australia, "has mostly been initiated by professional advocates who took the recommendations of the early expert reports on reducing the tobacco epidemic and the results of relevant local policy-relevant research and advocated for changes to be adopted" (Chapman and Wakefield 2001). While the same authors go on to assert that individuals and communities are increasingly involved in tobacco control advocacy, most efforts are still pursued by health NGOs and policy-oriented researchers (Chapman and Wakefield 2001). Regardless of the level of professionalism of the advocates, the greatest successes in achieving results in tobacco control advocacy have been seen in areas where there is an active, organized and well-coordinated effort.

> Advocacy is most likely to be successful when seemingly diverse chronic disease-related interest groups band together to circulate common messages and call for unified action. By combining their voices to deliver the powerful message that comprehensive and integrated action can stop the global epidemic of chronic disease, advocates can make a real difference. There is power in numbers. WHO (2006)

Case Study Three: Comprehensive Approach to Diverse Advocates: Health-Related Information Dissemination Amongst Youth in India

Health-Related Information Dissemination Amongst Youth (HRIDAY) is a voluntary organization of health professionals and social scientists engaged in activities aiming to promote health awareness and informed health activism among school and college students in India since 1992. HRIDAY has prepared a handbook for NGO personnel involved in tobacco control entitled *Effective Strategies for Tobacco Control Advocacy* (HRIDAY 2009). This document in itself is an interesting case study of the complex challenges facing an NGO in attempting to ensure that staff across a wide range of NGOs have consistent information, direction, motivation and support. The handbook has sections covering:

- The burden of tobacco globally and within India.
- Tobacco control legislation and litigation in India including a report of the FCTC implementation status in India.
- The role of civil society in tobacco control including information on advocacy, the role of coalitions, ways of broadening the tobacco control movement, behaviour change communication and how to use the Indian Right to Information Act for tobacco control.
- Case studies highlighting the use of celebrities, youth power, advocacy from a cancer foundation, mass media and legislation.

This comprehensive handbook provides evidence-based information in a consistent way that can be used by tobacco control workers across India. It highlights the laws that exist and creates a realistic sense of expectation in relation to enforcement with analysis of barriers to enforcement as well as opportunities for advocates to take to increase enforcement and compliance with tobacco control laws. It provides guidance for NGOs in relation to public interest litigation, research, advocacy, awareness, capacity building and operational research to implement programs and realise policies. The report provides guidelines for reporting legal violations, an observation checklist for violations of the Tobacco Control Act and information on the National Tobacco Control Programme (sic) in India.

The handbook does more than provide facts in the form of evidence; it provides advice on how organizations can work together and contribute to a more integrated and comprehensive tobacco control effort. It provides inspiration by giving examples of international best practice in smoke-free legislation and updates on litigation against tobacco companies in India. The handbook

explains the various articles of the FCTC and provides information on the status of implementation of each article. This helps NGOs to know where to focus their tobacco control advocacy efforts and highlights the articles that are further along in the implementation process.

The role of civil society and NGOs in tobacco control advocacy is clearly set out with discussion of dimensions of advocacy, steps in the advocacy process and a planning tool for developing strategic advocacy campaigns. The handbook then stresses the importance of organizations coming together to strengthen their voices and actions through the formation of coalitions. This section provides the arguments for collaboration, articulates characteristics of a successful coalition and indicates potential difficulties that may be faced by coalitions and networks.

The next section of the handbook provides advice on widening the tobacco control movement by engaging health professionals, using behaviour change communication and making use of Indian freedom-of-information legislation (known as the Right to Information Act). The case studies that conclude the document provide detailed information on how NGOs and civil society organizations have engaged the public, the media and political decision-makers in tobacco control advocacy including specific coverage of the development of media invitations and press releases. These case studies provide information, stimulation and inspiration to other organizations across India to take more concerted tobacco control action.

HRIDAY has produced a document in *Effective Strategies for Tobacco Control Advocacy* that gives organizations working toward tobacco control in India a better understanding of the breadth of issues that

(continued)

need to be covered in that country while at the same time providing these organizations with useful indicators of what other organizations are doing. The document supports organizations working alone as well as encouraging the development of more effective partnerships, networks and alliances. The breadth of information presented in this handbook is usually reserved to publications from the World Health Organization, regional offices of the WHO or large international NGOs. That such a detailed and comprehensive source could come from an NGO within one country is impressive. The relevance of Indian examples to the constituency of HRIDAY is critical for broader engagement with tobacco control advocacy in the world's largest democracy.

(Adapted from HRIDAY 2009)

Common Features of Tobacco Control Advocacy

The FCTC and its ongoing implementation are the obvious focus for tobacco control advocacy for the foreseeable future. This is due to the unique position of the FCTC as the world's only global public health treaty. It is useful to keep in mind, however, that the FCTC arose from decades of tobacco control advocacy that was supported by still-growing mountains of evidence, strong NGO and civil society support and dynamic leadership by people in powerful positions. There is no one-size-fits-all model for tobacco control advocacy. There are, however, some features of tobacco control advocacy that appear common to advocacy efforts.

In *Stop the epidemic of chronic disease: a practical guide to successful advocacy* (WHO 2006) a useful seven-step framework is articulated:

1. Define the situation
2. Establish goals and objectives
3. Identify your target audience
4. Develop key messages to influence the target audience
5. Develop and implement your advocacy plan
6. Engage media interest
7. Monitor and evaluate

These are common features called for in most "how-to" publications related to advocacy within the public health realm. The more tobacco-specific *Building Blocks for Tobacco Control: A Handbook* (WHO 2004) emphasises the importance of having a national focal point for coordination of tobacco control efforts and provides more advice on how to establish governmental structures to implement the FCTC. While this is a means of achieving tobacco control within a country, advocacy efforts are more likely to arise within the structures brought into partnership with the government to steer tobacco control activities. The handbook calls for the establishment of a structure that includes:

- Government ministries
- The private sector, including
  - Media
  - NGOs
  - Health professionals
  - Lawyers
  - Economists
  - Business, industry and labour unions
  - Other stakeholders such as rights, environmental, religious, consumer, youth, parent and teacher groups (WHO 2004)

Chapman and Wakefield (2001) emphasise the importance of tobacco control:

- Having upstream goals—being focused on the policy level rather than the service level of tobacco control
- Contesting debates—working to break down public and political inertia about an issue
- Being both opportunistic and responsive in advocacy campaigns
- Developing trust between government and NGO advocates
- Persevering despite setbacks

HRIDAY, an Indian coalition for health advocacy, stress the importance of blending science, politics and activism to generate public support for tobacco control activities (HRIDAY 2009). They also emphasise the importance of gathering and presenting information on:

- The health impact of tobacco
- Rates of tobacco use among various parts of the population (by gender, ethnicity, socio-economic status, education level, etc.)
- Economic arguments for tobacco control
- Situation analysis relevant to the specific region or area in which the tobacco control effort is to be conducted, conglomerated into a national report
- Barriers to tobacco control and strategies to overcome them, including de-bunking myths that may exist within populations or sub-populations
- Partners and potential partners who are engaged in tobacco control efforts or other public health efforts that may easily align with tobacco control objectives (NCDs, cancer-prevention, healthy settings, etc.)

Like WHO (2006), HRIDAY emphasise the importance of situation analysis and they articulate a role for tobacco control advocates in developing awareness, research and training, capacity building and looking outward to other tobacco control efforts for support and inspiration. There is also a call for documenting tobacco control advocacy and a strong emphasis on the value of litigation for tobacco control as a form of advocacy (HRIDAY 2009).

HRIDAY also encourage advocates to be clear and explicit about:

- Goals
- Intended audience for advocacy
- The specific message you are advocating
- The messenger who is most appropriate to deliver the message
- The most appropriate means of delivering the message
- The resources required to develop, deliver and monitor/evaluate the effectiveness of your advocacy effort
- Any gaps that exist in capacity, knowledge, funding, infrastructure, etc
- The initial steps to be taken
- The process and methods of evaluating the advocacy efforts

- The partnerships/alliances/coalitions necessary to achieve the best effort in the specific advocacy task (HRIDAY 2009)

The Public Health Advocacy Institute of Western Australia clearly support the idea that there is no prescribed method for advocacy in tobacco control. They emphasise the importance of context; capacity to advocate; human, information, infrastructure and financial resources; timing; and issue analysis in determining the appropriate course of advocacy action. They also emphasise the importance of:

- Data collection and verification
- Building credible partnerships
- Planning for and promoting small wins (not just big successes)
- Being clear about aims and objectives
- Being specific about the outcomes you seek to achieve
- Getting the timing right for tobacco control advocacy
- Being opportunistic
- Making issues local and relevant
- Framing the message in the evidence
- Compromising when necessary
- Knowing the enemy
- Keeping focused on the objectives
- Surprising and challenging the opposition
- Creating champions
- Evaluating (PHAIWA 2009)

The pattern that emerges from examination of advocacy guides or handbooks, regardless of the region of the world they are from, indicates a strong reliance on information; use of the media; the development and maintenance of partnerships across government and civil society/NGO sectors; clarity of objectives; persistence; and monitoring and evaluation.

As previously indicated, the context of tobacco control advocacy is a critical consideration when determining the appropriate course of action to take. Advocates must learn to gauge the political, economic and social factors that will work for them and against them. They must be ever mindful that they operate in an environment of tobacco industry opposition that may manifest itself in the most remarkable political, economic and social circumstances. But advocates can take comfort in the knowledge that they are not alone, that there is a growing body of evidence about what works and an ever-increasing body of expert tobacco control advocate organizations willing to share what they know, support other tobacco control advocates and help find solutions to complex tobacco control dilemmas.

Conclusion

The challenge of addressing the dramatically increasing rate of non-communicable diseases worldwide has been articulated and prioritised by the United Nations. The UN Political Declaration clearly recognised the importance of tobacco control and the utility of the World Health Organization FCTC as a critical step in addressing NCDs on a global scale. The development of the FCTC has given tobacco control advocates a clear and comprehensive set of objectives for which to advocate within countries. While the focus of the United Nations Political Declaration is on prevention of

disease more than health promotion, much of the language used in the Declaration is evocative of the World Health Organization's Ottawa Charter for Health Promotion (UN 2011; WHO 1986). Table 19.2 illustrates how health promotion principles and approaches from the Ottawa Charter are reflected in the FCTC.

This use of language is an endorsement of the ideas and concepts articulated in the Ottawa Charter and may be seen to be the application of contemporary health promotion thinking to a broader public health issue. The endorsement of policy-level approaches, reorientation of health services, capacity building at the individual and community level and the creation of supportive environments for NCD reduction all echo the action areas of the Charter. The call for partnerships, intersectoral action, inclusion of a broad range of stakeholders and broadening our understanding of NCD from solely a behavioural risk factor approach to a more social determinant-oriented approach are all consistent with the language and spirit of the Ottawa Charter (WHO 1986; UN 2011).

Table 19.2 Ottawa Charter reflected in the FCTC

Ottawa Charter	Framework Convention on Tobacco Control
Build healthy public policy	FCTC is a treaty (policy document) that requires signatories to implement tobacco control policies across numerous areas (see Table 19.1)
Create supportive environments	Article 8 is concerned with protection from exposure to tobacco smoke; Article 13 regulates tobacco advertising, promotion and sponsorship; Article 16 prevents sales to and by minors and prohibits giveaways, providing free tobacco products, and small packets, limits access of minors to vending machines
Strengthen community actions	Article 12 (education, communication, training and awareness) supports community action; Article 17 provides support for viable alternatives to tobacco workers, growers and sellers
Develop personal skills	Articles 9–11 (regulation of contents, product disclosure and packaging and labelling of products) contribute to individual capacity to make informed choices; Article 12 calls for training of health workers, community workers, social workers, media professionals, educators, decision-makers, administrators and other concerned persons
Reorient health services	Article 14 calls for the establishment of programs for diagnosis, counselling, prevention and treatment of tobacco dependence; Article 12 calls for training for health and community workers
Advocate (multiple targets for advocacy)	Articles 3 and 4 discuss the importance of political commitment, health, social, environmental consequences of tobacco use
Mediate (multi-sectoral approaches, whole of government, whole of society)	Article 4 calls for the participation of civil society; Article 5 calls for a national coordination mechanism; Articles 6–24 call for comprehensive multi-sectoral measures and responses including policy development across multiple sectors of government
Enable (information, life skills, opportunities to make healthy choices)	Article 12 calls for public awareness, education and communication on tobacco control, regulation of smoking in public places, development of counselling and cessation services

Challenges

While there are some impressive examples of tobacco control advocacy in some countries, there are many areas of the world where tobacco control has not achieved the same level of success. Due to legal and administrative structures in some countries, tobacco control is not consistently managed as a national issue. Different and in some cases conflicting regulations and practices mean that it may be possible to smoke in an indoor public space in one town and not in the neighbouring town. These circumstances may create additional challenges for tobacco control advocates as advocacy targets may need to be national, state/provincial and local. Rutter and Crossfield (2012) argue that strong national coordination of local governments and, in some cases, a sub-national tier of coordination effort can contribute to better tobacco control efforts while avoiding unnecessary duplication of effort. HRIDAY (2009) stress the success of state-based tobacco control cells in India that both build tobacco control capacity within the state and coordinate the initiatives of the tobacco control program.

Another challenge of contemporary tobacco control advocacy is that of marshalling expertise across the range of issues covered in the FCTC (WHO 2009; ACS CAN 2012; HRIDAY 2009). With provisions relating to taxation, public health, advertising, packaging and labelling, education, communication, training and public awareness as well as illicit trade, agriculture, legal liability and a range of scientific endeavours, it is clear that the FCTC expands beyond many of the traditional boundaries of advocacy for a health issue. The FCTC has created a holistic framework for tobacco control that, if done comprehensively, will necessarily involve multiple sectors of government, industry, NGOs and civil society. This is a manifestation of the holistic principles articulated in the Ottawa Charter for health promotion and can be seen as a concrete global example of these health promotion principles within the context of a public health concern.

Challenges facing tobacco control advocacy can be traced to a number of factors including the following:

- *Lack of political will*—It is important to distinguish between political will at the top of a hierarchy (President, Prime Minister) and within other critical parts of government. In some cases political will exists within the bureaucracy or among critical players such as the Minister for Health or the Minister for Finance. A key task for tobacco control advocates in environments of low political will is assessing where there is will and taking action to support and grow it (WHO 2006). In some cases where there is no political will advocates may find greatest success in generating demand for action in civil society (HRIDAY 2009). Beyond this, action may be needed to persuade political decision-makers of the magnitude of the tobacco problem and the effectiveness of interventions to address it (WHO 2004).

- *Lack of priority*—Developing countries may put greater emphasis on priorities such as primary health care, Millennium Development Goals or poverty alleviation (Lin 2010). Advocates operating in such an environment may gain from framing the benefits of tobacco control within the arguments for these other health priorities. Significant evidence exists to support tobacco control as a key contributor to multiple health issues (de Beyer et al. 2001; Esson and Leeder 2004; Beaglehole et al. 2008).

- *Negative influence of the tobacco industry*—When analysing the impact of tobacco control advocacy, it is critical to remember that the counter-advocacy efforts of the tobacco industry are formidable. Tobacco control advocates have to contend with not only the impact of highly addictive products, advertising, product placement and sponsorship (where they still exist) but also the consistent and well-funded efforts of global tobacco corporations to actively undermine tobacco control. Advocates must also counter efforts by the tobacco industry to discredit evidence, to break every restriction and to buy or coerce influence in political, social and policymaking spheres. The tobacco industry has produced false and misleading information at conferences and employed "experts" to make statements critical of impending tobacco control legislation (Corporate Accountability International 2008). The tobacco industry has also paid scientific consultants to question and create an atmosphere of doubt around research showing that second-hand smoke harms health, even going so far as to infiltrate the World Health Organization's International Agency for Research on Cancer (Global Smokefree Partnership 2008).

- *Lack of investment*—This may be investment at a national level due to lack of priority or simply due to lack of capacity to fund. In some countries funding for tobacco control is shared by national and state or provincial governments, and in some cases local authorities. A lack of priority or incapacity to fund tobacco control at any of these levels can lead to insufficient or uneven achievement of tobacco control objectives (Tauras et al. 2005). Advocacy to raise awareness of innovative funding within governments or external funds from philanthropic or developmental agencies may be required to address these issues (WHO 2004).

- *Lack of infrastructure*—In some parts of the world the appropriate funding, delivery, surveillance and reporting mechanism required for effective tobacco control simply do not exist. In countries where this is the case capacity building efforts and infrastructure development may necessarily be the priorities for tobacco control (WHO 2004; Stillman et al. 2006). Regional structures often play a supporting role in the development of appropriate infrastructure (Fleitmann 2000; El Awa 2010; SEATCA 2012). While infrastructure is usually thought of as the domain of governments, NGOs and civil society can be strong advocates for prioritising tobacco control infrastructure and developing the necessary human resource capacities (Reddy 2005; Open Society Institute 2007; HRIDAY 2009).

- *Relapse/lack of vigilance*—Once tobacco control policies have been adopted or legislation has been passed, there is an ongoing need for

ensuring ongoing enforcement of and compliance with the new policies and/or laws. Enforcement may be weak, and variable, or may change with a change in political climate (Crosbie et al. 2011).

Any combination of these factors can lead to what Lin (2010) refers to as lack of an enabling environment. Other factors contributing to this include low awareness or resistance to tobacco control measures by specific groups, the weak presence of NGOs, low awareness and support for tobacco control in the population, lack of expertise in tobacco control and an inadequate workforce (Lin 2010).

Advocates also have to be aware of two other potential issues that may affect the reception of advocacy messages: advocacy fatigue and "nannyism"—the myth that tobacco control is a result of a government arbitrarily restricting personal freedoms and fostering a "nanny state" through the proliferation of patronising public policy (Sparks 2011).

Advocacy fatigue relates to a lack of interest in tobacco control issues brought about by an overexposure to constant messages about tobacco control, or to waning interest in tobacco control due to a feeling that it "has been done" (MacKenzie and Chapman 2012). In countries where tobacco control is advanced, the challenge may be in making the focus of advocacy fresh and interesting. Creativity in approach is a critical aspect of ensuring that messages do not fall victim to advocacy fatigue (MacKenzie and Chapman 2012). Another relevant consideration in combating advocacy fatigue is the timing of advocacy efforts. It is difficult to create attention for tobacco control when numerous other serious issues are vying for media and public attention (Chapman and Wakefield 2001) or if efforts are out of sync with political or media timetables (PHAIWA 2009).

In relation to combating nannyism, the best weapon for tobacco control advocates is the evidence of harm done to human health by tobacco products and moral responsibility of governments to act in the best interest of the health and wellbeing of its citizens (Sparks 2011). Economic arguments can easily be made in relation to increased productivity, decreased payouts for exposure to tobacco smoke and reduced demand for treatment and care services (World Bank 2003). Increasingly the evidence is also mounting to counter the arguments that going smoke free is detrimental to restaurants, bars and the broader entertainment industry. Claims of nannyism can be countered with assertions of the responsibility of the state to protect its citizens and to be responsible with health-care spending (Winstanley et al. 2001; Cloud et al. 2011).

Tobacco control has always been a complex pursuit. The evidence of harms from tobacco use has evolved over decades. Rich and powerful tobacco interests have acted against advocates and attempted to thwart tobacco control efforts and develop and expand markets for their deadly products. The addictive nature of the substance, the allure of sophisticated marketing and ill-informed populations have all presented challenges to those who warn of the dangers of tobacco use.

The development of a global treaty, an FCTC, has provided a structured way of understanding and tackling tobacco issues on a national level. Tobacco control advocates have developed new ways of sharing expertise and experiences with one another and have formed new coalitions and alliances to support tobacco control in countries where it is in its most rudimentary stages. The challenges facing tobacco control advocates are great, and will remain great as long as the tobacco industry remains a large, wealthy, powerful force in the world. But the successful enactment of the world's first public health treaty gives cause for hope, a focus for activity and a measurable means of evaluating advocacy efforts.

References

American Cancer Society – Cancer Action Network (ACS CAN). (2012). *How do you measure up? A progress report on state legislative activity to reduce cancer incidence and mortality.* Atlanta, GA: American Cancer Society.

Arnott, D. (2012). Lessons from 50 years of tobacco control in the UK. In RCP (Eds.) *Fifty years since smoking and health: Progress, lessons and priorities for a smoke-free UK.* London: RCP.

Beaglehole, R., Epping-Jordan, J., Patel, V., Chopra, M., Ebrahim, S., Kidd, M., et al. (2008). Improving the prevention and management of chronic disease in low-income and middle-income countries: A priority for primary health care. *The Lancet, 372*(9642), 940–949.

Bureau of Health Promotion. (2011). *Taiwan tobacco control annual report 2011.* Taipei: Department of Health, Republic of Taiwan.

Centers for Disease Control and Prevention (CDC). (2006). *History of the surgeon general's reports on smoking and health.* Atlanta, GA: CDC.

Chapman, S., & Wakefield, M. (2001). Tobacco control advocacy in Australia: Reflections on 30 years of progress. *Health Education and Behaviour, 28*(3), 274–289.

Cloud, D. H., Islett, K. R., & Laugesen, M. (2011). *Mainstreaming public health in the Bloomberg administration: Processes for implementing reform. Proceedings of the 7th Transatlantic Dialogue on Strategic Management of Public Organizations.* Newark, NJ: Rutgers University.

Collishaw, N. (2009). *History of tobacco control in Canada.* Ottawa: Physicians for a Smoke-Free Canada.

Corporate Accountability International. (2008). *Protecting against tobacco industry interference: The 2008 global tobacco treaty action guide.* Boston, MA: Corporate Accountability International.

Crosbie, E., Sebrie, E. M., & Glantz, S. A. (2011). Strong advocacy led to successful implementation of smoke-free Mexico City. *Tobacco Control, 20*(1), 64–72.

de Beyer, J., Lovelace, C., & Yurekli, A. (2001). Poverty and tobacco. *Tobacco Control, 10*, 210–211.

Doll, R., & Hill, A. B. (1950). Smoking and carcinoma of the lung. *British Medical Journal, 2*(4682), 739–748.

Doll, R., & Hill, A. B. (1954). The mortality of doctors in relation to their smoking habits; a preliminary report. *British Medical Journal, 1*(4877), 1451–1455.

El Awa, F. (2010). The WHO framework convention on tobacco control as a tool for advancing health promotion: perspectives from the Eastern Mediterranean Region. *Global Health Promotion Supplement, 1*, 60–66.

Esson, K. M., & Leeder, S. R. (2004). *The millennium development goals and tobacco control: An opportunity for global partnership.* Geneva: WHO.

Farquharson, K. (2003). Influencing policy transnationally: Pro-and anti-tobacco global advocacy networks. *Australian Journal of Public Administration, 62*(4), 80–92.

Fleitmann, S. (2000). EU network promotes cross-border alliances against tobacco. *Global Health and Environment Monitor, 8*(2), 5.

Framework Convention Alliance (FCA). (2007). *Framework convention alliance on tobacco control annual report 07.* Geneva: Framework Convention Alliance.

Glantz, S., & Gonzalez, M. (2012). Effective tobacco control is key to rapid progress in reduction of non-communicable diseases. *The Lancet, 379*, 1269–1271.

Global Smokefree Partnership. (2008). *The framework convention on tobacco control article 8 toolkit.* Global Smokefree Partnership. http://www.globalsmokefree. com/gsp/ficheiro/toolkit.zip. Accessed 17 May 2013.

Health Related Information Dissemination Amongst Youth (HRIDAY). (2009). *Effective strategies for tobacco control advocacy.* New Delhi: HRIDAY.

Khanna, R., & Misra, B. (2000). *Presentation on behalf of voluntary organization in the interest of consumer education (Voice), New Delhi, India.* New Delhi: VOICE.

Kirk, R., Kirk, A., Sozanski, G., Heptonstall, S., Amuyunzu-Nyamongo, M., & Adebayo, A. (2009). *Focusing on community assets for health promotion: The role of NGOs and civil society in local empowerment. Proceedings of the 7th Global Conference on Health Promotion.* Geneva: WHO.

Lein, G., & DeLand, K. (2011). Translating the WHO framework convention on tobacco control (FCTC): Can we use tobacco control as a model for other non-communicable disease control? *Public Health, 125,* 846–853.

Lin, V. (2010). The framework convention on tobacco control and health promotion: strengthening the ties. *Global Health Promotion Supplement, 1,* 76–80.

Mackay, J., Eriksen, M. P., & Shafey, O. (2006). *The tobacco atlas* (2nd ed.). Atlanta, GA: American Cancer Society.

Mackenzie, R., & Chapman, S. (2012). Generating news media interest in tobacco control: Challenges in an advanced policy environment. *Health Promotion Journal of Australia, 23*(2), 92–96.

Mamudu, H. M., & Glantz, S. A. (2009). Civil society and the negotiation of the framework convention on tobacco control. *Global Public Health, 4*(2), 150–168.

Open Society Institute. (2007). *Taking on Goliath – Civil society's leadership role in tobacco control.* New York, NY: Open Society Institute.

Public Health Advocacy Institute of Western Australia (PHAIWA). (2009). *Advocacy in action: A toolkit for public health professionals* (2nd ed.). Perth: PHAIWA.

Reddy, K.S. (2005). *Role of civil society organizations in tobacco control: from research to policy to public health action.* Mumbai: Forum 9.

Roemer, R., Taylor, A., & Lariviere, J. (2005). Origins of the WHO framework convention on tobacco control. *American Journal of Public Health, 95*(6), 936–938.

Royal College of Physicians (RCP). (1962). *Smoking and health.* London: RCP.

Royal College of Physicians (RCP). (2012). *Fifty years since smoking and health: Progress, lessons and priorities for a smoke-free UK.* London: RCP.

Rutter, A., & Crossfield, A. (2012). Policy at the front line: the local, sub-national and national divide. In Royal College of Physicians (RCP) (Ed.), *Fifty years since smoking and health: Progress, lessons and priorities for a smoke-free UK.* London: RCP.

Southeast Asia Tobacco Control Alliance (SEATCA). (2012). *Catalyst for change.* Bangkok: SEATCA.

Sparks, M. (2011). Building healthy public policy: Don't believe the misdirection. *Health Promotion International, 26*(3), 259–262.

Sparks, M. (2012). Health promotion: Shaping and informing public health. In D. Juvinya & H. Arroyo (Eds.), *Health promotion, 25 years later.* Girona: Documenta Universitaria.

Stillman, F., Yang, G., Figueiredo, V., Hernandez-Avila, M., & Samet, J. (2006). Building capacity for tobacco control research and policy. *Tobacco Control, 15*(Supp 1), i18–i23.

Stratton, L., Shetty, P., Wallace, R., & Bondurant, S. (Eds.). (2001). *Clearing the smoke: The science base for tobacco harm reduction.* Washington, DC: National Academy Press.

Tauras, J. A., Chaloupka, F. J., Farrelly, M. C., Giovino, G. A., Wakefield, M., Johnston, L. D., et al. (2005). State tobacco control spending and youth smoking. *American Journal of Public Health, 95*(2), 338–344.

United Nations (UN). (2011). *Draft political declaration of the high-level meeting on the prevention and control of non-communicable diseases.* New York, NY: UN.

Wallack, L., Dorfman, L., Jernigan, D., & Themba, M. (1993). *Media advocacy and public health: power for prevention.* London: Sage.

Wallerstein, N. (1992). Powerlessness, empowerment and health: implications for health promotion programs. *American Journal of Health Promotion, 6,* 197–205.

Weiss, T. G. (1999). *International NGOs, global governance and social policy in the UN system. Globalism and social policy programme occasional paper 3/1999.* Helsinki: STAKES.

Winstanley, M., Woodward, S., & Walker, N. (2001). *Tobacco in Australia: Facts and issues.* Melbourne: Quit Victoria Council.

World Bank. (2003). *The economics of tobacco use and tobacco control in the developing world – A background paper for the high level round table on tobacco control and development policy.* Washington, DC: World Bank.

World Health Organization (WHO). (1979). *Controlling the smoking epidemic: Report of the WHO Expert Working Committee on Smoking Control: Technical Report Series No. 636.* Geneva: WHO.

World Health Organization (WHO). (1986). *The Ottawa Charter for health promotion.* Geneva: WHO.

World Health Organization (WHO). (2004). *Building blocks for tobacco control: A handbook.* Geneva: WHO.

World Health Organization (WHO). (2005). *WHO framework convention on tobacco control.* Geneva: WHO.

World Health Organization (WHO). (2006). *Stop the epidemic of chronic disease: a practical guide to successful advocacy.* Geneva: WHO.

World Health Organization (WHO). (2008a). *WHO report on the global tobacco epidemic, 2008 – The MPOWER package.* Geneva: WHO.

World Health Organization (WHO). (2008b). *WHO 2008–2013 action plan for the global strategy for the prevention and control of non-communicable diseases.* Geneva: WHO.

World Health Organization (WHO). (2008c). *Best practice in tobacco control – Regulation of tobacco products: Australian report.* Geneva: WHO.

World Health Organization (WHO). (2009). *History of the WHO framework convention on tobacco control*. Geneva: WHO.

World Health Organization (WHO). (2011). *Global status report on non-communicable diseases*. Geneva: WHO.

World Health Organization (WHO). (2012). *Parties to the WHO framework convention on tobacco control*. Resource document. World Health Organization.

Retrieved 8 August 2012 from http://www.who.int/fctc/signatories_parties/en/index.html.

Wynder, E. L. (1988). Tobacco and health: A review of the history and suggestions for public health policy. *Public Health Reports, 103*(1), 8–18.

Wynder, E. L., & Graham, E. A. (1950). Tobacco smoking as a possible etiologic factor in bronchiogenic carcinoma. A study of six hundred and eighty-four proved cases. *Journal of the American Medical Association, 143*, 329–336.

Evidence Synthesis to Inform NCD Prevention and Health Promotion

Tahna Pettman, Rebecca Armstrong, Belinda Burford, Jodie Doyle, Laurie Anderson, and Elizabeth Waters

Introduction

Making decisions about options for intervening to prevent NCDs and promote health implies a consideration of the likely balance between potential desirable and undesirable effects resulting from such interventions or strategies. This will be based in part on an understanding of what effect investments have had previously, why, for whom, under which circumstances, and at what cost. Over the past 20 years the generation of available information has increased markedly across the field, spanning fields of behavior change, improving environments for health, and reducing the burden of disease and injury. The sheer volume of information from primary research and evaluation studies, combined with a

T. Pettman, B.H.Sc., Ph.D. (✉) • R. Armstrong, M.P.H., Ph.D. • B. Burford, B.Sc. (Hons), Ph.D.
J. Doyle, Grad. Dip. Health Prom., M.P.H.
E. Waters, M.P.H., D.Phil.
Melbourne School of Population and Global Health, The University of Melbourne, 207 Bouverie Street, Carlton, Victoria 3010, Australia
e-mail: tpettman@unimelb.edu.au;
armr@unimelb.edu.au; belinda@burford.co;
jdoyle@unimelb.edu.au; ewaters@unimelb.edu.au

L. Anderson, M.P.H., Ph.D.
Department of Epidemiology, School of Public Health, University of Washington, 2838 Burnaby Park SE, Olympia, Washington, DC 98501, USA
e-mail: lmander@u.washington.edu

need to learn from what has gone before, means knowledge should be synthesized and summarized in an efficient, consistent and timely way, to better support decision-making in policy and practice (Armstrong et al. 2008).

This chapter intends to provide an overview of how we collect and synthesize knowledge, using the principles of transparency and reliability. Systematic review methodology is based on these principles and provides a framework for approaching a body of knowledge about what research has been undertaken in a particular area before. It involves articulating a question of interest, and searching comprehensively for information that can be appraised, synthesized, and interpreted to answer that question (Rychetnik et al. 2004). Understanding the key elements of the synthesis process is useful when using this form of evidence to inform decisions. Although interventions are the focus throughout this chapter in order to provide consistent examples, the processes outlined could be extrapolated to any knowledge that may inform decisions about NCDs and health promotion.

Systematic reviews differ from *rapid evidence reviews*; however, they share common features. Both aim to synthesize evidence on a clearly formulated question, using explicit methods to identify, select, and critically appraise relevant research, and a transparent process for analyzing and interpreting study findings (Higgins and Green 2006; Watt et al. 2008). However, they generally differ in breadth and depth: a rapid evidence review may ask a more narrow research question and conduct a truncated literature search. Both types of reviews can be useful in answering questions about whether an intervention produces a desired effect, but systematic reviews can arguably provide more information about how an intervention works, for whom, under what circumstances, and at what cost.

Systematic reviews also differ from a traditional literature review, which tends to be less comprehensive and transparent in identifying included studies and thus, are more prone to bias (Armstrong et al. 2008). Systematic reviews attempt to provide a summary of all well conducted studies and so reduce the reliance on single studies or studies of poor quality which may provide an incomplete or inaccurate picture of what works, for whom and why. Their methods are transparent, thus reducing the potential for bias in terms of the inclusion, appraisal and analysis of included studies (Oxman and Guyatt 1993; Higgins and Green 2006).

In the field of NCD prevention and management, systematic reviews address key questions relevant to policy and practice, and can include the following: (1) what determinants (including social, environmental) contribute to NCDs; (2) what interventions work (effectiveness); and (3) why interventions work (including how, for whom, under what circumstances, at what cost).

This chapter provides a brief overview of the process of *how* knowledge/evidence is synthesized in systematic reviews with the intent of supporting their use in NCD prevention and health promotion. This work has been developed in accordance with key international guidelines on synthesis of knowledge of health promotion interventions including the Cochrane Handbook (http://www.cochrane.org/resources/handbook/) and the CPHG Guide for Developing Cochrane Protocol (http://ph.cochrane.org/resources-and-guidance).

Planning to Engage with Evidence Syntheses

It is useful to understand how systematic reviews arise and are planned when consulting them to inform practice and policy decisions. Review questions may arise from a range of imperatives across research, practice and policy settings. For anyone engaging with the

evidence, key decisions need to be made about which interventions, populations, settings, and outcomes are to be addressed in order to meet the needs of practice or policy decision-making. Reviews of evidence should include this level of detail to allow you to assess their relevance to your context.

How Reviews of Health Promotion Evidence Are Planned

Review questions can originate from several sources, ranging from calls from government or a funding agency, one's own organization to guide future decision-making, or from an author's own personal or academic interest in a topic. However, in order for a review to be most useful, the question and the protocol for answering the question should reflect three main components: (1) a gap in the current evidence knowledge, (2) relevance to practitioners and decision-makers, and (3) sensible program logic.

1. *Understanding the current evidence base*
   Conducting an overall scoping of the existing evidence is a useful exercise to inform review topics by acknowledging current gaps and residual uncertainties. Presenting decision-makers and research funders with an outline of the state of the current evidence helps to identify the remaining need-to-know questions that could be informed by a well-conceived, quality-produced, systematic review of primary studies. Utilizing systematic review repositories and tapping into the knowledge of relevant stakeholders may be useful.

2. *Relevance to practitioners and decision-makers*
   Health promotion and public health interventions operate in a context that demands explicit acknowledgment of the political, logistical, and practical realities of those planning and implementing the interventions. Therefore, reviews of intervention evidence will be most useful to decision-makers if the provision of contextual and implementation information is a consistent thread that holds the review together (Waters et al. 2011b). More detail on what information should be included is provided in Chap. 25.

3. *Based on sensible program logic*

Logic models illustrate how a program is designed to achieve its intended outcomes, clarifying the review authors' reasoning by enhancing understanding of the theory of change underpinning programs or policies. In a review they can provide a framework for setting inclusion/exclusion criteria, for guiding the search strategy, for identifying relevant outcomes, and for examining differences among studies and along dimensions of interest (Anderson et al. 2011).

All three components here are served well by involving stakeholders in the planning stages of an evidence review. To ensure that the review question, the parameters set out in the review and the logic behind these decisions are congruent with stakeholders, individuals with a good working understanding of the nuances inherent in the research and policy environment should be recruited. This will help to ensure relevance of the evidence gathered and synthesized in the review.

Many review author groups choose to formalize collaboration with stakeholders by establishing review advisory groups. These groups can be very effective during the construction of the review question, helping to define the program logic (see below) and when deciding on the inclusion criteria or parameters (population/participants, intervention types, comparators and outcomes) for the review. For example, an author team currently reviewing the effects of involvement in conservation activities on various health outcomes (including intermediate outcomes of relevance to NCDs— well-being and physical activity levels) has recruited a "project reference group" comprising workers and participants in environmental enhancement/conservation activities from a wide range of key organizations volunteer groups, local authorities, and community advocates (Husk et al. 2013). The list was populated through direct author contacts, Web searches, and snowball contacting. The group contributed to:

- Sharing knowledge of organizations involved in relevant schemes and the nature of these activities.
- Ensuring that the author team had a comprehensive picture of the research and evaluations that have been undertaken in this area (especially the grey literature).

- Ensuring anticipated benefit for participation across different groups and how these are achieved (program theories) were well conceived.

Establishing a Framework for Drawing upon the Evidence

Asking an Answerable Question

After reviewers have scoped the gap in current knowledge and potential relevance of a review topic, the next stage is to formulate a specific question that the review seeks to answer. This process is commonly used not only in research settings, but also in practice and policy decision-making settings. Formulating an "answerable question" can facilitate the first steps of drawing upon evidence to inform health promotion planning and implementation. An answerable question enables searching for relevant research reports for decision-making purposes (Jackson and Baker 2005). This applies to situations where practitioners and policymakers wish to review evidence internally, or when engaging an external consultant or researcher to undertake an evidence review. The process of formulating an answerable question will help to clarify the expectations about the question to be answered among stakeholders. The process of formulating an answerable question may also assist when preparing to conduct or commission an evaluation of policy or practice (i.e., when generating practice-based evidence)—again this helps to clarify the expectations among stakeholders about what questions are to be answered within the evaluation.

Key concepts to be defined in an answerable question include population(s), intervention(s) and outcome(s). Further, depending on the question of interest, a comparison or control (C) may also be included (which may be no intervention, another intervention or standard practice). The PICO concepts are defined:

Population(s): In health promotion this may include whole populations, communities or individuals. You may also wish to consider whether there is value in limiting the population (e.g., street-connected young people, preschool-age children, etc.). Questions may also be limited to the effects of the interventions on disadvantaged populations in order to investigate the effectiveness of the interventions on reducing inequalities. Further information on addressing inequalities is provided later in this section.

Intervention(s): In your evidence search, you may wish to examine information on a number of different interventions to address one outcome (a lumped question), or you may wish to examine the effectiveness of one specific intervention (a split question). For example, you may wish to find all research about obesity prevention interventions (lumped) or you may wish to assess a specific intervention such as the effectiveness of nutrition policies in schools (split).

Another method may be consider examining "approaches" to health promotion rather than topic-driven interventions, for example relating to health behavior change you might wish to examine the effects of peer-led strategies, workplace interventions, or changes to the built environment. Additionally, you may wish to assess the effectiveness of a particular type of theory-based intervention (e.g., socio-ecological model; social-cognitive theory) for achieving certain health outcomes (e.g., improved dietary intake; smoking cessation).

Comparison(s): Comparison interventions may be no intervention, another intervention or standard (usual) practice or care. The choice of comparison or control has large implications for the interpretation of results. A question addressing one intervention versus no intervention is a different question to one comparing an intervention versus standard practice. This has relevance in health promotion and disease prevention particularly due to the nature of interventions and existing practices. For example, it is known that physical activity provides health benefits, so when searching on this topic you may find that some studies compare new physical activity interventions to an alternative or existing practice, rather than comparing the intervention to no treatment at all.

Outcome(s): The outcome(s) chosen for your question must be meaningful to your practice/decision-making and the population identified.

Health promotion interventions are inherently complex and therefore you would want to explore implementation processes of the intervention as well as its effects (outcomes). For example, implementation processes may include acceptability, adoption, appropriateness, cost, and reach or penetration (Proctor et al. 2011). Other outcomes to explore may include unintended effects (unexpected positive "ripple" effects, harms), cost-effectiveness, equity, and sustainability (Waters et al. 2011b).

Developing a clear question will reduce time and possible frustration when consulting with the evidence. An answerable question helps streamline the process of searching and assessing evidence. Having a question including the PICO concepts will facilitate an online search for evidence; and assessment of the relevance of the evidence retrieved, and application of the findings back to the original question. It may also be worthwhile considering the types (T) of evidence to answer such a question. A worked example for a PICO(T) question is shown in Box 1.

Box 1 Components of an Answerable Question: Example

As part of NCD prevention strategic planning, health promotion policymakers are interested in understanding what interventions had shown to be effective at increasing fruit and vegetable intake among children, in particular in socioeconomically disadvantaged communities. The question formulated is:

- *What community-based interventions are effective at enhancing access to fruit and vegetables among children 5–18 years old, particularly for those in socioeconomically disadvantaged areas?*

  The PICO(T) concepts defined within the answerable question are:

- Population: *Children 5–18 years old, socioeconomically disadvantaged communities.*
- Intervention: *Community-based interventions designed to increase fruit and vegetable access.*

(continued)

Box 1 (continued)
- Comparison or Control: *No intervention.*
- Outcomes: *Access to fruit and vegetables.*
- (Types of research studies/evaluations): *Randomized or quasi-randomized controlled trials (RCTs) and cluster RCTs, non-randomized studies, controlled before-and-after studies, and interrupted-time-series (ITS) (to assess changes that occur over time), and qualitative research emanating from included intervention studies to help contextualize the major findings, to help provide explanations (rather than causative understandings).*

As discussed in the previous section, an advisory group can be useful in the systematic review planning process. Similarly in a practice setting, even though you may ultimately be the only end-user of the answer to your question, acquiring advice from people with a range of experiences will ensure that your findings are relevant, generalizable and may even address the needs of other users. Hence, it may be valuable to establish an advisory group to assist in formulating a useful and answerable question. Members may include those who are familiar with the topic and include policy, funders, practitioners and potential recipients/community perspectives. Some examples of actual PICO questions developed in practice and policy settings that are likely to be generalizable to other users:
- *What interventions are considered "best practice" in promoting healthy eating and physical activity in schools?*
- *Do patient-targeted incentive interventions improve health behaviors and access to health services?*
- *Are mainstream health promotion interventions applicable and transferable to indigenous people?*

Questions About Health Inequalities

Health inequalities may be defined as "… differences which are unnecessary and avoidable but are also considered unfair and unjust" (Whitehead 1991). Many population-based disease prevention interventions may not be equally effective for all population subgroups (Lorenc et al. 2013). The effectiveness for the disadvantaged may be substantially lower.

To explore the evidence about interventions targeting disadvantaged groups or geographical areas, and to understand their outcomes on health equity, an answerable question can include key concepts to help facilitate a search. Evans and Brown (2003) suggest that there are a number of factors that may be used in classifying disadvantage, identifying categories of social differentiation, using the acronym PROGRESS-Plus (Kavanagh & Oliver 2008):

PROGRESS
- *Place of residence (e.g., rural or urban, area deprivation, housing characteristics)*
- *Race/ethnicity*
- *Occupation (e.g., professional, skilled, unskilled, unemployed)*
- *Gender*
- *Religion*
- *Education (e.g., level of education attained)*
- *Socioeconomic status*
- *Social capital (e.g., neighborhood, community, or family support)*

Plus additional categories such as:
- *Age*
- *Disability*
- *Sexual Orientation*
- *Other vulnerable groups (e.g., school non-attenders, young people in the criminal justice system, teenage parents, etc.)*
- *Socioeconomic status proxy measures (e.g., "IRSD" index of relative disadvantage* (Australian Bureau of Statistics 2006))

Examples of answerable questions including PROGRESS-Plus categories are shown in Box 2.

Searching for Literature Relevant to Preventing or Managing NCDs

Health promotion activities tend to be multifaceted, multidisciplinary, and increasingly cross-sectoral, which means that research and evaluation studies may be found in a wide range of electronic databases and online sources (Beahler et al. 2000; Grayson and Gomersall 2003; Jackson et al. 2005; Petticrew and Roberts 2006). Language and terminology

Box 2 Examples of Answerable Questions Developed for Decision-Making About Health Equity

- *What interventions are effective for promoting physical activity and healthy eating among people with disabilities and their carers?*
- *Are lay-person led chronic disease prevention interventions effective among culturally diverse groups?*
- *What is the effectiveness of obesity prevention interventions in pre-adolescents and adolescents in a rural or remote setting?*

around NCDs and health promotion frequently change, which adds to the complexity of searching for relevant literature. Also, many evaluations of health promotion interventions are never published in peer-reviewed journals. This information is referred to as "grey literature" and may be found in reports to or for government or nongovernment agencies, books, or chapters in books. This section provides both an overview of how literature is identified for inclusion in reviews, and a practical guide to finding reviews useful to health promotion decision-making.

How Health Promotion Evidence Is Identified for Reviews

A variety of approaches are used to evaluate health promotion activities (Nutbeam 1998; Raphael 2000; Nebot 2006) and as a consequence, the range of research studies included in an evidence review may vary considerably. For reviewers synthesizing evidence of health promotion interventions into reviews, finding all the relevant studies is much more complicated than retrieving clinical health studies, due to literature being scattered across a range of sources (Peersman and Oakley 2001). Reviewers need to use retrieval methods other than database searching to identify relevant studies. For example, a review promoting a shift from cars to

walking or cycling found only 4 of 69 relevant papers in major health databases such as Medline [34]. Difficulties also arise because terminology is imprecise and constantly changing [32].

As discussed in the previous section, a systematic review question should be carefully formulated and clearly written. Then, the types of study designs needed to answer the questions should follow naturally, rather than relying on a "hierarchy" of evidence to select study designs for inclusion in a review (Petticrew and Roberts 2003). For example, a question about the effectiveness of dietary salt restriction for preventing cardiovascular risk is best answered by systematic reviews, then randomized controlled trial (RCT) designs; whereas a question about the acceptability of nutrition policy in family day care settings is more likely to be answered by surveys or qualitative studies. Indeed, for many health promotion interventions, RCT-evaluations may not be available, due to issues of feasibility and ethics. An initial "scoping" search will assist in identifying study designs commonly used to address the question of interest in a particular topic area (Armstrong et al. 2007). In addition, depending on the purpose of the evidence review, the importance of including RCT-level evidence in an evidence review may vary (Moore and Moore 2011; Roberts et al. 2012). For example, a policy agency may have a broad question of interest, to be addressed by a broad scoping review. For instance, RCT-level evidence may not be considered important or relevant in addressing a question such as "What primary prevention programs have been implemented successfully in rural and remote communities?".

Qualitative studies are now more commonly included in systematic reviews of health promotion effectiveness studies, as qualitative research offers experiential information such as people's experiences (Evans and Fitzgerald 2002) or views (Harden et al. 2004). For example, qualitative research may be useful for exploring barriers and facilitators to breastfeeding among young mothers; or the applicability of chronic disease self-management programs among indigenous peoples.

When searching databases for a review, the key components of an electronic database search strategy should comprise *subject headings* and *textwords* to describe each element of the answerable PICO question. This is because subject headings may not be well developed for many of the topics we are interested in. The search strategy developed will not search the entire full-text of the article, therefore searching subject headings and textwords in the abstract will assist in finding relevant studies.

Hand-searching is important for reviewers in identifying further literature for a review due to the delay between publication of a journal and its appearance on an electronic database. There is little empirical evidence to confirm which journals are likely to retrieve the greatest number of high quality studies (Armstrong et al. 2005; Jackson et al. 2005). Sources to be hand-searched may be sourced from:

- Key journals in your area of interest that are not indexed in Medline/PubMed.
- Amedeo   http://amedeo.com/medicine/smo. htm (provides weekly literature overviews in some topic areas/journals related to health promotion).
- The Lamar Soutter Library list (Lamar Soutter Library 2004) (list of public health journals compiled by the University of Massachusetts Medical School contains 710 journals).
- The Core Public Health Journals list (Core Public Health Journal Project 2004) (list compiled by Yale University contains 644 journals).
- The Effective Public Health Practice Project (EPHPP) in Canada has found in the conduct of their reviews that the most productive journals to handsearch for health promotion articles are the following: *American Journal of Health Promotion, American Journal of Preventive Medicine, American Journal of Public Health, Canadian Journal of Public Health, BMJ.* Other useful journals include *Annual Review of Public Health, Health Education and Behavior (formerly Health Education Quarterly), Health Education Research, JAMA, Preventive Medicine, Public Health Reports, Social Science and Medicine.*

As discussed earlier, many health promotion intervention evaluations/studies are never published. Therefore, a range of other sources will need to be explored in order to identify relevant unpublished reports relevant to the review question, including:

- Trials registers and trials results registers, e.g., http://apps.who.int/trialsearch/
- Grey literature databases such as the System for Information on Grey Literature in Europe http://www.opengrey.eu/
- TRIP database http://www.tripdatabase.com
- Other sources of health promotion grey literature:
  - Relevant organizations that may hold reports, Government reports (which may contain relevant studies, or references to them)
  - Google Scholar http://scholar.google.com

In reviewing the evidence, a search needs to be *sensitive* and *specific* in order to retrieve all relevant studies and exclude irrelevant items. For example, when searching for articles on smoking cessation, a sensitive search would find every article that relates to smoking cessation, even though some of the articles may not be completely relevant; and a *specific* search excludes irrelevant articles. If the search results in too many results it is likely that your search is not *specific* (imprecise), but then there is less risk that relevant articles have been missed. If a search reveals too few studies, it may be due to the search being *too specific*, or there is simply a lack of evidence on that topic.

Locating Evidence Reviews Relevant to Health Promotion and NCD Prevention Policy and Practice

Before embarking on searching for individual research articles, it is important to determine if the topic has already been reviewed, which will save a lot of time in the evidence gathering process. Searching for primary studies on health promotion topics can be very time-intensive, as search strategies will need to be adapted for a number of

Table 20.1 Web sites containing evidence reviews relevant to health promotion and NCD prevention

Cochrane Collaboration	www.thecochranelibrary.com
	Also, a number of health promotion and public health topics are listed on the Cochrane Public Health Group Web site: www.ph.cochrane.org
Health-evidence (Canada)	http://health-evidence.org
The Evidence for Policy and Practice Information (EPPI) and Co-ordinating Centre (UK)	www.eppi.ioe.ac.uk
	Navigate to "Databases" to search the Database of Promoting Health Effectiveness Reviews (DoPHER); or browse by topic within "Knowledge library"
Centre for Reviews and Dissemination (UK)	www.york.ac.uk/inst/crd
Guide to Community Preventive Services (The Community Guide) (USA)	www.thecommunityguide.org
The National Library for Public Health (NLPH), National Institute for Health and Clinical Excellence (NICE) (UK)	http://www2.evidence.nhs.uk/search-and-browse
	http://www.nice.org.uk/guidance
The Campbell Collaboration	www.campbellcollaboration.org
Effective Public Health Practice Project (EPHPP) (Canada)	www.ephpp.ca/ourwork.html
Sax Institute (Australia)	www.saxinstitute.org.au
	Browse "Evidence check reviews"

databases, and broad searches using a wide range of terms may result in a large number of citations. In part, this is due to health promotion terminology being non-standardized, i.e., day-to-day words are often used to describe populations, interventions and outcomes.

There are a number of online sources of high quality, freely available systematic reviews of health promotion and NCD prevention interventions, which can be searched using simple keywords, or by a more advanced search. Whether using a simple or advanced search, the keywords should be guided by an answerable question including PICO concepts. A list of Web sites containing freely available reviews is shown in Table 20.1.

If you are unable to identify any reviews that address your particular question, you need to develop a search strategy to locate individual primary studies. More detailed information on how to conduct a systematic literature search of relevant literature can be found in a set of guidelines for conducting reviews of health promotion

and public health interventions by Armstrong and colleagues of the Cochrane Public Health Group Armstrong et al. (2007). It may also be useful to find the citations of key articles in PubMed (http://www.pubmed.gov/) and review the related articles suggested, to find other relevant studies that may help determine additional relevant subject headings and textwords. Conducting an advanced search in PubMed is also a good option where organizations and individuals do not have a paid subscription to electronic databases. A range of electronic databases may be consulted for identifying health promotion evidence such as those listed in Box 3.

Finding Evidence from Across Sectors and Countries

As described in Chap. 21 in the context of planning cross-sectoral programs, promoting health and preventing NCDs requires action across sectors in partnership. Success in health promotion interven-

Box 3 Electronic Databases Relevant to Public Health and Health Promotion

(Web sites listed for databases available freely via the Internet):

Psychology	PsycINFO/PscyLIT
Biomedical	CINAHL, LILACS (Latin American Caribbean Health Sciences Literature) http://www.bireme.br/bvs/I/ibd.htm, Web of Science, Medline, EMBASE, CENTRAL, Combined Health Information Database (CHID) http://chid.nih.gov/, Chronic Disease Prevention Database (CDP) http://www.cdc.gov/cdp/, SCOPUS
Sociology	Sociofile, Sociological Abstracts, Social Science Citation Index, Social Policy and Practice
Education	ERIC (Educational Resources Information Center), C2-SPECTR (Campbell Collaboration Social, Psychological, Educational and Criminological Trials Register)
	http://www.campbellcollaboration.org, REEL (Research Evidence in Education Library, EPPI-Centre) http://eppi.ioe. ac.uk
Transport	NTIS (National Technical Information Service), TRIS (Transport Research Information Service) http://ntl.bts.gov/tris, IRRD (International Road Research Documentation), TRANSDOC (from ECMT (European Conference of Ministers of Transport)
Physical activity	SportsDiscus
HP/PH	BiblioMap, TRoPHI (Trials Register of Promoting Health Interventions) and DoPHER (Database of Promoting Health Effectiveness Reviews) (EPPI-Centre) http://eppi.ioe.ac.uk, Public Health electronic Library (National Institute for Health and Clinical Excellence) http://www.phel.gov.uk/, Global Health
Other	Popline (population health, family planning)
	http://db.jhuccp.org/popinform/basic.html, Enviroline (environmental health)—available on Dialog, Toxfile (toxicology)—available on Dialog, Econlit (economics), NGC (National Guideline Clearinghouse) http://www.guideline.gov/
Qualitative	ESRC Qualitative Data Archival Resource Centre (QUALIDATA) (http://www.qualidata.essex.ac.uk), Database of Interviews on Patient Experience (DIPEX) (http://www.dipex.org)

tions that require multi-sectoral cooperation depends on a collaborative approach to gathering and applying evidence (Armstrong et al. 2006). Hence, when consulting with the evidence to inform decisions about health promotion implementation, information from a range of sectors and partners is necessary. Interventions and investments delivered in nonhealth sectors can have an important, measurable impact upon public health. For example, the effects of changes to street-scale urban design on population levels of physical activity (Heath et al. 2006; Giles-Corti et al. 2012). To capture this sort of evidence, searching for information from many sectors may be necessary including for instance urban planning, development, architecture, and engineering.

The use of multisectoral interventions also raises the issue of what should "count" as evidence for decision-making across sectors, and what part it plays in the decision-making process.

There may be challenges in using evidence when working across sectors, due to varying extent to which research evidence is valued and used among sectors outside health promotion and disease prevention settings (Armstrong et al. 2006; Roberts et al. 2012). Correspondingly, there may also be challenges in understanding how to integrate findings from research and evaluation with other types of evidence that are useful for decision-makers such as economic modelling.

There are a range of issues for low and middle income countries (LMICs) in preventing and managing NCDs, which will be described in Chap. 28. A key concern is about how evidence is developed and used in LMICs (McQueen 2001). Much of the research evidence and evidence reviews originate from resource-rich or predominantly English-speaking countries. A number of groups internationally are working towards building health promotion evidence to support LMICs, by developing guidelines for evidence reviews. For example The Cochrane Collaboration, The Campbell Collaboration, and other producers of systematic reviews are committed to ensure that all systematic reviews consider and address the needs of LMICs as much as possible. The Cochrane Public Health Group (Armstrong et al. 2007; Waters et al. 2011a) suggest measures including:

- Incorporation of multiple forms of evidence beyond randomized control trials
- A comprehensive search strategy including languages other than English and includes non-English publication sources
- Subgroup analyses—comparisons of outcomes across different population groups, e.g., low vs. high socioeconomic status
- Reporting of contextual and process related factor (such as cultural appropriateness of the interventions reviewed, skills and resources required to implement an intervention, characteristics of the target population (e.g., socioeconomic, cultural, literacy levels, place of residence)
- Cost and cost-effectiveness data.

Critical Appraisal and Strength of Evidence

How Individual Studies Are Appraised for Synthesis

The evidence synthesis process involves bringing together information from a range of sources. Do we treat all forms of evidence equally? What if studies addressing similar questions report conflicting findings? When using research studies/evaluations to inform decisions and recommendations, methodologically sound research should be used. Practice decisions should not be informed by findings from poorly designed studies/evaluations—the findings may not be trustworthy. Further, it cannot be assumed that because the study is published by a highly regarded journal or author, that the results of the study are trustworthy.

Critical appraisal is a term used to refer to the process of assessing individual studies using explicit, transparent methods to consider aspects of their methodological approach that are important for interpreting findings reliably. There are many terms used to describe parts or all of this process that are often used interchangeably which can lead to confusion (e.g., risk of bias assessment, quality assessment, trustworthiness, strength of evidence); however put most simply any critical appraisal of a research study should consider two dimensions of validity: internal validity and external validity.

Internal validity refers to how correctly the study answers its own research question. In other words, are the results or effects shown likely to be true? Would we expect to see the same results if the same study was conducted again in the same setting, population and context? Once a judgment is made about the internal validity of a study, it is just as important to consider the value/relevance of the research question and how likely it is that those outcomes would be achieved in another population, setting or context of interest. This is dependent on the intended purpose or application for which the research is being used.

For example, whether a group-based diabetes prevention program tested in a clinical research setting would be feasible and effective on a community scale, and/or in lower-income country contexts. Without internal validity, external validity is irrelevant. If a study is not internally valid, the question of whether not those findings can be applied in another context is immaterial, given we are not able to say with any confidence what the findings are.

The criteria used to appraise research evidence will depend on the type of research evidence being examined, in particular the study design. A list of critical appraisal tools is provided for users of research evidence and reviews in Box 4. Note that some tools are for appraising reviews and some

are for appraising individual studies, depending on what you are working with. Such tools are most commonly applied in the context of appraising published studies; however, the issues highlighted also apply to unpublished reports and many of these tools contain questions that are appropriate to consider when assessing such material.

Although many of the appraisal criteria commonly used for evaluating health promotion interventions have evolved from clinical contexts, alternative appraisal tools have been expanded to accommodate the nature of health promotion interventions and encompass the requirements of a credible and comprehensive evaluation of an intervention (Rychetnik et al. 2002). These tools appraise not only the internal validity of a research

Box 4 Critical Appraisal Tools	
Systematic reviews	health-evidence quality assessment tool for assessing systematic reviews: http://health-evidence.org (Navigate to "SEARCH" then "Our appraisal tools")
	CASP (Critical Appraisal Skills program)—ten questions to help make sense of reviews: http://www.casp-uk.net/wp-content/ uploads/2011/11/CASP_Systematic_Review_Appraisal_ Checklist_14oct10.pdf
Quantitative studies (interventions)	Cochrane Risk of Bias tool (for randomized controlled trials; see Chap. 8 of The Cochrane Handbook http://www.cochrane-handbook.org/)
	Cochrane EPOC Risk of bias tools for studies with a separate control group (randomized controlled trials, non-randomized controlled trials, controlled before-and-after studies) and interrupted time series http://epoc.cochrane.org/sites/epoc. cochrane.org/files/uploads/Suggested%20risk%20of%20 bias%20criteria%20for%20EPOC%20reviews.pdf
	CASP appraisal tools for quantitative study designs http://www. casp-uk.net/
	Effective Public Health Practice Project Quality Assessment tool for quantitative studies http://www.ephpp.ca/Tools.html
Qualitative studies	CASP appraisal tool for Qualitative Research http://www. casp-uk.net/wp-content/uploads/2011/11/CASP_Qualitative_ Appraisal_Checklist_14oct10.pdf
	Spencer L, Ritchie J, Lewis J, Dillon L. Quality in Qualitative Evaluation: A framework for assessing research evidence. Government Chief Social Researcher's Office. Crown Copyright, 2003. http://www.civilservice.gov.uk/wp-content/ uploads/2011/09/a_quality_framework_tcm6-38740.pdf

reported, but they also consider the application to health promotion practice. These tools will be explored in Chap. 21 within applicability.

As the goal of evidence synthesis is to consider a body of evidence to answer a question, there is a need to move beyond appraising individual studies to consider the collection of individual studies as a whole, in order to make overall recommendations. The most widely accepted method for evaluating a body of evidence of the effectiveness of interventions is the Grades of Recommendation, Assessment, Development, and Evaluation (GRADE) (http://www.gradeworkinggroup.org/index.htm). The GRADE method is designed to incorporate considerations of internal validity (study design, methodological quality) with external validity (consistency, directness) and combine these into a judgment about the overall quality of the evidence in terms of "the extent of our confidence that the estimates of effect are correct" (Balshem et al. 2011). The strength of recommendation for action is considered separately based on the anticipated desirable and undesirable consequences, quality of evidence, values/preferences, and resource use (Guyatt et al. 2008), meaning that a low quality body of evidence can still give rise to a strong recommendation and vice versa. Another advantage to using systematic reviews as opposed to individual studies to inform policy and practice is that systematic reviews will consider the overall body of evidence.

Trustworthiness of Health Promotion Evidence Reviews

Systematic reviews normally include a critical appraisal step so that the evidence included within them has been appraised; however, a systematic review is a form of research and there will be variations in methodological quality, relevance, and value. As for individual studies, we can find systematic reviews posing similar questions that may present differing conclusions about the evidence. It is important to examine how these differences might arise if review findings are to be applied

in practice and policy. This means that the evidence user will also need to appraise systematic reviews when using them to inform decisions. As with individual studies, there are tools available to guide appraisal of systematic reviews.

In Box 4, we have included two critical appraisal tools that can be used for appraising systematic reviews. In Box 5, we provide an example of a completed version of one of those tools: the Health Evidence quality assessment tool. The value of this tool is that it is relatively quick and easy to complete and the questions are a helpful guide for evidence review users to consider important elements of the review process that may differ between reviews. Health Evidence (www.health-evidence.org) maintains an online repository of systematic reviews that are accompanied with evidence summaries of what each review shows as well as quality assessment ratings.

Conclusion

To understand the effectiveness of NCD prevention and health promotion initiatives that have been previously evaluated, reviews of the evidence are a useful resource for research users and researchers alike. This chapter has provided you with an overview of the key elements of the systematic review process. We have identified the links between these steps; so the way in which a question is asked will drive the search for evidence which will in turn impact on the scope of studies included and synthesized. Using systematic reviews should always be a priority for those making decisions, including those relevant to NCDs, as they synthesize a body of evidence they provide an overarching picture of the current state of available evidence. Systematic reviews also incorporate an appraisal of the potential risk of bias which gives a sense of how trustworthy a body of evidence and so give insight in to its scope for further application. Systematic reviews are one form of evidence likely to be used in NCD decision-making processes. Understanding how they are developed is useful in understanding the contribution they might make to your practice.

Box 5 Example of a Completed Health-Evidence Quality Assessment Tool for Appraising Systematic Reviews

Quality Assessment Tool		
Criterion	Yes	No
1. Did the authors have a clearly focused question [population, intervention (strategy), and outcome(s)]?	Yes	
2. Were appropriate inclusion criteria used to select primary studies?	Yes	
3. Did the authors describe a search strategy that was comprehensive? (Check all strategies used) ☑ Health Databases ☐ Hand Searching ☑ Psychological Databases ☑ Key Informants ☑ Social Science Databases ☑ Reference Lists ☐ Educational Databases ☑ Unpublished Other:	Yes	
4. Did search strategy cover an adequate number of years?	Yes	
For question 5, 6 and 8, please choose the column relating to the appropriate methodology. *Only fill out the column that applies.*		
5. *Quantitative reviews:* Did the authors describe the level of evidence in the primary studies included in the review? ☐ Level I (RCTs only) ☑ Level II (non-randomized, cohort, case-control studies) ☐ Level III (uncontrolled studies) 5. *Qualitative reviews:* Do the authors provide a clear description of the range of methods in each of the primary studies included in the review?	Yes	
6. *Quantitative reviews:* Did the review assess the methodological quality of the primary studies including: (minimum requirement: 4/7 of the following) ☑ research design ☑ study sample ☐ participation rates ☑ source of bias(confounders, respondent bias) 6. *Qualitative reviews:* Did the review assess the methodological quality of the primary studie including: (minimum requirement: 4/7 of the following) ☐ suitablity of methodology/paradigm to the research question ☐ sampling (selection of participants/settings/documentation) ☐ clear description of context, data collection, and data analysis	Yes	

Box 5 (continued)

□ data collection (measurement of independent/dependent variables) ☑ follow-up/attrition rates □ data analysis	□ rigor: □ i) audit trail □ ii) some coding by 2 or more coders, if appropriate □ iii) deviant case analysis (negative cases) □ iv) respondant validation (member checking) □ triangulation □ reflexivity (researcher and research process) □ relevance (credibility, consistency, applicability, transferability)		
7. Are the results of the review transparent?		Yes	
8. *Quantitative reviews:* Was it appropriate to combine the findings of results across studies?	8. *Qualitative reviews:* Is there a description of how reviewers determined results were similar enough across studies to compare or combine them?	Yes	
9. Were appropriate methods used for combining or comparing results across studies?			No
10. Does the data support the author's interpretation?		Yes	
TOTAL SCORE = 9			

References

Anderson, L. M., Petticrew, M., Rehfuess, E., Armstrong, R., Ueffing, E., Baker, P., et al. (2011). Using logic models to capture complexity in systematic reviews. *Research Synthesis Methods, 2*(1), 33–42.

Armstrong, R., Doyle, J., Lamb, C., & Waters, E. (2006). Multi-sectoral health promotion and public health: The role of evidence. *Journal of Public Health, 28*(2), 168–172.

Armstrong, R., Jackson, N., Doyle, J., Waters, E., & Howes, F. (2005). It's in your hands: The value of handsearching in conducting systematic reviews of public health interventions. *Journal of Public Health, 27*(4), 388–391.

Armstrong, R., Waters, E., Roberts, H., Anderson, L., Oliver, S., & Petticrew, M. (2008). Systematic reviews in public health. In K. Heggenhougen & S. Quah (Eds.), *International encyclopedia of public health* (Vol. 1, pp. 297–301). San Diego, CA: Academic Press.

Armstrong, R., Waters, E, Jackson, N, Oliver, S, Popay, J, Shepherd, et al. (2007). *Guidelines for systematic reviews of health promotion and public health interventions.* http://ph.cochrane.org/sites/ph.cochrane.org/files/uploads/Guidelines%20HP_PH%20reviews.pdf. Accessed 1 Sept 2012.

Australian Bureau of Statistics. (2006). 2039.0—Information paper: An introduction to socio-economic indexes for areas (SEIFA). B. Pink. Canberra: Australian Bureau of Statistics. Commonwealth of Australia. http://www.abs.gov.au.

Balshem, H., Helfand, M., Schünemann, H. J., Oxman, A. D., Kunz, R., Brozek, J., et al. (2011). GRADE guidelines: 3. Rating the quality of evidence. *Journal of Clinical Epidemiology, 64*(4), 401–406.

Beahler, C. C., Sundheim, J. J., & Trapp, N. I. (2000). Information retrieval in systematic reviews: Challenges in the public health arena. *American Journal of Preventive Medicine, 18*(4), 6–10.

Core Public Health Journal Project. (2004). *Core public health journal project (Ver 0.9)*. Retrieved March 18, 2005, from www.med.yale.edu/eph/library/phjournals.

Evans, D., & Fitzgerald, M. (2002). The experience of physical restraint: A systematic review of qualitative research. *Contemporary Nurse, 13*(2–3), 126–135.

Evans, T., & Brown, H. (2003). Road traffic crashes: Operationalizing equity in the context of health sector reform. *Injury Control and Safety Promotion, 10*(1–2), 11–12.

Giles-Corti, B., Ryan, K., & Foster, S. (2012). Increasing density in Australia: Maximising the health benefits and minimising harm. *Melbourne, Report to The National Heart Foundation of Australia*. www.heartfoundation.org.au.

Grayson, L., & Gomersall, A. (2003). *A difficult business: Finding the evidence for social science reviews*. London: ESRC UK Centre for Evidence Based Policy and Practice, Queen Mary University of London. Working paper 19.

Guyatt, G. H., Oxman, A. D., Kunz, R., Falck-Ytter, Y., Vist, G. E., Liberati, A., et al. (2008). Going from evidence to recommendations. *British Medical Journal, 336*(7652), 1049–1051.

Harden, A., Garcia, J., Oliver, S., Rees, R., Shepherd, J., Brunton, G., et al. (2004). Applying systematic review methods to studies of people's views: An example from public health research. *Journal of Epidemiology and Community Health, 58*(9), 794–800.

Heath, G. W., Brownson, R. C., Kruger, J., Miles, R., Powell, K. E., Ramsey, L. T., & the Task Force on Community Preventive Services. (2006). The effectiveness of urban design and land use and transport policies and practices to increase physical activity: A aystematic review. *Journal of Physical Activity and Health, 3*(Suppl 1), S55–S76.

Higgins, J. & Green, S., (Eds.). (2006). Cochrane handbook for systematic reviews of interventions. In *The cochrane library*. Chichester: John Wiley & Sons, Ltd.

Husk, K., Lovell, R., Cooper, C., & Garside, R. (2013). Participation in environmental enhancement/conservation activities for health and well-being in adults (Protocol). *Cochrane Database of Systematic Reviews, 2*.

Jackson, N., & Baker, P. (2005). *Evidence based practice in public health: Workbook, Central Area Population Health Services, and Cochrane Public Health Group*. http://ph.cochrane.org/workshops-and-events.

Jackson, N., Gupta, S., Howes, F., Armstrong, R., Brunton, G., Rees, R., et al. (2005). *Handsearching for health promotion and public health trials and systematic reviews*. XIII Cochrane Colloquium, Melbourne, Australia.

Kavanagh, J., & Oliver, S. (2008). Reflections on developing and using PROGRESS-Plus. *Equity update: Cochrane Health Equity Field and Campbell Equity Methods Group*. Ottawa, ON, Cochrane Health Equity Field 2.

Lamar Soutter Library. (2004). *The Lamar Soutter Library*. Retrieved March 2005, from http://library.umassed.edu/ebpph.

Lorenc, T., Petticrew, M., Welch, V., & Tugwell, P. (2013). What types of interventions generate inequalities? Evidence from systematic reviews. *Journal of Epidemiology and Community Health, 67*(2), 190–193.

McQueen, D. V. (2001). Strengthening the evidence base for health promotion. *Health Promotion International, 16*(3), 261–268.

Moore, L., & Moore, G. F. (2011). Public health evaluation: Which designs work, for whom and under what circumstances? *Journal of Epidemiology and Community Health, 65*(7), 596–597.

Nebot, M. (2006). Health promotion evaluation and the principle of prevention. *Epidemiology and Community Health, 60*(1), 5–6.

Nutbeam, D. (1998). Evaluating health promotion—Progress, problems and solutions. *Health Promotion International, 13*(1), 27–44.

Oxman, A., & Guyatt, G. (1993). The science of reviewing research. *Annals of the New York Academy of Sciences, 703*, 125–133.

Peersman, G., & Oakley, A. (2001). Learning from research. In S. Oliver & G. Peersman (Eds.), *Using research for effective health promotion*. Buckingham: Open University Press.

Petticrew, M., & Roberts, H. (2003). Evidence, hierarchies, and typologies: Horses for courses. *Journal of Epidemiology and Community Health, 57*(7), 527–529.

Petticrew, M., & Roberts, H. (2006). *Systematic reviews in the social sciences*. Oxford: Blackwell Publishing Ltd.

Proctor, E., Silmere, H., Raghavan, R., Hovmand, P., Aarons, G., Bunger, A., et al. (2011). Outcomes for implementation research: Conceptual distinctions, measurement challenges, and research agenda. *Administration and Policy in Mental Health and Mental Health Services Research, 38*(2), 65–76.

Raphael, D. (2000). The question of evidence in health promotion. *Health Promotion International, 15*(4), 355–367.

Roberts, H., Petticrew, M., Liabo, K., & Macintyre, S. (2012). 'The Anglo-Saxon disease': A pilot study of the barriers to and facilitators of the use of randomised controlled trials of social programmes in an international context. *Journal of Epidemiology and Community Health, 66*(11), 1025–1029.

Rychetnik, L., Frommer, M., Hawe, P., & Shiell, A. (2002). Criteria for evaluating evidence on public health interventions. *Journal of Epidemiology and Community Health, 56*(2), 119–127.

Rychetnik, L., Hawe, P., Waters, E., Barratt, A., & Frommer, M. (2004). A glossary for evidence based public health. *Journal of Epidemiology and Community Health, 58*(7), 538–545.

Waters, E., Armstrong, R., Doyle, J., Pettman, T., Hall, B., Priest, N. et al. (2011a). 7: Evidence in public health. In H. Keleher & C. MacDougall (Eds.), *Understanding health promotion*. South Melbourne, VIC: Oxford University Press.

Waters, E., Hall, B. J., Armstrong, R., Doyle, J., Pettman, T. L., & de Silva-Sanigorski, A. (2011b). Essential components of public health evidence reviews: Capturing intervention complexity, implementation, economics and equity. *Journal of Public Health, 33*(3), 462–465.

Watt, A., Cameron, A., Sturm, L., Lathlean, T., Babidge, W., Blamey, S., et al. (2008). Rapid reviews versus full systematic reviews: An inventory of current methods and practice in health technology assessment. *International Journal of Technology Assessment in Health Care, 24*, 133–139.

Whitehead, M. (1991). The concepts and principles of equity and health. *Health Promotion International, 6*(3), 217–228.

Tahna Pettman, Rebecca Armstrong, Belinda Burford, Jodie Doyle, Laurie Anderson, and Elizabeth Waters

Introduction

In planning for implementation of NCD prevention and health promotion initiatives, a range of factors are at play in practice and policy contexts including for example resources, political climate, and public or community views. However, critical to the success and safety of health promotion interventions is the application of evidence, that is, knowledge about what past investments *work*, for *whom* and *why*, under which circumstances, and at what cost. Although it may be challenging to integrate research evidence within a contemporary knowledge of population factors, views, politics, and other contextual information, it is not impossible. An example from the field of NCD prevention that most clearly demonstrates this is tobacco control-successful interventions

T. Pettman, B.H.Sc., Ph.D.(✉) • R. Armstrong, M.P.H., Ph.D. • B. Burford, B.Sc. (Hons), Ph.D.
J. Doyle, Grad. Dip. Health Prom., M.P.H.
E. Waters, M.P.H., D.Phil.
Melbourne School of Population and Global Health, The University of Melbourne, 207 Bouverie Street, Carlton, Victoria 3010, Australia
e-mail: tpettman@unimelb.edu.au;
armr@unimelb.edu.au; jdoyle@unimelb.edu.au;
belinda@burford.co;
ewaters@unimelb.edu.au

L. Anderson, M.P.H., Ph.D.
Department of Epidemiology, School of Public Health, University of Washington, 2838 Burnaby Park SE, Olympia, Washington, DC, 98501, USA
e-mail: lmander@u.washington.edu

and activities have been adapted and implemented according to context and politics whilst underpinned by theory and strong empirical evidence. This process of combining different types of evidence (empirical, experiential, tacit, etc.) is the hallmark of what may be referred to as *evidence-informed* decision-making. Building upon recognised models of evidence-based practice (Dawes et al. 2005), evidence-informed decision-making in health policy and practice involves the incorporation of best available evidence in the context of all other political and organizational factors (Jewell and Bero 2008).

As the calibre and timeliness of monitoring and evaluation of interventions increase, the body of knowledge about health promotion effectiveness grows incrementally. Views on the type of evidence and corresponding debates have masked the essential need to understand *how* and *why* strategies work, and what information is essential to decision-makers in making the best decision in relation to changes that have emerged in population health across the globe. Not only are governments and non-government organizations keen to make decisions that are likely to be beneficial, but increasingly health promotion and public health practitioners are being asked to demonstrate that their work has measurable benefits to the public (McQueen 2002). Similarly, it is important to know that interventions do not cause harm (Macintyre and Petticrew 2000).

The volume of information generated from research and evaluation has increased markedly across the NCD prevention and health promotion field, spanning behaviour change, improving environments for health, and reducing the burden of disease and injury foci. The amount of primary research and evaluation studies drives a need for this knowledge to be synthesised and summarised in an efficient, consistent and timely way, to better support decision-making in policy and practice (Armstrong et al. 2008). The challenge of evidence-informed decision-making in the fields of NCD prevention and health promotion is the drawing together of a diverse range of evaluations that use different types of research methods, from various research paradigms and contexts, to help answer a question (Rychetnik et al. 2002). This is where it becomes useful to consider reports that synthesise multiple research/evaluation studies in order to provide overall conclusions—known as *reviews* of evidence.

For several reasons, many of which were explored in Chap. 20 and are further illustrated in this chapter, systematic reviews of the effects of interventions provide a powerful tool for supporting decision-making about future NCD prevention and health promotion investments. Systematic reviews have long been recognised as a tool for health-care decision-making (The Cochrane Collaboration 2012) and more recently have begun evolving to meet the needs of *public health* decision-making contexts. Systematic reviews provide an essential tool for users of evidence, which aims to make the *decision to use evidence* more efficient. This chapter describes important elements of information to scan for when accessing systematic reviews, these elements representing information that is often required by decision-makers to inform decisions, planning, and implementation. It is hoped that, over time, more systematic reviews of NCD prevention and health promotion initiatives will include all the elements described.

It is also acknowledged that systematic reviews may not yet provide the answers to all the pressing issues in contemporary public health policy and practice. In the fields of health promotion and NCD prevention and management, the

types of questions are many and varied. Thus, a range of types of evidence will be necessary in decision-making. For simplicity, this chapter focuses on three key questions that may arise most frequently, which may be *answered* with different types of evidence: (1) What determinants (e.g. social, environmental) contribute to NCDs? (2) What interventions work (effectiveness)? (3) How do interventions work (including why, for whom, under what circumstances, at what cost)? Further, questions may relate to evidence on specific interventions (for instance, a review of the impact of school-based health promotion programs) or a broader range of interventions addressing specific problems (such as a review of interventions for type 2 diabetes prevention). A range of international research institutions and government agencies (such as The Cochrane Collaboration, the Centre for Reviews and Dissemination, the National Institute for Clinical Excellence) are broadening the scope of health promotion evidence by synthesising knowledge about complex interventions, from across sectors, to support policy and practice decision-making. Examples of recent Cochrane reviews of relevance to prevention and health promotion are provided at the end of this chapter. This chapter also proposes some key steps that practitioners can take to engage with and *use* research evidence, to inform and support their planning and implementation.

Essential Components of Evidence Reviews Relevant to NCDs

In order to be most useful for practice and policy decision-making, a range of information on process and outcomes should be included in systematic reviews, in order to answer questions about what investments and interventions work, why, for whom, under which circumstances, and at what cost (Waters et al. 2011). This section describes from a decision-making perspective what elements to look for in evidence reviews (and other research reports), as this information will assist in combining sources of evidence for decision-making for policy and practice.

Pathways Operating and Theoretical Underpinnings: Theoretical Frameworks/Logic Models

Health promotion and NCD prevention interventions are inherently complex-they are multifaceted and delivered in multiple settings targeting individuals, groups, organizations, and environments and systems. Take for example an intervention to reduce alcohol-related harm by limiting outlet density in a community. Initially it may sound like a simple intervention with one key component. However, consider that such an initiative would also comprise multiple components and engage a range of stakeholders in order to manage outlet-owner perceptions, change local government licensing procedures, align with state government regulations, gain support from the general public, respond to industry opposition, and develop responsible beverage service skills.

As interventions like these become more multifaceted, and thus more complex, it is important to reflect on the role theory plays. Health promotion and NCD prevention interventions are usually (and should be) based on a particular theory. However controversy remains about whether or not theory makes a difference to intervention effectiveness. Theories relevant to health promotion seek to explain mediators of change such as the following:

- Individual behaviour—examples include Stages of Change model (Prochaska and DiClemente 1982), Health Belief Model (Rosenstock 1974), Theory of Reasoned Action (Ajzen and Fishbein 1980), and Social cognitive theory (Bandura 1998)
- Interpersonal influences—examples include Social Learning Theory (Bandura 1971)
- Activities throughout communities—community organization theories, Organizational Change Theory, Diffusion of Innovations Theory (Rogers 1962), social-ecological theory (McLeroy et al. 1988)

A contemporary example of how interventions are informed by theory might be the application of the social-ecological model to community-based obesity prevention: applying this theory to practice in the "real world" acknowledges the complex interactions between individuals' behaviour and their broader environments that influence access to food and physical activity. Hence, the range of environments (physical, social, financial, political) would be considered, which would lead to a range of settings and stakeholders (e.g. child-care centres, recreation spaces and transit routes, food outlets) to be included in a multi-strategic intervention approach.

Where relevant theories are not available, logic models are useful in understanding intervention pathways. Logic models have long been used in understanding complex programs to improve health and social outcomes (McQueen 2001). Logic models may also be referred to as theoretical or conceptual frameworks and are a pictorial illustration of how an initiative (e.g. service, policy, or program) is designed to achieve its intended activities and outcomes. Logic models are important tools for program planning, evaluation, and more recently logic models have been acknowledged for their usefulness in synthesising public health evidence (Baxter et al. 2010; Anderson et al. 2011; Zaza et al. 2005).

When consulting with research evidence for decision-making, a logic model or a theoretical framework may or may not be explicitly stated. Rather, parts of theories may be used in conjunction with others, a dominant theory may be used with or without others, or a range of theories may be used to explain different intervention components. The impact of theory on intervention processes and impacts may not be formally collected. However, authors may reflect on the impact of theory within the intervention (Armstrong et al. 2007).

Program Implementation

Health promotion and disease-prevention initiatives often operate in contexts demanding recognition of political imperatives, service systems, funding flows, changes and shortages, intervention staff skills and competencies, and multi-strategic partnership approaches. The gap between information generated by research effectiveness studies versus policy and practice-relevant implementation knowledge needs to be overcome. Researchers involved in implementation research in health have been developing relatively simple approaches in order to understand the complexities within large-scale, "real-world" research studies and evaluations so that meaningful answers to important policy and practice questions can emerge (Waters et al. 2011). Quite often, questions in a practice or a policy setting are not about *what* works but *how* it works, *why*, for *whom*, and in what *circumstances*. For example, questions about implementation may look like the following:

- If healthy eating policies are likely to be effective at improving child nutrition status, *how* would this be implemented across a range of children's settings?
- If interpersonal violence is a determinant of health, *how* would we act upon this at the community level? *Who* would interventions target, and *what* would a multi-strategy approach look like?
- If we wish to change the built environment to promote walking and cycling, *how* do we modify existing urban planning laws at different levels of government to allow changes to take place?

Journal reporting standards such as the CONSORT guidelines and the TREND Statement call for intervention content to be described, but do not provide direction on what information should be collected about underlying theory or causal mechanisms, program or policy components and processes, or contextual factors (Moher et al. 2001; Des Jarlais et al. 2004). When consulting evidence reviews or original research to make decisions about the *how*, *why*, or *who* questions, there are a range of factors that reviews and research studies may have reported on in their process evaluations. These factors are summarised in Box 1 and are discussed in further detail in Applicability and Transferability of this chapter, to illustrate how this information can inform decision-making in policy and practice.

Applying Evidence to Health Promotion in Policy and Practice Settings

As mentioned briefly in appraising research evidence, the use of evidence for decision-making requires you to consider the context in which you are working. The following section introduces you to some approaches to assessing the relevance of research evidence to your setting and some options for dealing with the multiple sources of evidence that are characteristic of complex health promotion decisions.

Assessing Applicability and Transferability: The Importance of Context

Evidence reviews provide a summary of the evidence of effectiveness and will often try to provide detail about the implementation of these studies to aid replication. Information about implementation is often limited as it is not usually well described in primary studies. For example, in the childhood obesity review, only seven studies out of 55 included information about the cost of programs. This information is important for decision-makers.

There are a number of issues to consider when considering the applicability and transferability of research evidence from either reviews or primary studies to your setting. Variations in culture, geography, workforce skill, human resource capacity, and financial resources are to be expected. However, we know that it can be useful to consider evidence beyond that generated in our own neighbourhood, community, or country. This helps to drive the innovation that is characteristic of health promotion.

The use of research evidence to support decision-making requires consideration of both the applicability and transferability of that evidence to your setting. Applicability, or feasibility, refers to the *potential* of the implementation of an intervention. For example, a worksite capacity building program to promote health and safety

Box 1 Implementation factors that may be measured and reported in health promotion evidence (Armstrong et al. 2007; Proctor et al. 2011; Brownson et al. 2012)

- Acceptability (whether the characteristics of interventions are satisfactory or agreeable among the target population and related stakeholders)
- Adoption (uptake of the intervention in the relevant setting(s))
- Appropriateness (whether interventions are relevant to address a health issue)
- Cost (for participants, for implementation)
- Feasibility (suitability or practicability of the intervention to the setting(s), stakeholder readiness)
- Integrity or fidelity (whether the intervention was delivered as intended)
- Penetration (levels of spread of the intervention, e.g. through organizations, levels of policymaking)
- Reach (participation in the intervention)

Understanding Outcomes

NCD prevention and health promotion interventions have the potential to improve population health, and systematic reviews can determine the effectiveness of these interventions collectively in achieving their desired outcomes. Effectiveness and cost-effectiveness may be the most commonly measured outcomes of interventions. Well-intentioned interventions may cause harm and increase health inequalities unintentionally. Additionally, an intervention may be considered effective, but depending on the time over which evaluation occurs, the extent to which the intervention can be maintained or sustained beyond the intervention period may be unknown. Hence, equity, ethics, and sustainability are critical outcome issues for health promotion evidence.

Equity and Ethics

When reviewing the evidence on effectiveness of interventions for decision-making, outcomes of equity and ethical considerations should be taken into account. As a general rule, intervention effectiveness is measured in terms of the total number/population who benefit from the intervention. However, this takes no account of the distribution of those benefits (Hawe and Shiell 1995), and therefore does not address issues of health equity outcomes. For example, in reporting outcomes of population-level tobacco control interventions, overall improvements in smoking prevalence may be observed; however this may mask the differences among groups of the population such as young people and those who are socio-economically disadvantaged (Hiscock et al. 2012).

Even well-intentioned interventions may actually increase inequalities or cause harm (Macintyre and Petticrew 2000). To examine whether interventions address equity outcomes, evidence to look for includes:

- A valid measure of the health outcome (or change in health outcome)
- A measure of disadvantage (i.e. definitions of socio-economic position, urban/rural)
- A statistical measure for summarising the differential effectiveness

When seeking specific interventions that are reported to be effective or potentially effective at reducing inequalities, the evidence should define the interventions as:

- More effective for disadvantaged groups compared to advantaged groups
- Equally effective across the socio-economic spectrum (*potentially* effective reducing health inequalities due to the higher prevalence of health problems among the disadvantaged)
- Targeted only at disadvantaged groups and is effective

(continued)

(continued)

Systematic reviews of the evidence are uniquely placed to determine if the evidence exists for effective interventions to reduce global health inequity (Tugwell et al. 2010). As discussed in Chap. 20 in the context of formulating an answerable question to guide an evidence review, the acronym PROGRESS (Place, Race, Occupation, Gender, Religion, Education, Socioeconomic status, Social status) provides a relatively straightforward approach to standardising the way in which determinants of equity are examined and reported as outcomes (Kavanagh et al. 2008). Whether or not primary research studies have addressed equity explicitly in their outcome reporting, the PROGRESS framework can be used to facilitate searching and extracting this information from primary research during an evidence review.

To date, very few systematic reviews have focused on the effect of interventions on inequalities in health (Millward et al. 2001) although this is now starting to change, with the establishment of groups such as the Campbell and Cochrane Health Equity Methods Group (http://equity. cochrane.org/), and the Cochrane Public Health Group (http://ph.cochrane.org)

Sustainability

The long-term outcomes of NCD prevention programs and health promotion are often not fully realised due to factors affecting maintenance of the intervention's benefits, integration into settings, communities and systems, or a lack of capacity building in recipient settings (Shediac-Rizkallah and Bone 1998). Too often, health promotion practitioners are faced with short-term funding models for delivering programs and the sustainability of the initiative frequently goes unevaluated for this reason. Hence, evidence to inform decisions about what interventions are sustainable, why, and how is lacking.

Most often, sustainability is measured through the continued use of specified intervention components, beyond the time that external support or funding is terminated (Shediac-Rizkallah and Bone 1998; Brownson et al. 2012). For example, beyond the completion of a funded school-based healthy eating intervention, sustainability may be measured as the continuation of a canteen/tuck-shop food policy, fruit and vegetable "breaks" in classrooms, and professional development for school staff and teachers. Other outcomes of sustainability in health promotion interventions may include continued partnerships (e.g. across organizations, or communities), and policies or procedures becoming routinised.

Sustainability outcomes may be measured and reported in various ways in evidence reviews. A recent review identified 125 studies focusing on sustainability of new programs and innovations, finding that approximately half of the studies relied on self-reports to assess sustainability (or elements that influence sustainability), using both qualitative and quantitative methods, but that few studies employed rigorous methods of evaluation (e.g. objective evaluation, judgement of implementation quality, or fidelity) (Wiltsey Stirman et al. 2012). Influences on sustainability included organizational context, capacity, processes, and factors related to the new program or practice themselves. When using evidence for decision-making, it is useful to acknowledge the length of the studies or evaluations represented in the evidence, and consider how initiatives can be made more sustainable, to increase health outcome improvements.

among restaurant workers may not be feasible in some settings without first gaining support from restaurant owners, unions, and resources to support practice change. We are also interested in assessing the transferability or generalisability of study findings. That is, if we implemented a workplace health promotion program to improve cardiovascular health that was evaluated in a small-scale research setting, would we get the same results as were presented in the research evidence if applied to a larger scale community setting? Table 21.1 provides a useful set of questions to aid the consideration of applicability and transferability.

Combining Different Types of Evidence in Decision-Making: What to Consider

Combining a range of sources of evidence to inform decisions about NCD prevention is crucial. Systematic reviews will not provide all of the information we need to plan and implement programs. Approaches to combining different types of evidence require consideration of the type of decision and the partners involved.

Generally, when making decisions, you will be faced with three common questions:

- *What is the issue* (health problems/issues, priorities)?
- *What works* (what interventions are effective, cost-effective, equitable)?
- *How to implement* (processes of intervention implementation, barriers and enablers, experiences)?

These questions are applicable to a range of scenarios such as new funding rounds, emerging health priorities, emerging research evidence, and political imperatives. See Box 2.

Conclusions

In order to be certain that NCD prevention and health promotion initiatives are likely to be effective and do not cause harm, decisions should be informed by the best available research evidence. Systematic reviews are a powerful and mostly reliable tool to assist in this process as they summarise all high-quality evidence that addresses key practice questions. However, in order for systematic reviews and other types of research evidence to be useful to those working in NCD prevention and health promotion, essential information about theory, implementation, and outcomes is required. Applying evidence to practice and policy is challenging but can be made more efficient with the assistance of concepts of applicability and transferability, and by considering options for combining different types of evidence

Table 21.1 Considering context: The importance of applicability and transferability

Applicability

Does the political environment of the local society allow for this intervention to be implemented?

Is there any political barrier to implementing this intervention?

Which organization will be responsible for the provision of the intervention in the local setting? Is there any possible barrier to implementing this intervention due to the structure of that organization?

Would the general public and the targeted (sub) population accept this intervention? Does any aspect of the intervention go against local social norms? Is it ethically acceptable?

[a]Does the target population in the local setting have sufficient means (for example, educational, financial, social, geographical) to receive the contents of the intervention?

Can the contents of the intervention be tailored to suit the local culture?

Does the provider of the intervention in the local setting have the skill to deliver this intervention? If not will training be available?

Are the essential resources for implementing this intervention available in the local setting? (A list of essential resources may help to answer this question)

Transferability

What is the baseline prevalence of the health problem of interest in the local setting? What is the difference in prevalence between the study setting and the local setting?

Are the characteristics of the target population comparable between the study setting and the local setting? With regard to the particular aspects that will be addressed in the intervention, is it possible that the characteristics of the target population, such as ethnicity, socio-economic status, and educational level, will have an impact on the effectiveness of the intervention?

Is the capacity to implement the intervention comparable between the study setting and the local setting in such matters as political environment, social acceptability, resources, organizational structure, and the skills of the local providers?

[a]This question has been modified from the original question that appears in Wang et al. (2006)

Box 2 Combining different types of evidence in practice and policy settings— examples of scenarios

1. *After a period of extensive community consultation, you have decided to focus on healthy eating initiatives to address diabetes prevalence in your next strategic plan.*

   What works? You would need to consider systematic reviews, comparative intervention studies, and local evaluations.

   How to implement? Hypothetically you may find that healthy food policies and workforce capacity building initiatives *work* best; hence you would need evidence about how to implement such changes including training required, resources, settings to target, and infrastructure such as facilities for food outlets, policy templates, etc.

2. *A new funding round has been released to address social connections to improve health among isolated groups, and your organization is keen to work with people with a disability. You do not know much about this population group.*

   What is the issue? You would need to find data, surveys, or qualitative information describing the social issues experienced by people with an intellectual, physical, or psychiatric disability, and how this affects their physical and mental health.

   What works? You would need to find systematic reviews, comparative intervention studies, and local evaluations describing what programs and services have been evaluated to increase social connections and which have demonstrated health and well-being outcomes.

3. *You and your colleagues have just come across a research paper which talks about lowering speed limits in residential areas to prevent pedestrian injuries. It looks interesting, because it also suggests that this intervention may promote increased physical activity through walking.*

   What works? You would need to find systematic reviews describing the effectiveness of reducing speed limits on injuries and physical activity, compared with other traffic calming interventions.

4. *At a community meeting organized by the local council, a number of people suggest that changes be made to the walking tracks to encourage people to use them. Your manager asks you to consider options to bring back to the group.*

   What works? You would need to find systematic reviews describing the effectiveness of enhancing access to walking trails. Other options described in the evidence may include building exercise facilities, informational outreach, and providing access to existing local facilities.

   How to implement? Hypothetically you may find that a multi-strategy approach is most effective at enhancing access to walking tracks and hence you would need evidence about how to implement such changes to the built and natural environments, infrastructure required, cost, and associated social marketing/promotional efforts required.

Combining Different Types of Evidence in Decision-Making: Processes

Given that processes for decision-making vary considerably across organizations it is difficult to identify the "best" approach to assist in combining different types of evidence to inform decisions. Ideally, decisions should be transparent so that it is

(continued)

(continued)

clear that the various forms of evidence have at least been considered. Answering these three questions (as relevant) will aid this transparency. Some examples of generic organizational processes where asking these questions of the evidence could be incorporated are listed below:

- Team meetings
- Partnership meetings (e.g. when working across sectors and settings)
- Internal organization/staff meetings
- Strategic planning sessions
- Strategic plan/action plan/project plan templates
- Stakeholder consultations

There may also be merit in drawing on deliberative dialogue processes (face-to-face discussions where diverse individuals exchange and weigh ideas and opinions about the evidence on a topic for which they share an interest), and considering the value of a facilitator in these processes.

in decision-making. Organizational processes and systems are proposed, which are likely to be important in facilitating evidence-informed decision-making.

Further Reading: Selected Cochrane Reviews of Relevance to NCD Prevention and Health Promotion

As at September 2012. All reviews are available online at http://www.thecochranelibrary.com.

Child Health

- Community-based interventions for the prevention of burns and scalds in children
- Community-based supplementary feeding for promoting the growth of children under 5 years of age in low- and middle-income countries
- Group-based parent-training programmes for improving emotional and behavioural adjustment in children from birth to 3 years old
- Household interventions for preventing domestic lead exposure in children
- Individual- and group-based parenting programmes for improving psychosocial outcomes for teenage parents and their children
- Interventions for tobacco use prevention in indigenous youth
- Outreach strategies for expanding health insurance coverage in children

Consumer and Communication Strategies

- Email for clinical communication between health-care professionals
- Internet based interventions for smoking cessation
- Mobile phone messaging reminders for attendance at health-care appointments

Community Health

- Dietary advice with or without oral nutritional supplements for disease-related malnutrition in adults
- Electric fans for reducing adverse health impacts in heatwaves
- Exercise for improving balance in older people
- Increased consumption of fruits and vegetables for the primary prevention of cardiovascular diseases
- Interventions for preventing falls in older people living in the community
- Interventions for promoting physical activity
- Interventions to promote the wearing of hearing protection
- Reduced or modified dietary fat for preventing cardiovascular disease
- Transtheoretical model for dietary and physical exercise modification in weight loss management for overweight and obese adults

Effective Practice/Health Systems

- Audit and feedback: effects on professional practice and health-care outcomes
- Collaboration between local health and local government agencies for health improvement
- Decision aids for people facing health treatment or screening decisions
- Integration of HIV/AIDS services with maternal, neonatal, and child health, nutrition, and family planning services
- Interventions to improve the use of systematic reviews in decision-making by health system managers, policymakers, and clinicians
- Training health professionals in smoking cessation

Injury Prevention

- Home safety education and provision of safety equipment for injury prevention
- Safety education of pedestrians for injury prevention

Mental Health

- Group-based parent training programmes for improving parental psychosocial health

Oral Health

- Interventions for tobacco cessation in the dental setting

Pregnancy and Childbirth

- Antenatal breastfeeding education for increasing breastfeeding duration
- Antenatal dietary advice and supplementation to increase energy and protein intake
- Effect of restricted pacifier use in breastfeeding term infants for increasing duration of breastfeeding

- Intermittent oral iron supplementation during pregnancy
- Interventions for preventing excessive weight gain during pregnancy
- Optimal duration of exclusive breastfeeding
- Support for healthy breastfeeding mothers with healthy term babies
- Vitamin D supplementation for women during pregnancy
- Zinc supplementation for improving pregnancy and infant outcome

Tobacco Control

- Enhancing partner support to improve smoking cessation
- Interventions for tobacco cessation in the dental setting
- Mass media interventions for smoking cessation in adults
- Training health professionals in smoking cessation

References

Ajzen, I., & Fishbein, M. (1980). *Understanding attitudes and predicting social behaviour*. Englewood Cliffs, NJ: Prentice Hall.

Anderson, L. M., Petticrew, M., Rehfuess, E., Armstrong, R., Ueffing, E., Baker, P., et al. (2011). Using logic models to capture complexity in systematic reviews. *Research Synthesis Methods, 2*(1), 33–42.

Armstrong, R., Waters, E., Jackson, N., Oliver, S., Popay, J., Shepherd, J., et al. (2007). Guidelines for Systematic reviews of health promotion and public health interventions. http://ph.cochrane.org/sites/ph.cochrane.org/files/uploads/Guidelines%20HP_PH%20reviews.pdf. Accessed 1 Sept 2012

Armstrong, R., Waters, E., Roberts, H., Anderson, L., Oliver, S., & Petticrew, M. (2008). Systematic reviews in public health. In: K. Heggenhougen and S. Quah, (Eds.), *International encyclopedia of public health*, (pp. 297–301). San Diego, USA: Academic Press

Bandura, A. (1971). *Social learning theory*. New York: General learning corporation.

Bandura, A. (1998). Health promotion from the perspective of social cognitive theory. *Psychology & Health, 13*(4), 623–649.

Baxter, S., Killoran, A., Kelly, M. P., & Goyder, E. (2010). Synthesizing diverse evidence: The use of primary qualitative data analysis methods and logic models in public health reviews. *Public Health, 124*(2), 99–106.

Brownson, R. C., Colditz, G. A., et al. (Eds.). (2012). *Dissemination and implementation research in health. Translating science to practice.* New York, NY: Oxford University Press.

Dawes, M., Summerskill, W., Glasziou, P., Cartabellotta, A., Martin, J., Hopayian, K., et al. (2005). Sicily statement on evidence-based practice. *BMC Medical Education, 5*(1), 1.

Des Jarlais, D., Lyles, C., & Crepaz, N. (2004). Improving the reporting quality of nonrandomized evaluations of behavioral and public health interventions: The TREND statement. *American Journal of Public Health, 94*(3), 361–366.

Hawe, P., & Shiell, A. (1995). Preserving innovation under increasing accountability pressures: The health promotion investment portfolio approach. *Health Promotion Journal of Australia, 5*(2), 4–9.

Hiscock, R., Bauld, L., Bauld, L., Amos, A., & Platt, S. (2012). Smoking and socioeconomic status in England: The rise of the never smoker and the disadvantaged smoker. *Journal of Public Health, 34*(3), 390–396.

Jewell, C. J., & Bero, L. A. (2008). Developing good taste in evidence: Facilitators of and hindrances to evidence-informed health policymaking in state government. *The Milbank Quarterly, 86*(2), 177–208.

Kavanagh, J., Oliver, S., & Lorenc, T. (2008). Reflections on developing and using PROGRESS-Plus. Equity update: Cochrane Health Equity Field and Campbell Equity Methods Group. Ottawa, Ontario, Cochrane Health Equity Field. 2. http://equity.cochrane.org/Files/Equity_Update_Vol2_Issue1.pdf. Accessed 1 Sept 2012.

Macintyre, S., & Petticrew, M. (2000). Good intentions and received wisdom are not enough. *Journal of Epidemiology and Community Health, 54*(11), 802–803.

McLeroy, K. R., Bibeau, D., Steckler, A., & Glanz, K. (1988). An ecological perspective on health promotion programs. *Health Education & Behavior, 15*(4), 351–377.

McQueen, D. V. (2001). Strengthening the evidence base for health promotion. *Health Promotion International, 16*(3), 261–268.

McQueen, D. V. (2002). The evidence debate. *Journal of Epidemiology and Community Health, 56*(2), 83–84.

Millward, L., Kelly, M., & Nutbeam, D. (2001). *Public health interventions research: The evidence.* London: Health Development Agency.

Moher, D., Schulz, K., & Altman, D. (2001). The CONSORT statement: Revised recommendations for improving the quality of reports of parallel-group randomised trials. *Lancet, 357*(9263), 1191–1194.

Prochaska, J. O., & DiClemente, C. C. (1982). Transtheoretical therapy: Toward a more integrative model of change. *Psychotherapy: Theory, Research & Practice, 19*(3), 276–288.

Proctor, E., Silmere, H., Raghavan, R., Hovmand, P., Aarons, G., Bunger, A., et al. (2011). Outcomes for implementation research: Conceptual distinctions, measurement challenges, and research agenda. *Administration and Policy in Mental Health and Mental Health Services Research, 38*(2), 65–76.

Rogers, E. M. (1962). *Diffusion of innovations.* New York, NY: The Free Press.

Rosenstock, I. (1974). Historical origins of the health belief model. *Health Education Monographs, 2*(4).

Rychetnik, L., Frommer, M., Hawe, P., & Shiell, A. (2002). Criteria for evaluating evidence on public health interventions. *Journal of Epidemiology and Community Health, 56*(2), 119–127.

Shediac-Rizkallah, M. C., & Bone, L. R. (1998). Planning for the sustainability of community-based health programs: Conceptual frameworks and future directions for research, practice and policy. *Health Education Research, 13*(1), 87–108.

The Cochrane Collaboration. (2012, March 7, 2012, 9:55). Evidence-based health care and systematic reviews. Retrieved September 18, 2012, from http://www.cochrane.org/about-us/evidence-based-health-care

Tugwell, P., Petticrew, M., Kristjansson, E., Welch, V., Ueffing, E., Waters, E., et al. (2010). Assessing equity in systematic reviews: Realising the recommendations of the Commission on Social Determinants of Health. *BMJ, 341.*

Wang, S., Moss, J. R., & Hiller, J. E. (2006). Applicability and transferability of interventions in evidence-based public health. *Health Promotion International, 21*(1), 76–83.

Waters, E., Hall, B., Armstrong, R., Doyle, J., Pettman, T., & de Silva-Sanigorski, A. (2011). Essential components of public health evidence reviews: Capturing intervention complexity, implementation, economics and equity. *Journal of Public Health, 33*(3), 462–465.

Wiltsey Stirman, S., Kimberly, J., Cook, N., Calloway, A., Castro, F., & Charns, M. (2012). The sustainability of new programs and innovations: A review of the empirical literature and recommendations for future research. *Implementation Science, 7*(1), 17.

Zaza, S., Briss, P. A., & Harris, K. W. (2005). *The guide to community preventive services. What works to promote health?* New York, NY: Oxford University Press.

The Health Promotion Argument: NCDs and Public Health

22

David V. McQueen

Introduction

Concern with health and disease at the population level has historically been the primary focus of public health. While epidemiology as a primary subject area of public health concentrated on the etiological origins of disease and their distribution, the rest of the public health enterprise had broader interests. This was particularly true in what Rosen aptly called the "industrialism and the sanitary movement from 1830 to 1875" (1958). This was the period of the politicization of public health by such champions as Rudolph Virchow, Louis-René Villermé, and Edwin Chadwick. Regrettably, from a health promotion perspective, after such a population focus much of public health thinking and practice that followed into and including most of the twentieth century focused more on the individual. This was partly as a result of the rise of a bacteriological theory of disease etiology (cf. Chapters VII and VIII in Rosen), but can also be viewed as a political inheritance from the European colonialism concerns with hygiene and tropical medicine. From time to time, particularly from the mid twentieth century onwards, there was also a

modest interest in community and social medicine, notably in Britain. Towards the end of the twentieth century and in recent decades there has been increasing interest in noninfectious etiologies and chronic diseases in public health. An American manifesto of this broader interest was the creation at the public health agency CDC in 1988 of a National Center for Chronic Disease Prevention and Health Promotion (NCCDPHP).

While often discussed in public health circles as chronic diseases, in recent years the term "noncommunicable diseases" (NCDs) has become a globally acceptable term for this broader area. As remarked in numerous chapters of this handbook the term NCD is somewhat clumsy, often differently defined, but has been marketed as the term of choice particularly by WHO. The World Health Assembly adopted an *Action Plan for the Global Strategy for the Prevention and Control of Noncommunicable Diseases in 2008* (WHO 2008). The use of the term NCD has gained significant recognition through recent efforts by WHO to engage the United Nations General Assembly to address NCDs in 2011 in New York (cf. Chaps. 25 and 27). Further, WHO through multiple documents and with the support of many NGOs globally have reiterated the consequences of NCDs as a major source of global deaths, suffering, and economic challenges, termed by many as the "burden" argument (cf. Chapter 6 and others). While the terminology has shaped a more narrow argument for population health resulting in

D.V. McQueen (✉)
2418 Midvale Court, Tucker, GA 30084, USA
e-mail: davidmcqueen07@gmail.com

D.V. McQueen (ed.), *Global Handbook on Noncommunicable Diseases and Health Promotion,*
DOI 10.1007/978-1-4614-7594-1_22, © Springer Science+Business Media, LLC 2013

institutional interpretations that have a reductionist view of the scope of NCDs, many public health researchers and practitioners accept that the terminology is imperfect and that work on NCDs includes many areas of public health work including mental illnesses, injury, environmental challenges, and contextual factors in health and disease. NCDs, from a general public health perspective, whether seen more broadly, as in the work of the WHO Commission on the Social determinants of Health (WHOCSDH 2008) or narrowly as in the Rio Declaration on the Social Determinants of Health (WHO 2011), are a critical area for pubic health action. This is even more critical because of the financial and social hardships NCDs place on low- and middle-income countries (Ebrahim and Smeeth 2005).

Despite the well-recognized burden of NCDs, most governmental institutions (whether international, national, or local) of public health have been slow to acknowledge two critical challenges related to NCDs. The first relates to capacity; the second relates to ideology. The failure to recognize the potential and important role and contribution of the field of health promotion in reducing the burden of NCDs globally is closely related to the lack of acknowledgement of these two challenges. This unfortunate situation persists in the second decade of the twenty-first century.

A broad conception of resources and capacity is useful to understand issues related to the challenge of global capacity to address NCDs. Resource commitments in public health institutions are not distributed in relationship to the burden of NCDs. In institutions across the globe, the budgetary commitments to work on NCDs are a proportionally small percentage of budget resources when compared with the allocations to communicable diseases (cf. WHO Program budgets in recent years). More critically, the number of positioned public health researchers and practitioners with responsibilities for working on NCDs is not in proportion to the demand of NCDs and the opportunities to prevent and control NCDs. Not only is this a pressing problem for low- and middle-income countries where the public health infrastructure is often weak, but it also holds for many high-income countries. This problem will be very difficult to solve in a period where economies are challenged and growth of public health resources is not seen as a priority. It could be asserted that an equitable redistribution of the currently available resources devoted to public health, that adequately addressed both NCDs and infectious diseases to reflect the real burdens, would leave public health damaged, particularly if there are no additional resources added. Thus the argument needs to be made that, independent of the infrastructure of public health institutions, more general funds may be the only practical and sufficient solution to address the needs of public health. Public health institutions and NGOs will have to address this challenge urgently. The capacity issue is critical to support a more comprehensive approach to NCDs that addresses those areas that are beyond the scope of the narrow focus introduced above.

The ideological challenge is equally fraught with difficulties. To a large extent this challenge is one of differing relevant disciplinary approaches that need to be taken into account, each disciplinary area having its own ideological base. The present infrastructure of public health institutions favors biomedical disciplines and individual models over social ones in terms of its approach to public health. This holds true for work on the NCDs as well, despite recent efforts to champion the role of social determinants in health and the recognition of the so-called causes of the causes in disease etiology in such undertakings as the WHO Commission on the Social Determinants of Health. The Commission presented clear arguments that many of the causes of morbidity and mortality in populations rested on a foundation of poverty, inequity, social injustice, and poor health policy. This viewpoint was hardly unknown prior to the work of the Commission; these relationships were well understood by those working in social epidemiology and the sociology of medicine since the later half of the twentieth century (cf. McQueen and Siegrist 1982). What the Commission added was the recognition by the premier international health organization of an apparent causal chain between social factors such as poverty, inequity, and social justice, leading to behavioral causes leading to unfortunate health outcomes particularly in the NCDs. Furthermore, this line of observed correlations held true regardless of the level of economic development. Among the many implications of this work, one of the most obvious is that many of the attributed causes cited by the Commission represent areas of work that lie outside of the disciplinary background and training of many who research and practice public health. Importantly, many of the Commission's conclusions imply that backgrounds in the social and political sciences are needed to effectively address the causes. The growing field of social epidemiology is an effort within the current public health sphere to address these fundamental causes (cf. Krieger 2011). Nevertheless, despite the efforts of many social epidemiology is still bounded by its biomedical theoretical base.

The area of public health that has a salient role in dealing with these challenges is health promotion. " NCDs present a complex picture of associated risk factors, causes, and causes of the causes in social contexts that are highly varied and complicated to understand. They present the kind of patterning that the field of health promotion has long recognized, understood, and tried to address with limited funding, limited capacity, and little support from governmental and international agencies across the globe " (McQueen 2011). A distinguishing feature of health promotion is that it focuses on actions directed at strengthening and developing the capabilities of people, acting individually and/or collectively to improve health at both the individual and population levels. Health promotion efforts involve changing those contextual conditions, whether social, environmental, or economic, that impact health. This work is carried out with special attention to equity and social justice. Thus, health promotion views itself as a primary action component for global social progress. Many in health promotion regard it as an area of public health work that engages in efforts to empower people to control their own health through collective efforts to address the determinants of health, notably those that relate to people's everyday life conditions. There is recognition that many of these conditions are shaped by and are the result of public policies and therefore an understanding of the political processes in every cultural context is a feature of health promotion practice and research.

However, the field of health promotion has its own burdens; it also lacks resources globally and it has a decidedly undeveloped global capacity and infrastructure. It is generally agreed that the NCD area is unrepresented in the public health infrastructure of most LMICs; by comparison, health promotion has even less a part of such infrastructures. Yet, it is the area of public health that is most concerned with addressing broad health issues and focusing public health toward the social context of health. It is the area of public health that has a salient role in dealing with these challenges in health promotion. It focuses on actions directed at strengthening and developing the capabilities of people to improve health at both the individual and population levels. Health promotion involves changing contextual conditions, whether social, environmental, or economic, that impact health. Further, it is carried out with an emphasis on equity and social justice. Thus, health promotion views itself as a primary action component for global social progress. Health promotion is the spiritual home for those sociologists, anthropologists, and political and social scientists that wish to not only prevent disease but also promote health. Particularly in the area of NCDs where many of the causes and solutions lie outside the area of clinical medicine, health promotion with its emphasis on social action would seem to be the logical partner to the disease-oriented specialists. In addition, the ideology of health promotion is driven by the values of equity, social justice, and a concern with health as a human right within the guidelines laid out by the United Nations and enshrined in the WHO constitution. Health promotion does not seek to just describe the social determinants of health; it wishes to take action to change those determinants with the end goal of improving health. These actions are taken on the basis of values.

Values, Health Promotion, and Action on NCDs

It may be claimed that values in health promotion stem mostly from a contextual position and perspective; they are not independent from those who define them. Thus if health is a value, it is because health promoters, or someone, or some institution say it is. There is no value for health independent of the entity that says so. By defining health as a value, public health and health promotion incorporate the idea of values as fundamental to the conduct of public health. It is not just health as a value; it opens the door for the incorporation of ideas such as equity as a value, social justice as a value, and women's rights as a value. Since the 1980s and the Ottawa Charter, the notion that health promotion was driven by values has been largely accepted (McQueen and de Salazar 2011). This primal emphasis on values distinguishes health promotion from more technical and biomedical approaches to health. Further, this emphasis opened the door for a discussion of values that could bring in the perspectives of such key thinkers as Amartya Sen (1979, 1999) and Jennifer Ruger (2006, 2010) as well as the incorporation of a contextual value-based ethics as elaborated by Rawls and others (Rawls 1971; Venkatapuram 2011).

Equity is one of the key value concepts that characterize present-day health promotion thinking. Equity has been a subject of considerable debate and discussion globally (cf. Braveman 2006). The precise definition of health equity remains elusive, but the idea has focused on discussions around health disparities, inequalities, and other forms of apparent maldistribution of health resources in populations. What is most salient about equity is that it is shaped by government structures and policies and therefore becomes a particular challenge for governance. In most countries health inequities are highly related to systematic decisions by government actors to distribute resources unequally in the population, thus favoring some components of the population over others in terms of the experience of health and disease (McQueen 2012).

The concept of health equity owes much to the writings of Sen, who in his Tanner Lecture of 1979 laid out most of the essential components of equity in terms of equality in moral philosophy. Sen examined the predominant types of equality, namely, utilitarian equality, utility equality, and Rawlsian equality. Rawlsian equality argued, "each person is to have an equal right to the most

extensive basic liberty compatible with a similar liberty for others" (Rawls 1971, p. 60). Sen, as an economist, introduced concepts of equality based on welfare economics. This critical turn moved the considerations of equality out of the more classical philosophical realm and into economic ideology. This approach would be replicated later by the adaption of the idea to the world of health, health economics, and ultimately health promotion. At the time that health promotion was embracing cross discipline thinking in health, Sen moved to a "capabilities approach" that would tie resources to the individual and group efforts to distribute these resources in an ethically driven effort to equitable distribution. At the same time these efforts created a paradigm shift that would tie together equity with human and economic development. This shift in thinking accelerated in the new millennium and ties health to development (cf. UNGA 2011).

From a health promotion perspective the current efforts of those trying to incorporate the social determinants of health and the NCD burden argument into broad policy goals such as the MDGs are traceable to the fundamental shifts in value concepts arising from the 1980s and the subsequent discussion on inequalities and health. That this value discussion was clearly in the thinking of many of those in health promotion is well documented in the Ottawa Charter and its background documents and carried forward in numerous global health promotion meetings (WHO/EURO 1984, 1998; WHO 1986, 2009). The extension of the value concept of health equity leads inevitably to discussions on living a full, lengthy, and relatively disease-free life and fits well into the current ideology for the practice of health promotion.

Rawls' approach should be considered further. John Rawls wrote in the early seventies what was and still is considered by many as the definitive treatise on social justice (Rawls 1971). Entitled *A Theory of Justice*, this seminal work ties the political process into the value concept of equity. He argued from a notion of "original position" that individuals acting in a group, without awareness of the resources of the others in the group, would move to an egalitarian position of distributive justice.

The point here is not to delve into the thought processes that would lead to such an outcome, but to note that this type of thinking has influenced the equity discussion to this day. Rawls was certainly not naive and he modified the egalitarian perspective to accept that there would, in the real world, be both liberty and difference resulting in some real and perceived inequities. However the value is still to minimize the impact of the differences. The critical point arising from Rawls is that social justice and hence equity are tied to agency and thus become an ethical concern.

The development of the discussions around the works of Sen and Rawls and their explication over recent years pinpoint the classical concerns with the interaction of structure and agency. It is not the role of this chapter to delve into the complicated sociological debate between structure and agency; Chap. 5 by Frohlich has already explored this. However it is important for one to keep in mind that a value concept such as health equity usually resorts to a discussion of structural change (e.g., distribution of government resources) versus agency (e.g., actors, individuals, and civil society). This is perhaps one reason why health promotion may be seen as a radical approach by some in public health. Furthermore, the structure versus agency discussion introduces the question of whether those concerned with health equity should focus on values or on ethics in an effort to improve human health. Jennifer Ruger has over the last decade taken up this discussion of social justice in detail and successfully linked it to health and health care (2004, 2010). Her work further integrates the work of Sen and political theory and provides considerable guidance for health policy.

Finally, a major question to consider is individual versus social values. In essence it can be argued that values belong only to the individual. This is part of the larger philosophical question of whether values exist independently from a conscious mind that can conceptualize values. This is not a trivial question as witness the recent US Supreme Court decision that a corporation can be considered an individual thus implying that an institution is conceptually an individual

(2010). In the consideration of values related to health, the issue is whether values are only within individuals, or whether groups can have shared values, whether societies can have shared values, and finally whether a government can actually have values. There are no fixed solutions to this query, but many would argue that organizations do have social values as long as there are individuals or groups that validate those values.

It may be argued that much of this value orientation in health promotion derives from Western philosophical traditions. Nonetheless, the question arises as to whether there are differences in different Western heritages. For example, is the United State's value heritage critically different from that of Western Europe? The answer is neither obvious nor simple and demands a lengthy historical and philosophical treatise. Undoubtedly, in health promotion practice and research, there are aspects that are peculiarly American and distinguish it from other regions of the world. Nonetheless, it is probably equally true that there is great variation on values within and across Europe. Certainly, by analogy, few would have difficulty in recognizing that the values with regard to health in a North America containing Canada, the United States, and Mexico might have considerable variation. Indeed much has been written about the particular role of values in health in the Canadian context (Giacomini et al. 2001) where the health care system itself is seen as a core Canadian value. In an apposite way of thinking in the United States there has been an ongoing debate for decades on whether health, and by implication health care, is a human right or a privilege.

Science, Values, and Health Promotion

One can assert confidently that belief in science is a strongly held value in Western thought. Indeed modern scientific thinking has its deep structure firmly embedded in Western history, notably since the seventeenth century. Above all, science seeks clear explanations of what works and why. Insofar as medicine is seen as a science and public health as a science-driven field of work, these disciplines are held accountable to the rigors of scientific proof. Health promotion, as well, seeks to build its practice on a scientific base (McQueen and Jones 2007; Rootman et al. 2000). Almost parallel to the rise of such value concerns as equity and social justice in the world of health has been the rise of accountability framed in terms such as "evidence-based medicine" and "effective" knowledge translation (this is discussed in further detail in Chap. 3). At first glance these scientific expectations could also be framed as values and would appear to be in line with the chief values that have been discussed above; however, these "science" values have imbedded methodological and measurement theories that are rarely found in the discussion of value concepts. The underlying epistemology of values such as equity and social justice is to be found in moral philosophy. Further it could be argued that the idea of "health" as a value is also embedded in this same epistemology. Hoverer, evidence has its underlying epistemology in the philosophical traditions of logic and science. These epistemological sources are distinct traditions and ones that have often been at odds in Western history. The eighteenth-century Scottish philosopher David Hume wrote that all assumptions of value involve projections of one's own sentiments onto whatever is said to have value (2007).

The choice between values and science depends on one's context. There is no law that says that science and values need to be in agreement nor in conflict; both outcomes are possible. However, at various times choices involving science and values need to be taken. Unfortunately for decision-taking efforts such choices are often not transparent and are often confusing. For example, value choices are implied in many aspects of the WHO Commission's Report on Social Determinants. In the Report the scientific, epidemiologically based, evidence clearly lays out the correlational connections between values such as health equity, social justice, education, and human dignity and good health. Despite a long history in public health of knowing the strong relationship between contextual factors and good health, it was the Commission's Report that solidified this knowledge to a position beyond doubt scientifically. However knowledge is not enough for effective action on the value-related causes of poor health. It is only the precursor to action. The science of how effectively to change these causes is highly problematic and in reality significant changes in the attributable causes may imply political philosophies tied to values that may not be in concert with those of the underlying values that relate to good health. Very basic value concepts such as freedom of choice and public democracy may in themselves be inimical to addressing some key causal values. It is not the point to debate this here, but merely to lay out why considerations to deal with such problems of health inequities face such extraordinary challenges. As a field of action, health promotion has to deal with values and must sort out the conflicts that exist. For example, health promotion argues for recognition and valuing the concept of diversity, but at the same time argues for the value of equality. These two values need not always stand in contradiction to each other, but at times they do. Similarly, freedom of choice is seen as an important value, but sometimes such freedoms may be in conflict with what is seen as good for the population. When one sees value conflicts, one also observes criticisms such as health promotion leading to the so-called nanny-state as one current example. Perhaps an even more telling value conflict is found in the debates on gun control in the United States. Unlike the epidemiological perspective that can center its focus on description of a problem, health promotion, by its very nature, must be concerned with action and change.

Conclusion

The public interest in NCDs and the field of health promotion are highly related to public health areas and both would benefit greatly by a recognition of this relationship and a future that builds on the strengths of these two areas to support each other. The area of NCDs brings to health promotion an area of public health that is replete with nonmedical issues and problems. Whether conceived of as "chronic diseases" or chronic diseases plus injury or some other formulation, the key causal components of NCDs remain social and contextual, especially when these causes are conceived of in terms such as the "causes of the causes" and the fundamental areas of work relate to the social context of health. This context is exactly where the main focus of health promotion conceptual thinking is found and it is the abundant source of approaches to intervention.

While the importance of health promotion to develop interventions for changes in broad areas such as health equity is clear, there is also a key role for health promotion in understanding needed innovations in classical and routine public health practices. As discussed in detail in Chap. 4, surveillance is one such area. Routine social and behavioral risk factor surveillance can monitor over time the changes that are occurring in particular risk factors and can serve as a way to see if health promotion actions are making a difference. Thus the evidence question can be addressed as to whether or not health promotion interventions are working. Such measurements and analyses in turn provide the information for planning further interventions and policy with regard to NCDs.

It is unfortunate that, at the time of this writing, those concerned with NCDs and those working in health promotion do not work more closely together. It is perhaps a problem of acceptance of both parties on the need to work more closely together. Both parties share an intense interest in reducing the burden of disease and promoting the healthiest populations obtainable. However, on a hopeful note, the recent UN effort to address NCDs (cf. Chaps. 18, 25, and 27) was met by a strong advocacy approach from the International Union on Health Promotion and Education (IUHPE 2011). In particular the IUHPE advocated: "The adoption of a strategy that reflects the fact that reducing NCDs will require action across a number of areas. This includes tobacco control, improving food supply and systems and environments for physical activity, reducing hazardous alcohol intake and delivering cost-effective and affordable essential drugs and technologies."

Further in terms that relate to the value component of health promotion the statement was made that "equity forms a central part of the NCD prevention and control agenda and disproportionate attention and resources are needed to be allocated to addressing the needs of disadvantaged groups. Risk factors are clustered in disadvantaged populations and communities, and those in these communities often have the poorest access to health services, healthy environments, and health promotion programs" which formed a part of the health promotion position. These approaches were and remain very much in alignment with many groups pursuing the reduction of the NCD disease burden globally (cf. NCD Alliance at their Web site: http://www.ncdalliance.org/). In conclusion, there is a strong and compelling argument for the role of health promotion as both an area of action and as a component of modern public health in addressing global NCDs.

References

Braveman, P. (2006). Health disparities and health equity: Concepts and measurement. *Annual Review of Public Health, 27*, 167–194.

Ebrahim, S., & Smeeth, L. (2005). Non-communicable diseases in low and middle-income countries: A priority or a distraction? *International Journal of Epidemiology, 34*(5), 961–966.

Giacomini, M., Hurley, J., Gold, I., Smith, P., & Abelson, J. (2001). *Values in Canadian health policy analysis: What are we talking about?* Ottawa: Canadian Health Services Research Foundation.

Hume, D. (2007). *An enquiry concerning human understanding. P. Millican (Ed. and intro.). Hume's book first published 1748.* Oxford: Oxford University Press.

IUHPE. (2011). *Advocating for health promotion approaches to NCD prevention: Key messages from the International Union for Health Promotion and Education in the up to the United Nations High Level Meeting on NCDs in New York, Sep. 2011.* Paris: IUHPE.

Krieger, N. (2011). *Epidemiology and the peoples health.* New York, NY: Oxford Univ. Press.

McQueen, D. V. (2011). A challenge for health promotion. *Global Health Promotion, 18*, 8–9.

McQueen, DV. (2012). *Value base, ethics and key challenges of health governance for health protection, prevention and promotion, expert background paper for the WHO/EURO document Governance for health in* the 21st century: A study conducted for the WHO Regional Office for Europe. /RC61/Inf.Doc./6.

McQueen, D. V., & De Salazar, L. (2011). Health promotion, The Ottawa charter and developing personal skills: A compact history of 25 years. *Health Promotion International, 26,* 194–201.

McQueen, D. V., & Jones, C. M. (Eds.). (2007). *Global perspectives on health promotion effectiveness.* New York, NY: Springer Science & Business Media.

McQueen, D. V., & Siegrist, J. (1982). Sociocultural factors in the etiology of chronic disease. *Social Science and Medicine, 16*(4), 353–367.

Rawls, J. (1971). *A theory of justice.* Cambridge: The Belknap Press of Harvard University Press.

Rootman, I., Goodstadt, M., McQueen, D., Potvin, L., Springett, J., & Ziglio, E. (Eds.). (2000). *Evaluation in health promotion: Principles and perspectives.* Copenhagen: WHO (EURO).

Rosen, G. (1958). *A history of pubic health.* New York, NY: MD Publications.

Ruger, J.P. (2004). Health and Social Justice, *The Lancet, 364,* 1075–1080

Ruger, J. P. (2006). Ethics and governance of global health inequalities. *Journal of Epidemiology and Community Health, 60*(11), 998–1002.

Ruger, J. P. (2010). *Health and social justice.* New York, NY: Oxford University Press.

Sen, A. (1979). *Equality of what?" The Tanner lecture on human values,* delivered at Stanford University, May 22, 1979.

Sen, A. K. (1999). *Development as freedom.* New York, NY: Knopf.

U.S. Supreme Court. (2010). *Citizens united, Appellant v. Federal Election Commission.* Docket nos.08-205 Citations: 558 U.S. 310.

UNGA. (2011). *United Nations General Assembly. Political declaration of high level meeting of the general assembly on the prevention and control of noncommunicable diseases. Rep noA/66/L.* New York, NY: United Nations General Assembly.

Venkatapuram, S. (2011). *Health Justice: An argument from the capabilities approach.* Cambridge, UK: Polity.

WHO. (1986). *Ottawa charter for health promotion.* Geneva: WHO.

WHO. (2008). *Action plan for the global strategy for the prevention and control of noncommunicable diseases.* Geneva: WHO.

WHO. (2009). *Milestones in health promotion: Statements from global conferences.* Geneva: WHO. cf. http://www.who.int/healthpromotion/Milestones_Health_Promotion_05022010.pdf.

WHO. (2011). *Rio political declaration on social determinants of health.* Geneva: WHO.

WHO (EURO). (1984). *Health promotion: A discussion document on the concepts and principles.* Copenhagen: WHO (EURO).

WHO (EURO). (1998). *Health promotion evaluation: Recommendations to policymakers.* Copenhagen: WHO (EURO). cf. http://whqlibdoc.who.int/euro/1998-99/EUR_ICP_IVST_05_01_03.pdf.

WHOCSDOH. (2008). *Closing the gap in a generation. Health equity through action on the social determinants of health.* Geneva: WHO.

Public Health, NCDs, Health Promotion, and Business Partnering: Benefits, Concerns, Remedies, and Moving Towards Creative Partnering

23

Becky H. Lankenau and Maria D. Stefan

Introduction

The UN High-Level Meeting on Non-Communicable Diseases (NCDs), in September 2011, officially focused long overdue world attention on NCDs and commanded the attention of countries to take action to stop this burgeoning epidemic and its potentially catastrophic economic consequences. Preceding and subsequent guidance documents such as The Toronto Charter and the World Health Organization (WHO) 2008–2013 Action Plan for the Global Strategy for the Prevention and Control of NCDs (Global Advocacy Council 2010; WHO 2008) have consistently advocated for collaboration with the private sector, and partnerships across sectors, as essential components of identifying solutions to the complex problem of NCDs and helping countries implement proven, scalable, culturally relevant, economically viable interventions with the potential to affect positive, sustainable change. The recent global financial crisis, and resulting escalating challenges to governments to ade-

quately fund social agendas, has increased the partnership imperative. The intent of this chapter is to suggest creative partnering as a means to maximize scarce resources and find sustainable solutions to NCDs. It addresses the benefits and concerns of developing partnerships, suggests remedies to alleviate concerns, offers approaches to establishing partnerships, and provides examples of multi-sectoral partnership efforts from around the world.

Benefits

At the Third International Congress on Physical Activity and Public Health (ICPAPH) held in Toronto in May 2010, three of the Symposia focused on various aspects of building partnerships which can be applied to the problem of NCDs in general beyond just combating physical inactivity. In "Powerful Partnering: Courting New Realms to Boost Physical Activity Promotion" (Lankenau et al. 2010), the following examples were given of benefits to be derived from establishing partnerships:

1. Enhanced political commitment and policy support to physical activity. (For example, working with domestic legislative groups or partnering with leading financial organizations such as the World Bank on in-country initiatives.)
2. Increased societal acceptance and perception of added value of physical activity promotion.

B.H. Lankenau (✉)
Centers for Disease Control and Prevention (CDC) (Retired), PO Box 941190, Atlanta, GA, 31141, USA
e-mail: eaglebird1119@gmail.com

M.D. Stefan (✉)
CHASEAMERICA GROUP, 1800 J.F.K. Blvd, Suite 300, Philadelphia, PA, 19103, USA
e-mail: maria@chaseamericagroup.com

D.V. McQueen (ed.), *Global Handbook on Noncommunicable Diseases and Health Promotion*,
DOI 10.1007/978-1-4614-7594-1_23, © Springer Science+Business Media, LLC 2013

(For example, parks and recreation partnerships to expand green spaces, potentially increasing adjacent property values.)

3. Expanded dissemination reach for physical activity messages. (For example, working with large companies having extensive domestic and global office networks, as well as disease research and prevention organizations such as the American Heart Association and World Heart Federation.)

4. Marketing expertise to formulate creative physical activity communications approaches. (Private sector partnerships.)

5. Scientific consensus on important issues such as physical activity guidelines. (Collaboration with professional organizations such as the American College of Sports Medicine (ACSM) and international organizations such as the WHO.)

6. Manpower resources for training activities such as domestic and international courses. (For example, academic institutions and nongovernmental organizations (NGOs).)

7. Manpower resources for technical assistance on domestic and international projects. (Follow-up on development of national physical activity plans in selected countries by partners in academic institutions and NGOs.)

8. Expanded entry points to effective physical activity promotion. (Working with the International Olympic Committee (IOC) and the World Federation of the Sporting Goods Industry (WFSGI) on Sport For All conferences and other activities to encourage population-based participation in physical activity rather than only elite sport.)

9. Concentrated focus on various determinants and barriers to physical activity. (Urban planning groups designing safer walking and cycling environments.)

10. Proactive dialogue to anticipate changing contexts in which to promote physical activity most effectively. (For example, financial institutions may suggest shifting from a purely health focus to economic development.)

11. Funds for conference support, research and program implementation. (Working

with foundations such as Gates and Robert Wood Johnson, as well as the private sector.)

Expanding engagement between the public health and private sector can also lead to new learning and knowledge transfer, access to specific populations, and implementation and promotion of work, school, family, and community activities.

Concerns

Government and voluntary agencies, in particular, have often been hesitant to develop partnerships with other organizations. Even seemingly benign collaboration, with other scientific organizations or academic institutions, can be stymied by territoriality concerns regarding credit for joint achievements. Nontraditional partnering, especially with the private sector, raises additional red flags that have frequently immobilized potentially valuable partnership efforts. The public health and private sector have tended to be ill at ease with each other, and contemplation of partnering has often been characterized by suspicion, mistrust, lack of respect, and sometimes downright animosity. Since the training, motivations, and cultures of the two sectors are quite divergent, it is not surprising that fruitful collaborations are not easily accomplished. Types of concerns can generally be summarized as follows:

1. Exclusivity—Pursuing a partnership with a single entity to the exclusion of other potentially direct competitors

2. Product placement—Concern that a product manufactured by a partnering company is not consistent with public health messaging

3. Manipulation of scientific integrity—Concern that a private sector partner will take advantage of a collaboration to inappropriately influence various scientific positions of the public health partner

4. Implied endorsement—Concern that simply by associating in a partnership collaboration, the public health partner is sanctioning an organization, company, and/or product lines

Remedies

Four actions that can help alleviate the most common concerns of partnering with the private sector are the following:

1. A written agreement can be prepared detailing a mutual understanding of the goals and objectives, roles and responsibilities, as well as the context and limitations of the collaborative relationship. The formality of this document can range from a simple memorandum of understanding (MOU) to a more stringent, legal instrument.
2. Round tables of multiple groups from the same industry can be organized to diffuse the exclusivity issue, for example a pharmaceutical or a food and beverage round table.
3. Corporate attribution can be limited to discrete recognition in program booklets, signs at conference gatherings, introductory/closing remarks by public health representatives, and/or follow-up thank-you notes.
4. Visibility of potentially contentious products can be minimized by disallowing sample giveaways and focusing on only the most healthful among multiple product lines.

Initiating Private Sector Partnering

In the "Powerful Partnering" symposium at the ICPAPH (Lankenau et al. 2010), Culhane presented key leadership practices and a framework for convening conversations that can help foster innovation and new partnerships:

1. Curiosity: Pursue genuine interest in others and other perspectives, world views.
2. Creative orientation and current reality: Focus on the vision you want to achieve and develop an accurate understanding of what currently and really exists.
3. Value my voice and our collective voice; speak your truth, at the same time you value and tap the wisdom of others.
4. Balance inquiry and advocacy: Contribute powerful questioning and learning towards exploration, at the same time you communicate your perspective in a way that can be heard.

5. Use divergent and convergent thinking: Invite different viewpoints and disruption to invent new possibilities as well as build powerful decisions, resolution, and commitment.
6. Serve as learner and expert: Seek new capability and freely share your experience and knowledge.

With the key leadership practices as a foundation, the steps to convening productive conversations include the following:

1. Engage: Clarify intention, examine current reality, identify shared purpose, and plan for inquiry.
2. Inquire: Explore stories and experience, consider interests, and investigate multiple perspectives.
3. Invent: Identify options, disrupt old thinking, and co-create.
4. Commit: Outline action, build agreement, and capture learning.

These principles are valuable in establishing a positive mindset prior to initiating a private sector partnership. Once the potential benefit of a partnership is acknowledged, there are two critical steps to approaching a private sector partner, as outlined by Stefan in her commentary, "Powerful Partnering: engaging the best to do the most in courting new realms to boost physical activity" (Stefan 2011):

1. Identify the purpose of a strategic alliance or collaboration. Is it to build awareness, seed a social movement, educate and change behavior, create engagement opportunities, foster development or sustainability platforms, reduce costs, increase amenities, build champions, advance public policy, build organizational competencies, and create volunteers or a mix of strategies? The public health sector can activate a dialogue with the private sector using any of these platforms.
2. Once the purpose has been defined, investigate whether a company has a corporate mission, value, or social responsibility statement that speaks to a health or a sustainability platform. If such a statement exists, that facilitates building a dialogue about shared values. If it does not, there can still be an examination of where there might be common ground.

A second symposium from the ICPAPH was entitled "Public Private Partnerships in Physical Activity and Sport: Principles for Successful, Responsible Partnerships" (Murumets et al. 2010). A draft protocol was presented by representatives of a multi-sectoral Steering Committee as part of a research project which included, for example, an extensive literature review, secondary study of best practices in partnerships involving sport and physical activity, and technical consultations. The Protocol reiterates that embarking on public/private sector partnerships involves a three-phased approach of (1) assessing potential partners; (2) building the partnerships; and (3) managing the partnership. The management phase is further elaborated to include project definition, planning, initiation execution, close, evaluation, and communication.

Organizations, such as the WHO and Red Actividad Fisica de las Americas/Physical Activity Network of the Americas (RAFA/ PANA), have also studied partnership issues, acknowledged and promoted their value, and published cautionary guidance documents for public health practitioners (RAFA 2009; WHO 2008).

Rules of the Road for Building Public–Private Partnerships

If the public health sector can embrace a collaborative mindset, it will open infinite possibilities to expand reach, revenue, and engagement in building sustainable shared values with the private sector in the fight against NCDs. As articulated in the third of the partnership symposia at ICPAPH, Professor Ilkka Vuori stated: "Too often the selling arguments have focused too much on the interests of ourselves and not those more relevant to the other parties. These weaknesses can be decreased by finding the needs, goals, and motives of the partners, and by building a win-win strategy on this basis" (Vuori et al. 2010). With that in mind, here are some rules of the road for how the public health sector can engage the best in the private sector to do the most:

- Understand that many businesses are moving beyond promotional relationships and want to establish collaborations that capture sustainability, social responsibility, and networks.
- Establish a story to open a dialogue, and set out the need and rationale for the collaboration and what is to be achieved.
- Identify public health roles, responsibilities, and partnership deliverables.
- Identify business targets by sector, reviewing their goodness strategies through their mission/value statements, current programs and platforms, and ethical codes of conduct.
- Identify business units that have responsibility for programs currently being funded.
- Define the core resources, capacities, and competencies that public health can bring to an engagement to either boost the current programs or create new opportunities.
- Define stakeholder value creation.
- Outline the communication process: Who will be affected by the partnership internally and externally; who will have the responsibility for communicating to and engaging stakeholders and through what channels; how will communication between partners be managed; and what is the external communications strategy and program.
- Define how the partnership will be institutionalized in each organizational architecture so that should people who are advocates leave, there is a collaborative continuum (Stefan 2011).

Partnering Tasks

The benefits to be gained by selective partnering are substantial. However, successful partnering requires time and commitment and, therefore, has staff resource implications. Important tasks of partnering include, but are not limited to, the following:

- Maintain timely, positive, constructive, ongoing dialogue.
- Study the language, culture, and incentives of potential partners in order to most attractively propose the areas of mutual interest for collaboration.

- Proactively study shifts in priorities of potential partners in order to propose projects in the most acceptable context.
- Develop attractively produced marketing materials to enhance dialogue with potential partners in person or by mail.
- Develop and maintain a current "wish list" of proposals in order to enable opportunistic response to new collaborative opportunities.
- Approach the challenge of building partnerships with an open mind and a sense of humor.

Making the Case for PPPs

The public's health has become the key social issue of the twenty-first century, and is the metaphor for a brave new worldview of how the public sector and private sector must think about their relationships to each other and the world.

Confronted by a toxic combination of poor social policies, weak government health care capacity, recessionary economics and impacts from rapid urbanization, aging populations, and twenty-first century lifestyles, a chronic disease epidemic is causing skyrocketing health care costs that is impacting the "fitness" of nations, companies, and individuals, especially in low- and middle-income countries.

The dominant driving force for private sector involvement in global health can be laid at the doorstep of global economics, as governments, alone, cannot provide all that is required for peoples' health and well-being. The dimensions of global health are too broad, complex, and costly to be solved by any one actor. According to the Institute for Health Metrics and Evaluation, the total annual value of money and goods donated to global health from all sources, public and private, has risen from less than $8 billion in 1995 to almost $27 billion in 2010—with most of that increase occurring since 2002 (Institute for Health Metrics and Evaluation 2010).

A study in 2008 estimated that no fewer than 40 bilateral donors, 26 United Nations agencies, 20 global and regional funding mechanisms, and 90 distinct initiatives—such as the rapidly proliferating "public–private" and "product–development" partnerships—were involved in collecting and delivering assistance for health programs in poor countries, to say nothing of the uncountable number of smaller scale initiatives and civil-society, community-based, and individually supported efforts (McColl 2008).

While public money still makes up much of total health aid, the private sector plays an increasingly large and important role in funding projects, shaping policies, and determining courses of action. The Gates Foundation's $1 billion of yearly giving on global health is essentially equivalent to the WHO's entire annual budget; then there is the Rockefeller Foundation and the Clinton Global Initiative, without even accounting for smaller scale foundations and NGO grants.

Yet the recent study by the University of Washington's Institute on Health Metrics and Evaluation concluded that the percentage of development assistance for health spent on NCDs was less than 1 %, while others have calculated this as less than 3 % (Nugent and Feigl 2010).

In addition, WHO notes that many countries, even those with heavy disease burden from NCDs, lack adequate surveillance mechanisms to take account of illness prevalence and trends (Beaglehole et al. 2011).

The old, mechanist, and determinist Newtonian view of the world no longer functions. Global health issues are not top-down. They cut across sectors and stakeholders. They require approaches, investments, and solutions that are relational, multidimensional, and collaborative, and that are built on a platform of accountability, with shared values and shared commitments at the center, whose interconnected participants depend on each other for their mutual effectiveness and sustainability. With the recognition that the "future ain't what it used to be," public/private partnerships have come of age and continue to evolve. Multi-sector and multi-stakeholder partnerships, as advocated by the United Nations, are no longer simply additive to core organizational missions: they are essential to success.

There is no one definition of public/private sector partnerships, nor one model of PPPs that can be characterized as "best." The United Nations defines PPPs as "voluntary and collaborative relationships between various parties, both public and nonpublic, in which all participants agree to work together to achieve a common purpose or undertake a specific task and to share risks, responsibilities, resources, competencies and benefits" (United Nations General Assembly 2007).

The scope and reach of partnerships vary, from local, national, and global to whom the actors are: governments, NGOs, companies, individuals, and to levels of commitment and objectives of the partnership. As Jane Nelson suggests in her book on building UN-business partnerships that was commissioned by the Global Compact, a key feature distinguishing PPPs from other interactions with the private for-profit sector is the "shared process of decision making" (United Nations 2010).

The Interdependence of the Public and Private Sectors

The success of PPPs is to a great extent determined by the quality, vision, and persistence of leaders from the public and private sectors, recognizing that together they can achieve more than separately. Experience has shown that positive results depend on the careful management of specific issues related to accountability, governance and oversight, risk management, and multiplier effects of capacity building. Expanding engagement between the public and private sector can lead to a convergence of new learning, market knowledge, research transfer, and increased workforce and financial capacities. This convergence can result in the development of "best practices" for delivering effective and cost-efficient health-based interventions, health promotion messaging, and increased training and education capacity-building opportunities.

The public health and private sector working together allows us to identify each of our organizational core capacities and where the needle movers are in creating behavior change; where we can leverage and impact different sectors and

different stakeholders to maximize capacity building; how to best separate out immediate issues from three-to-five-year policy shifts, and identify where the system blocks are; and how we can collaborate to create systemic change while developing national and/or global platforms around metrics to show evidence-based results for optimizing health and wellness (American College of Sports Medicine 2011).

Strategic engagement has to be rooted in a stakeholder relationship management system. This is not a new moral code, but a business model that realizes as Einstein famously said: "A problem cannot be solved by the same consciousness in which it arose." Elements of business and the public sector are realizing that they operate in an ecosystem no different than nature, and that for every action there is a reaction (Stefan 2011).

It is important to recognize that the interest in public/private partnerships is not solely dependent on the need of the public health sector. The private sector is a willing partner in bringing human, financial, knowledge, and communications resources to the global public health table. In return for its investment, it gets increased influence in global policy making, enhanced corporate authority and legitimacy, better public image, opportunity to identify new, scalable innovations, expanded sales and marketing penetration, increased profits, and healthier employees and customers. The public sector gets increased expertise, human and financial resources, and knowledge and delivery capacities, otherwise difficult to acquire.

In "Global Health's Private Sector Revolution," Josh Michaud, writes:

"On the recipient side, private actors—in supply chains, logistics, management and accounting, and program-implementation—are filling the longstanding gaps in capacity at developing countries' Ministries of Health. Failures or gaps in public-sector delivery capacities have some looking for solutions from private industry, either through funding private-sector activities with public money, or seeking to convince public officials of the business case for private involvement—especially in planning, management and other relevant areas.
In addition, there is increasing buy-in and understanding of the links between better health and

positive economic and development impacts. This has engendered broader thinking about constraints and solutions to health problems, drawing in professionals from fields outside those traditionally associated with medicine and public health. As a result, lawyers, MBAs and economists are complementing the doctors, nurses and pharmacists that practically wholly comprised health-program implementation in previous decades. Beginning with the World Bank's landmark 1994 World Development Report focused on health as a vehicle for economic growth and disease as a barrier to development, and in the wake of similar findings in the high-profile 2001 WHO-sponsored Commission on Macroeconomics and Health report, it has become conventional wisdom that individual and country-level health status is a determinant of—and is determined by—economic development." (Michaud 2010)

On the horizon is also an "mHealth" revolution, catalyzed by the private sector that will utilize the vast and still-growing mobile phone market to transform how poor country populations access health information and seek out and interact with health care systems.

The WHO Commission on Social Determinants of Health made an aspirational call for closing the health gap in a generation. To ensure that the call is fulfilled, focused research, coherent policies, and multi-sectoral partnerships for action are required to expand the evidence base and implement interventions that show evidence of effectiveness in combating heart disease, lung disease, certain cancers, and respiratory ailments that are cause for 80 % of premature deaths, especially among those who do not have resources to pursue health choices easily (WHO Commission on Social Determinants of Health 2008).

Scale of Need for NCD PPPs

In further making the case for NCD public/private partnerships, the scale of need speaks for itself as reported in the WHO Global Status Report on Noncommunicable Diseases 2010:

- Evidence now shows that the poor may begin life with increased vulnerability to NCDs; are then exposed to additional risks throughout life; and as a consequence are more likely to die prematurely from NCDs. NCDs do not affect only the elderly: many who develop NCDs in developing countries do so at a relatively young age—a recent study of 23 low- and middle-income countries found that 43 % of NCD deaths were among those aged under 70, or nearly 50 % of the working-age population is affected.

- Death rates from NCDs rose from 59 % globally in 2001 to 67 % in 2010. Much of that increase is from developing countries. According to the WHO, over 80 % of cardiovascular deaths, 90 % of deaths from respiratory disease, and 67 % of all cancers occur in developing countries.

- Between 2008 and 2030, NCD deaths as a share of total deaths are projected to rise by 1 % in high-, 12 % in middle-, and 45 % in low-income countries. For the 15–59-years-of-age population, these projections include a decrease of −5 % in high-income, and increases of 12 % in middle- and 32 % in low-income countries. In absolute terms, deaths from NCDs in middle- and low-income countries are projected to rise by over 50 %, from an estimated 28 million in 2008 to 43 million by 2030. The change will be particularly substantial in Sub-Saharan Africa, where NCDs will account for 46 % of all deaths by 2030, up from 28 % in 2008, and in South Asia, which will see the share of NCD deaths increase from 51 to 72 % over the same time frame.

- New trends suggest that many developed countries could be entering a fifth as-yet-unnamed phase of epidemiological transition, characterized by an epidemic of obesity and diabetes prevalence. In two decades, obesity has grown by almost 400 %. According to the WHO, worldwide, more than 1 billion adults are overweight, and 300 million are clinically obese.

- In 2006, the number of overweight people in the world overtook the number of malnourished, underweight people for the first time. In China, overweight rates doubled from 13.5 to 26.7 % between 1991 and 2006, with diabetes reaching a level similar to the USA at over 92 million. It is now the most important underlying cause of death in the Pan American region and the range of consequent illnesses is wide among those who survive. Even more disturbing are increases in childhood obesity, which lead to large increases in diabetes and hypertension (WHO Global Status Report on Noncommunicable Diseases 2010a).

A near tripling of ischemic heart disease and stroke mortality in Latin America is expected over the next two decades (PAHO, "Health in the Americas". Volume 1, 2002). And the fact that such a high proportion of CVD burden occurs earlier among adults of working age in developing countries can lead to a large impact on a developing country's economic viability. More than half the people in the world live in urban environments where investments in green space, recreational facilities, and active transport systems are not a priority, contributing to greater health disparities, environmental degradation, and social inequities among the most vulnerable—women, children, disabled, aging, and poor.

- Thirty-five million people in the Latin American region are currently affected by diabetes; WHO forecasts an increase to 64 million by 2025 (Barcelo et al. 2003).
- In India, it is predicted that by 2025, 57.2 % of the population will have diabetes (PriceWaterhouseCoopers 2007).
- Cardiovascular diseases (CVD) are already a major cause of death and disability and a main driver of South Asia's NCD epidemic. Indeed, the average age of first-time heart attack sufferers is 53, lower by 6 years than in the rest of the world. In the Middle East and North Africa, NCD prevalence is increasing amongst women and adolescents, driven by factors unrelated to age, such as increasing rates of obesity and smoking (Mahal et al. 2010).

Costs of NCDs and Their Impact on Economies, Health Systems, and Individuals

The World Economic Forum's (WEF) "Global Risks" project has identified NCDs as being one of the greatest threats to the global economy in

2010, with only risks such as asset price collapse being seen as both more likely and with the potential for greater economic loss (WHO 2008).

- The global economic impact of the five leading NCDs—CVD, chronic respiratory disease, cancer, diabetes, and mental ill health—could total USD 47 trillion over the next 20 years, according to the WEF study. The study concludes that the cumulative costs of CVD, chronic respiratory disease, cancer, and diabetes in low- and middle-income countries are estimated to surpass USD 7 trillion in 2011–2025, an average of nearly USD 500 billion per year, causing significant loss of life, capital, and labor during people's most productive years.
- Although the disease burden and the societal and health care costs of CVD are high, the resources devoted towards health care are extremely scarce. The gross national income (GNI) per capita of developed countries ($27,000) is nearly 25-fold that of developing countries ($1,100). Furthermore, developed countries devote twice as much of their GNI (10 %) to health care compared with low- and middle-income countries (6 %). This results in about a 40-fold difference between developed and developing countries in funds devoted to health care (Gaziano 2005).
- The sharp rise of NCDs in emerging market economies such as Russia, India, and China is particularly worrying. Experts say that between 2005 and 2015 these countries could lose $200 billion to $550 billion of national income due to the effects of NCDs on their populations. On average, 10 days are lost per employee per year due to NCDs and injuries in the Russian Federation (Suhrcke et al. 2007).
- Annual income loss from NCDs, arising from days spent ill and in caregiving efforts, amounted to US$ 23 billion (0.7 % GDP) in India in 2004.
- (WHO World Health Report 2010b).

In the Province of Taiwan, China, the probability of being in the labor force was reduced by 27 % by CVD and 19 % by diabetes (Mete and Schultz 2002). Studies in China showed that tobacco use increased the odds of sick leave by between 32 and 56 % (Tsai et al. 2005).

The World Health Report 2010 states that each year, 100 million people are pushed into poverty because they have to pay directly for health services; in some countries, this may represent 5 % of the population forced into poverty each year. Financial hardship is not restricted to low- and middle-income countries: almost four million people in six OECD countries (Greece, Hungary, Mexico, Poland, Portugal, and the Republic of Korea) reported forms of financial hardship caused by paying for health care. The report indicates that direct out-of-pocket payments still represent more than 50 % of total health expenditures in a large number of low- and middle-income countries.

The rise of NCDs among younger populations is cause for particular concern because it will diminish the ability of these countries to capitalize on the opportunities that would otherwise be provided by their demographic dividend, that is, the economic benefits generated during the period when a relatively larger portion of the population is of working age. During that period, one would expect higher economic output per capita, which allows greater wealth generation and more resources to be channeled into savings and productive investments. The significance of missing out on the demographic dividend will become all too apparent when many countries are confronted with the rapid aging of their populations. The proportion of people over 65 years of age is expected to double over a period of 21 years in Brazil, 25 years in India, and 26 years in China. In many high-income countries, the same demographic transition took more than a century. With NCD levels also rising, many developing countries will face a compound challenge of rapid and unhealthy aging that threatens to place significant pressure on their economic and social structures while compressing the timeline available for effective adaptation.

In the World Bank Report on the *Growing Danger of Non-Communicable Diseases*, it notes: "The challenge of confronting NCDs at a lower level of economic development can converge with related policy challenges. For example, rising food prices may persist, reflecting structural changes in the global economy, and could exacerbate the NCD challenge. Higher food prices will heighten risk factors related to poor diets and malnutrition, and poor families affected by NCDs will find it harder to meet their basic needs. Some middle-income countries will be confronted with increasing NCD burdens in the face of already existing dependency ratio and social welfare system challenges, which will make effective response even more challenging" (World Bank 2011).

Specific examples of economic impact include the following:

- China: Reducing cardiovascular mortality by 1 % per year between 2010 and 2040 could generate an economic value equivalent to 68 % of China's real GDP in 2010 or over PPP US$10.7 trillion.
- Egypt: NCDs could be leading to an overall production loss of 12 % of Egypt's GDP, as the country's labor supply is estimated to be 19 % below its potential due to lost employment of those suffering from chronic disease conditions.
- Brazil: Costs of NCDs between 2005 and 2009 could equal 10 % of Brazil's 2003 GDP.
- India: Eliminating NCDs could have, in theory, increased India's 2004 GDP by 4–10 %.

The magnitude of the challenge to health systems is undeniable in diagnosis and treatment, as NCDs require multiple patient interactions, frequently in more expensive inpatient settings and over long time periods.

H. E. Mr. Ban Ki-moon, former United Nations Secretary General, has stated:

"The United Nations and business need each other. We need your innovation, your initiative, your technological prowess. But business also needs the United Nations. In a very real sense, the work of the United Nations can be viewed as seeking to create the ideal enabling environment within which business can thrive." (United Nations General Assembly 2007).

"Poverty is something that no one should endure. Markets can flourish only in societies that are healthy. And societies need healthy markets to flourish. That is why we have to boost our private-public alliance. We need to bring knowledge, resources and innovation together in a way that links sustainability with opportunities for growth." (Ki-moon 2008).

Differing Perspectives About PPPs

The UN recognized the need for partnership in the Millennium Development Goals. The WHO emphasized in its Global Strategy on Diet, Physical Activity and Health that "the private sector can be a 'significant player' in promoting healthy diets and physical activity." The WHO's 2008–2013 Action Plan for the Global Strategy for the Prevention and Control of Noncommunicable Diseases includes as one of its six major objectives the need to "promote partnerships" in NCDs. The World Bank paper, *"Effective Responses to Noncommunicable Diseases: Embracing Action Beyond the Health Sector,"* explores the scope for response in greater depth, and considers the role that actors from various sectors—including health, education, urban planning, agriculture, transport, and industry—can play in preventing NCDs.

Conflicts of Interest Versus Shared Values

Yet, with all of the evidence before us, there remains a vocal segment of civil society and public health that have a problem with the growing acceptance of public/private sector partnerships in the NCD area. Activists point to the policy actions of the tobacco, food and beverage, pharmaceutical, and mining industries, in developing countries, as examples, where there has been a lack of goodwill and trust. They believe that governments have an obligation to care for its citizens and not be co-opted by the largesse of companies whose product lines, pricing, and general shareholder business model present a conflict of interest to societal general well-being and the promotion of healthy people and healthy behaviors.

The public sector's underlying concerns are not only the need for transparency and legitimacy but also stewardship, shaped by new rules of engagement. Over 100 NGOs and medical groups signed a petition in July 2011, saying that there needed to be a code of conduct with industry, as there was a "lack of clarity of roles for the industry sector in UN health policy setting and shap-

ing." They are concerned about the imbalance of power that currently exists and lack of safeguards, especially when company interests are tightly linked to the political process, and that their business model, not just their philanthropy, actually provides societal, stakeholder, and ecological benefits. While one cannot make companies into civil society organizations or charities, it is ironic that companies originally were vested with corporate charters only to the extent that their businesses actually benefited society (Conflicts of Interest Coalition. Statement 2011).

Others engaged in public/private partnership building are more pragmatic and see a new organic worldview taking shape, where shared values and shared commitments are producing greater returns than the risk of doing nothing. They point to companies reporting to shareholders and stakeholders about how their actions in the marketplace contribute to general health and well-being, and see partnerships as something more than window-dressing and "blue-washing," generating scalable, long-term innovation and sustainable value for both business and society. They are taking ownership of their impact.

Importantly, global academic, social, political, and development forces are coming together in search of effective, cost-affordable, culturally salient, and politically viable opportunities to simultaneously prevent and treat disease and promote health-enabling lifestyles and environments.

The UN High-Level Meeting on NCDs, among a host of other major initiatives related to urban health and child development, has shined a light on the fact that for the first time in human history, the numbers of obese people match the number of hungry people, creating a double burden of disease. Additionally, whereas 80 % of diseases are NCDs, and 20 % are communicable diseases, 80 % of the dollars to fund interventions are going towards the communicable disease side of the equation.

Issues of Human and Social Capital

The recent dramatic increase in PPPs reflects broader changes in the aid paradigm, reflecting perceived failures of top-down economic aid and an increased concern with issues of human and social capital, as well as the strengthening of civil society organizations.

Public medical facilities, and systems at large, are overwhelmed and underresourced. Health facilities are overcrowded and the few physicians who are available are often not able to spend the time with patients necessary to fully inform them of their choices for treatment and disease management. The private sector can play a valuable role by augmenting public services with additional patient education.

Policy-makers at all levels of government are facing tough choices among funding priorities. However, nations do not have to experience this gloomy future. The chronic diseases causing these cost increases are preventable. Health systems strengthening measures and creating health-enabling environments that foster social integration and reduce health disparities are possible. Creating policy change in institutional settings like schools, in child and aftercare settings, and in corporate environments is possible. And, developing a "health-in-all" policies prevention approach across the "whole of government" is doable.

A few years ago, Timberland CEO, Jeffrey Swartz, accepted a friend's invitation to spend half a day in a teen halfway house. His friend promised him that his life would never be the same. After answering the troubled teen's question about what he did ("I'm responsible for the global execution of strategy at Timberland)," Jeff asked the teen what he did. The response: "I work at getting well." Swartz said later that the teen's answer trumped his own answer and changed his life and that of his company "to make the world a better place" (Sisodia et al. 2007).

These days, concepts such as "emotional intelligence" and "servant leadership" are in vogue. Where once corporate philanthropy was an obligation, it is fast becoming viewed as a competitive advantage for attracting and retaining top talent and for remaining competitive in the market. Where corporate responsibility was once an oxymoron, today it is becoming ingrained as part of corporate mission. In today's global economy, companies are less inclined to objectify customers as "targets" and employees as

"human resources." They are taking a more societal view, forming relationships with customers, employees, and other stakeholders that further the fulfillment of everyone's agenda in much the same way a healthy natural ecosystem works. Business leaders are beginning to regard the term "survival of the fittest" not in terms of who is the most competitive and strongest, but who is the most collaborative and adaptable.

The Economics of National and Worksite Performance

The issue of NCDs and morbidity and mortality trends matter to global companies as cost containment and value-enhancing productivity and performance issues. Big picture: Companies need stable environments in which to operate. They also need healthy customers and healthy employees. According to companies like Johnson & Johnson, the body is now being viewed as business relevant … physically, mentally, socially. This triple bottom line on an individual basis translates into a triple bottom line for companies, as it affects employee performance, corporate financial performance, and contribution to community health and wellness.

As national and global economies are important to business, the NCD issue affects economies through reduced labor supply, labor outputs, and lower tax revenues that result in corresponding increased insurance and productivity costs to employers and increased public health and social welfare expenditures that are bankrupting countries. Health care costs in the USA have grown at more than slightly twice the pace of the GDP. In the USA, chronic disease costs the economy more than US$1 trillion annually. Simultaneously, public funds are paying for a larger and larger share of these costs through medicare and medicaid. This means there is less money to support other needed programs. Additional projections indicate that, for example, India could lose $237 billion (US) over the next few years due to health-related costs (DeVol and Bedroussian 2007).

In order to reduce costs, employers need to be aware of both their employees' health needs and their access to health care because this access can affect overall workforce health. In China, the lack of access to affordable care is a serious issue. Most Chinese citizens are uninsured: 45 % of urban populations and 79 % of rural populations pay out of pocket for health insurance (Hew et al. 2006).

Despite the daily feed of large-font headlines calling our attention to corporate sins, companies and trade associations are involved in a realignment of beliefs and value systems with an emergent change in their worldview that signals a more human face and involvement with their employees and the communities in which they live, work, learn, and play.

For example, in partnership with the Chinese Ministry of Health, Medtronic has opened a Patient Care Center in Beijing to provide patients with the information they need to make informed decisions about their care and treatment. The center also provides physicians with therapy and product training. In many countries the shortage of health care providers severely restricts the population's access to treatments. Medtronic has trained 30,000 physicians on new medical devices and solutions, increasing access to life-savings therapies like smart implants to actively manage chronic diseases (Butel 2011).

Over the past 3 years, the World Economic Forum's Worksite Health Alliance has committed to building health sustainability in the workplace, creating tools and processes to engage corporate decision-makers and show the impact of wellness initiatives. They also document how NCDs limit employee performance capacity through absenteeism, premature death, and presenteeism (underperformance on the job), with costs for a US company reaching as much as $70 million annually, based on the medical expenditure of picking up employee health care, lost time, and lost productivity (World Economic Forum 2012).

Social Investment and Transparency

Because the private sector can be more nimble and take greater risks than the public sector, they have an essential role in advancing the NCD agenda and supporting advancements in chronic

disease management. Businesses have great capacity for, and expertise in, market research, and can also provide funding and share their skills to help to build a knowledge base in developing countries. Private sector involvement in research has been specifically called for in, for example, the *Grand Challenges in Chronic Noncommunicable Diseases*, published in Nature in 2007. Private companies who invest in aggressive research and development agendas and in scaling up promising technologies can increase profits and significantly impact the quality of life of those living with chronic diseases.

Public/private partnerships represent the convergence of a perfect storm, with opportunities for integrated interventions and systemic change, the positive outcome. During the past two decades many people in the social investment, accountability, and activist communities have worked hard to develop a responsibility assurance framework (principles and standards, monitoring and certification, and standardized reporting for nonfinancial issues). Peer pressure from other corporations and media attention have contributed to these developments. This system of "soft law," while it can mandate nothing, can place considerable pressure on companies to become more responsible, accountable, and transparent. Add the increasing importance of reputation to companies, combined with a growing population of more sophisticated consumers and employees who care about responsibility, and you have a ratcheted-up set of expectations, especially for big companies.

A 2006 review of global public–private health partnerships by Buse and Harmer notes that many global health partnerships (GHPs) engage in activities related to the development of policy and norms, creating potential conflicts of interest if for-profit organizations have a role in policy setting (Buse and Harmer 2007).

A GHP for NCDs would need clear guidelines that include an ethical framework and code of conduct, to manage conflicts of interest and to firewall policy development. However, with these measures in place, it is important to recognize that the private sector has an important role in the prevention and control of NCDs and can contribute towards many of the actions outlined in the Political Declaration, such as increased access to quality-assured and affordable medicines and technologies, reduction of salt content in foods, and implementing measures on restricting marketing of unhealthy foods to children.

The Sixty-third World Health Assembly in May 2010 endorsed a policy on WHO engagement with global health partnerships and hosting arrangements (World Health Organization 2010c):

"Pursuit of the public-health goal takes precedence over the special interests of participants. Risks and responsibilities arising from public–private partnerships need to be identified and managed through development and implementation of safeguards that incorporate considerations of conflicts of interest.

The partnership shall have mechanisms to identify and manage conflicts of interest. Whenever commercial, for-profit companies are considered as potential partners, potential conflicts of interest shall be taken into consideration as part of the design and structure of the partnership."

Additionally, guidelines used by existing mechanisms such as *Partnership for Maternal, Newborn and Child Health (PMNCH) and Roll Back Malaria* could be used as a basis for discussions on a policy for a GHP for NCDs (Harding et al. 2010).

Lessons can also be learned from the experiences of platforms such as *PMNCH*, which has been successful in harnessing the capabilities and resources of the private sector through its Partners Forum towards implementation of the UN Secretary General's Global Strategy for Women and Children's Health while also guarding against potential conflicts and retaining independence in policy formulation (Roll Back Malaria 2007).

An evolution of change is now in process. Today, there are 7,700 companies registered with the UN Global Compact, committed to adopting principles of meaning that put this culture of change into practice on the human rights and environmental fronts. Well over 82,000 transnational corporations do business today, compared to about 37,000 in 1990. Operating with about 810,000 foreign affiliates, they employ more than 77 million people, and feed into millions of sup-

pliers and distributors operating along their global value chains (UNCTAD 2009).

Public/Private Sector Partnership Models and Key Partnership Trends

UN Agencies, Funds, and Programs are PPP Pioneers in working to meet the targets of the UN Millennium Development Goals. According to the UN *Coming of Age* Report, "The U.N. has had the greatest positive impact when it has focused on using its convening power instead of taking a lead role in technical advice or setting policy goals that conflict with the members' interests. The most successful partnerships have been those where the UN has brought leading businesses, NGOs, governments, research institutes and multilateral bodies to the same table to work out solutions" (Hoxtell et al. 2010).

UN Development Program (UNDP) is a partnership leader in developing business and cultivating inclusive markets. The "Business Call to Action" platform and the Growing Sustainable Business Initiative are some of its recent successful multi-stakeholder partnership initiatives to encourage innovative business models that create economic and developmental benefits.

UNHCR (Office of UN High Commissioner on Refugees) spearheads UN–business cross-fertilization on the organizational level to raise public awareness of displaced people and help UNHCR become a more efficient and effective organization.

World Food Program (WFP) has been leading the way in developing partnerships which harness contributions of corporate core competencies, products, and services to achieve development results that benefit both parties, for example through its Moving the World partnership with TNT. TNT offers four forms of support to the WFP: Knowledge transfer: sending out specialist employees all over the world to transfer skills and knowledge; hands-on support: supporting WFP in the field to improve on distribution and logistics during emergency operations; awareness and fund-raising: raising awareness and funds for WFP through public information activities, marketing campaigns, and employee fund-raising initiatives; and transport for good.

UNAIDS is considered the leader in advocacy partnerships and developing funding mechanisms.

Below are key partnership trends cited by The *Coming of Age* Report, along with examples of NCD PPPs that we have resourced to showcase these trends in action:

Core Business and Value Chain Partnerships

These enterprise solutions accelerate and sustain access by the poor to needed goods and services and/or employment and livelihood opportunities. They also include behavior change strategies that promote the availability of "healthy" product choices and lifestyles.

- The *International Federation of Pharmaceutical Manufacturers and Associations*, in cooperation with the Commonwealth Business Council, has reported out significant multi-sector partnerships between its members, NGOs, and government, in areas of providing access to medicines, strengthening health systems, and educating the public about diabetes and CVD. A list of partnerships can be accessed at http://partnerships.ifpma.org/.

- The *Global Business Coalition* boasts a membership of nearly 200 companies, including multinationals such as the Coca-Cola Company, Exxon Mobil, and Pfizer, which heretofore has concentrated efforts on stopping TB, malaria, and AIDS, and is now turning its attention to NCDs with members developing public/private partnerships that create capacity building training and education programs, public awareness, and cash and in-kind donation programs. Their tools and resources for promoting *Healthy Women, Healthy Economies* are easily translatable to NCD issues of lifestyle and the need for work, education, and empowerment partnerships built around reducing health disparities and increasing gender equity and social integration, www.gbchealth.org.

- In 2008, the *International Food and Beverage Association*, comprising eight major international food and nonalcoholic beverage companies, made voluntary global public commitments to action in support of continuing efforts to implement the 2004 WHO Global Strategy on Diet, Physical Activity and Health. These commitments include reformulating and introducing new products to provide consumers with options they can use in building sensible, balanced diets; providing easy-to-understand and meaningful, fact-based nutrition labeling and information; changing how and what the industry advertises to children; supporting nutrition education and physical activity programs; and participating in national and regional efforts with governments, NGOs, and professional organizations to promote healthy lifestyles in the workplace and in communities (The International Food and Beverage Alliance Letter to WHO Director General in May, 2008; www.ifballiance.org).

- *The Global Alliance for Improved Nutrition, GAIN*, has a number of public/private partnerships for delivering nutrition fortification in developing countries, www.gainhealth.org.

- The *Consumer Goods Forum*, a global network of more than 650 retailers, manufacturers, service providers, and other stakeholders across 70 countries, works together to address consumer health and wellness. CGF has adopted resolutions to address three primary areas: availability of products and services that support healthier diets and lifestyles; transparent, fact-based information that helps consumers make informed choices; and communication and educational programs to raise awareness and inspire healthier lifestyles, www.theconsumergoodsforum.com.

Advocacy and Public Policy Engagement

These partnerships promote awareness and improve the health-enabling environments through advancement of legislative policies and regulations, multi-sector network alliances, and media/public education strategies, including regional and national government, civil society, and private sector examples.

- The *PAHO Partners Forum for Action on NCDs* was created by PAHO, in collaboration with the International Business Leaders Forum (IBLF), the Pan American Health and Education Foundation (PAHEF), the WEF, and in consultation with the CARMEN network, the WHO Collaborating Centers, international NGOs, and Consumers International, as a catalyst for multi-sector partnerships that drive direct social, environmental, and policy action to prevent three million deaths over the next ten years in the Americas, www.paho.org/panamericanforum/.

- The *American College of Sports Medicine, Exercise Is Medicine Global Initiative* is a multi-stakeholder coalition dedicated to encouraging health care professionals to assess the physical activity of their patients and prescribe physical activity interventions to prevent, treat, and manage NCDs while also providing education and training interventions that connect the clinical world to the world of the public health community, www.exerciseismedicine.org.

- *SUSTRANS*, a UK program, is a very influential health promotion program that delivers a range of environmental and behavioral interventions with several thousand partners, including schools, clubs, local authorities, health sector, community groups, and business to get children and young people walking and biking. Similarly in the USA, the "Safe Routes to School" program supported by the US Department of Transportation is a national partnership program with state and regional networks who also promote the use of joint resources, www.sustrans.org.uk.

- *The WEF, through its Healthy Living workstream, is* focused on preventing and treating NCDs through advocacy, dialogue, partnerships, and "best practices" that engage world leaders in shaping global, regional, and industry agendas to achieve targeted health outcomes. Deliverables to date include the

Workplace Wellness Alliance which has 150 members and covers 4.5 million workers worldwide; a milestone report galvanizing the economic burden of NCDs; the establishment of a Civil Society Task Force which was used as a conduit for critical input to the process of developing the UN Political Declaration on Prevention and Control of NCDs; and the launch of the "Wellness Week" in September 2011 in New York City and ten other cities in Latin America, www.weforum.org.

- The *NCD Alliance* is a good example of a network of more than 900 national member associations in over 170 countries to address the need for a global framework for reducing NCDs, with established targets and indicators. Recognizing the need for concerted action and in response to the UN General Assembly call for a High Level Meeting on NCDs, in May 2010, the NCD Alliance was founded by a coalition of four global NGOs: the International Diabetes Federation (IDF), International Union Against Cancer (IUCC), World Heart Federation (WHF), and International Union Against Tuberculosis and Lung Disease. The Alliance also includes a "special interest group" of more than 230 NGOs spanning a diversity of 10 NCD-related interests and sectors. This represents a single voice to advocate for the five major diseases and the four primary risk factors, tobacco, alcohol, unhealthy diet, and physical inactivity, www.ncdalliance.org.

- *US First Lady Michelle Obama's signature program, "Let's Move,"* is an example of a government multi-sector/multi-stakeholder effort engaging numerous civil society, professional organizations, companies, and local municipalities in reducing childhood obesity in cities and towns, schools, and health care institutions across the nation. The campaign has made great strides to engage the private sector in constructive ways. For example, the campaign has partnered with Walmart to reduce sugar, sodium, and trans fats in thousands of its products, and lower fruit and vegetable prices to increase access to healthy food choices, www.letsmove.gov.

- *Healthy Caribbean Coalition's Get the Message* campaign has utilized mobile phone and social media platforms to demonstrate and generate support for the UN HLM on NCDs. The effort cooperated with two large mobile phone providers and had mobile subscribers in 17 Caribbean countries texting (free of charge) Caribbean leaders on the importance of voting in support of the UN Political Declaration on NCDs, www. healthycaribbean.org.
- *Designed To Move:* A Physical Activity Action Agenda, represents a social movement involving 70 experts and nearly 100 global organizations from sports, fitness, sports science, physical education, sport development, and public health disciplines, who are champions committed to creating early positive experiences for children and integrating physical activity into every day life, through development of advocacy, communications, and leadership best practices that can be modeled, measured and evaluated to reverse the global physical inactivity epidemic. www.designedtomove.org.

Scaling Social Investment and Philanthropy

New financing approaches represent significant potential for positive change. The private sector provides different types of support, including traditional philanthropy, social venture funds, and hybrid or blended-value financing mechanisms.

- Foundations, such as the *Robert Wood Johnson Foundation*, are addressing the issue of childhood obesity from a public health perspective and have contributed millions of dollars to projects dedicated to helping reduce the rates of childhood obesity by 2015. Their "Healthy Kids, Healthy Communities" is a national RWJF program that is helping nearly 50 communities across the country reshape their environments to support healthy living and prevent childhood obesity. The RWJF Active Living Network creates and nurtures a network of professionals, advocates, and organizations to support and promote the creation of active, healthy communities. Some 70 organizations—from such diverse disciplines as planning, design, transportation, parks and recreation, local government, and public health—had signed on as network partners as of December 2007.
- *Cause-related marketing collaborations* have the potential to generate significant benefits through promotional campaigns in which companies pledge a share of sales revenues to their public partners. Models include the following:
  - Companies contributing a percentage of credit card purchases to designated projects. *Target's* "Take Charge of Education" is an example whereby consumers linked their Target credit card to a K-12 school of their choice. Since 1997, schools have received donations twice a year to use funds for anything they need, for a total of $324 million donated (Designed to Move 2012).
- *Corporate Licensing* programs that pledge a share of profits from sales of products, like in the *PRODUCT RED* trademark campaign, which has transferred more than US$150 million to the Global AIDS Fund (Sprott et al. 2010).
- *Celebrity-driven initiatives*, like *LIVESTRONG*, a cancer advocacy organization founded by Lance Armstrong has undertaken a comprehensive social media strategy across a number of platforms and campaigns, achieving high volumes of participants from across the globe and raising more than $100 million in the fight against cancer, www. livestrong.org.
- *Government multi-sector initiatives* in Latin America are generating funding for large-scale initiatives to channel innovation and financing into programming focused on children and youth at risk.
  - The *Inter-American Development Bank* partnership, "Paving the Way" Alliance for Sports and Development, between the

IDB, FC Barcelona, NBA, VISA, and Colgate, the municipality of Rio de Janeiro, and community NGOs has invested more than $20 million since 2005. The Alliance's goal is to promote the social inclusion of 4,000 disadvantaged youth in Rio's favelas through sports programs, www.designedtomove.org (2012).

– *Academia Da Saude Project in Brazil*, a national program of the Brazilian Ministry of Health, has committed to a $1 billion investment in building 4,000 community gyms across the country by 2015, backed up by a cross-national and transdisciplinary collaboration (the GUIA Project) between the CDC, the Prevention Research Center in St. Louis, PAHO, and the Federal University in Sao Paolo, among others. The effort is a physical activity intervention aimed at reducing health disparities among the most vulnerable, reducing NCDs, and increasing social integration through creation of health-enabling environments. *The GUIA Project, Prevention Research Center, St. Louis (2005),* www.projectguia.org.

  – *Using fiscal measures through tax incentives and spending to support community health and development is another financing mechanism at work:*Examples are exempting medicines and foods from sales tax and imposing an excise tax on cigarettes and alcohol. A wide range of countries and local jurisdictions tax tobacco, with acknowledged success in reducing consumption (Nugent and Feigl 2010).

Conclusion

Global health partnerships should not be viewed as ends in themselves. Without a clear global plan of action that includes key performance indicators, targets, resource requirements, and commitment from relevant actors to implement, a partnership may lack effectiveness and entail high transaction costs.

The world that today's public health community and companies face is tumultuous and increasingly connected. Each depends on three interconnected systems for their success: the natural environment, the social and political environment, and the global economic environment. The fact that many corporations control more resources than do many countries can create fear and, with the changing worldview, suggests a need for new mechanisms of governance. One study in 2000 found that of the 100 largest revenue producers in the world, 51 were companies rather than countries (Anderson and Cavanagh 2000).

"To engage the best to do the most" in the immediate term means you have done your homework:

• Performed a stakeholder analysis
• Defined constituencies and communities important and aligned to your organization and brand values
• Documented needs and assessed potential partner interests and influence
• Pinpointed those best to help build capacity, identified roles, responsibilities, and expected commitments of each partner
• Checked for problematic conflicts of interest attached to the arrangement and mechanisms for addressing them
• Developed the mutual win/win–lose/lose scenarios for each
• Assessed the scope, reach, and resources needed from both—for convening, advocacy, communications, research, capacity building, and funding to affect sustainability and effectiveness.

At the end of the day, public/private partnerships can play an important role in fostering global health equity and keep public health at the center of the relationship. If we change our worldview from an "either/or" framework to a collaborative mindset that celebrates "the and," we open ourselves up to infinite possibilities, including one where public/private partnerships can be the linchpin for expanding reach, revenue, and trusted engagement in building sustainable shared values and a "culture of health for all" that achieves a better balance between "me" and "we."

References

American College of Sports Medicine (2011) Stefan, M., *U.N. side event report on physical activity and NCDs, September*. www.acsm.org/unsideevent

Anderson, S., & Cavanagh, J. (2000). *Top 200: Rise of Corporate Global Power*. Washington, DC: Institute for Policy Studies.

Barcelo, A., Aedo, C., Raipathak, S., & Robles, S. (2003). The cost of diabetes in Latin America and the Caribbean. *Bulletin of the World Health Organization, 8*(1), 19–28.

Beaglehole, R., Bonita, R., Horton, R., et al. (2011). Priority actions for the non-communicable disease crisis. *Lancet, 377*(9775), 1438–1447.

Buse, K., & Harmer, A. (2007). Seven habits of highly effective global public-private health partnerships: Practice and potential. *Social Science & Medicine, 64*, 259–271.

Butel, J. (2011). *Executive Vice President and Group President, International at Medtronic, NCD Series*, Center for Strategic and International Studies http://csis.org/event/tackling-global-ncd-epidemic

Conflicts of Interest Coalition. (2011). Statement of concern on lack of clarity on role of industry for June *UN interactive hearing and September UN High Level Meeting* (2011). http://info.babymilkaction.org/node/458. Accessed Sept 14, 2012.

Designed to Move. (2012). NIKE, ACSM, ICCSPE (co-authors).

DeVol, R., & Bedroussian, A. (2007). *An unhealthy America: The economic burden of chronic disease (No. 2010)*. Santa Monica, CA: Milken Institute. Retrieved from http://www.milkeninstitute.org/pdf/chronic_disease_report.pdf.

Gaziano, T. A. (2005). *Cardiovascular disease in the developing world and its risk management*. Cardiology Rounds, Cardiovascular Division of Brigham and Women's Hospital, Boston, MA.

Global Advocacy Council for Physical Activity, International Society for Physical Activity and Health. (2010). *The Toronto charter for physical activity: A global call to action*. www.globalpa.org.uk

Harding, A., Axelson, H., & Bustreo, F. (2010). *Child Health and the Missing Link*: Working with the private sector for better results. The partnership of maternal, newborn and child health.

Hew, C., Yu, D. Y., & Li, N. P. (2006). *Health care in China*. Retrieved April 12, 2010, from http://www-935.ibm.com/services/us/imc/pdf/g510-6268-healthcare-china.pdf

Hoxtell, W., Preysing, D., & Streets, J. (2010). *Coming of age: UN private sector collaboration since 2008*. http://unglobalcompact.org/docs/news_events/8.1/Coming_of_Age.pdf

Institute for Health Metrics and Evaluation. (2010). *Financing global health: Development assistance and country spending: In: Chapter1: Tracking development assistance for health*.

Ki-moon, B. (2008). *Remarks to the 1st private sector forum on the millennium development goals* [speech] Sept 24, 2008, New York.

Lankenau, B., Culhane, D., & Stefan, M. (2010). Powerful partnering: Courting new realms to boost physical activity promotion. *Journal of Physical Activity and Health, 7*(Suppl 3), S356–S357.

Mahal, A., Karan, A., & Engelgau, M. (2010). *Global status report on NCDs: Monitoring NCDs and their risk factors*.

McColl, K. (2008). Europe told to deliver more aid for health. *The Lancet, 371*(9630), 2072–2073. doi:10.1016/S0140-6736(08)60901-0.

Mete, C., & Schultz, T. P. (2002). *Health and labour-force participation of the elderly in Taiwan*. New Haven, CT: Yale University.

Michaud, J. (2010). *Global health's private sector revolution*, World Politics Review

Murumets, K., O'Reilly, N., Tremblay, M. S., & Katzmarzyk, P. T. (2010). Public private partnerships in physical activity and sport: Principles for successful, responsible partnerships. *Journal of Physical Activity and Health, 7*(3), S349–S351.

Nugent, R. & Feigl, A. B. (2010). *Where have all the donors gone? Scarce donor funding for noncommunicable diseases*. Working Paper No. 228. Center for Global Development; Washington, DC.

PAHO (2002). *Health in the Americas*, Volume 1. http://www.aho.org/hq/index.php?option=com_content&view=article&id=6436&Itemid=1723&lang=en.

Physical Activity Network of the Americas (RAFA-PANA). (2009). RAFA-PANA guidelines for approaching industry partners. Accessed at www.rafapana.org.

Prevention Research Center, St. Louis, (2005). www.projectguia.org.

PriceWaterhouseCoopers. (2007). *Working towards wellness - an Indian perspective*."

Roll Back Malaria. (2007). *Conflict of Interest Guidelines*. http://www.rbm.who.int/docs/constituencies/RBMcoiPolicy.pdf

Sisodia, R. S., Wolfe, D. B., & Sheth, J. N. (2007). *Firms of endearment, How world-class companies profit from passion and purpose*. Upper Saddle River, NJ: Wharton School.

Sprott, M., Hoxtell, W., Preysing, D. & Strakhova, M., (2010). Review of global cause-related marketing activities, Coming of age report, [internal UNICEF study], Berlin.

Stefan, M. (2011). Powerful partnering: Engaging the best to do the most. *IUHPE Journal of Global Health Promotion, 18*, 27–30. doi:10.1177/1757975911412404.

Suhrcke, M., et al. (2007). *Economic consequences of noncommunicable diseases and injuries in the Russian Federation*. Geneva: World Health Organization.

Tsai, S., et al. (2005). Workplace smoking related absenteeism and productivity costs in Taiwan. *Tobacco Control, 14*, i33–i37.

UNCTAD. (2009). *World investment report 2009: Transnational corporations, agricultural production and development* (p. 22). New York & Geneva: UNCTAD.

United Nations General Assembly. (2007). *Toward global partnerships. Resolution A/C.2/62/L.33/Rev.1, para.2.*

United Nations Global Compact. (2010). A global compact for development. Adapted from Jane Nelson and Dave Prescott *Business and millennium development goals: A framework for action 2003–2008.*

Vuori, I., Blair, S., Bull, F. C., & Katzmarzyk, P. T. (2010). More collaboration-more power in combating ill health. *Journal Of Physical Activity And Health, 7*(Suppl 3), S359–S360.

WHO. (2008). *2008–2013 Action plan for the global strategy for the prevention and control of noncommunicable diseases* http://www.who.int/nmh/publications/9789241597418/en/index.html.

WHO. (2010a). *Global Status Report on NCDs*, Editor: Dr. Ala Alwan, Assistant Director-General, NCDs and Mental Health. ISBN 978 92 4 068645 8 (PDF) http://www.who.int/nmh/publications/ncd_report_full_en.pdf. *Analysis by region uses WHO updated esti-mates for 2008 and baseline projections for 2030; analysis by income group uses WHO 2008–2030 baseline projections.* Sources: World Bank analysis by the authors, based on the WHO Global Burden of Disease estimates and projections and the World Bank regional/income country groupings.

WHO. (2010b). World Health Report. *Health systems financing: the path to universal coverage.* http://www.who.int/whr/2010/en/index.html

WHO. (2010c). *Partnerships report by the Secretariat. Sixty-third world health assembly. document A63/44.* Geneva: World Health Organization 22 April 2010. http://apps.who.int/gb/ebwha/pdffiles/WHA63/A6344-en.pdf

WHO Commission on Social Determinants of Health. (2008). http://www.who.int/social_determinants/thecommission/finalreport/en/index.html

World Bank. (2011). *The growing danger of noncommunicable diseases.*

World Economic Forum. (2012). Workplace health alliance. *Investing in a sustainable workforce*

Section IV

Institutions and Organizations

Framing International Trade and Chronic Disease

24

Ronald Labonté, K.S. Mohindra, and Raphael Lencucha

Background

The nature and magnitude of the burden of chronic disease in low- and middle-income countries (LMICs) are now well understood, as are their impacts on health systems and national economies (World Health Organization [WHO] 2010; Mathars and Loncar 2006; Hossain et al. 2007; Alwan et al. 2010; Dans et al. 2011). What is less clear is how we should address chronic disease in LMICs, although doing so will require actions at both local and global levels (de-Graft Aikins et al. 2010). At the global level, international trade, despite bringing potential health

benefits through economic growth (a point we return to), is one of the major driving factors of a growing chronic disease burden. Trade's effects on chronic disease risk occur *progressively* along multiple pathways. It is the intent of this chapter to explicate those pathways.

Trade is not a new phenomenon: Human societies have long histories of trade with each other and one might even describe barter and exchange as inherently human social qualities (Labonté 2010). What is new is the volume of trade in goods and services, which has reached unprecedented levels over the past century, and the global scale at which trade now occurs. Also, the pattern of trade has morphed into an unequal playing field, where international trade rules tend to benefit disproportionately high-income countries (Birdsall 2006; Gallagher 2007; Polanski 2006; Sundaram and von Arnim 2009). The rise in global production chains, liberalization of global financial flows, and stark inequalities in countries' political and bargaining power are at the heart of many of the contentions concerning contemporary global trade.

Health concerns associated with trade have been a feature of national and global policy debate since the establishment of the World Trade Organization (WTO) in 1995 and its extensive suite of trade treaties aimed at progressively liberalizing the cross-border flow of goods, services, and finance. Such concerns are far from new. Disease has long followed trade routes, from infectious pandemics of past eras to SARS

This chapter draws upon earlier work by the three coauthors, including Mohindra, K. S., Lencucha, R., and Labonté, R., "Reaching behind borders: international trade and chronic disease," in T. Schrecker (ed.) *Research Companion to the Globalization of Health*, Toronto: Ashgate, 2012; and Labonté, R., Mohindra, K., and Lencucha, R. "Framing International Trade and Chronic Disease," *Globalization and Health* 21(3):273–87, 2011.

R. Labonté (✉) • K.S. Mohindra
Institute of Population Health, University of Ottawa, 1 Stewart Street, Room 216B, Ottawa, Canada K1N 6N5
e-mail: rlabonte@uottawa.ca; katia.mohindra@gmail.com

R. Lencucha
Faculty of Health Sciences, University of Lethbridge, 4401 University Drive West, Lethbridge, Alberta, T1K3M4, Canada
e-mail: raphael.lencucha@uleth.ca

in more recent times. The link between trade and infectious disease has been well documented (Fidler 2003; Saker et al. 2004; Kimball 2006); and there is now an emerging evidence base that global trade is also linked with the rise of chronic disease in many LMICs. This linkage is associated, in part, with the global diffusion of unhealthy lifestyles and health-damaging products (Beaglehold and Yach 2003), posing a particular challenge to countries still facing high burdens of communicable disease.

The existing literature on trade and chronic disease has tended to focus on certain health problems, such as diabetes and overnutrition (Hawkes 2006; Yach et al. 2006). Lacking is an understanding of how such trade affects chronic disease more generally and through multiple pathways. To address this knowledge gap, we developed a generic framework which depicts the determinants and pathways connecting global trade with chronic disease. We then applied this framework to three key risk factors for chronic disease: unhealthy diets, alcohol, and tobacco, or what are sometimes referred to as "risky commodities." This led to specific "product pathways," which we propose can be further refined and used by health policy-makers to engage with their country's trade policy-makers around health impacts of ongoing trade treaty negotiations, and by researchers to continue refining an evidence base on how global trade is affecting patterns of chronic disease. We focused our evidence gathering primarily on Latin America, sub-Saharan Africa, and Asia, where the impact of international trade agreements in the global flow of these products has been subject of greatest health comment and concern.

Trade-Related Globalization Chronic Disease

There are at least six interrelated ways in which trade-related globalization affects NCD pathways:
1. *Rising incomes.* Extreme poverty (USD 1.25/ day) has decreased globally since the era of liberalized trade, as outsourcing created more

employment in LMICs (Labonté and Schrecker 2009), improving (at least some) people's social stratification, especially for women in patriarchal societies who obtain work in export processing zones. Rising incomes in LMICs create new and exploitable markets for "risky commodities" (processed food, sugary drinks, tobacco, and alcohol) by the global food, beverage, and tobacco transnationals (Lawrence 2011; Labonté et al. 2011).
2. *Persisting poverty.* The rising tide of globalization's economic growth has not lifted people very far. Poverty at the USD 2.50/day level has increased by almost the same number as the decline in the more extreme rate (Chen and Ravallion 2008). This places pressure on somewhat better-off but still poor households to obtain caloric energy in cheaper, less nutritious food, now more readily available, increasing their vulnerabilities to NCDs. Falling incomes for manual and industrial workers in high-income countries (HICs) made redundant by outsourcing has much the same effect.
3. *Urbanization.* These pressures in LMICs are exacerbated by globalization's influence on migration from rural agricultural to urban wage-labor livelihoods. This migration is attributed, in part, to the rise in global food production chains, export-oriented agricultural policies, and forced displacements of rural populations to permit energy (oil, hydroelectric) or mineral (mining) extractions. Urban living decreases physical activity and exposes populations to unhealthy commodities and lifestyles (Food and Agriculture Organization [FAO] of the United Nations 2002; Chow et al. 2009; Subramanian and Davey 2006; Agyemang et al. 2005). Rapid urbanization in LMICs is further characterized by informal settlements ("slums") where overcrowding and lack of open space compound difficulties in active living, and access to fresh or healthy foods is more difficult.
4. *Labor market insecurity.* Despite the new employment opportunities in LMICs created by globalization, much of this work is insecure or part-time with few or no benefits, a problem

of longer and worsening standing in wealthier countries (Schrecker and Labonté 2010). Across Latin America two-thirds of the urban population lives below the poverty line competing for an insufficient supply of jobs, with almost 60 % of all employment in the insecure, informal sector (Inter-American Development Bank [IADB] 2011). This insecurity, generalizing to other life domains such as housing and food, is associated with increased CVD and possibly other NCD risks (Cornia et al. 2007; Wilkinson and Marmot 2003).

5. *Nutrition transition.* For decades researchers have argued that economic development in LMICs is accompanied by an overall shift from under- to overnutrition, with well-documented trends in increased consumption of oils and fats in such emerging economies as China, India, Brazil, Russia, Mexico, and South Africa (Popkin 1994, 1997, 2002). It is now also occurring in low-income countries and at rates that exceeded similar transitions in today's HICs, partly an effect of liberalization and the growth of global food trade. Bad foods are good global commodities with high profits; good foods are bad global commodities with low profits (Caraher and Cowburn 2005).

6. *Financial crises.* Liberalized financial markets, banking deregulation, and digital technologies have fuelled numerous currency crises since the 1990s. The health-harmful effects of these episodic financial meltdowns in developing county regions resulting from unemployment, poverty, and dramatic cuts to health and social spending were experienced first and worst by those most vulnerable and least responsible for their making (Floro and Dymski 2000; Parrado and Zentento 2001). The 2007 global crisis that erupted with the collapse of the US real estate bubble has similarly increased unemployment and poverty in much of the world, and has been followed by an "austerity agenda" in which worst affected countries are being required to cut spending, reduce public sector employment, and privatize remaining public assets: that is, to continue with and deepen the neoliberal globalization project that most analysts

thought had been discredited by the banking failures (Labonté 2012). In the short term, declining incomes arising from the crisis may lead to a drop in alcohol and tobacco consumption, although they also lead to increased consumption of unhealthy, low-priced foods (Stuckler et al. 2011). Spending cuts under the austerity agenda are reducing access to health services (several countries are increasing user-fees in their public health systems), and will likely reduce the abilities of governments to undertake NCD prevention programs.

All of the above effects of trade-related global market integration have essentially made NCD risk factors "communicable" (with food, tobacco, and alcohol consumption serving as "vectors"), blurring the conventional distinction between communicable and non-communicable diseases. International trade takes place outside of, as well as within, the reach of enforceable trade treaties; our concern in this chapter is primarily with trade treaties and their rules, and how these limit governments' policy flexibilities (policy space and capacity).

Policy Space, Policy Capacity, Trade Treaty Rules, and Risks of Chronic Disease

"Policy space" describes "the freedom, scope, and mechanisms that governments have to choose, design and implement public policies to fulfill their aims" (Koivusalo et al. 2009, p. 7). "Policy capacity" refers to the fiscal ability of states to enact those policies or regulations, which depends upon their ability to capture sufficient revenue through taxation for this purpose. Both space and capacity can be affected by trade treaties. One concern with trade treaties is their "behind-the-border" shrinking of policy space by prohibiting a range of "trade-related" domestic regulatory options that could be used to promote healthy habits or, conversely, to restrict unhealthy ones. The primary purpose of all trade treaties is to reduce barriers to cross-border trade. One of the key principles underlying this purpose is *national treatment*: foreign goods or committed services covered by a trade treaty must be treated the same as the identical or "like" domestic good or service. Internal tax and regulatory measures must be applied equally to imported and domestic goods or committed (scheduled) services in order to avoid trade disputes. To protect population health found to be in violation of trade agreements (the so-called *health defense*), governments have to prove that these policies are "necessary" and "consistent" with the norms of trade openness and nondiscrimination. Past and ongoing disputes over regulations governing tobacco imports and additives, alcohol products, and food items highlight the stringency with which this requirement is pursued (Mitchell and Voon 2011). Further limitations on the health defense include requirements that domestic regulations that could discriminate against foreign imports, even if treated no differently than national goods, must be based upon international standards or scientific risk assessments (Labonté 2010). These trade principles constrain policy space.

Policy capacity, in turn, refers to the resources states have to monitor or enforce regulations that they are able to promulgate. The issue of capacity is of considerable importance to LMICs, many of which have excellent laws "on the books" but lack effective enforcement measures. The policy capacity trade issue is that liberalization requires progressive reductions in tariffs (border taxes). Developing countries rely more heavily upon tariffs for their tax revenue than do developed nations. Although developing countries are granted more latitude in retaining higher tariff levels, they are under considerable political pressure to lock in and reduce their tariffs, in both multilateral WTO negotiations and notably in bilateral and regional trade treaties. In theory, developing country governments should be able to shift their tax bases from tariffs to sales or income taxes, assuming that their economies grow with increased liberalization. In reality, many developing, and most low-income, countries subject to tariff reductions as conditions for loans from the international financial institutions (the World Bank and IMF) have been unable to do so (Baunsgaard and Keen 2010; Glenday 2006), partly as a result of inadequate institutions to implement alternate tax regimes (Aizenman

and Jinjarak 2009). For a majority of these countries there has been a net decline in overall public revenues (Labonté et al. 2008)—a loss in policy capacity—with implications for spending in health, education, or public regulations that can affect primary and secondary prevention of chronic disease.

Governments still retain substantial policy flexibilities within existing WTO Agreements, although these flexibilities continue to be eroded through ongoing treaty negotiations. Of considerable concern is the dramatic increase in bilateral or regional trade treaties, an outcome of stalled negotiations in the more multilateral WTO forum. Many of these bilateral and regional treaties, especially those involving the US or European Union (EU) and LMICs, include liberalization commitments, intellectual property rights protection, and agreements on government procurement that go beyond those in existing WTO trade treaties, and which can limit policy space to a much greater extent than WTO trade rules (Lynch 2010; Thangavelu and Toh 2005; Dahrendorf 2009). Finally, it is important to grasp that the intent of a government regulation "plays a very limited role in determining whether a measure violates a prohibition" of a trade treaty (McGrady 2011, p. 127). Arguing that the regulatory purpose was to protect public health holds little weight if, even unintentionally, it violates a trade rule—even a government invokes the health defense. Where this is of concern with respect to NCD risks is in how trade rules affect four of the key NCD control strategies:

- Demand reduction (e.g., pricing, taxation)
- Supply reduction (e.g., bans, import restrictions, regulation of distribution outlets)
- Reduced risk exposure (e.g., smoking restrictions, rules over alcohol content or salt/fat content)
- Informing consumers (e.g., labeling requirements)

Generic Framework

Figure 24.1 provides a generic framework of the linkages between chronic disease and international trade. Trade can be broadly segmented into

General framework: Trade and chronic disease

Legend:

⟶ Financial flows

- - - -➤ Trade of goods

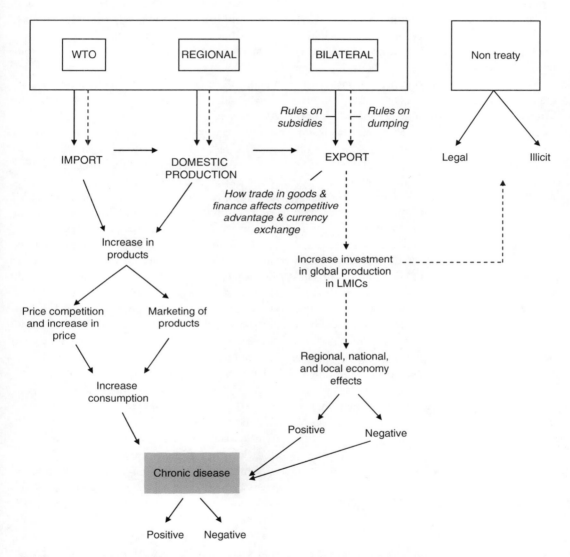

Fig. 24.1 A generic framework of the linkages between chronic disease and international trade

two categories: treaty, which includes bilateral, regional, or multilateral under the WTO and non-treaty, which includes both legal (but non-treaty) and illicit trade. Trade treaties can affect trade in goods in two main ways: increased trade in raw or finished products (depicted with solid arrow lines) and increased foreign investment in domestic production, manufacturing, and distribution (depicted with dotted arrow lines). Increased imports and domestic production result in increased domestic availability of a particular product. Greater quantity and availability, in turn, increase price competition (lower prices) and marketing and (generally) promotion of the product, both of which lead to increased product consumption. Increased consumption can have positive or negative consequences on chronic diseases depending on whether it is a health-promoting (e.g., nutritious food) or health-damaging (e.g., highly processed food) product. Increased foreign investment in a particular product can also lead to economic growth which, if adequately taxed, can contribute to revenues for health and other health-promoting social programs. However, if this product has harmful effects (e.g., tobacco), increased consumption is more likely to lead to poorer health outcomes, burdening health systems and offsetting any economic gains. Moreover, increased imports and foreign investment can displace domestic producers and manufacturers, which can reduce local revenues and food security (if local food crops are displaced) and increase dependency on foreign companies, making it more difficult to introduce regulations constraining their market growth or raising corporate taxes. Non-treaty trade in products has similar effects apart from legally binding constraints on a country's tariffs or domestic policies. Illicit trade is difficult to document for most products and is not discussed further in this chapter.

Specific Pathway Products

Tobacco Trade and Health

Trade liberalization in tobacco products is a concern for its potential to offset declining use in developed countries by penetrating new markets in developing nations. Trade can increase the disease consequences of tobacco consumption through two main pathways: trade and investment liberalization, and the impact of trade rules on government policy space.

Liberalization of International Tobacco Trade and Investment

Trade liberalization has led to increased tobacco consumption in LMICs (Taylor et al. 2000) through a combination of tariff reduction, liberalization in FDI, and minimal national tobacco control measures, all of which preceded tobacco control measures in many countries. This combination of factors increases competition in domestic markets, and contributes to a reduction in the prices of tobacco products and an increase in advertising and promotion expenditures, all of which lead to increases in tobacco consumption. As one example market liberalization led to a 1-year increase in the US tobacco products in Japan from 16 % in 1986 to 32 % in 1987 and a corresponding stall in the decline of tobacco consumption among adults and an increase in the level of consumption among adolescent girls (Honjo and Kawachi 2000). When South Korea opened its domestic market to the US tobacco product imports there was an 11 % increase in smoking among males and an 8 % increase among females in just 1 year (United States General Accounting Office [USGAO] 1992). Similar liberalization requirements have taken place in bilateral trade agreements, including an agreement between the USA and China in which China was required to cut tariffs on imported cigarettes. Consumption patterns corresponded with the abolition of tariffs, expanded sales networks, and removal of advertising and marketing restrictions, all policy strategies explicitly pursued by tobacco transnational companies to increase LMIC consumption rates (Bialous and Shatenstein 2002).

While using trade treaties to lower tobacco tariffs has been one strategy pursued by tobacco companies to increase LMIC consumption, an arguably more critical one has involved using financial market liberalization to control domestic tobacco industries worldwide. Referring to a now famous trade dispute in 1990 between Thailand and the USA, Callard and colleagues (2001) speculate that transnational tobacco companies (TTCs) sought to buy out or enter into a joint venture with the Thai Government's tobacco monopoly in order to enhance their economic foothold in a large market and, more importantly, to increase their political influence with the goal of weakening Thailand's tobacco control legislation (Callard et al. 2001). WTO's General Agreement on Trade in Services (GATS) mode 3 (commercial presence) facilitates such investment when countries have committed different facets of their domestic tobacco industry to liberalization, although the explosive growth in bilateral investment treaties likely plays an even greater role. Philip Morris, an American TTC, draws over half of its cigarette profits from overseas (Weissman and Hammond 2000). Less than 10 years ago it was estimated that British American Tobacco controlled 50 % of all Latin American cigarette sales (Bialous and Shatenstein 2002). In the Dominican Republic, Philip Morris became the sole owner of cigarette division *Industria de Tabaco León Jimenes SA* and as a report of this buy-out suggests:

> Philip Morris could benefit and increase its market share in the Dominican Republic through more aggressive marketing now that it has complete control over the cigarette division. Philip Morris also could benefit from DR-CAFTA (Central American Free Trade Agreement) by exporting the products it manufactures in the Dominican Republic to Central America (Euromonitor 2009).

A World Bank study estimated that cigarette production in LMICs rose from 40 to 70 % in the past few decades (Jha and Chaloupka 1999), the result primarily of the movement of TTCs into such countries through domestic company acquisition and foreign direct investment. In Argentina, for example, approximately 90 % of the tobacco market is now controlled by two TTCs (Philip Morris Corporation and British American Tobacco), neither being domestically owned (Sawaya et al. 2003). In South Africa, British American Tobacco owns 94 % of the tobacco market (Mejia and Perez-Stable 2006). Foreign investment, in turn, is associated with increased consumption: amongst former Soviet Union republics, those countries that received foreign direct investment from TTCs between 1991 and 2001 saw an increase in tobacco consumption of 51 % compared to a 3 % drop in those that did not (Van Walbeek 2006).

Trade Rules and Government Policy Space

Tobacco products generally fall under the WTO's General Agreement on Tariffs and Trade (GATT), concerned primarily with the reduction of import taxes, and the Agreement on Technical Barriers to Trade (TBT), which covers nontariff barriers to trade (Taylor et al. 2000). Tobacco production is also governed by the Agreement on Agriculture (AoA) with respect to allowed versus prohibited subsidies to tobacco farmers: of health-promoting benefit if tobacco subsidies were successfully challenged under the AoA, but a potential limitation if subsidies to former tobacco growers shifting to food crops were deemed impermissible. Tobacco marketing is covered by both the GATS, with respect to advertising and distribution services, and TRIPS, with respect to regulatory restrictions that might encroach on cigarette logos as "intellectual property rights." The WTO system makes tacit reference to health as an interpretative principle (Bloche 2002); and there are explicit exceptions that allow countries to avoid trade rule compliance if it is "necessary to protect human, animal or plant life and health" (GATT article XX(b); GATS XIV(b)). Dispute panels have generally interpreted the "necessity test" to these exceptions quite narrowly, requiring that countries provide sufficient evidence that particular health measures (such as Thailand's attempt to restrict imports of foreign tobacco products to reduce supply, successfully challenged by the USA in 1989) are essential to protect the health of the population, and that there is no other "less trade-restrictive" option available (in the Thai–USA case, nondiscriminatory taxation and advertising bans that could have the same effect).

Trade treaties enable tobacco and tobacco products to cross borders more easily. On the one hand, trade negotiations have been used by TTCs as opportunities to ensure that domestic regulations do not seriously imperil their penetration into LMIC markets (Shaffer et al. 2005); on the other, the Framework Convention on Tobacco Control (FCTC), negotiated under the WHO system, is seeking to strengthen national tobacco control through a global agreement obliging tobacco control policies to be pursued by all

WHO member states that ratify the treaty. Whether and how the FCTC will be utilized in tobacco-related trade disputes is only now becoming a public health concern.

The FCTC, for example, encourages use of taxation and restrictions on duty-free imports as tobacco control measures (Article 6(2)). Although nondiscriminatory domestic taxes would be permitted under WTO law, GATT rules prevent a country from using import taxes (tariffs) to restrict tobacco supply beyond their existing "bound" level. All countries, including LMICs, are supposed to lock in and reduce these levels over time, thereby gradually eroding this potential tobacco control tool. Moreover, outside of the WTO system, "nearly every investment and trade agreement negotiated by the United States eliminates or reduces trading partners' tobacco tariffs and protects US tobacco companies' overseas manufacturing and investment" (Bollyky and Gostin 2010, p. 2637). The USA remains one of the few countries to not ratify the FCTC.

The FCTC contains specific provisions that, assuming foreign tobacco products are treated the same as domestic ones (the nondiscrimination standard of the WTO), a country's tobacco control measures should not be subject to a trade dispute. But it is not always clear if this will be the case. GATS provisions could affect restrictions on tobacco advertising (one of the control measures identified in the FCTC, Article 13(2)) and tobacco distribution systems. Advertising bans, if they focus solely on the content (tobacco products), are nondiscriminatory (apply to all forms of tobacco) and do not simply attempt to restrict the amount of advertising, and may be able to fend off a dispute challenge (McGrady 2011). Efforts to restrict distribution services (such as number or location of retail outlets) are more vulnerable to a trade challenge. This would apply only to WTO member countries that have committed to liberalize these sectors under GATS, and to do so without restriction. If faced with a challenge, these countries could argue that the health exception applied, whether this would be accepted by a dispute panel is unknown. Or they could "invoke the FCTC itself as an independent defence, although this would be

controversial" (Mitchell and Voon 2011, p. 2). All WTO member countries face negotiating pressure to continue the "progressive liberalization" commitment of GATS and to expand the sectors to which they commit, including advertising and distribution. Their best option if liberalizing these sectors is to exempt from them all tobacco products, which would be a permissible option under GATS.

A recent case involving the USA and Indonesia highlights the importance of taking account of WTO rules on national treatment (nondiscrimination). To comply with domestic legislation restricting flavors in cigarettes to prevent adolescent smoking, the USA banned imports of clove cigarettes. Indonesia argued that the domestic legislation, by exempting "menthol" from the list of flavors, discriminated against its clove cigarettes in favor of the US-manufactured menthol cigarettes. This constituted a violation of the TBT Agreement and its national treatment (nondiscrimination) obligation. Indonesia also argued that there were "less trade-restrictive" ways to meet the public health goal of reducing adolescent smoking than a ban on clove cigarette imports. The WTO dispute panel ruled with Indonesia on the first argument (nondiscrimination) but with the USA on the second (agreeing that a ban was a necessary public health policy).[1] The panel also referenced the FCTC in its decision, which leaves the door open to bans on clove

---

[1] Indeed, the stringency of this necessity test may be changing. A recent dispute settlement involved Brazil's ban on retread tires from the EU on the grounds that huge stockpiles of such tires were mosquito-breeding grounds which increased the risk of infectious disease. The dispute panel accepted the public health necessity of this measure (even though it was not a direct cause of disease) and that although other, less trade-restrictive measures could have been used, these other measures did not negate the public health importance of the ban. Unfortunately, because other regional trade agreements allowed small amounts of used tire imports from neighboring countries, the WTO panel ruled in favor of the EU, until Brazil is able to affect a totally nondiscriminatory ban. These dispute panel findings indicate that there may now be somewhat greater flexibility for domestic regulations affecting tobacco, alcohol, and food imports using the health defense if the regulations are defended on very specific public health grounds (McGrady 2011).

cigarettes *if* the USA also extended this ban to menthol cigarettes (which also happen to be the tobacco product of choice for most young American smokers) (McGrady 2012). Similar concerns, but not yet disputes, have been expressed about Canada's ban on flavors (again excluding menthol) and other additives in cigarettes, which has the effect of banning imports that contain burley tobacco, which is not used by Canada's domestic tobacco industry. What these disputes highlight is the importance of ensuring that tobacco control policies are, intentionally or otherwise, protectionist policies.

TTCs are using trade treaties to argue against other tobacco control measures, including packaging requirements. Article 11 of the FCTC makes the explicit provision that warning labels on cigarette packages must be "50 % or more of the principal display areas" with 30 % as an absolute minimum (WHO 2005a, p. 10). Measures that exceed the minimum standards set forth by the FCTC are being challenged under the WTO system and bilateral investment treaties, the latter permitting private companies to directly sue national governments for perceived expropriation of their property and earnings (real or potential). In a recent case, Philip Morris challenged Uruguay's decision to implement larger warning labels on tobacco packages than the minimum referenced in the FCTC. It used rules set out in a Swiss–Uruguay investment treaty, arguing that such warning labels violated its intellectual property rights by reducing the space in which it could feature its "brand" name and logos (Lencucha 2010). Philip Morris is also challenging Australia's plain-packaging law (another of the FCTC's recommended control strategies), using a bilateral investment treaty between Australia and Hong Kong; the ability of TTCs to search out such treaties is known as "forum shopping." Canada's earlier attempt to require plain-packaging was abandoned after Philip Morris threatened a similar suit using the investor-state provisions of North American Free Trade Agreement (NAFTA)—a "regulatory chill" that the threat of a suit alone can cause. Three other tobacco companies (British American, Japan, and Imperial) have joined the legal battle against

the Australian regulation; and at least two tobacco-producing countries (Honduras and the Ukraine) have launched WTO disputes under the TRIPS Agreement, which is considered to be a potentially more serious challenge than those brought under bilateral investment treaties because the specific trade rules covering such protection remain ambiguous and difficult to interpret (McGrady 2004). The fact that countries that are parties to the FCTC are nonetheless challenging tobacco control measures consistent with the FCTC's intent attests to an ongoing lack of policy coherence between domestic public health and international trade.

Alcohol Trade and Chronic Disease

Concerns are also rising about the impact of numerous WTO agreements on liberalized trade in alcohol, and the extent to which some of the recommended actions in the 2010 WHO Global Strategy to Reduce the Harmful Use of Alcohol (restricting alcohol outlets, availability and marketing, using taxation and prices to reduce consumption) may run afoul of trade rules. As with tobacco products, trade and investment liberalization affect alcohol-related chronic diseases through two principle pathways: increased availability, affordability, and marketing, and decreased flexibilities in alcohol control policies.

Increased Availability, Affordability, and Marketing of Alcohol

The production, distribution, and marketing of alcohol are becoming increasingly globalized. Most alcoholic beverages are largely purchased in the country of production, although cross-border trade in spirits (primarily those produced in HICs) has become subject to disputes over differential tax regimes (primarily exercised by LMICs). More importantly, and as with tobacco, international alcohol brands are now being produced industrially in plants owned, co-owned, or licensed by multinational corporations (Jernigan 2000). The penetration of transnational alcohol corporations in LMIC markets has increased the availability, affordability, and marketing of alcohol products (Grieshaber-Otto et al. 2000; Jernigan 2009), all of which affect consumption rates.

Greater diversity of alcohol products made available through reduced tariffs on imports can increase overall alcohol consumption as these products can target a variety of tastes and preferences, although in some cases consumers may simply shift from domestic to foreign products (Gould and Schacter 2002). Many of the new foreign beverages contain higher alcohol content compared to domestic products (Grieshaber-Otto et al. 2000; Room and Jernigan 2000), which has become a focus of several trade disputes discussed shortly. As alcohol companies "thirst for new markets" (Jernigan 1997), intensive marketing practices are adopted as a means to increase consumption of alcohol, particularly in LMICs (Gould and Schacter 2002). The role of advertising is a critical factor in differentiating between "globalized" and other types of alcohol (Jernigan 2009). Whereas traditional local alcoholic products are marketed based on availability, quality, and price, a global alcohol product is "synonymous with its imagery … represents a culture of its own" (Jernigan 2000, p. 471). Alcohol is being marketed through increasingly sophisticated avenues, including direct marketing (e.g., podcasting, cell phones), mainstream media, and via sporting and cultural events. The EU and the USA in current GATS negotiations are aggressively pursuing unlimited liberalization commitments in advertising; and "the World Spirits Alliance has described the Doha Round as offering 'an excellent opportunity for the international distilled spirits industry to create new opportunities to expand its exports to world markets,'" identifying "liberalisation of restrictions on services, including distribution and advertising" as one of its top five priorities for the new trade round (Gould 2005, p. 367). An existing dispute under European Union trade rules has already found that a Swedish advertising ban on alcohol, even though nondiscriminatory since it applied to all alcohol products, was still ruled a de facto discrimination because domestic brands were better known to the public than were imported products (Zeigler 2006). As with tobacco, and with reference to GATS negotiations, the best strategy for WTO member countries under pressure to liberalize these sectors is to exempt all alcohol advertising and distribution services from their commitments.

Decrease Alcohol Control Policies

Many of the alcohol control policies that can help reduce alcohol-related harm (e.g., tariffs, taxes, licensing, labeling, regulation of the size of alcoholic beverage containers, identifying certain brands as "noxious" or "injurious") are considered to be barriers to trade under several WTO trade agreements (Gould and Schacter 2002).

Reducing the control of state monopolies and enterprises is a key element of many trade treaties. Researchers have observed an increase in alcohol consumption and alcohol-related problems following their elimination; the Nordic countries are a case in point. Since the early twentieth century, Finland, Norway, and Sweden had state monopolies on production and wholesale, import and export, and off-premise retail monopolies—all with the overarching goal of reducing individual and social harm from alcohol consumption (Nordlund 2007). Following integration into the European Union and the European Economic Area (EEA), these countries have yielded to pressure to undertake trade activities that adopt the principles of national treatment or nondiscrimination. Alavaikko and Österberg demonstrated that following Finland's entry into the European Union in 1995, the country's markets opened and the state alcohol monopoly company, Alko, lost its traditional capacity for alcohol decision-making policy (Alavaikko and Österberg 2000). Mäkelä and Österberg observed that alcohol consumption increased 10 % in 2004 and levels have remained higher ever since (Mäkelä and Österberg 2009). The EU for years has argued that Canada's liquor board monopolies which operate in many of the country's provinces function to impose restriction on European alcohol imports. A 2003 WTO trade policy review attempted to pressure Canada to liberalize these state monopoly boards (Zeigler 2006), although so far without success.

Another key element of trade treaties is a greater "harmonization" of taxes and duties on alcoholic beverages (Grieshaber-Otto et al. 2000).

In particular, national alcohol taxation systems have been directly affected by the application of the national treatment requirement. A few years ago, the EU requested the WTO to examine the Philippine's excise tax regime, which includes a higher tax rate on imported spirits than domestic spirits (International Centre for Trade and Sustainable Development [ICTSD] 2009). The EU claimed that this provided unfair market competition, whereas the Philippines defended the law on the grounds that it provided support to indigenous communities who produced spirits from their raw materials, like coconut and sugarcane. In 2011 the WTO agreed with the EU (since the tax was clearly discriminatory) (European Commission 2011), with the Philippines committed to reducing its import taxes to comply with the ruling, a policy that will almost certainly lead to increased consumption in the Philippines.

Similarly, complaints brought by Canada, the USA, and the EU against Japan's higher tax rate for vodka than *shochu* (its domestic "like" product) were successful in an earlier 1996 WTO ruling. *Shochu*, however, typically contains between 25 and 40 % alcohol, whereas vodka contains between 35 and 50 %. A similar ruling was made against Korea's higher tax on higher alcohol content imported spirits, than its domestic spirits (McGrady 2011). The effect will be higher overall alcohol consumption. In both cases, however, the public health arguments for reducing overall alcohol consumption were not as prominent in the policy as they might have been which may have weakened the ability of the two Asian countries to invoke a health defense.

Simply put, when health arguments are not specifically invoked it is unlikely Chile, for example, levied a disproportionately high tax rate on spirits that had alcohol content higher than 40 %, which was successfully challenged by the EU (Gould and Schacter 2002). But, like Japan and Korea before it, Chile did not invoke public health arguments, instead relying on the argument that the policy was nondiscriminatory since it applied to all alcohol products, both domestic and imported. The EU, in this dispute, countered that most varieties of *pisco*, the domestically pro-

duced spirit, by law was required to have an alcohol content below 35 %, whereas most imported spirits had alcohol content of 40 % or above, thus having the effect of providing unfair tax advantage to the domestic product. The WTO agreed, although noting in its ruling that "members of the WTO are free to tax distilled alcoholic beverages on the basis of their alcohol content and price." Taxing on the basis of alcohol content is one of the WHO's recommended alcohol control strategies. This particular WTO ruling thus appears to conform with this health argument; but it also added that such a policy would only be permissible "as long as the tax classification is not applied so as to protect domestic production over imports," meaning that a discriminatory tax on alcohol content, even if designed for public health purposes, could still be found in violation of trade treaty obligations (World Trade Organization [WTO] 1999).

While some trade analysts argue that policies that are motivated purely by health interests may have more flexibility under trade law than what is often perceived (Baumberg and Anderson 2008), the ruling in the Japan–EU dispute over alcohol was clear that the intent of the policy did not matter, only whether or not it was unnecessarily trade-restrictive. The implication for alcohol control policies is that extreme care needs to be taken in crafting the policies to ensure that there is no hidden import discrimination, and that the health goals of the policy are explicit and defensible as having no other options by which they might be achieved (referred to in trade talk as ensuring that the policy can pass the "aims-and-effects test").

Even with this caution, nondiscriminatory alcohol control policies could still be challenged by different trade treaty provisions. In a pre-WTO GATT case brought by the USA against Canada's minimum pricing for beer products, the panel ruled that, even if the minimum price applied to all beers (domestic and imports), if it prevented imports from selling at a lower price it was a de facto discrimination (McGrady 2011). This could have implications for price controls as a means of managing overall alcohol consumption levels. The TBT Agreement, in turn, has provisions related to "technical regulations" which include packaging and labeling requirements. Thailand in 2010 announced a number of new health warning labels that it will require on alcohol products. These warnings are quite explicit, even dramatic; and several WTO members have expressed concerns about them citing the TBT. At the time of writing (2013) it is not known how this issue will unfold. The Agreement on Sanitary and Phytosanitary Measures (SPS), for different reasons related to the need to justify regulations by reference to international standards or scientific risk assessments, could also be used to challenge what some alcohol-exporting countries might regard as "excessive" labeling or other control policies.

Food Trade and Chronic Disease

There are three general pathways linking trade and foreign direct investment from food to chronic disease, related to changes in the food system: growth of transnational food corporations (TFCs); liberalization of international food trade and investment; and global food advertising and promotion.

Growth of Transnational Food Corporations

Food production, distribution, and retailing have been consolidated into a small number of TFCs. Food retailers in particular have undergone an intense and rapid transformation; changes that occurred in regions such as Latin America between 1990 and 2000 took place in the USA over a period of 50 years (Reardon and Berdegue 2002). In 2003, the top 30 food retailers controlled almost 30 % of the market in Latin America and 19 % in Asia and Oceania (Hawkes et al. 2009). Reardon and his colleagues have labeled the retail transformation beginning in the early 1990s as a "take-off" period (Reardon et al. 2009), launching a "supermarket revolution" and the rapid spread of fast-food chains. The growth of supermarkets during the 1990s can be attributed to demand side factors, notably urbanization, the entry of women into the workforce, and economic growth (Reardon and Berdegue 2002),

as we noted earlier in this chapter. The supply side is driven by trade liberalization and foreign direct investment (FDI). Conditions for FDI were facilitated initially through the easing on investment regulations as part of structural adjustment programs, and subsequently through a variety of bilateral and regional trade agreements. FDI has played a critical role in the diet transition as it has especially targeted highly processed foods (Hawkes 2004). In Latin America, between 1988 and 1997, FDI in food industries grew from USD 222 million to USD 3.3 billion (Rayner et al. 2007). Hawkes and her colleagues, meanwhile, reviewed the available evidence on the links between international trade and dietary patterns (Hawkes et al. 2009). They found supporting evidence, notably from India and the Pacific Islands, that the increase in international trade has shifted dietary patterns from local, "healthy" diets to the consumption of fattier diets (see Box 1).

Box 1 From Tuna to Turkey Tails

The Federated States of Micronesia (FSM) has rights over the richest tuna fishing grounds in the world. Prior to its integration within global markets and economic dependency (partly arising from US aid projects in the 1960s and 1970s) it relied upon fish stocks for its protein source. As its economy "developed" from an agriculture and fishing to wage-labor, FSM became more reliant on trade and foreign investment. Part of this reliance came in the form of selling its tuna fishing rights to countries like Japan, as it lacked the infrastructure to engage commercially with the global tuna trade. Meanwhile, the USA, until 1986 the "administering authority" of FSM and under terms of trade within that authority, began exporting to FSM turkey tails, the high-fat, gristle, and heavily salted part of a turkey deemed inedible in its own country. Overweight and obesity rates rose in tandem with this dietary shift (Cassels 2006).

(continued)

Box 1 (continued)

Western Samoa has a ban on turkey tails, although not on "mutton flaps" (high-fat, low-quality cuts of lamb). Like other South Pacific Island nations whose diets have become globalized, it is experiencing high rates of overweight and obesity though at a slightly lower rate than those countries with no turkey tail bans (Cassels 2006). In its bid to become a member of the WTO, however, Western Samoa had to agree to eliminate its turkey tail ban within 12 months of accession. A "transitional" period of two additional years would be allowed, during which time the country could impose a domestic ban on the sale of turkey tails (though imports would still be allowed). After this period, the ban would have to be removed. According to the WTO accession agreement, the "transitional" period is intended "to allow time to develop and implement a nation-wide programme promoting healthier diet and life style choices" (WTO 2011)—a revealing glimpse at how the global economy prefers control of NCDs at the level of individual choice rather than at economic source. Moreover, while some South Pacific nations are now contemplating a ban on turkey tails and mutton flaps, their ability to do so may be challenged under the SPS Agreement, its requirements for scientific risk assessments, and "consistency" in defining the appropriate level of protection against risks to health (meaning that unless all domestic high-fat food risks to health were banned, even if consumed only occasionally, an import ban could be found to be discriminatory) (McGrady 2011).

Liberalization of International Food Trade and Investment

Liberalization of trade—eliminating quotas, reducing tariffs, and privatizing state trade agencies—was adopted by many LMICs either voluntarily or as a condition of structural adjustment loans from the international financial institutions initiated in the 1980s, with a quickening pace during the 1990s as many countries entered into global, regional, and bilateral trade agreements (Hawkes et al. 2009). Food was first represented in multilateral trade treaties with the formation of the WTO in 1995 and adoption of the AoA. Before this time, agricultural trade existed largely outside of formal trade treaties, and developing countries did not have to reciprocate in granting greater market access to developed country exports. With the WTO's trade rules and dispute settlement procedures, developing countries are under increasing obligation and ongoing negotiation pressures to lower tariffs, export subsidies, and domestic agriculture support (AoA), as well as to open themselves to FDI in food-related sectors they may have committed under GATS. Alongside a growing number of bilateral and regional treaties, such as the NAFTA, the Central American Free Trade Agreement (CAFTA), and the Southern Common Market (MERCOSUR), regulation of international food trade and investment is increasingly governed by trade treaty rules. A specific example of trade treaty effects on health-related food policies includes the long-standing dispute between the European Union and several countries over the EU ban on hormone-treated beef; the ban violates requirements for scientific risk assessments under the WTO SPS Agreement (Labonté et al. 2010).

While international trade of food and food products has increased, so have the level of subsidies provided to agricultural producers in HICs (notably the USA, the EU, and Japan) with much of their produce (particularly American and European) going to export markets. This has led some trade policy analysts to argue that the high level of subsides can be viewed as dumping (Anderson et al. 2001), defined in trade terms as goods entering a foreign market at less than "normal" prices and impermissible under the WTO's GATT Agreement. These subsidies are due to be reduced under the terms of the AoA (which gave WTO member nations a 10-year moratorium from trade disputes related to agriculture, which expired on December 31, 2004), although both the USA and the EU have been altering slightly the terms of their subsidies to allow them to still qualify under the AoA's complex set of "boxes" permitting some, but disallowing other, supports to domestic producers. Much prevailing criticism of subsidies is that they damage the value of food exports from developing countries by suppressing world prices. From a public health vantage, eliminating production subsidies on unhealthy food products (such as fats, sugars, or high fructose corn syrup) is likely to do more health good than harm for all countries. But their elimination on healthier and essential food products could do more harm than good to many low-income countries which have become net-food importers—as a result of population growth, loss of arable land, and years of advice to shift from food products for domestic consumption to nonfood cash crops (cotton, coffee, tobacco) for export (Labonté et al. 2008; FAO 2006).

The AoA does retain considerable policy flexibilities with respect to managing food-related NCD risks. Although there is negotiating pressure to reduce tariffs on all food products, countries can choose to reduce tariffs on healthier imports first while retaining tariffs on unhealthy foods. A problem may arise if both healthy and unhealthy foods are "like" each other and differ only in, for example, the amounts of salt, fat, sugar, or trans fat they contain, and especially if the country retaining a stiff tariff on what it considers to be an obesogenic food allowed such foods to be produced and sold domestically. Some domestic subsidy space remains which countries could apply to healthier food production (fruits, vegetables) while removing subsidies for production of foods that are higher in fat (dairy, animal). These flexibilities, however, depend on countries having the financial resources to make use of them (Atkins 2010), and may still be liable to a trade challenge unless the domestic subsidies to fruits and vegetables did not lead to imported fruits and vegetables losing market share (Fidler 2010). Trade challenges under the AoA on export subsidies (which the AoA discourages but permits) could be made on unhealthy foods (fats, oil, sugar, dairy, and livestock), although this would require coherence within challenging countries between their health and economic development sectors, the latter of which may very well want to encourage such

unhealthy food imports or be subsidizing such exports themselves.

FDI in food-related production, processing, and retailing, enhanced by reducing investment barriers, has increased the presence of TFCs in most developing countries. This presence can increase food availability through reduction in retail prices following the removal of import barriers on food, depending on the dynamics of international and domestic prices. Food retail prices can also be lowered by the reduction of investment barriers since TFCs often purchase agricultural products at lower cost and promote economies of scale, but they also benefit from the lower agricultural cost of their own products. Hawkes and Thow demonstrate these effects in their analysis of the Central America—Dominican Republic—Free Trade Agreement (Hawkes and Thow 2008), which the authors argue will likely lead to greater consumption of highly processed food, meat, and other nontraditional foods in Central America. As another example, FDI in Eastern Europe after the fall of the Berlin Wall increased dramatically but with the bulk of it going towards sugar and confectionary, followed by soft drinks, milk/dairy, and other processed foods, very little went into fruits or vegetables (Lobstein 2010).

Impacts on food trade and invest liberalization on domestic production raise concerns about short- and longer term food security. A recent study by the United Nations Food and Agriculture Organization (FAO) examined trade liberalization and food security in fifteen small and large developing countries (Chile, Guatemala, Guyana, Peru, Cameroon, Ghana, Kenya, Malawi, Morocco, Nigeria, Senegal, Tanzania, Uganda, China, and India). Their key finding was that "trade reform can be damaging to food security in the short to medium term if it is introduced without a policy package designed to offset the negative effects of liberalization" (FAO 2006, p. 75).

Global Food Advertising and Promotion

Advertising and promotion marks the third pathway through which trade is affecting food systems and NCDs. In order to dominate in competitive food retailing markets, corporations employ aggressive marketing techniques. Spending on food advertising is now higher than it is for tobacco (Chopra and Darnton-Hill 2004); and billions are spent annually advertising soft drinks (Rayner et al. 2007). The global food advertising has been steadily growing and the advertisement market is controlled by a few communications networks (Hawkes et al. 2009). Processed food, especially targeted to children, has been the main focus of promotion and advertising (Hawkes et al. 2009). Advertising and product marketing have contributed to changing cultural expectations of food (Rayner et al. 2007) and the "systematic molding of taste by giant corporations" (Chopra and Darnton-Hill 2004, p. 1559). Marketing has been especially targeted to youth. During the late 1990s, soft drink companies targeted school children by selling products in attractive combination packages in schools in Mexico and Colombia, which led to a 50 % increase in soft drink sales among children (Hawkes et al. 2009). Evidence from industrialized and developing countries found that children engage with food advertising and that there is clear link between advertising to children and the consumption of these products (Hastings et al. 2007; Institute of Medicine 2006).

Consistent with the WHO's Global Strategy on Diet, Physical Activity and Health, several countries have begun to legislate restrictions on advertising to children, although most countries still rely upon formal or informal encouragement of corporate self-regulation (Hawkes and Lobstein 2011). As countries move towards enforceable regulatory approaches, the threat of a trade dispute arising from such restrictions could be reduced. However, as with tobacco and alcohol, commitments to liberalize advertising services under GATS could precipitate a trade dispute, if advertising restrictions disadvantaged foreign advertisers that specialized in the child or the youth market. The same risk exists if a country wished to restrict advertising for certain unhealthy foods, since that is where most FDI in advertising is directed (Sawaya et al. 2003). Similar advice thus follows (and applies equally to services with respect to food distribution systems): Exempt food products from GATS advertising and distribution commitments to preserve maximum domestic policy space for regulating food marketing and availability.

Finally, there is some concern with the potential impact the SPS Agreement could have on countries' food regulations. The SPS, as a general rule, requires that any trade-distorting food policy, even if it is nondiscriminatory, should be based on either an international standard (to which it defers to *Codex Alimentarius*) or, in the absence of a standard or if the requirement exceeds that in *Codex*, that it be based on a scientific risk assessment (McGrady 2011). *Codex* is actively developing standards relevant to the WHO's global diet strategy (L'Abbé et al. 2010), but has long had concerns expressed about the extent to which it is dominated by food industry scientists, both as members of "bingos" (business-interested NGOs) and as part of national government delegations, and always in numbers disproportionate to public interest groups or researchers (Baby Milk Action 2011a, b). Two issues exist here. The first is that *Codex* standards may, for some countries, be considered too low for their food policy purposes, and thus vulnerable to an SPS trade dispute. The second is that labeling requirements that do not conform to international standards could also be challenged.

Conclusion

This chapter has reviewed some of the extant evidence on the role that trade and financial liberalization has played in increasing the global diffusion of risk factors for NCDs. There is some potential for trade treaties to aid in reducing the global diffusion of risk factors, such as enforcing an end to domestic subsidies for agricultural exports harmful to health (e.g., sugars, fats, tobacco) or removal of tariffs on the import of drugs used to treat NCDs—although the continued expansion of intellectual property rights in bilateral and regional trade treaties could price this NCD treatment option out of range for many LMICs. Indeed, as this chapter has elaborated, there remains considerable actual or potential health harm in trade treaties when such treaties are driven by liberalization as the policy end and with only minimal regard to the health consequences.

This potential has been noticed in the run-up to the UN Summit on Non-Communicable Diseases that took place in September 2011. A meeting of African health ministers in early April 2011 issued a declaration on NCDs stating, *inter alia*, that "although globalization, trade and urbanization are important in human development, they are also major external drivers responsible for widening health inequities within and between countries and populations" demanding "the integration of health in all policies across sectors in order to address NCD risk factors and determinants" (WHO 2011a). This declaration repeats a theme woven throughout the WHO's *Global Status Report on Non-Communicable Diseases 2010*, which noted that "the rapidly growing burden of NCDs in developing countries is not only accelerated by population ageing; it is also driven by the negative effects of globalization, for example, unfair trade and irresponsible marketing" (WHO 2011b, p. 33). WHO Director-General, Margaret Chan, was even more forceful in her comments to the April 2011 First Global Ministerial Conference on Health Lifestyles and Non-Communicable Disease Control convened in Moscow, regarded as an agenda-setting event for the September UN Summit:

> Today, many of the threats to health that contribute to noncommunicable diseases come from corporations that are big, rich and powerful, driven by commercial interests, and far less friendly to health. ... Today, more than half of the world's population lives in an urban setting. Slums need corner food stores that sell fresh produce, not just packaged junk with a cheap price and a long shelf-life (Chan 2011).

While not referencing trade *per se*, the outcomes Chan cites are logically and empirically linked to trade and the globalized food, tobacco, and spirits industries. Yet, notwithstanding the exclusion of the tobacco industry from the Moscow Conference, many of these same globally trading corporations were present to participate in the Conference. Press reports of the Conference quote some of these corporate representatives complaining that companies are "unfairly blamed for consumer's choices" or that "the overfed are voluntarily overfed" (Englund 2011), reinforcing a concern implicit in the Conference's emphasis on "healthy lifestyles"

that intervention strategies for NCD control could take the easy path of regulating individual health behaviors rather than corporate economic or social practices.

The UN NCD Summit partly affirmed this concern. The Political Declaration that emanated from the Summit did contain several references to the social determinants of health, an inclusion to be applauded and seized upon by health promoters and public health practitioners. At the same time, much more was made of health behaviors, fueling worries that we are experiencing "lifestyle drift" where the focus is returning to individual behaviors and away from corporate actors. The Political Declaration was particularly conciliatory in this regard, using the language of partnership (rather than regulation) to urge companies to "consider producing and promoting more food products consistent with a healthy diet" and to "take measures ... to reduce the impact of the marketing of unhealthy foods and non-alcoholic beverages [soft drinks] to children." This soft selling reflects the political influence of the food and beverage industry in the run-up to the Summit, and its hard selling of the ideas of corporate social responsibility and voluntary action. But social responsibility has a way of evaporating when it affects profit and market share. A few months before the Summit, Pepsi Co, which had let its soft drink advertising budget lag in order to promote its healthier products, lost ground to rival Coca-Cola, resulting in an about-face and a plan to massively increase its soft drink promotion budget (iStockAnalyst 2011). The US-based Campbell's Company, seen as a leader in voluntarily reducing salt in some of its products, similarly announced in just prior to the Summit an almost 50 % increase in the salt of one of its previous low-sodium soup brands due to flagging market sales, a move welcomed by The Salt Institute as a cautionary tale to companies wanting to cut sodium in their products (Weeks 2011).

Paralleling this acquiescence to corporate power, the Political Declaration contained only one (very much passing) mention of trade and none of investment liberalization. Yet, as this chapter has argued, trade and investment treaties have become weapons of choice for companies fighting new restrictions on their global hawking of unhealthy products. Health promoters must begin to understand better trade and investment policy, and to engage more effectively with the foreign affairs departments of their national governments negotiating such treaties, if they wish to put some brakes on these very communicable characteristic of non-communicable diseases.

References

Agyemang, C., Redekop, W. K., Owusu-Dabo, E., & Bruijnzeels, M. A. (2005). Blood pressure patterns in rural, semi-urban and urban children in the Ashanti region of Ghana, West Africa. *BMC Public Health, 5*, 114.

Aizenman, J., & Jinjarak, Y. (2009). Globalisation and developing countries - A shrinking tax base? *Journal of Development Studies, 45*(5), 653–671.

Alavaikko, M., & Österberg, E. (2000). The influence of economic interests on alcohol control policy: A case study from Finland. *Addiction, 95*(Suppl. 4), 565–579.

Alwan, A., MacLean, D., Riley, L., d'Espaignet, E. T., Mathers, C. D., Stevens, G. A., et al. (2010). Monitoring and surveillance of chronic non-communicable diseases: Progress and capacity in high-burden countries. *Lancet, 376*(9755), 1861–1868.

Anderson, K., Dimarananb, B., Francois, J., Hertel, T., Hoekman, B., & Martin, W. (2001). The cost of the rich (and poor) country protection to developing countries. *Journal of African Economies, 10*, 227–257.

Atkins, V. J. (2010). Agricultural trade policy instruments to promote health diets in developing countires: An Assessment of the opportunities within the framework of the WTO agreement on agriculture and the Doha development agenda. In C. Hawkes, C. Blouin, S. Henson, N. Drager, & L. Dubé (Eds.), *Trade, food, diet and health: Perspectives and policy options* (pp. 264–278). Oxford: Wiley-Blackwell.

Baby Milk Action. (2011, April 27). *WHO global forum in Moscow: Tackling food-related diseases: Voluntary measures or regulation - carrot or stick?* Press release. Baby Milk Action. http://info.babymilkaction.org/press-release/pressrelease01may110. Accessed May 9, 2012.

Baby Milk Action. (2011, November 12–18). *The Business of malnutrition: Breaking down trade rules to profit from the poor.* Press release. Baby Milk Action. http://info.babymilkaction.org/sites/info.babymilkaction.org/files/Codex%20PR%20THURS3.pdf. Accessed May 1, 2012.

Baumberg, B., & Anderson, P. (2008). Health, alcohol and EU law: Understanding the impact of European single market law on alcohol policies. *European Journal of Public Health, 18*(4), 392–398.

Baunsgaard, T., & Keen, M. (2010). Tax revenue and (or?) trade liberalization. *Journal of Public Economics, 94*(9–10), 563–577.

Beaglehold, R., & Yach, D. (2003). Globalisation and the prevention and control of non-communicable disease: The neglected chronic diseases of adults. *Lancet, 362*(9837), 903–908.

Bialous, S. A., & Shatenstein, S. (2002). *Profits over people: Tobacco industry activities to market cigarettes and undermine public health in Latin America and the Caribbean.* Washington, DC: Pan American Health Organization. http://www.paho.org/English/DD/PUB/profits_over_people.pdf. Accessed May 8, 2012.

Birdsall, N. (2006). *The world is not flat: Inequality and injustice in our global economy* (WIDER Annual Lecture 9). Helsinki: World Institute for Development Economics Research. http://www.wider.unu.edu/publications/annual-lectures/en_GB/AL9/_files/78121127186268214/default/annual-lecture-2005.pdf. Accessed May 8, 2012.

Bloche, M. G. (2002). WTO deference to national health policy: Toward an interpretive principle. *Journal of International Economic Law, 5*, 825–848.

Bollyky, T. J., & Gostin, L. O. (2010). The United States' engagement in global tobacco control. *Journal of the American Medical Association, 304*(23), 2637–2638.

Callard, C., Chitanondh, H., & Weissman, R. (2001). Why trade and investment liberalisation may threaten effective tobacco control efforts. *Tobacco Control, 10*(1), 68–70.

Caraher, M., & Cowburn, G. (2005). Taxing food: Implications for public health nutrition. *Public Health Nutrition, 8*(8), 1242–1249.

Cassels, S. (2006). Overweight in the Pacific: links between foreign dependence, global food trade, and obesity in the Federates States of Micronesia. *Globalization and Health, 2*(10). doi: 10.1186/1744-8603-10.

Chan, M. (2011, April 27). *The rise of chronic noncommunicable diseases: An impending disaster.* Opening remarks at the WHO Global Forum: Addressing the challenge of noncommunicable diseases, Moscow, Russian Federation. http://www.who.int/dg/speeches/2011/global_forum_ncd_20110427/en/index.html. Accessed May 8, 2012.

Chen, S., & Ravallion, M. (2008). *The developing world is poorer than we thought, but no less successful in the fight against poverty* (World Bank Policy Research Working Paper 4703). Washington, DC: World Bank. http://papers.ssrn.com/sol3/papers.cfm?abstract_id=1259575. Accessed May 7, 2012.

Chopra, M., & Darnton-Hill, I. (2004). Tobacco and obesity epidemics: Not so different after all? *BMJ, 328*(7455), 1558–1560.

Chow, C., Lock, K., Teo, K., Subramanina, S. V., McKee, M., & Yusuf, F. (2009). Environmental and societal influences acting on cardiovascular risk factors and disease at a population level: A review. *International Journal of Epidemiology, 38*(6), 1580–1594.

Cornia, G. A., Rosignoli, S., & Tiberti, L. (2007). *Globalisation and health: Impact pathways and recent evidence.* Santa Cruz: University of California, Center for Global, International and Regional Studies. http://escholarship.org/uc/item/2358z815. Accessed May 8, 2012.

Dahrendorf, A. (2009). *Global proliferation of bilateral and regional trade agreements: A threat for the World Trade Organization.* Maastricht, Netherlands: Universiteit Maastricht.

Dans, A., Ng, N., Varghese, C., Tai, E. S., Firestone, R., & Bonita, R. (2011). The rise of chronic non-communicable diseases in Southeast Asia: Time for action. *Lancet, 377*(9766), 680–689.

de-Graft Aikins, A., Unwin, N., Agyemang, C., Allotey, P., Campbell, C., & Arhinful, D. (2010). Tackling Africa's chronic disease burden: from the local to the global. *Globalization and Health, 6*(5). doi: 10.1186/1744-8603-6-5

Englund, W. (2011, April 29). WHO takes on chronic disease. *The Washington Post.* http://articles.washingtonpost. com/2011-04-29/world/35231015_1_chronic-diseases-chronic-illnesses-account-unhealthy-food. Accessed May 9, 2011.

Euromonitor. (2009). *Tobacco in Dominican Republic.* Euromonitor International. http://www.euromonitor. com/Tobacco_in_Dominican_Republic. Accessed August 20, 2009.

European Commission. (2011). Questions and answers on the final WTO panel report in the case brought by the EU and the US against the Philippines over discriminatory taxation of distilled spirits. European Commission. http://trade.ec.europa.eu/doclib/ press/ index.cfm?id=735. Accessed May 8, 2012.

Fidler, D. (2003). Emerging trends in international law concerning global infectious disease control. *Emerging Infectious Diseases, 9*(3), 285–290.

Filder, D. (2010). The impact of international trade and investment rules on the ability of governments to implement interventions to address obesity: A case study from the European charter on counteracting obesity. In C. Hawkes, C. Blouin, S. Henson, N. Drager, & L. Dubé (Eds.), *Trade, food, diet and health: Perspectives and policy options* (pp. 279–297). Oxford: Wiley-Blackwell.

Floro, M., & Dymski, G. (2000). Financial crisis, gender and power: An analytical framework. *World Development, 28*(7), 1269–1283.42.

Food and Agriculture Organization of the United Nations (FAO). (2002). The developing world's new burden: Obesity. FOCUS. http://www.fao.org/FOCUS/E/obesity/obes1.htm. Accessed May 8, 2012.

Food and Agriculture Organization of the United Nations (FAO). (2006). *Trade reforms and food security: Country case studies and synthesis.* Rome: Food and Agriculture Organization of the United Nations.

Gallagher, K. (2007, March). *The political economy of the Doha round: Shrinking benefits and real costs for developing countries.* Paper presented at the International Studies Association 48th Annual Convention, Chicago.

Glenday, G. (2006). *Toward fiscally feasible and efficient trade liberalization.* Durham: Duke Center for Internal Development.

Gould, E. (2005). Trade treaties and alcohol advertising policy. *Journal of Public Health Policy, 26*(3), 359–376.

Gould, E., & Schacter, N. (2002). Trade liberalization and its impact on alcohol policy. *SAIS Review, 22*(1), 119–139.

Grieshaber-Otto, J., Sinclair, S., & Schacter, N. (2000). Impacts of international trade, services and investment treaties on alcohol regulation. *Addiction, 95*(Suppl. 4), 491–504.

Hastings, G., McDermott, L., Angus, K., Stead, M., & Thomson, S. (2007). *The extent, nature and effects of food promotion to children: A review of the evidence.* Geneva: World Health Organization.

Hawkes, C. (2004). The role of foreign direct investment in the nutrition transition. *Public Health Nutrition, 8*(4), 357–365.

Hawkes, C. (2006). Uneven dietary development: linking the policies and processes of globalization with the nutrition transition, obesity and diet-related chronic diseases. *Globalization and Health, 2*(4). doi: 10.1186/1744-8603-2-4.

Hawkes, C., Chopra, M., & Friel, S. (2009). Globalization, trade, and the nutrition transition. In R. Labonté, T. Schrecker, C. Packer, & V. Runnels (Eds.), *Globalization and health: Pathways, evidence and policy* (pp. 235–262). New York: Routledge.

Hawkes, C., & Lobstein, T. (2011). Regulating the commercial promotion of food to children: A survey of actions worldwide. *International Journal of Pediatric Obesity, 6*(2), 83–94.

Hawkes, C., & Thow, A. (2008). Implications of the Central America-Dominican Republic-Free Trade Agreement for the nutrition transition in Central America. *Pan American Journal of Public Health, 24*(5), 345–360.

Honjo, K., & Kawachi, I. (2000). Effects of market liberalisation on smoking in Japan. *Tobacco Control, 9*(2), 193–200.

Hossain, P., Kawar, B., & El Nahas, M. (2007). Obesity and diabetes in the developing world – A growing challenge. *The New England Journal of Medicine, 356*(3), 213–215.

Institute of Medicine. (2006). *Food marketing to children and youth: Threat or opportunity?* Washington, DC: National Academies.

Inter-American Development Bank (IADB). (2011). *Urban sustainability in Latin American and the Caribbean.* Inter-American Development Bank. http://idbdocs.iadb. org/wsdocs/getdocument.aspx?docnum=35786014. Accessed May 8, 2012.

International Centre for Trade and Sustainable Development (ICTSD). (2009, August 5). EU takes legal action on Philippine liquor tax. *Bridges Weekly Trade News Digest, 13*(29). http://ictsd.org/i/news/ bridgesweekly/52476/. Accessed May 8, 2012.

iStockAnalyst. (2011, June 28). Pepsi goes back to its roots with Pepsi-Cola marketing. iStockAnalyst. http://www.istockanalyst.com/finance/story/5258994/ pepsi-goes-back-to-its-roots-with-pepsi-cola-marketing. Accessed May 8, 2012.

Jernigan, D. (1997). *Thirsting for markets: The global impact of corporate alcohol.* San Rafael: The Marin Institute for the Prevention of Alcohol and Other Drug Problems.

Jernigan, D. (2000). Applying commodity chain analysis to changing modes of alcohol supply in a developing country. *Addiction, 95*(Suppl. 4), 465–475.

Jernigan, D. (2009). The global alcohol industry: An overview. *Addiction, 104*(Suppl 1), 6–12.

Jha, P., & Chaloupka, F. J. (1999). Curbing the epidemic: governments and the economics of tobacco control. Washington, DC: The World Bank. http://www.usaid.gov/policy/ads/200/tobacco.pdf. Accessed May 8, 2012.

Kimball, A. M. (2006). *Risky trade: Infectious disease in the era of global trade*. Aldershot: Ashgate.

Koivusalo, M., Schrecker, T., & Labonté, R. (2009). *Globalization and policy space for health and social determinants of health* (Globalization Knowledge Network Research Papers). Ottawa: University of Ottawa, Institute of Population Health. http://www.globalhealthequity.ca/electronic%20library/Globalisation%20and%20policy%20space%20for%20health%20and%20social%20determinants%20of%20health%20Koivusalo%20May%202009.pdf. Accessed May 9, 2012.

L'Abbé, M. R., Lewis, J., & Zehaluk, C. (2010). The potential of the codex alimentarius to promote healthy diets worldwide – the Canadian experience of implementation. In C. Hawkes, C. Blouin, S. Henson, N. Drager, & L. Dubé (Eds.), *Trade, food, diet and health: Perspectives and policy options* (pp. 238–263). Oxford: Wiley Blackwell.

Labonté, R. (2010). Liberalized trade and the public's health: What are the linkages? What is the evidence? What are the healthy options? In A. den Exter (Ed.), *International trade law and health care: In search of good sense* (pp. 9–36). Rotterdam: Erasmus University Publishers.

Labonté, R. (2012). The austerity agenda: how did we get there and where do we go next? *Critical Public Health, 22*(3), 257–265.

Labonté, R., Blouin, C., Chopra, M., Lee, K., Packer, C., Rowson, R., et al. (2008). *Towards health-equitable globalisation: Rights, regulation and redistribution* (Globalization and health Knowledge Network: Research Papers). Ottawa: University of Ottawa, Institute of Population Health. http://www.globalhealthequity.ca/ electronic%20library/GKN%20Final%20Jan%208%202008.pdf. Accessed May 8, 2012.

Labonté, R., Blouin, C., & Forman, L. (2010). *Trade, growth and population health: An introductory review*. Ottawa: Collection d'études transdisciplinaires en santé des populations/Transdisciplinary Studies in Population Health Series.

Labonté, R., Mohindra, K. S., & Lencucha, R. (2011). Framing international trade and chronic disease. *Globalization and Health, 7*(1), 21.

Labonté, R., & Schrecker, T. (2009). Introduction: Globalization's challenges to people's health. In R. Labonté, T. Schrecker, C. Packer, & V. Runnels (Eds.), *Globalization and health: Pathways, evidence and policy* (pp. 1–33). New York: Routledge.

Lawrence, F. (2011, November 23). Alarm as corporate giants target developing countries. *The Guardian*. http://www.guardian.co.uk/global-development/2011/nov/23/corporate-giants-target-developing-countries. Accessed May 8, 2012.

Lencucha, R. (2010). Philip Morris versus Uruguay: Health governance challenged. *Lancet, 376*(9744), 852–853.

Lobstein, T. (2010). Tackling childhood obesity in an Era of trade liberalisation. In C. Hawkes, C. Blouin, S. Henson, N. Drager, & N. Dubé (Eds.), *Trade, food, diet and health: Perspectives and policy options* (pp. 195–218). Wiley-Blackwell: Oxford, UK.

Lynch, D. (2010). *Trade and globalization*. Plymouth: Rowman & Littlefield.

Mäkelä, P., & Österberg, E. (2009). Weakening of one or more alcohol control pillar: A review of the effects of the alcohol tax cuts in Finland in 2004. *Addiction, 104*(4), 554–563.

Mathars, C., & Loncar, D. (2006). Projections of global mortality and burden of disease from 2002 to 2030. *PLoS Medicine, 3*(11), 2011–2030.

McGrady, B. (2004). TRIPs and trademarks: the case of tobacco. *World Trade Review, 3*(1), 53–82.

McGrady, B. (2011). *Trade and public health: The WTO, tobacco, alcohol, and diet*. New York: Cambridge University Press.

McGrady, B. (2012). *Tobacco product regulation and the WTO: Appellate Body Report, US – Clove Cigarettes* (Briefing paper). O'Neill Institute for National & Global Law. http://www.oneillinstitutetradeblog.org/wp-content/uploads/2012/04/briefing-paper.pdf. Accessed May 7, 2012.

Mejia, P., & Perez-Stable, E. J. (2006). Tobacco epidemic in Argentina: The cutting edge of Latin America. *Prevention and Control, 2*(1), 49–55.

Mitchell, A., & Voon, T. (2011). Implications of the World Trade Organization in combating non-communicable diseases. *Public Health, 125*(12), 832–839.

Nordlund, S. (2007). The influence of EU on alcohol policy in a non-EU country. *Journal of Substance Use, 12*(6), 405–477.

Parrado, E. A., & Zentento, R. M. (2001). Economic restructuring, financial crises and women's work in Mexico. *Social Problems, 48*(4), 456–477.

Polanski, S. (2006). *Impact of the Doha round on developing countries*. Washington, DC: Carnegie Endowment for International Peace.

Popkin, B. (1994). The nutrition transition in low-income countries: An emerging crisis. *Nutrition Reviews, 52*(9), 285–298.

Popkin, B. (1997). The nutrition transition and its health implications in lower-income countries. *Public Health Nutrition, 1*(1), 5–21.

Popkin, B. (2002). The shift in the states of the nutrition transition differ from past experiences! *Public Health Nutrition, 5*(1A), 205–214.

Rayner, G., Hawkes, C., Lang, T., & Bello, W. (2007). Trade liberalization and the diet transition: A public health response. *Health Promotion International, 21*(1), 67–74.

Reardon, T., Barrett, C., Berdegue, J., & Swinnen, J. (2009). Agrifood industry transformation and small farmers in developing countries. *World Development, 37*(11), 1717–1727.

Reardon, T., & Berdegue, J. (2002). The rapid rise of supermarkets in Latin America: Challenges and opportunities for development. *Development Policy Review, 20*(4), 371–388.

Room, R., & Jernigan, D. (2000). The ambiguous role of alcohol in economic and social development. *Addiction, 95*(Suppl. 4), 523–535.

Saker, L., Lee, K., Cannito, B., Gilmore, A., & Campbell-Lendrum, D. (2004). *Globalization and infectious diseases: A review of the linkages (social, economic and behavioural research. Special Topics No. 3)*. Geneva: World Health Organization.

Sawaya, A., Martins, P., & Martins, V. (2003). *Impact of globalization on food consumption, health and nutrition in urban areas: A case study of Brazil*. Rome: Food and Agriculture Organization of the United Nations. http://www.guardian.co.uk/global-development/2011/nov/23/corporate-giants-target-developing-countries. Accessed May 8, 2012.

Schrecker, T., & Labonté, R. (2010). Globalization. In D. Vlahov, J. I. Boufford, C. Pearson, & L. Norris (Eds.), *Urban health: Global perspectives* (pp. 13–26). San Fransisco: Jossey-Bass.

Shaffer, E. R., Waitzkin, H., Brenner, J., & Jasso-Aguilar, R. (2005). Global trade and public health. *American Journal of Public Health, 95*(1), 23–34.

Stuckler, D., Basu, S., Suhrcke, M., Coutts, A., & McKee, M. (2011). Effets of the 2008 financial crisis on health: A first look at European data. *Lancet, 378*(9876), 124–125.

Subramanian, S., & Davey Smith, G. (2006). Patterns, distribution and determinants of under and over-nutrition: a population based study of women in India. *American Journal of Clinical Nutrition, 84*(3), 633–640.

Sundaram, J. K., & von Arnim, R. (2009). Trade liberalization and economic development. *Science, 323*(5911), 211–212.

Taylor, A., Chaloupka, F. J., Guindon, E., & Corbett, M. (2000). The impact of trade liberalization on tobacco consumption. In P. Jha & F. J. Chaloupka (Eds.), *Tobacco control in developing countries* (pp. 343–364). Oxford: Oxford University Press.

Thangavelu, S. M., & Toh, M.-H. (2005). Bilateral 'WTO-Plus' free trade agreements: The WTO trade policy review of Singapore 2004. *The World Economy, 28*(9), 1121–1128.

United States General Accounting Office (USGAO). (1992). *Advertising and promoting US cigarettes in selected asian countries*. Washington, DC: USGAO.

Van Walbeek, C. (2006). Industry responses to the tobacco excise tax increases in South Africa. *South African Journal of Economics, 74*(1), 110–122.

Weeks, C. (2011, July 17). Campbell's adding salt back to its soup. *Globe and Mail*. http://www.theglobeandmail.com/life/health/new-health/health-news/campbells-adding-salt-back-to-its-soups/article2097659/. Accessed May 9, 2012.

Weissman, R., & Hammond, R. (2000, October). International tobacco sales. Foreign policy in focus. http://www.fpif.org/reports/international_tobacco_sales_revised_oct_2000. Accessed May 8, 2012.

Wilkinson, R., & Marmot, M. (2003). *Social determinants of health: The solid facts*. Geneva: World Health Organization.

World Health Organization (WHO). (2010). *Global strategy to reduce harmful use of alcohol*. Geneva: World Health Organization. http://www.who.int/substance_abuse/alcstratenglishfinal.pdf. Accessed May 8, 2012.

World Health Organization (WHO). (2011a). *The Brazzaville declaration on non-communicable diseases prevention and control in the WHO African region*. Geneva: WHO.

World Health Organization (WHO). (2011b). *Global status report on noncommunicable diseases 2010*. Geneva: WHO.

World Trade Organization (WTO). (1999). *Chile – Taxes on alcoholic beverages*. Report of the Appellate Body. http://www.worldtradelaw.net/reports/wtoab/chile-alcohol(ab).pdf. Accessed May 9, 2012.

World Trade Organization (WTO). (2011, October 28). *Working party adopts Samoa's membership package*. World Trade Organization. http://www.wto.org/english/news_e/news11_e/acc_wsm_28oct11_e.htm. Accessed May 8, 2012.

Yach, D., Stuckler, D., & Brownell, K. D. (2006). Epidemiologic and economic consequences of the global epidemics of obesity and diabetes. *Nature Medicine, 12*(1), 62–66. doi:10.1038/nm0106-62.

Zeigler, D. W. (2006). International trade agreements challenge tobacco and alcohol control policies. *Drug and Alcohol Review, 25*(6), 567–579.

Addressing NCDs Through Multilateral Engagement at the United Nations: The Role of WHO

25

Sylvie Stachenko

The Scale of the Non-communicable Disease Challenge

Non-communicable diseases (NCDs) have become a global challenge. Thirty-six million deaths in 2008 were due to NCDs as estimated by the World Health Organization (WHO). The "big four" NCDs—cardiovascular diseases, cancer, diabetes and chronic lung diseases—share the four main risk factors historically associated with socio-economic development. These include unhealthy diet, physical inactivity, tobacco use and harmful use of alcohol. Tobacco use is considered the most avoidable risk factor and is responsible for one sixth of NCD deaths globally, with an estimated one billion people consuming tobacco products daily (Beaglehole et al. 2011). Unhealthy diets characterized by consumption of foods high in saturated and trans fats, salt and sugars and patterns of low fruit and vegetable consumption are responsible for approximately 40 % of NCD deaths annually. Excessive alcohol consumption accounts for 2.3 million deaths annually and over half of these deaths relate to cancer, cardiovascular disease and liver cirrhosis. Finally, physical inactivity accounts for 3.2 million deaths each year. Although insufficient inactivity is highest in high income country, it is increasingly prevalent in middle income countries especially in women (WHO 2010).

Mortality from NCDs is expected to increase by 17 % from 2005 to 2015, accounting for 69 % of deaths in 2030 (WHO 2010). Evidence suggests that illness and death from cardiovascular diseases in developing countries are occurring at a younger age cutting in the productive years (Beaglehole et al. 2007). It is clear that the economic impact of the rising burden of NCDs is widespread affecting governments, national economies, businesses and individuals and families. NCDs have important indirect costs including reduced workforce participation and increased job turnover which negatively affect economies (Olusoji et al. 2007). Consequently, NCDs have widespread costs for both the health and non-health sector. In fact, a recent World Economic Forum report identifies NCDs as one of the top ten most severe global risks (World Economic Forum 2010).

The WHO and its Global Status Report on NCDs released in 2011, have played a critical role in exposing the threat posed by rapidly increasing rates of diabetes, cancer, cardiovascular and chronic lung diseases. WHO suggests that NCDs are also a growing barrier to development, given that 80 % of total deaths caused by NCDs in 2010 occurred in developing countries.

S. Stachenko (✉)
Centre for Health Promotion Studies,
School of Public Health, University of Alberta,
3-262 Edmonton Clinic Health Academy,
11405-87 Avenue, Edmonton, AL, Canada T6G1C9
e-mail: sylvie.stachenko@ualberta.ca

D.V. McQueen (ed.), *Global Handbook on Noncommunicable Diseases and Health Promotion*,
DOI 10.1007/978-1-4614-7594-1_25, © Springer Science+Business Media, LLC 2013

Moreover, WHO highlights that the rising prevalence of NCDs and their risk factors adversely impact progress towards achieving the Millenium Development Goals (WHO 2010).

While the proximate behavioural risk factors are well known, the underlying determinants are global and complex in nature. Some of these factors include the growing urbanization, marketing practices of the food industry, the growing concentration of global food manufacturers, trade practices that adversely affect the pricing and availability of healthy foods, the rapid growth of supermarkets (WHO 2005a, b, c). In this regard, it is increasingly acknowledged that NCDs are part of a complex web of interdependence and as such, require a global collective response to address the determinants that have become increasingly transnational in scope (Koplan et al. 2009).

Towards a Global Political Partnership and Leadership Role of WHO

The global community has only recently begun to respond to NCDs through collective action. In this regard, over the last decade, WHO has played an important role in highlighting the urgency for responding to the NCD threat worldwide and has led the development of the FCTC (WHO 2003) as well as the *Global Strategy on Diet, Physical Activity and Health* (WHO 2004).

More recently, WHO launched the NCD Action Plan which emphasizes the importance of international cooperation and collaboration to "lead and catalyze an intersectoral and multilevel response" to NCDs (WHO 2008a, b, c). The NCD Action Plan was written for the community of international development partners, as well as those in government and civil society concerned with urgent action to address the rapidly increasing burden of NCDs in low- and middle-income countries and its serious implications for poverty reduction and economic development. The First global ministerial conference on healthy lifestyles and NCD control in April, 2011 and the resulting Moscow Declaration similarly emphasized the importance of whole of society approaches at all levels and across a number of sectors.

Six Regional Offices operate within the WHO and most of them have developed their own NCD plan aligning with the global NCD plan with a focus on practical, cost-effective and evidence-based interventions that Member States can implement. In some Regions, there have been significant political leadership to advance the global NCD dialogue. For example, in 2007 a Summit on NCDs of the Caribbean Community (Caricom) Heads of Government was held in Trinidad and Tobago. The summit was a catalyst for raising the priority accorded to NCDs within the international community, recognizing the issue as one that requires both health and non-health sector input and solidifying high level government commitment for action (Kirton et al. 2011a, b).

The recent emergence of numerous initiatives relevant to the goals of NCD prevention and control points to the urgent need for an overarching global response. The landscape for Global Health has become more populated and diverse than before. Increasingly, global health players also include regional organizations such as among others, the European Union, the African Union and the Association of South Asian Nations. In addition, donor governments have launched major bilateral global health efforts. All these official actors share space with a burgeoning number of non-governmental organizations and foundations dedicated to advancing global health. As a result, the effectiveness in players and resources is often diluted by an uncoordinated and incoherent system.

The global health community continues to look to WHO as the leading global health technical agency. WHO is unique in that it combines the necessary institutional mandate, legal authority and public health expertise to be the lead international organization for the prevention and treatment of NCD, but does require support from other global organizations. Opportunities for multi-sectoral and multi-stakeholder collaboration under prevention and control of NCDs will likely require a broader policy for dealing with an increasing number and variety of stakeholders including the private sector (Magnusson 2010).

A positive development in this regard was the global summit convened by the UN and attended by Heads of State and Governments to curb the

NCD epidemic afflicting both the developed and developing countries. After several months of active negotiations, the UN General Assembly unanimously adopted on September 16, 2011 a Political Declaration that acknowledged the global scope of the crisis and identified the key components of a "whole-of-government" and "whole-of-society" response (United Nations General Assembly 2011).

The Political Declaration presents a highly focused agenda for strengthening a coherent international response in support of national and regional programmes and specifically requests WHO to undertake particular actions and initiatives. The main actions highlighted in the Political Declaration specifically for WHO leadership, include:

- Setting norms and standards:
  - To develop a global monitoring framework (paragraph 61) and recommendations for a set of voluntary global targets, building on the Secretariat's ongoing work, through the governing bodies of WHO in 2012 (paragraph 62).
  - To collaborate with the United Nations Secretary-General in submitting a report to the General Assembly at its sixty-seventh session (in 2012) on options for strengthening and facilitating multi-sectoral action through effective partnership (paragraph 64).
- Exercising a leading and coordinating role within the United Nations system:
  - By establishing and institutionalizing strong collaborative links with United Nations agencies, funds and programmes (paragraphs 13, 43, 45, 46, 51 and 61–64).
- Developing an Implementation plan for the outcome of the High-level Meeting:
  - By preparing, in consultation with Member States and organizations in the United Nations system an updated 6-year action plan (2013–2018), taking into account the outcomes of the High-level Meeting.
- Expanding technical competence and resources:
  - By providing support to WHO's Member States in developing national plans and policies for prevention and control of NCDs (paragraphs 43(e), 45 and 51) in the areas of normative functions, technical collaboration, and strengthening and facilitating multi-stakeholder action.

The response of WHO to the follow-up of the Declaration has been very timely. The 130th Session of the WHO Executive Board in January 2012 had on its Agenda a report on WHO leadership role in the outcomes of the high level meeting on prevention and control of NCD. One of the follow-up tasks for the WHO was to develop effective ways of strengthening and facilitating multi-sectoral actions through partnerships and to take a coordinating role in the prevention of NCDs with UN Agencies Funds. A list of proposed areas for joint collaboration was developed at the first meeting of the UN Funds, Programs and Funds (WHO 2011: 4).

UNDP and WHO in response to the political declaration also proposed in march 2012 that the United Nations Country Teams integrate, according to country context and priorities, NCDs into the United Nations Development Assistance Framework (UNDAF) design processes and implementation, with initial attention being paid to the countries where UNDAF roll outs are scheduled for 2012–2013 as well as into the post 2015 development agenda.

While the effectiveness of the High Level Meeting in ensuring that NCDs become a priority within various agency programs is not known at this time, it did facilitate dialogue between health and non-health global actors in advancing the NCD agenda. There have been discussions to establish similar high level dialogue among prominent regional institutions in some Regions such as in the Americas to advance multi-sectoral action for the prevention and control of NCDs.

As noted above, the Declaration also called for the development of a Global Monitoring Framework. In May 2012, at the 65th World Health Assembly (WHA), there was broad commitment by the Member States to the target of reducing cardiovascular diseases, cancers, diabetes and chronic respiratory diseases by 25 % by 2025. This agreement does mark an important step in the NCD global policymaking process. For the first time, there was a move away from aspirational goals to an action-based approach that would be anchored in quantifiable targets. This could signal the beginning of the development of global standards in surveillance with a requirement to report on progress in implementing policies on NCDs. Reporting provisions can help maintain commitment in tackling the NCDs. Periodic reporting could also provide a focal point for the participation of civil society.

A global and regional consultation process on the NCD Global Monitoring Framework has been launched and it is expected that the other NCD related targets will be adopted at the 66th WHA including the four targets relating to risk factors including tobacco use, harmful use of alcohol, unhealthy diet and physical inactivity. Other potential targets also include raised blood pressure and salt/sodium, obesity, fat intake, alcohol, cholesterol, and healthy system responses such as availability of essential medicines for NCDs.

Building on Experience: The Global Policy Challenges in Addressing NCDs

It is vital that we examine WHO led international experiences to draw out the key lessons in supporting effective international action to address NCD (WHO 1997). To date, the conceptual framework for global action on "lifestylerelated" NCD is largely embodied in two WHO initiatives: the FCTC and GSDPAH. A feature of both diet and tobacco-related NCD diseases is the presence of powerful multinational corporations and the challenge of regulating their products. WHO has adopted a treaty-based approach with tobacco but a facilitative, advocacy-based approach for diet and physical activity.

Under the leadership of its Director General, WHO prioritized tobacco control and began negotiations towards a framework convention. The treaty based approach was a strategic choice because of the evolving concerns about loss of sovereignty of national governments in the face of World Trade Agreements (Zacher 2007). Participation of the NGOs and their ongoing input into the conference of the parties was a critical success factor (Hammond and Assent 2003) that highlights the importance of non-state

actors. The move towards using policy tools such as legislation or regulations represents an explicit cultural shift from individual to social responsibility on the issue of tobacco smoking.

WHO's most significant achievement has been the Framework Convention on Tobacco Control (FCTC) which was the first convention adopted under Article 19 of the WHO Constitution which came into force in 2005. The FCTC has focused global attention around this problem and enhanced WHO's standing. Some of the partnerships to support tobacco control efforts in low and middle income countries such as the Bloomberg and Bill and Melinda Gates foundations are emerging as major contributors to the WHO FCTC implementation. Such partnerships have been critical in resisting the influence of the tobacco industry at the country level.

WHO's Global Strategy on Diet, Physical Activity and Health (GSDPAH) in 2004, established a broad coalition of agencies including and stakeholders working with countries and the food industry to advance implementation but to date progress has been slow.

The GSDPAH did identify an important role for WHO in close cooperation with other UN agencies such as the FAO, the WTO, the World Bank, other development banks and the Codex Alimentarius Commission. However, one of the criticisms of the GSDPAH is that it offered a purely voluntary menu of policy options for governments (WHO 2004). The GSDPAH also prompted controversy from companies concerned about adopting restrictions on marketing certain foods and beverage products.

There are clear opportunities for WHO to stimulate the development of global standards and provide a baseline for responsible transnational corporate behaviour. In fact, the European Charter on Counteracting Obesity (WHO 2006) specifies that governments should adopt specific regulatory measures to substantially reduce the extent and impact of commercial promotion of energy dense food, moving towards an international code of practice in this area.

In 2006, a study of global food manufacturers, retailers and food service companies concluded that only a minority had altered their business practices in response to the GSDPAH. Of the 25 corporations studied, ten had taken action on salt, five on sugar, four on fat and eight on trans fats, but only two on portion sizes (Lang et al. 2006). In Europe, the *EU Platform for Action on Diet, Physical Activity and Health* has, since March 2005, provided a forum for the food industry, as well as NGOs, medical and consumer groups, to make public commitments on measures to reduce obesity and to improve diet and physical activity. In this regard, nine soft drink makers have undertaken not to advertise soft drinks to children *aged 11 or less* (European Union 2006).

Global Interdependence and the Challenge of Addressing the Global Determinants of NCD

The challenge of NCDs calls for a profound rethinking of the international agencies capable of modifying the global conditions that influence the NCD determinants. According to the WHO Constitution (WHO 1946), the WHO's objective is "the attainment by all peoples of the highest possible level of health." In order to achieve that objective, among the functions of the WHO shall be "to promote, in co-operation with other specialized agencies where necessary, the prevention of accidental injuries" and "to promote, in co-operation with other specialized agencies where necessary, the improvement of nutrition, housing, sanitation, recreation, economic or working conditions and other aspects of environmental hygiene (WHO 1946).

Health determinants are modified by policies and interventions beyond health. And, at the global level, the policies, guidance, and cooperation by and among multilateral agencies (such as WHO, UNDP, UNICEF, UNESCO, ILO, UN-Habitat, FAO, ECLAC, WTO, the multilateral banking system, and UNEP) are profoundly influencing the risks and protective factors for NCDs.

However, it will require major efforts among those institutions to link their actions. A good example has been the Intergovernmental panel on climate change (which includes UNEP and WMO), or the well-established Codex Alimentarius (which includes FAO, WHO, and other institutions). Still, many international organizations are ill prepared for the complex processes of multi-stakeholder diplomacy (Kickbush 2011). The capacity to build these cooperative mechanisms has to be greatly expanded, towards a focus on NCDs.

There have been and continues to be good momentum to dialogue with multilateral agencies to establish coherent actions on NCDs through four major global conferences including the United Nations High-level Meeting (UN-HLM) on NCD prevention and control, in New York City, in September 2011, the Global Conference on Social Determinants of Health, in Rio de Janeiro, in October 2011, the UN Conference on Sustainable Development ("Earth Summit 2012") in Rio de Janeiro, in June 2012, and the 8th Global Conference on Health Promotion, in Helsinki, in June 2013, addressing the "Health in All Policies" approach.

Currently NCDs are not present in the Millenium Development goals which represent a high profile global partnership embracing goals to be achieved collectively within a 15 year timeframe (2005–2015) to address poverty (United Nations General Assembly 2010). There are many lessons from the achievement of the Millenium Development Goals which translated these goals into a global coherent work program requiring periodic reporting and establishing milestones against which Multilateral Organizations could be measured (United Nations 2000).

There is debate whether adequate attention has been given to the broader social determinants in the field of NCD given the clear relationship between poverty and NCD. In many countries, much of the focus continues to be directed at lifestyle factors to address the rise in NCDs and inadequate attention is placed on factors such as rapid unplanned urbanization, unhealthy transport systems, or insecure jobs. A failure to assert the SDH could weaken policy support for the multilevel, multi-sectoral measures needed to effectively address NCDs, or space for countries to implement the public health regulation and market controls needed to address these SDH in a liberalized global economy.

It is worth noting the World Bank has acknowledged that NCDs have become a critical challenge due to an epidemic of tobacco consumption and obesity in many middle and low income countries World Bank Strategy for Health, Nutrition and population health (2006). It has become an important global health policy actor through its global experience, strong country presence, capacity to engage with all government sectors and capacity to engage finance ministries. This gives the Bank the unique capacity to engage with the broader determinants of NCDs.

Action on the global determinants of NCDs will be a long term challenge which will require the establishment of international legal instruments capable of regulating the global determinants of tobacco, poor diet and alcohol abuse. The development of global norms and strategies is an intensely political process, as the FCTC and GSDPAH illustrated. In this regard, leadership from coalitions and stakeholders could be important in mobilizing political power and commitment to address NCD prevention.

The Changing WHO Context

The WHO was founded to attain higher levels of health for all people, but the world in which the WHO operates today is very different from that of six decades ago. While this overriding aim is still guiding the WHO's work, the strategies and the context in which the WHO strives to pursue this goal have certainly changed in today's highly complex—multilevel, multifactor, multi-issue—global governance system

The UN system and WHO need to adapt to the new geopolitical context. The inter-mingling of economic, health and other issues within the NCD Agenda points to an important theme for the future governance of NCDs. Notwithstanding the leadership WHO has shown through the FCTC and Global NCD Strategy, it remains true that multi-sectoral influence and change at country level— not to mention progress in addressing global health determinants—require coalitions of international agencies, INGOs, governments, food manufacturing and retail companies, and other stakeholders.

No single international institution has the financial resources, technical capacity, credibility, or legal or political mandate to drive the complex changes that are needed to reverse the global and country-level determinants of NCDs. Successful action requires a collective response to the *global* determinants that undermine national health sovereignty.

One step towards a global response to NCDs was the formation of a Global Noncommunicable Disease Network (NCDnet). NCDnet is a WHO-sponsored initiative and include the participation of the World Bank, the World Economic Forum, and leading INGOs. By uniting disease-specific NGOs with health stakeholders active in tobacco control, healthy diets and physical activity, NCDnet aimed to "raise the priority accorded to noncommunicable diseases in development work" and to "catalyze effective multi-stakeholder action at global and country levels."

Clearly, transnational factors that impact on health but are beyond the control of national governments should be addressed by horizontal initiatives that call on the financial, normative and political power of international agencies and forums. A collective global response to NCDs requires initiatives by coalitions of stakeholders capable of exercising transnational influence, as well as a coordinating mechanism to provide leadership across all initiatives. In this regard, WHO's leadership is vital and is more critical now than ever before.

In this regard, WHO has undergone a reform process which should pave the way for WHO to maintain its critical role as the world's leading technical authority on health in at the global level According to the WHO Director-General Report A 64/4, the reform framework aims to provide: (1) a greater coherence in global health, with the WHO playing a leading role in enabling the many different actors to play an active and effective role in contributing to the health of all peoples; (2) improved health outcomes, with the WHO meeting the expectations of its member states and partners in addressing agreed global health priorities, focused on the actions and areas where the organization has a unique function or comparative advantage, and financed in a way that facilitates this focus; and (3) an organization which pursues excellence.

Discussion of the capacity for multilateral processes to advance NCD global health goals raises debate over the extent to which WHO merely provides a framework for action, or whether it retains an independent capacity to influence global policy in its own right. In this regard, WHOs constitutional mandate for leadership in the development of global health norms and standards is unique but often underutilized.

Some critics suggest that WHO needs to regain its role in the contemporary architecture for global health governance. In many instances, it had handed down its strategic responsibilities to others including the Global Fund, the World Bank, Gavi and the Bill and Melinda Gates Foundation. In addition, an important concern is the lack of alignment between the WHO's objectives including NCDs and its funding priorities. Much of the current funding structure is dominated by voluntary contributions which are earmarked. A key challenge for WHO is to focus on a few critical functions and delivering those to the highest possible quality (Horton 2012).

The Importance of Civil Society

Historically, NGOs have been an important catalyst for the development of a number of major instruments in global health. Global campaigns by NGOs and transnational advocacy networks have been effective in focusing attention on a broad range of social issues. Two relevant examples of effective mobilization are offered by the global response to poverty reduction and HIV/AIDS prevention and reduction. Both are significant global health and development challenges that require a concerted global response. Global attention was only focused on these issues as a result of sustained and coordinated action by civil society, both within countries and internationally.

Since 2000, the global development agenda has been driven in large part by the anti-poverty Millennium Development Goals (MDGs). The three health-related goals relate to child and maternity health (MDGs 4 and 5) and HIV/AIDS,

malaria and tuberculosis (MDG 6): NCDs are absent and therefore not as yet identified as a priority for international development partners. While an increasing number of developing countries are requesting support to address the growing impact of NCDs, donors are currently reluctant to divert resources away from the extant MDGs, which remain a high priority. Civil society institutions should be an important influence on the debate about the place of NCDs in the development agenda.

The global response to HIV/AIDS prevention and control was also very much transformed by a Special Session of the United Nations General Assembly in 2001, and civil society played a significant role in supporting that process. National AIDS Council and Commissions were created in many countries to facilitate cross sector interventions and could provide valuable lessons for the current NCD movement. Typically, NGOs, the private sector, various ministries and academics participated in these commissions which guided the development of national strategic HIV/AIDS frameworks and plans.

To date, civil society institutions have played an important role in the prevention and control of NCDs at both country and global level, in particular nongovernment organizations (NGOs), academia, and professional associations. Within countries, these groups help to shape the policy response, and also support or deliver prevention and treatment programmes. These same institutions provide important support to the WHO technical and normative functions and for the implementation of regional and country-level NCD action plans.

Over recent years, civil society organizations have increasingly worked together to address NCD prevention and control (NCD Alliance 2010). Civil society organizations coalesced to form the Framework.

Convention Alliance during the negotiation process for the WHO Framework Convention on Tobacco Control (WHO FCTC). This pooling and coordination of expertise and resources became a powerful force during the negotiation process, including acting as a strong counterforce to the tobacco industry, and has continued to play a strong and effective role in supporting and monitoring the implementation of the WHO FCTC. Importantly, it also facilitated participation at a global level by civil society institutions from the developing world and, in turn, helped to strengthen the capacity and capability of these institutions. This has had benefits at the national level by increasing their effectiveness in influencing the development, implementation and monitoring of NCD prevention and control policies.

More recently, a number of civil society institutions, in particular NGOs, have come together to coordinate more effectively their contribution to global NCD prevention and control. A significant milestone was the establishment of the NCD Alliance, a formal alliance of four international federations of NGOs representing the four main NCDs outlined in the Action Plan for the Global Strategy for the Prevention and Control of NCDs—cardiovascular disease, diabetes, cancer, and chronic respiratory disease, as a mutual platform for collaboration and joint advocacy.

The value of these "collective" civil society organizations is considerable. By working together, unified key messages can be agreed and then delivered to a range of audiences and through a range of means, in particular through the wide "grassroots" networks that each NGO has in individual countries. Further more, it also facilitates participation at a global level by civil society institutions from the developing world and, in turn, helps to strengthen the capacity and capability of these institutions. This has had benefits at the national level by increasing their effectiveness in influencing the development, implementation and monitoring of NCD prevention and control policies.

Such alliances in NCD prevention and control are also forming within countries and are having similar benefits. Aside from a united voice around key messages, there is a wider base of community support for advocacy and resource mobilization. The pooling of resources allows a greater degree of participation than might be possible by individual organizations. History demonstrates the importance of social mobilization in catalyzing social and economic change, and this is true also for NCD prevention and control.

Civil society institutions have already played a significant role globally and nationally in the NCD agenda, and this role will need to be strengthened. There are new avenues for civil society institutions to play a broader role by pressuring the private sector for access to healthier food, sharing information and influencing consumers directly in ways that could influence market demand.

Research and Monitoring Challenges

WHO has invested heavily in the development of global burden of disease data (Lopez et al. 2006), and this has strengthened the case for action. Ultimately, however, it is policies and programs, not only data, that will improve health outcomes.

Evaluating the impacts of the multi-sectoral set of policies needed in order to respond effectively to NCDs could not take the form of randomized controlled trials. Nevertheless, the world is a laboratory, and as populations are exposed to new policies, one function that deserves to be further strengthened at the global level is that of the "policy observatory" engages with governments, funders, advocates and researchers, identifying evidence-based best practices, promising policies, novel yet untested strategies, and failed policies.

Initiatives such as the Policy Observatory on NCDs co-hosted by the Pan American Health Organization (PAHO), and the WHO Collaborating Centre on Noncommunicable Disease Policy within the Public Health Agency of Canada. Monitoring of policies and policy outcomes may be useful in sharing lessons learnt across the globe.

Few global health interventions are evidence-based; what works in one place may not work elsewhere. More knowledge about interventions costs and cost-effectiveness is critical. What works and what doesn't work in health policy design and implementation also require more examination.

WHO research function certainly includes providing training and support. For example, in countries with limited resources, global partnerships for research can build national capacity in policy development and program delivery, and seed national leadership In this regard, WHO has also developed a *Prioritized Research Agenda for Prevention and Control of NCDs*. The *Research Agenda* seeks to strengthen national NCD research systems by ensuring that decisions about the implementation of policies and programs are grounded in evidence, to identify knowledge gaps, and to encourage research in areas that respond to priority health needs.

Transnational research partnerships can also increase the diversity of data, and give added legitimacy to policy responses at the country level. The *global* public health research function for WHO could include evaluating different models of interventions It is the capacity to analyze responses to NCDs across countries and in diverse environments that is most likely to lead to WHO's goal of developing a core package of policy interventions, and of primary care interventions, that are evidence-based and also well adapted to different contexts.

Partnership Challenges

The NCD challenge requires new ways of thinking and responses, and thus enhanced and creative collaboration. The United Nations with its universal membership has been moving towards new models for facilitating and coordinating international engagement. In this regard, a number of partnerships, alliances and networks, and collaborations exist and are dedicated to health issues such as the Global Fund to fight AIDS, Tuberculosis and Malaria.

With regard to NCD, the UN Economic Commissions partnered with WHO in the lead-up to the UN High Level Meeting in September 2011, by convening various regional dialogues on NCDs. Given the breadth of UN agency engagement in development, there are ample opportunities to secure continued involvement in and support for NCDs and specific multi-sectoral action.

In this regard, WHO is leading a process to identify means to better coordinate such efforts. In addition, through its country level leadership in health, WHO is working with UN Country Teams

to introduce coherent actions to tackle NCDs including introduction of NCDs into UNDAFs. Explorations are underway to explore a possible UN Multi-donor Trust Fund for NCDs or to use existing ones for related multi-sectoral action.

The partnerships underway at the national, regional, and global levels employ a range of models to achieve a diversity of goals. Lessons-learned from existing multi-sectoral partnerships that may inform the global response to NCDs activities, or alternatively could be brought into and combined with new, broader efforts.

The challenges associated with an effective response to NCD will require expanded partnerships to access to expert input and advocacy from policy partners, greater communication of policy goals, and greater opportunity for engaging at country level beyond traditional WHO-Health Ministry relationships.

WHO does have certain policies and procedures applicable to handling conflict of interest issues, the opportunities for multi-sectoral and multi-stakeholder collaboration on the prevention and control of NCDs will in all likelihood require a broader policy for dealing with the increasing number and variety of stakeholders, including the private sector. The United Nations has operated its outreach with the private sector through the UN Global Compact which was launched in 2000 to help in achieving the Millenium Development Goals. This could provide a starting point whereby the private sector can work alongside UN agencies if they commit to the principles and guidelines of the Global Compact. In fact, the business sector has come to play a significant role in many global partnerships and in the governance of organizations such as the Global Fund to fight AIDS, Tuberculosis and Malaria. The benefits and constraints of corporate social responsibility are widely debated but are viewed by some as initial steps towards changing the role of business beyond philanthropy into a whole of society approach to health (Porter and Kramer 2011).

In contrast to the tobacco industry, WHO has welcomed the food industry and other business sectors as partner. To this end, the WHO has begun to explore new platforms for multi-stakeholder governance. At the Regional level, the Pan-American Health Organization (PAHO) Partners Forum on Chronic Disease in the Americas (PAF-NCD) has implemented a novel approach to fostering multi-sector engagement (Hospedales and Jane-Llopis 2011). As a multi-sectoral platform, the PAF-NCD engages government, civil society, the private sector and academia to support the implementation of PAHOs Regional Strategy for NCDs and National NCD action plans. Some of the benefits derived from such a partnership approach include resource pooling, greater access to technical expertise, dissemination of health information and better awareness of health issues, particularly outside of the health sector (Magnusson 2010).

WHO can lead the development of innovative approaches to harness the power of the complete range of business players and the rich diversity of stakeholders from community and civil society, each of which invest resources and competencies into a global NCD effort. It is argued that such innovative partnerships for whole of society approaches should form the basis for the new governance for health in the twenty-first century (WHO 2012). For the WHO, the main challenge is the fine balance between opportunities and risks associated with the participation of private interests. The mandate given by member countries stipulates that credibility, independence, objectivity, integrity, and impartiality must be assured at all times.

Conclusion

Economic globalization and trade liberalization are driving forces for NCDs. Flows of information on the Internet, transnational networks are emerging expressions of the increasingly complex interconnections in the modern era. Not surprisingly, there is a patchwork of institutional mandates, activities, authority, and resources that characterize global health initiatives without a clear vision to tackle the broad determinants of NCD, In addition, WHO leverage at national level is mitigated by the fact that its links are with health ministries, rather than finance ministries.

The rise of an increasingly global economy no longer firmly rooted in nation states demands new forms of global governance In this regard, the response to the global burden of chronic disease will require a strategic assessment of the *global processes* that are likely to be most effective in encouraging the implementation of effective policies at country level, and in influencing the multinational corporations. Possible processes for driving policy change may include international legal instruments creating legal obligations on signatories to implement certain policies, economic incentives and innovative partnerships between global and national stakeholders for the advancement of shared policy objectives. Coherence among the various sectors is essential for effective action and will also require seamless coordination from local to global level by making use of the various levels of WHO.

The global governance of NCD will require a dynamic relationship between the complete set of civil society, private sector, non-governmental organization, nation-state and other national and transnational institutional responses. Despite the shared goal of reducing the burden of NCDs, global initiatives are competing for resources and political attention, and whether or not any particular form of institutional arrangements achieves precedence in setting the agenda and mapping the contributions of others in the field remains to be seen.

Regardless of the precise institutional mechanisms that exist for coordinating the global response, *there are unique global public health functions* that need to be discharged by WHO. In this regard, it is clear that WHO must play a central role and it will be important that NCD prevention should become, as far as possible, a shared project of the international community, rather than another branch of WHO's activities. The institutional arrangements needed to ensure an effective global response to NCDs will therefore need to manage this tension between providing coherence and global leadership, while nevertheless encouraging new initiatives, and sharing ownership in order to benefit from the unique strengths of other partners.

References

Beaglehole, R., Ebrahim, S., Reddy, S., Voûte, J., & On behalf of the chronic disease action group. (2007). Prevention of chronic diseases: A call to action. *Lancet, 370*(9605), 2152–2157.

Beaglehole, R., et al. (2011). Priority actions for the non-communicable disease crisis. *Lancet, 377*, 1438–1447.

Fifth report of Committee A (Draft). 64 World Health Assembly A64/61. WHO. (2011, May 23). First Meeting of UN Funds, Programmes and Agencies on the Implementation of the Implementation of the Political Declaration of the High-level Meetin of the General Assembly on the Prevention and Control of NCDs (New York, December 8, 2011)

Global Risks. (2010). *A global risk network report*. Rep no 201209, Geneva: World Economic Forum

Hammond, R., & Assent, M. (2003). The framework convention on tobacco convention on tobacco control: Promising start, uncertain future. *Tobacco Control, 12*, 241–242.

Horton, R. (2012). Offline: Can WHO survive? *The Lancet, 380*, 1457.

Hospedales, J., & Jane-Llopis, E. (2011). A multistakeholder platform to promote health and prevent non communicable diseases in the regions of the Americas: The Pan American Health Organization Partners Forum for Action. *Journal of Health Communications, 16*, 194–196.

Kickbush, I. (2011). Global health diplomacy: How foreign policy can influence health. *British Medical Journal, 342*, d3154.

Kirton, J., et al. (2011). Controlling NCDs through summitry: The CARICOM case. Global Health Diplomacy Program, Munk School of Global Affairs, University of Toronto. Version of June 17, 2011. Pan American Health Organization.

Koplan, J., Christopher Bond, T., Merson, M., et al. (2009). Towards a common definition of global health. *Lancet, 373*(9679), 1993–1995.

Lang, T., Rayners, G., & Kaolin, E. (2006). The food industry, diet, physical activity: A review of reported commitments and practice of 25 of the worlds largest food companies. London: Centre for Food Policy City University. Retrieved October, 2012 from http://www.city.ac.uk.

Lopez, A., Mathers, C., Ezzati, M., Jamison, D., & Murray, C. (2006). *Global burden of disease and risk factors*. New York/Washington, DC: Oxford University Press/World Bank.

Magnusson, R., (2010). Global health governance and the challenge of chronic, non-communicable disease. Sydney Law School Legal Studies Research Paper, No. 10/123

NCD Alliance. (2010). UN votes yes for NCD summit. May 10. www.ncdalliance.org/node/80 (March 2012).

Olusoji, A., Smith, O., & Robles, S. (2007). *Public policy and the challenges of chronic noncommunicable diseases*. Washington, DC: The International Bank for Reconstruction and Development/The World Bank.

Porter, M., & Kramer, M. (2011). Creating shared value. *Harvard Business Review, 89*, 62–77.

United Nations General Assembly. (2010). Keeping the promise: United to achieve the millennium development goals. September 17. www.un.org/en/mdg/summit2010/pdf/mdg%20outcome%20document.pdf (October 2012).

United Nations General Assembly. Political declaration of high level meeting of the general assemblyon the prevention and control of noncommunicable diseases. Rep noA/66/L. United Nations General Assembly.

WHO. (1997). Jakarta Declaration on leading health promotion into the 21st century. *Fourth International Conference on Health Promotion: New Players for a New Era—Leading Health Promotion into the 21st Century, Jakarta*. Geneva: World Health Organization.

WHO. (2003). *Framework convention on tobacco control*. Geneva: World Health Organization.

WHO. (2004). *Global strategy on diet physical activity and health*. Geneva: World Health Organization.

WHO. (2005a). *Preventing chronic diseases: A vital investment. WHO global report*. Geneva: World Health Organization.

WHO. (2005b). WHO framework convention on tobacco control. WHA56.1.

WHO. (2005c). Bangkok Charter for health promotion in a globalized world. *Sixth Global Conference on Health Promotion, Thailand*. Geneva: World Health Organization.

WHO. (2006). Constitution of the World Health Organization Basic Documents, Forty-fifth edition, Supplement.

WHO. (2006). European charter on counteracting obesity. Retrieved May 2013 from http://ww.euro.who.int/data/assets/pdffile/005/87458/E89568.pdf.

WHO. (2008a). *World health statistics*. Geneva: WHO.

WHO. (2008b). *2008–2013 Action plan for the global strategy for the prevention and control of noncommunicable diseases*. Geneva: WHO.

WHO. (2008c). *The global burden of disease: 2004 update*. Geneva: World Health Organization.

WHO. (2010). *Global strategy to reduce the harmful use of alcohol*. Geneva: World Health Organization.

WHO. (2011). *Global status report on non-communicable diseases 2010*. Geneva: World Health Organization.

WHO. (2012). Regional office for Europe. In I. Kickbush & D. Gleicher (Eds.), *Governance for health in the 21st century*. Copenhagen: World Health Organization. ISBN 9789289002745.

WHO Reform: Governance: Promoting engagement with other stakeholders and involvement with and oversight of partnerships. Retrieved August, 2011 from http://apps.who.int/gb/ebwha/pdf_files/EB130/B130_5Add4-en.pdf. *Health Diplomacy Monitor, 2*(4).

World Bank Strategy for Health Nutrition and Population Results. (2006, May 30). *Background note for a briefing to the committee on development effectiveness on the preparation of the New Bank HNP strategy*. Washington DC: World Bank

World Health Organization. (WHO 2011c). Definition of region groupings. Retrieved August 25, 2011, from http://www.who.int/healthinfo/global_burden_ disease/definition_regions/en/index.html.

World Health Organization/World Economic Forum. (2008). Preventing noncommunicable diseases in the workplace through diet and physical activity: WHO/ World Economic Forum report of a joint event. ISBN 978 92 4 159632 9.

Zacher, M. (2007). The transformation in global health collaboration since the 1990s. In A. Cooper, J. Kirton, & T. Shrecker (Eds.), *Governing global health: Challenge, response, innovation* (pp. 15–27). Aldershot, UK: Ashgate.

Governance, Policy, and Institutions

David V. McQueen

Governance

In present day public health the term "governance" has become widely used in recent years. However, there are many definitions of governance, samples of which can be found in many documents (cf. Dodgson et al. 2002; Finkelstein 1995; Hufty 2011; Rosenau 1995, 1999; World Bank 1991). In addition, discussions and definitions continue to abound (cf. the Web site of the Council on Foreign Relations (http://www.cfr.org/issue/global-governance/ri23). Whatever definition one wishes to work with the key consideration is that the word "government" is a noun and is an institutional word, of which more later in this chapter. Governance is more of a verbal concept, it is what a government or governmental type entity does. It might be a geopolitical government (nation-state), a corporate government (business entity), a sociopolitical government (tribe, family, etc.), or any number of different kinds of government, but governance is the physical exercise of management power and policy. The term government is also used more abstractly as a synonym for governance, as in the phrase, "Peace, Order and Good Government" found in

Section 91 of the 1867 Canadian Constitution Act, as well as in a number of Commonwealth Country documents. In any case most definitions deal with the process by which decisions are made, the exercise of political authority, how institutions collaborate and delegate resources, and, in other words the management of power by institutions. From its beginnings public health has been involved with governance and it remains a key area for public health research and understanding (cf. McQueen et al. 2012a).

Health Governance

As a notion, governance for health has been around since ancient times; however, as a modern concept that is at the heart of current public health approaches it is relatively recent (Kickbusch 2007, 2010). A recent WHO study considered the concept in detail and tied it to many of the new issues relevant to present day public health: *New approaches to governance are driven by the changing nature of the challenges faced by twenty-first century societies, of which health is only one and which is not always given priority. Most of these challenges, however, have significant health impacts, which have so far not been considered sufficiently. The challenges include systemic shocks, such as natural disasters and disease outbreaks, as well as longer-term processes, such as urbanization, epidemiological and demographic transitions, food insecurity, climate change and*

D.V. McQueen (✉)
2418 Midvale Court, Tucker, GA 30084, USA
e-mail: davidmcqueen07@gmail.com

D.V. McQueen (ed.), *Global Handbook on Noncommunicable Diseases and Health Promotion*,
DOI 10.1007/978-1-4614-7594-1_26, © Springer Science+Business Media, LLC 2013

widening economic disparities. Unique to our times are the synergistic global interconnections among these large-scale challenges (and opportunities) and the interdependence of most of the solutions. The complexity of these so-called "wicked problems" calls for systems approaches and networked responses at all levels and will force policy-makers to move out of their silos compartments (WHO EURO 2011a, p. vi).

In almost all discussions of present day health governance several key notions continue to be emphasized. Some of the notions relate to the nature of present society. The concept of globalization is well accepted. Society is viewed a complex. That is, the operations of society cannot be reduced to simply understanding the functions and operations of a single part. The whole is greater than the sum of the parts and means that every component is interdependent with another. There is the belief that the whole is at the same time systematic but also somewhat chaotic, giving rise to so-called "wicked" problems. The recognition that problems in policy can be dealt with but not solved with any finality is a hallmark of present day thinking on health policy. Strangely enough, this recognition has long been a hallmark of the so-called hard sciences such as physics and astronomy and has come to be accepted as part of the standard approach to understanding. In the health sciences there have been movements towards finding solid evidence and understanding through research (cf. Chap. 3). In health policy and governance this search for evidence and understanding has gradually yielded to the same realization as in the hard sciences. That is, that an evidence-based understanding of governance and policy has to give way to a simpler view of evidence informed policy (Bowen and Zwi 2005).

Given this complexity and the recognition that policy is a wicked problem, the other key notions follow. A major notion is the importance of basing health policy on a new metrics as Kickbusch and others have asserted: "The whole of government and the whole of society must become more familiar with the complex dynamics of health and its determinants in order to govern better (WHO EURO 2011a, p. 73)." This approach makes the development of policies to address NCDs and in

particular the social determinants of health much more plausible, because it implies the necessary changes in the institutions of health themselves. Not only do internal governmental institutional structures, such as departments, agencies, bureaus, and civil services structures need to be changed, but also the relationships between these institutional structures and the organizational entities residing outside of the governmental institutions, such as NGOs, civil society, and the business sector. Health policy for governance now becomes a whole of society approach that requires a major shift from twentieth century structures (McQueen et al. 2012).

Global Health Governance

With regard to global health governance an elaborate conceptual review was undertaken and presented in a discussion paper by Dodgson, Lee, and Drager for the WHO Department of Health and Development in 2002. This paper succinctly lays out the key concepts and the arising issues that concern governance. One of the important aspects that they review is the distinction between the idea of "global health governance" and "international health governance." Essentially, governance is a general idea that "can be defined as the actions and means adopted by a society to promote collective action and deliver collective solutions in pursuit of common goals. Thus, the broad term that is encompassing of the many ways in which human beings, as individuals and groups, organize themselves to achieve agreed goals (Dodgson et al. 2002, p. 6)." A more narrow concept is that of health governance. However, health governance is seen by some as "international health governance (IHG)" and by others as "global health governance (GHC)." Essentially, as developed historically, IHG was related to governance actions carried out by agreement between two of more countries and by actions of their governments.

However, globalization (cf. Chap. 24) has fundamentally changed the way we look at global health governance in that the role of the social determinants of health have become critically important. This fact is coupled with the additional complexity added by the need to understand the role of inequalities and institutions and the conclusions of what to do down the governance's path, even as they are expressed in more biomedical terms (WHO 2011). Thus, the impact of globalization has taken the idea of health governance away from just being the processes and bureaucratic operations of higher level governmental institutions and placed it firmly onto the subject matters of governance as opposed to the institutions of governance. This is a fundamental change and at the essence of global health governance. What Held et al. succinctly stated about global governance involving "not only the formal institutions and organizations through which the rules and norms governing world order are (or are not) made and sustained—the institutions of the state, intergovernmental cooperation and so on—but also those organizations and pressure groups—from MNCs, transnational social movements to the plethora of non-governmental organizations—which pursue goals and objectives which have a bearing on transnational rule and authority systems (1999, p. 50)" clearly applies as well to the current state of health governance. The whole discussion of governance and health governance in particular is that the concept now includes all the dimensions of governance, ranging from ethical considerations, to ideas about leadership, and ultimately to a comprehension of global health systems. Thus, health governance not only is faced with complexity but is also intertwined with all the other wicked problems facing contemporary public health. The implications of this are great and undoubtedly reveal that we are probably just at the beginning of trying to more fully understand the role of health governance, what it is and how it works.

Considerable elaboration, discussion and scholarly materials on global health governance already exist and are available at the Web site http://blogs.shu.edu/ghg/about-global-health-governance/. This is the site of the peer reviewed, open access, scholarly journal on the topic, *Global Health Governance*. A seminal article to be read from this source is that by Nora Y. Ng and Jennifer Prah Ruger entitled Global Health

Governance at a Crossroads (2011). This comprehensive review brings up to date many of the issues that have arisen in Global Health Governance in the past decade. They point out that the concept of global health governance is more complex than the older notion of international heath governance, and this is a result in particular of the influence of globalization (cf. Chap. 24). They allude also to the much discussed post-Westphalian concept that has developed in political science, arguing that the old structure of nations that were held together as an international group following the Peace of Westphalia in the seventeenth century no longer holds. In short, national boundaries have become much less relevant than in the past. They also make the point that the new global health governance area lacks structure and is ill defined as a concept. It is also notable that the traditional international players have moved into the global concept even as their institutional structures, bound by national politics, often remain locked in a nationalistic past. This is particularly true for the major health organizations and especially the World Health Organization with its close structural ties to national member states. This outmoded and dated structure affects the health action areas of health promotion and efforts on NCDs profoundly. Non-governmental organizations (NGOs) also play a major part in questions of global governance (cf. Chap. 10) as well as public private partnerships (PPPs) (cf. Chap. 23). What these types of organizations bring to the table are considerable degrees of freedom of movement in dealing with specific health issues. They can be concerned with governance without being a part of formal government structures and can more easily work across national boundaries. Examples of such NGO work are abundant. For example the Carter Center's work to eliminate malaria and lymphatic filariasis in the Caribbean (http://www.cartercenter.org/health/hispaniola-initiative/index.html), or CARE's work on maternal health Programs in sub-Saharan Africa (http://www.care.org/campaigns/mothersmatter/index.asp), or the many preventive health programs funded by the Gate's Foundation. Nonetheless, despite the many success stories and the changing nature of global health governance, Ng and Ruger note that there are still major issues and challenges that remain. Perhaps the major issue is one that involves the way for all the various institutions and governments to cooperate with each other. Cooperation generally depends upon mechanisms to make this possible and historically most institutions, whether governments or NGOs have little experience in creating or managing such mechanisms. Other non-technical problems are commonplace. Turf wars are common as well as entrenched attitudes about who has what role to play. Given all this difficulty to engage in cooperative work, NCDs present a particular challenge because most of the historically successful public health programs attempting to address diseases have been those with "vertical" success, especially where there is a single highly visible disease involved such as smallpox or Guinea worm. NCDs involve much more variegated disease with loose definition characteristics. For example, heart diseases (cf. Chap. 17) offer a very complex set of approaches to a great many disease categories that are part of the heart disease spectrum. Unfortunately, the success of vertical programs often diverts governments and agencies into bypassing the complexities of NCDs. This results in spiking of resources in some areas over others, as in the case of the particular attention given to HIV. Nonetheless there are efforts that concentrate on underlying broad based concerns such as health systems strengthening. Ng and Ruger note that "Non-communicable diseases (NCDs) are receiving more attention now that the globalization of unhealthy diets and sedentary lifestyles is making them both more common and more deadly … Observers urge action, particularly through multisectoral partnerships;" (Ng and Ruger 2011 p. 13).

Governance and HiAP

Governance is a verbal concept related to the idea of agency. It is an active term that implies some capacity of actors to change or manipulate structure, in the case of governance the structure of government. Thus, health in all policies, HiAP, is an outcome of governance and agency. Nonetheless, governance is conducted through the use of structures that are built into government. As is usually the case structures, e.g., committees, legislatures, agencies, etc. are easier to see than agency, which is the activity of or in the structures. This visibility is undoubtedly why there is so much more literature on structures rather than on agency. We have a surfeit of documents, statements, declarations, agreements, charters, and other such written texts (Ståhl et al. 2006); what we lack is an understanding as to how these documents are made active or given agency.

The concept of HiAP is basically a political idea without any carefully argued theoretical underpinnings. Of course it does relate to those historical dimensions of a public health discussed in detail in Chap. 22. However, it resides more in that part of public health that is concerned with power and politics. It also is a concept that in its ideological statement asserts that health belongs in all of the political power process. It is in that sense presumptive and aggressive as a concept. One sees this aggressiveness in statements such as "all ministers are health ministers." While presumptive, such statements echo the sentiments of Virchow and others who injected power politics into the health arena. What is notable is how non-threatening the statements around HiAP appear. Perhaps this itself is the result of the concept being primarily ideological and in itself not seen as a threat. What is clear as that the concept of HiAP is a move away from the individual centered, biomedical view of public health that dominated the twentieth century. This concept of HiAP fits nicely into what Kickbusch has called the "expansion of the territory of health." She writes: "The risk profile of late modernity implies that solutions need to be found beyond the medical health system and that health policy needs to concern itself with investments in other parts of society" (2007, p. 151).

One may regard the notion of HiAP as one of late modernity and as representative of a newly emerging broader scope for public health. Part of that broader scope is the emergence of the recognition of contextual factors, both social and cultural, as helping to define an area of legitimacy for public health (cf. Chap. 6).

Once contextual factors are seen as a legitimate area for public health action, the political implications follow. They follow because most of the contextual factors are in the political rather than the medical realm. And it follows on that issues such as inequity become important both politically and from a health standpoint. It also follows that health promotion as an activity of public health becomes salient; one does not prevent inequity, one promotes equity. HiAP is a health promotion response to this renewed critical thinking.

In most advanced economies governance occurs in all sectors of society and it operates at all levels of government from national to local. In reality most areas of governance are mundane (sewers, transportation, energy, education, etc.). In highly developed societies these areas operate continuously, bureaucratically and with little relation to the politics of the time. While politics plays a role in these activities, one does not expect the supply of potable water to be dependent on whether the government is politically left leaning, centrist, or right wing. Nonetheless the politically formed institutions of government related to HiAP play a role in the public's health. They comprise the institutions for action in the HiAP approach. Furthermore some seemingly mundane areas such as housing policy may become hot political items. Health considerations can enter into the field of debate and discussion. How these considerations enter may be highly contextual, variable, parochial, local, or national. For example, potable drinking water may seem rather nonpolitical until it becomes an issue of water resources and supplies that may cross political boundaries. HiAP has historically had a role in governance and has been highly politicized. An example of this is the reconstruction of Paris under Napoleon III. "When Baron Haussmann set out to "straighten" the streets of Paris and create the great boulevards of today the rationale may have been largely for defense of the Monarchy, but the outcome was the clearing of bad housing, reduction of pollution and highly improved sanitation for the Parisians. It was, from another perspective, a major effort to address the social determinants of health by changing the social and physical landscape. That this was carried out as an act of governance is

without doubt, even if it was a monarchial government. One can see similar countless examples in many movements that combined governance and civil society to address large-scale urban infrastructure, most notably the creation in most Western cities, particularly in America, of vast and extraordinary park systems. The ethos may have been to create place or beauty and leisure, but this is easily translated into today's notions of healthy cities. Most of these and other efforts to improve the commons were the result of governance actions…"(McQueen et al. 2012, p. 8).

Value Driven Governance

In recent years a values discussion has entered heavily in to thinking about public health and health promotion (Mayes and Oliver 2012; Gostin et al. 2004; Gostin and Madison 2006). The subject of values in health related governance draws upon millennia of philosophical discussion by ancient and modern philosophers. While many of the conceptual components are ancient, many are found in the current debates on health, health policy, and health governance. What is also clear is that the discussion is often without clarity in definition and terms. Perhaps this is not surprising as many of those who discuss values in health are not trained philosophers or skilled logicians. Also the discussions are often highly contextual, reflecting the biomedical view of the participants. Chief among the oft-discussed value concepts are notions such as equity, social justice, dignity, and human rights. These values are reflected in numerous health promotion documents and notably in those associated with the WHO Commission on the Social Determinants of Health, (WHOCSDOH 2008). These documents, in general, show a bias towards a Western philosophical tradition reflecting the discussions in moral philosophy that characterized Western thinking historically. While the philosophical discussion of values is ancient the academic discourse is more recent. This base, extensively reviewed by writers such as Joas (2000) and Kuhn (1975), stems from the writings of key German figures such as Hermann Lotze, Immanuel Kant, and in particular the works of

Friedrich Nietzsche. Nietzsche, in particular, emphasized the contextual or contingency nature of values. Much of this nineteenth century discussion related back to medieval debates over realism and nominalism, which in turn related to classical debates between an Aristotelian or Platonic perspective. The focus of debate was whether values are fundamental concepts that exist independently of human thought (Platonic, realist) or whether they are highly contextual and bound to changing human interpretations (Aristotelian, nominalist). On examination one would conclude that the discourse on values and ethics in governance is relegated more to the pragmatic and less to the realm of deep moral philosophy. In many ways the elaborate work and discussion of values in health in the past three decades has been the effort to pull the deeper philosophical debate on values into the realm of the pragmatic. And that pragmatic is the field of governance. Much of the discourse now is cantered on values such as dignity, liberty, democracy, equality, rule of law, human rights; pluralism, tolerance, justice, solidarity, and non-discrimination. Despite widespread Western identification of these values, they are subject to possible value-conflicts when working on health across sectors and within subpopulations in all countries. This, in turn, may result in value trade-offs in the policy translation process. It is this trade off and translation that moves the value based ideology into the realm of ethical actions taken by institutions ad governments regarding health, health prevention and health promotion. Further these potential value conflicts lead inevitably to confrontation with parallel values such as accountability and civil participation.

Ethics and Governance

Ethics are involved in taking decisions on values. Most ethical considerations in public health involve normative ethics. Normative ethics is concerned with how to act taking into account value-concepts. Normative ethics is largely a prescriptive effort, or as some would term it applied ethics. Ethical decisions are seldom straightfor-

ward. It is complex to judge what is right or wrong in actions and this in turn has led to considerations of partial rightness, a concept that was historically quite developed in ethical writings. However, the influence of the work of John Rawls (1971) tended to move the focus in health directly to moral arguments underpinning action.

In public health, when actions are taken to protect the health of a population, to prevent the spread of a disease, to promote the health of a community, to reduce poverty that leads to poor health, to increase health literacy, then ethical value laden efforts are being undertaken. These efforts to effect change link values and ethics directly to governance; it is the action component of government structure. This apparent fact is undoubtedly not disconnected from the common concerns of public health prevention and health promotion that arose chiefly out of a Western philosophical tradition. This tradition is made explicit with the use of value concepts such as equity and social justice in the efforts to address the social determinants of health and NCDs in the work of the WHO SDOH Commission (WHOCSDOH 2008).

The Mixture of Policy, Governance, and Values in Public Health, NCDs, and Health Promotion

Policy discussions of health at the highest levels may be viewed as aspirational or visionary. Major policy documents of international organizations, e.g., UN agencies such as WHO, and those stemming from the ministries of governments belong to this category (UNGA 2011; WHO 2009). Of course, in reality they are generally statements derived from the collective work of staffers, bureaucrats and political appointees. As such they are usually crafted after many hours of debate and dialogue among the writers and assigned no explicit authorship beyond that of the institution itself. The policy documents produced are given titles such as statement, resolution, charter, agreement, etc. They draw on value principles rather than ethics because they are primarily visionary and rarely state the ethical means by which the vision is to be carried out. Often goals (recommendations) are stated, but without specification of means. Because the statements are at such a visionary level those outside the visionary process may consider them as somewhat vague. The challenge for policy at this level is how to translate this vision into collective action. That process is generally left to others, often petty bureaucrats and to broader collectives such as civil society. The bureaucrats may be well positioned within governmental institutions and charged with the governance responsibility implied by the policy. Whereas civil society residing outside direct government must argue policy from direct merits to those taking action.

The process of taking high level policy to action is hardly simple and often lacking in the long run. Those composing policy are generally not the same people that would put policy into action. In addition, substantive resources for action are often lacking. In recent years the role of civil society in creating the impetus for visionary statements has been well recognized and appreciated by those studying policy. That recognition has been often less understood by institutionalized policy makers. Nonetheless, civil society and in particular those more formal NGOs comprising part of civil society, have pushed back at governmental institutions with their own sets of values. Indeed, sometimes the NGO will be organized specifically around a value that directly relates to health or health promotion. That is the NGO's raison d'être is in itself to persuade standing governmental institutions to adopt value based visionary statements in their area of interest (cf. Chaps. 10 and 27). Governance relates to policy in myriad ways. Often it is difficult to distinguish when the primary operation is one of policy or governance, but the expressions of governance and policy within government are seen in the day to day operations of management, legislation, procurement, resource allocation, communication and the other categorical operations of the institution we call government. In brief, policy, governance and the institutions of government ultimately tie back to the value concepts that underlie the functioning of government. In essence the role of government is to make values explicit in the governed.

Evidence and Policy

At the present time there is considerable focus in public health on governance, policy and health in all policies. Two implications are notable. The first is that once one moves to a broad policy perspective one is no longer just in the health arena. Rather, all the dimensions of policy and how it is developed and implemented become part of the discussion revealing a large literature of relevance; the narrow field of health policy is superseded by the broad area of policy in general. The second has to do with the question of evidence. That is, what is the evidence basis for making policy? What is the evidence basis that policy makes any difference? What is the scientific basis, if any, for advocating health in all policies? Those in public health may be comfortable with the ideological and value basis for health in all policies, but the comfort level for the evidence of the effectiveness of health in all policy is much more in question (Brownson et al. 2009; Macintyre 2012).

This is not a new concern, in the USA a 1978 National Research Council report, Knowledge and Policy: The Uncertain Connection (NRC 1978) stated that the state of knowledge with regard to systematic evidence of policy effectiveness was not good. As a result, more recently The Committee on the Use of Social Science Knowledge in Public Policy was charged by the National Research Council "to review the knowledge utilization and other relevant literature to assess what is known about how social science knowledge is used in policy making… [and] to develop a framework for further research that can improve the use of social science knowledge in policy making." (NRC 2012) Remarkably, this 2012 report, Using Science as Evidence in Public Policy, also showed that the evidence base is weak or nonexistent and concluded that a research approach that leads to an understanding needs major revision. One summation from the report is most applicable to policy related to health: "Science has five tasks related to policy: (1) identify problems, such as endangered species, obesity, unemployment, and vulnerability to natural disasters or terrorist acts; (2) measure their magnitude and seriousness; (3) review alternative policy interventions; (4) systematically assess the likely consequences of particular policy actions—intended and unintended, desired and unwanted; and (5) evaluate what, in fact, results from policy. Across all of these tasks, there are political and value considerations that are outside the scope of science." (p. 4).

The efforts to develop health policy and notably the idea of health in all policies face significant challenges when it comes to reviewing alternative policy interventions. To date many of the policy oriented statements still reflect interventions that address behavioral factors in the causation of NCDs. Alternative policy areas have been proposed for some time. Ron Labonte has made the case in detail with regard to issues related to globalization and has provided specific alternative proposals (cf. Chaps. 6 and 24); Hillary Graham has made the case for addressing inequalities (Graham 2009); and Arline Geronimus the case for addressing structural influences on the health of urban populations (2000). Other researchers have proposed numerous alternative policy areas, but the key factor here is what policies institutions such as the WHO take up. In general they take up more narrow policies and narrow policies do not fit well with the concept of health in all policies.

When it comes to systematically assessing the likely consequences of particular policy actions—intended and unintended, desired and unwanted and evaluating what, in fact, results from policy, the public health area is on very weak ground. There are recent endeavors such as that from the European Observatory (McQueen et al. 2012) that provide insight into some of the specific processes and organizational mechanisms that tie structure to agency in policy actions as well as the excellent report from the expert group meeting in Liverpool on how can the health equity impact of universal policies be evaluated? Insights into approaches and next steps (WHO EURO 2011b). They noted, following extensive discussion and efforts to delineate the challenges in policy evaluation, several promising approaches such as systems approaches, innovative uses of natural experiments, cross-national comparative policy analyses using policy typologies, historical analyses, and drawing insights from complexity theory. There are other efforts to assess policy, such as discussed by Ruetten et al. in Chap. 9, but there is a need for many studies to fully understand the evaluative components of policy. Despite these valiant initial efforts to deal with large-scale policy evaluation, significant challenges remain to fully understand policy impact systematically. At the output end of evaluation, that is where policy translates into results on the ground, locally, nationally, or globally there is relatively little available evaluation. Unless and until more resources in public health are given over to evaluation of policy, health policies will be based largely on persuasion rather than on any scientific basis.

Institutions

Throughout this chapter and book there have been many discussions about and references to "institutions." Like so many everyday words used in public health this word denotes many different ideas. In general, when I use the term the meaning can be either structural or functional, or, an entity that has both a physical and personnel structure as well as an acting or agency component. For example, the Centers for Disease Control (CDC) and Prevention, is a US federal agency under the Department of Health and Human Services headquartered in unincorporated DeKalb County, Georgia, in Greater Atlanta. As such, the CDC has many buildings, bricks and mortar, thousands of employees working in many centers, divisions, and branches charged with the mission to be an agency for public health in the USA. It is noteworthy that this huge institution is regarded as an agency, because that wording means that its structure is designed for intervention. However, the concept of institution also carries the more ephemeral notion of an entity that exists independent of structure and agency, such as when it is used in a phrase such as "the institution of democracy." In recent years the whole subject of institution has become a focus of social science examination.

Geoffrey Hodgson in his definitive article What Are Institutions? (2006) first defines them as such: "we may define institutions as systems of established and prevalent social rules that structure social interactions." This, of course, is a very broad and conceptual definition that seems somewhat distant from the notion of a brick and mortar agency. Part of the solution in defining the common usage in public health is the use of the word institution when, in fact, it is an organization that is being discussed. However, that organization may operate, de facto, as an institution under the above definition. This is a conundrum that has faced social science since the early work by Thorsten Veblen and others on organizational theory. Hodgson finally describes organizations as "special institutions that involve (a) criteria to establish their boundaries and to distinguish their members from nonmembers, (b) principles of sovereignty concerning who is in charge, and (c) chains of command delineating responsibilities within the organization." (p. 18).

In recent years, the debates in political science and sociology around the nature of institutions have led to an ongoing and critical discussion of what is termed the "new institutionalism." For the public health researcher concerned with NCDs and health promotion this somewhat arcane discussion of new institutionalism may be quite distant. However, the discussion has revealed some of the key considerations that operate in our consideration of public health institutions and/or organizations. Ellen Immergut, in her work on "The Theoretical Core of the New Institutionalism" (1998), delineated some of the chief ideas that one has to keep in mind with regard to institutions. First, institutions may be seen as collective organizing bodies to carry out political will through actions. This is at the heart of the agency idea and ties into earlier discussions of governance. Second, are what Immergut calls the "contextual logics of causality" that can be stretched to apply to the area of causality related to the NCDs and their so-called social determinants. This notion relates to the idea that institutions themselves determine the specific variables that are chosen for action. In a most comprehensive review of the new institutionalism Peter Hall and

Rosemary Taylor discuss the various forms of institutionalism and give examples of this in organizational entities (1996). They review the work on the sociological perspective on institutions; one quotation seems particularly pertinent to health institutions dealing with NCDs and health promotion: "…the problematic that sociological institutionalists typically adopt seeks explanations for why organizations take on specific sets of institutional forms, procedures or symbols; and it emphasizes how such practices are diffused through organizational fields or across nations. They are interested, for instance, in explaining the striking similarities in organizational form and practice that Education Ministries display throughout the world, regardless of the differences in local conditions… (p. 947)."

There are a considerable number of dimension of institutions that could be elaborated at this point, but this is a monograph on NCDs and health promotion in public health. The point here is that there are many dimensions of institutionalism that appear to be relevant to understanding why institutions in public health are formed as they are and act as they do. It also reveals the need to better understand the role of these institutional interpretations in discussions of governance and health policy. But above all it reveals a need to understand why our institutions address the contextual factors in health as they do and why health promotion has been rather unsuccessful at providing an appropriate institutional response to the problems of public health.

Conclusion

The world and literature related to governance, policy, and institutions related to public health, NCDs, and health promotion is not only vast but also one of increasing interest and diversity. Many topics relevant to this area have not been covered in this chapter, partly because some are covered elsewhere in this book, and partly because they would require a more extensive search and analysis of the growth in this area. As an example of just a subcomponent of this area that has recently received attention consider the area of intersectoral governance for health in all policies covered in the recent publication from IUHPE, WHO (EURO) and the European Observatory on Health Systems and Policies (McQueen et al. 2012). This document concentrates just on the structures, actions and experiences inside of governmental institutions in developing HiAP. The revealed structures and actions are highly complex, highly cultural, and in many cases highly related to national political structures. The point is that the whole policy area of public health is very complex. A response to this fact by the Canadian government was the establishment in 2005 of six National Collaborating Centres (NCCs) to strengthen and renew the public health system in Canada. The National Collaborating Centres for Public Health's mission is to translate relevant evidence produced by academics and researchers so that it can be used by public health practitioners and policy-makers. Notably one of the most active and productive centers is the National Collaborating Centre for Healthy Public Policy, located in the province of Quebec, whose mission is to increase the expertise of public health actors across Canada in healthy public policy (http://www.ncchpp.ca/en/). The establishment of such an institutional response to the need for careful examination of the research on health public policy is a tribute to the foresight of the Canadian government. Finally this area continues to grow in importance for all the issues discussed relevant to NCDs and health promotion in this book. It seems clear that if the burden of NCDs and necessary health promoting actions are to be taken globally, it will be because good governance and a healthy public policy has done its work.

References

Bowen, S., & Zwi, A. B. (2005). Pathways to "evidence-informed" policy and practice: A framework for action. *PLoS Medicine, 2*(7), e166. doi:10.1371/journal.pmed.0020166.

Brownson, R. C., Chriqui, J. F., & Stamatakis, K. A. (2009). Understanding evidence-based public health policy. *American Journal of Public Health, 99*, 1576–1583.

Dodgson, R., Lee, K., & Drager, N. (2002). *Global health governance: A conceptual review*. London: WHO/London School of Hygiene & Tropical Medicine. Discussion Paper No. 1. http://www.bvsde.paho.org/texcom/cd050853/dodgson.pdf

Finkelstein, L. (1995). What is global governance? *Global Governance, 1*, 367–372.

Geronimus, A. T. (2000). Mitigate, resist, or undo: Addressing structural influences on the health of urban populations. *American Journal of Public Health, 90*, 867–872.

Gostin, L. O., Boufford, J. I., & Martinez, R. M. (2004). The future of the public's health: Vision, values, and L.O. strategies. *Health Affairs, 23*(4), 96–107.

Gostin, L. O., & Madison, P. (2006). What does social justice require for the public's health? Public health ethics and policy imperatives. *Health Affairs, 25*(4), 1053–1060.

Graham, H. (2009). Tackling health inequalities: The scope for policy. In H. Graham (Ed.), *Understanding health inequalities* (pp. 199–218). New York, NY: McGraw Hill.

Hall, P. A., & Taylor, R. C. R. (1996). Political science and the three new institutionalisms. *Political Studies, 44*:936–957. Article first published online: December 22, 2006. DOI: 10.1111/j.1467-9248.1996.tb00343.

Held, D., McGrew, A., Goldblatt, D., & Perraton, J. (1999). *Global transformations: Politics, economics and culture*. Stanford: Stanford University Press.

Hodgson, G. M. (2006). What are institutions? *Journal of Economic Issues, 40*, 1–25.

Hufty, M. (2011). Investigating policy processes: The governance analytical framework (GAF). In U. Wiesmann & H. Hurni (Eds.), *Research for sustainable development: Foundations, experiences, and perspectives. Perspectives of the Swiss National Centre of Competence in Research (NCCR) North-South, University of Bern* (Vol. 6, pp. 403–424). Bern, Switzerland: Geographica Bernensia.

Immergut, E. (1998). The theoretical core of the new institutionalism. *Politics and Society, 26*, 5–34.

Joas, H. (2000). *The genesis of values*. Chicago: University of Chicago Press.

Kickbusch, I. (2007). Health governance: The health society. In D. McQueen & I. Kickbusch (Eds.), *Health and modernity: The role of theory in health promotion*. New York, NY: Springer.

Kickbusch, I. (2010). Health in all policies: The evolution of the concept of horizontal governance. In I. Kickbusch & K. Buckett (Eds.), *Implementing health in all policies*. Adelaide: Government of South Australia.

Kuhn, H. (1975). Werte—eine urgegebenheit. In H.-G. Gadamer & P. Vogler (Eds.), *Neue anthologie* (Vol. 7, pp. 343–373). Stuttgart: Thieme.

Macintyre, S. (2012). Evidence in the development of health policy. *Public Health, 126*, 217–219.

Mayes, R., & Oliver, T. R. (2012). Chronic disease and the shifting focus of public health: Is prevention still a political lightweight? *Journal of Health Politics Policy and Law, 37,* 181–200.

McQueen, D. V., Wismar, M., Lin, V., Jones, C. M., & Davis, M. (Eds.). (2012). *Intersectoral governance for health in all policies: Structures, actions and experiences.* Copenhagen: WHO Regional Office for Europe on behalf of the European Observatory on Health Systems and Policies.

Ng, N. Y., & Ruger, J. P. (2011). Global health governance at a crossroads. *Global Health Governance, 3*(2), 1–37.

NRC, National Research Council. (1978). *Knowledge and policy: The uncertain connection.* Washington, DC: The National Academies Press.

NRC, National Research Council. (2012). Using science as evidence in public policy. Committee on the use of social science knowledge in public policy. In K. Prewitt, T. A. Schwandt, & M. L. Straf (Eds.), *Division of behavioral and social sciences and education.* Washington, DC: The National Academies Press.

Rawls, J. (1971). *A theory of justice.* Cambridge: The Belknap Press of Harvard University Press.

Rosenau, J. N. (1995). Governance in the twenty-first century. *Global Governance, 1,* 13–43.

Rosenau, J. N. (1999). Toward an ontology for global governance. In M. Hewson & T. Sinclair (Eds.), *Approaches to global governance theory.* Albany: Suny Press.

Ståhl, T., Wismar, M., Ollila, E., Lahtinen, E., & Leppo, K. (Eds.). (2006). *Health in all policies: Prospects and potentials.* Helsinki, Finland: Ministry of Social Affairs and Health.

UNGA United Nations General Assembly. (2011). *Political declaration of high level meeting of the general assembly on the prevention and control of noncommunicable diseases. Rep noA/66/L.* New York, NY: United Nations General Assembly.

WHO. (2009). *Milestones in health promotion: Statements from global conferences.* Geneva: WHO. (cf. http://www.who.int/healthpromotion/Milestones_Health_Promotion_05022010.pdf)

WHO. (2011). *Global status report on noncommunicable diseases 2010.* Geneva: World Health Organization.

WHO (EURO). (2011a). Governance for health in the 21st century: A study conducted for the *WHO Regional Office for Europe.* EUR/RC61/Inf.Doc./6. Copenhagen: WHO EURO.

WHO (EURO). (2011b). How can the health equity impact of universal policies be evaluated? Insights into approaches and next steps: Synthesis of discussions from an Expert Group Meeting. In B. Milton, M. Moonan, D. Taylor-Robinson, & M. Whitehead (Eds.), A joint publication between the WHO European Office for Investment for Health and Development, Venice, Italy and the Liverpool WHO Collaborating Centre for Policy Research on Social Determinants of Health Held at the University of Liverpool, November 2010. Copenhagen: WHO EURO

WHOCSDOH. (2008). *Closing the gap in a generation. Health equity through action on the social determinants of health.* Geneva: WHO.

World Bank. (1991). *Managing development: The governance dimension.* A Discussion Paper. No. 34899. Washington, DC: The World Bank.

NCDs and Civil Society: A History and a Roadmap

Johanna Ralston and Sania Nishtar

On May 26, 2012 Member States of the World Health Assembly approved a global target of 25 % reduction in premature mortality from non-communicable diseases (NCDs) by 2025 (WHO 2012). That means 2 % per year reduction in under-70 mortality from cardiovascular disease, cancer, diabetes, chronic respiratory disease. This is excellent news for the NCD community and takes the Political Declaration of the UN High Level Meeting on Noncommunicable Diseases in September 2011 from rhetoric to action. While a series of additional and more specific targets will be approved by the end of the year, including proposed targets on reducing salt, physical inactivity, and daily tobacco smoking, the overall mortality target is a critical turning point and a testament to successful advocacy across many civil society organizations and evidence that was first promoted by WHO in 2005. Most important, the success of this target and the Summit itself are due in no small part to successful advocacy and collaboration by the NCD community, which itself has emerged as cohesive whole only in very recent years, when individual

groups dedicated to risk factors and specific diseases including cancer and CVD started to join forces to address the emerging NCD pandemic in low and middle-income countries.

The challenges in reaching the target and ensuring realization of the goals set forth in the Political Declaration are several, and include:

1. Funding pressures, including those related to the continued economic downturn that has most recently affected Europe and a lack of funding sources for NCDs.
2. The degree to which action will be driven by NCD organizations—both public and NGOs—and the degree to which individual disease and risk factor groups will carry forward the charge.
3. The absence of a legitimate and accepted framework for working across sectors and limited explicit ownership of the NCD issue outside of health.

Given these goals, it is useful to look back on how NGOs played a key role in the period leading up to the UN HLM and approval of the mortality target, and what role they will play moving forward.

The role of global NGOs in the NCD space is a relatively recent phenomenon. While a handful of membership organizations have been working in global cancer, cardiovascular disease, diabetes, CRD, and other diseases, and other groups such as IUHPE focusing on health promotion issues globally, the absence of recognition of NCDs as a matter of global urgency has been strangely

J. Ralston (✉)
World Heart Federation, 7 Rue des Battoirs, Case postale 155, 1211 Geneva 4, Switzerland
e-mail: johanna.ralston@worldheart.org

S. Nishtar, S.I., F.R.C.P., Ph.D.
Heartfile, One Park Road, Chak Shahzad, Islamabad, Pakistan
e-mail: sania@heartfile.org

D.V. McQueen (ed.), *Global Handbook on Noncommunicable Diseases and Health Promotion*,
DOI 10.1007/978-1-4614-7594-1_27, © Springer Science+Business Media, LLC 2013

lacking. A study by Center for Global Development that was released in 2010 viewed this weak prioritization in terms of funding; an analysis of official development assistance for health in 2008 revealed that an astonishing 97 % of health-related ODA went to communicable diseases and other health issues, with only 3 % dedicate to NCDs (Nugent 2012). In trying to understand why and how this occurred, the absence of NCDs in the Millennium Development Goals is a clear driver. At the time that the MDGs were being developed, the data on NCDs were starting to become available, but the strong evidence as outlined in Global status Report on NCDs (WHO 2010), and the World Bank report on Curbing the Epidemic were either not yet available or widely disseminated and thus not translating into policy. In particular, while Curbing the Epidemic looked at cost, in general there was limited research on either the burden or consequent cost of the emerging NCD epidemic in low and middle-income countries.

At the time, there was strong evidence of the financial and security risks associated with HIV/AIDS in LMICs and, both because of burden and because of the need to avoid distorting health budgets and aid flows (Hulme 2009), malaria and tuberculosis were also added as explicit targets. Anecdotal evidence indicates that NCDs were considered but dismissed as a lower priority, again because of the focus on no more than eight priorities as critical for global development. In addition to absence of data, NCDs continued to be perceived as largely afflictions of high income and middle aged or older populations, and linked to personal choice, with policy interventions dismissed as the state acting as a nanny. For example, the Economist as recently as 2006 noted that Margaret Chan, then newly elected Director General of the World Health Organization, should "cure the agency's addiction to noisy campaigns against obesity, smoking and other non-infectious ailments… Many of these afflictions arise from personal choice, and are not contagious."

The era of advocacy for NCDs has important roots in the tobacco control advocacy movement and in particular in the successful alliances that led to the development of the Framework Convention on Tobacco Control. The impetus for the FCTC came from increased activity in the mid-1990s to look at concerted policy efforts around tobacco control across borders; tobacco as a multinational issue was starting to be understood as one that would require a supranational approach since the drivers of the devastating health consequences of tobacco were trade and economics rather than the traditional disease vectors of communicable diseases. The increased evidence for action in tobacco control, as well as accelerated activity by the tobacco industry brought on by the facilitating market access measures of globalization, coincided with the arrival at WHO of Director General Gro Harlem Brundlandt, who was supportive of a WHO-led treaty process to enlist the commitment of all Member States in a set of evidence based tobacco control policy measures. From a civil society perspective, the FCTC was critical in bringing together actors outside of health, including consumer rights organizations, women's groups, environmental advocates concerned with the consequences of secondhand smoke, and important for the later development of the NCD movement, disease groups that had not necessarily collaborated before including cancer, cardiovascular and respiratory disease organizations. The lobbying work leading up to the FCTC, and since 2003 in ensuring ratification and support for implementation at the Conference of Parties meetings and at country level, required this broad base of organizations—many of which continued their commitment to FCTC implementation through membership and action in the Framework Convention Alliance—to define common asks and messages.

While health groups had previously worked in alliances—e.g., the Global Alliance for Vaccine Initiative and the Global Fund for AIDS, Tb, and Malaria—the opportunities presented by FCTC and the unique attributes of a multi-sectoral alliance created a foundation for advocacy that became an essential building block for the NCD movement. For cardiovascular, cancer and respiratory disease groups, a precedent was established around joint advocacy as each element of the FCTC was refined at the policy level and then implemented at country level (diabetes groups also played a role though the impact of tobacco on diabetes was less powerful than for CVD, cancer and CRD). Thus there were county level alliances in place that served as an important framework for broader NCD engagement. Country examples of civil society leadership emerged during this time, more broadly focused on NCDs. In Pakistan Heartfile not only advocated for but also led the process of developing an integrated national plan of action, which addressed the four diseases with common risk factors: The National Action Plan for the Prevention and Control of Non-communicable disease and Health Promotion in Pakistan (Nishtar 2010; Nishtar et al. 2006). This was structured as a public-private partnership between the Ministry of Health, WHO and Heartfile (Heartfile MOU 2003).

At the same time, there was increasing recognition in other ways that a single disease focus had its limitations in an increasingly crowded global health space. Under the advocacy leadership of Professor Martin Slinik, the International Diabetes Federation was successful in securing a WHO declaration on diabetes in 2006 (UN Resolution 61/225). While an important marker for mobilizing IDF members around a policy ask, the following years saw frustration at the lack of traction around translation of a global WHO declaration into effective policy at the global or country levels. This was a driver behind the appointment of Ann Keeling as CEO of the International Diabetes Federation in 2009, given her extensive experience in women's rights and advocacy. In 2009 she approached the then-CEOs of World Heart Federation and the Union for International Cancer Control (UICC), both in Geneva, to explore forming an alliance around shared risk factors and the potential for a political instrument such as a UN Summit to galvanize action of NCDs as a development issue. All the CEOs agreed to form the NCD Alliance and this was formalized by their respective board presidents: to include NCDs in the Millennium Development Goals, to secure a UN Summit on NCDs, to ensure access to essential NCD meds in LMICs, and to integrate NCD prevention and control into health systems.

The unique strength of the federations was their role as single disease organizations with member bases that extended to almost every country, meaning there could be efficiency in having three (and

eventually four) groups with a reach of close to 1,000 member organizations. In 2010, recognizing that a group dedicated to chronic respiratory disease was missing; the Alliance invited Nils Billo, Director of the Union for International TB and Lung Disease ("the Union") to join, which also added a dimension of tobacco control and strong operations research in key countries. Meanwhile the UICC and WHF had new CEOs with backgrounds in the private sector and global cancer, respectively, and the group was finalized. Another important moment was the launch of the World Economic Forum Global Risks report in 2010, which showed chronic disease (as NCDs were described) as the third leading cause of risk in the world, far ahead of communicable diseases and providing a business and economic argument for addressing NCDs.

A critical external opportunity was presented when Caribbean health ministers met to address the growing NCD burden and call for UN action. Sir George Alleyne, Director Emeritus of PAHO, was instrumental in securing this meeting; while he had great credibility in infectious diseases, he increasingly recognized that NCDs were the critical new issue and his credibility brought increased attention to this issue. From the NCD Alliance perspective, the Caricom meeting presented an opportunity for concerted advocacy among members, and member organizations in the Caribbean such as the Jamaican Heart Foundation were further mobilized to work together. Dr. Trevor Hassel, then vice president of the World Heart Federation, was instrumental in launching the Healthy Caribbean Coalition to bring together civil society stakeholders across the region to increase policy and public attention on the burden of NCDs. The Caribbean region was also important in calling for a UN summit because of the power of numbers; a critical mass of Member States in a relatively small geographic region could mobilize support with speed and unity of message. The Caricom countries also able to mobilize additional blocs of support through the Pacific island nations and eventually, the Commonwealth states.

The Summit was approved in May 2010 and the NCD Alliance and its members quickly mapped out a plan for the next 15 months. As NCDA founding

Chair Ann Keeling has noted, "we asked for a Summit and thought it would take 5 years to come about; instead it happened in 15 months." With no time to lose, the Alliance launched a business plan to secure funding to hire a small team in Geneva and to carry out key campaign activities leading up to the Summit. At the Clinton Global Imitative meeting in September in New York, Medtronic Foundation announced a $1 million grant to the Alliance for activities leading up to the Summit, and a Partners group was also launched, comprising the larger members of the federations, such as Livestrong and American Heart Association, as well as stakeholders including FCA and the Global Health Council. The Alliance launched an advocacy mechanism of core targets and common messages to members of the federations, as well as political mapping to identify priority states and staffing in New York (including in kind support from the American Cancer Society) to build relationships with UN Missions who would have eventual responsibility for drafting the outcomes document for the Summit, the vehicle for specific commitments by Member States. The Alliance also joined forces with the Lancet NCD Action Group to produce an advocacy and evidence piece in advance of the Moscow Ministerial meeting in April 2011, where health ministers from across the globe gathered in Moscow in what became an important gathering pre-Summit, at which the Moscow Ministerial Declaration on Healthy Lifestyles was produced. The joint Lancet-NCD Alliance document, Priority Actions for the NCD Crisis, was published online in April 2011 and in print in May, and served as an important tool in advocacy with UN Missions and through wide dissemination across membership. In addition, the NCD Alliance released its own Proposed Outcomes Document outlining 34 key asks across the disease groups and under the broad categories of leadership, support, prevention and care, among others (NCD Alliance 2012).

In June of 2011 the zero draft of the outcomes document was released, and the Alliance immediately mobilized its members to call on their ministers of foreign affairs and ministers of health to ask for specific language to be included. Led by longtime tobacco control advocate Judith Watt, language was successfully advocated.

More notable, while the UN had expected the process of approving the zero draft to take a week or so, strong language from G77 countries and the actions of civil society meant negotiations were drawn out over 6 weeks before being suspended for three and half weeks in early August. At that time the NCD Alliance made an extra push to draw attention to the outcomes document (by then referred to as the political declaration) and secured media coverage in the Financial Times, Economist, and other key outlets. It is believed that this media coverage helped to secure key language and the final document was approved on the first day of the HLM, September 19.

The role of NGOs outside of the NCD Alliance has a mixed history, with some striking successes including the important cost study produced by the World Economic Forum (http://www3.weforum.org/docs/WEF_Harvard_HE_Global EconomicBurdenNonCommunicableDiseases_2011.pdf) as well as challenges including the demise of the Global Health Council, the struggle to gain traction by organizations such as the Oxford Health Alliance, and the continued lack of clear models on engaging with the private sector, which has been a critical funder of NCD efforts to date. While the Clinton Global Initiative hosted a session on NCDs following the Summit and has been a core partner of the Global Smokefree Worksite Initiative, a concrete partnership to bring smokefree worksites to companies and governments across the globe, further engagement by NGO coalitions has been fairly limited. Among WHO regions there have been notable successes in attempting to put NCD policy into practice, most recently with the launch of PAHO's partnership forum that brings together private sector, the public sector and NGOs around common NCD targets.

Recommendations for the Way Forward

The most pressing issues for the NGO movement including NCD Alliance will be ensuring that they are included in partnership mechanisms,

Table 27.1 Structures implementing paragraph 64

Type	Simple affiliation	Lead partner(s)	Secretariat	Joint venture
Key features	No formal structure Ideal for informal collaboration with limited and short term goals	One or several partners assume lead role Ideal for small number of partners	Quasi-formal alliance with secretariat, Board, and staff Centralized funding, focused on partner coordination	Separate entity with major financial resources and financing or implementation capacity Strong central authority over partners
Examples[a]	Uniting to Combat Neglected Tropical Diseases NCDNet	Pink Ribbon Red Ribbon Partnership Clinton Health Access Initiative	PMNCH Global Health Workforce Alliance Global Alliance for Clean Cookstoves Global Road Safety Partnership	GAVI STOP TB

[a]For illustrative purposes

finding common ground across sectors, and working in productive and ethical ways with both private sector and public sector stakeholders. On the issue of partnership, NCD Alliance has looked at the four broad organizational structures common to GSPs which Member States may consider in evaluating options for implementing paragraph 64 of the Political Declaration These range from loose affiliations with no formal structure, to large joint ventures. Table 27.1 outlines these structures.

Nongovernmental organizations in general and the NCD Alliance in particular can bring significant value to the set of actions that are now mandated through the UN Political Declaration, which has been described at WHO meetings as the "roadmap" for NCDs leading to 2025. The NCD Alliance represents the combined strength of apex NGOs, thousands of foundations, societies, and professional associations across the globe. These need to be part of any global action or coordinating mechanism for NCDs. NGOs can help implement the policy directions stated in the Political Declaration through creating awareness, garnering support, catalyzing action, helping with technical solutions, and assisting with monitoring and evaluation in an environment where accountability in the development domain is fast gaining traction. Policies, systems, and tools need to be created to harness the potential of NGOs.

References

Heartfile. (2003). *Memorandum of understanding—national action plan on NCDs*. Retrieved from http://www.heartfile.org/napmou.htm

Hulme, D. (2009). *The millennium development goals (MDGs): A short history of the world's biggest promise*. Manchester: University of Manchester.

NCD Alliance outcomes document. (2012). Retrieved August 6, from 2012 http://www.ncdalliance.org/proposed_outcomes_document

Nishtar, S. (2010). *National action plan for prevention and control of non-communicable diseases and health promotion in Pakistan*. Retrieved from http://www.heartfile.org/pdf/NAPmain.pdf

Nishtar, S., Bile, K. M., Ahmed, A., Faruqui, A. M. A., Mirza, Z., Shera, S., et al. (2006). Process, rationale, and interventions of Pakistan's national action plan on chronic diseases. *Preventing Chronic Disease, 3*(1), A14.

Nugent, R. (2012). *Where have all the donors gone? Scarce donor funding for non-communicable diseases*. Retrieved August 6, from 2012 http://www.cgdev.org/files/1424546_file_Nugent_Feigl_NCD_FINAL.pdf

World Diabetes Day. (2012). Retrieved August 6, 2012 from http://www.worlddiabetesfoundation.org/media%283892,1033%29/UNR_media_kit_0407.pdf

World Health Organization. (2010). *Global status report on non-communicable diseases*. Geneva: World Health Organization.

World Health Organization. (2012). EB130.R7: Prevention and control of non-communicable diseases: Follow-up to the high-level meeting of the United Nations General Assembly on the Prevention and Control of Non-Communicable Diseases, ninth meeting.

Developing Health Promotion Workforce Capacity for Addressing Non-communicable Diseases Globally

Margaret M. Barry, Barbara Battel-Kirk, and Colette Dempsey

Introduction

Developing workforce capacity to address non-communicable diseases (NCDs) is recognized universally as being a key strategy in tackling the burden of NCDs. A sufficient, well-distributed, adequately trained, organized and motivated health workforce is identified in the *Global Status Report on Noncommunicable Diseases* (WHO 2010a) as being at the core of an effective response to NCDs. The importance of a skilled workforce was also recognized in the World Health Organization report on implementation of the NCD global strategy (WHO 2008a, b) and the Institute of Medicine 2010 report on *Promoting Cardiovascular Health in the Developing World* (IOM 2010). The Political Declaration of the High-level Meeting of the General Assembly on the Prevention and Control of Non-communicable Diseases (United Nations 2011) underscored the scale of the NCD crisis and the urgent need for action. Addressing the health inequities that contribute to and result from the

M.M. Barry (✉) • C. Dempsey
Health Promotion Research Centre, National University of Ireland Galway, University Road, Galway, Ireland
e-mail: margaret.barry@nuigalway.ie; colette.dempsey@nuigalway.ie

B. Battel-Kirk
BBK Consultancy, 47 Triq Gheriexem, Rabat, RBT 1909, Malta
e-mail: bbkconsultancy@eircom.net

burden of NCDs calls for the building and strengthening of public health capacity, including effective intersectoral action on the social determinants of health, as emphasized in the Rio Political Declaration on Social Determinants of Health (WHO 2011a). Developing workforce capacity is, therefore, a central plank of effective action on the prevention and control of NCDs.

The argument for a health promotion approach to addressing NCDs globally has been well developed in other chapters in this book. Effectiveness in reducing the global burden of NCDs depends on a workforce that is equipped with the core skills to implement current health promotion knowledge, policies and practices, yet is flexible and adaptable to change (IUHPE 2011). In practical terms, there is a need to develop workforce capacity for sustainable, ethical, and effective health promotion action to target NCDs at all levels—globally, regionally, nationally, and locally.

The level of capacity and infrastructure to support health promotion action varies within and across countries. There is, however, a particular concern regarding insufficient capacity to meet NCD challenges in low and middle-income countries (LMICs). This includes health workforce and infrastructure capacity, as well as sustainable funding, for the implementation of policies and strategies that promote population health. Among the recommendations made by the IUHPE (2011) to the United Nations High Level Meeting on NCDs in September 2011, in their document

D.V. McQueen (ed.), *Global Handbook on Noncommunicable Diseases and Health Promotion*,
DOI 10.1007/978-1-4614-7594-1_28, © Springer Science+Business Media, LLC 2013

"Advocating for Health Promotion Approaches to Non-communicable Diseases" was the following:

- That the relevant workforce is equipped with the core health promotion competencies to implement current knowledge, policies and practices to contribute effectively in reducing the global burden of NCDs
- That the domains of core competency for health promotion should inform the supply of an expanded and skilled workforce of health promotion specialists (Allegrante et al. 2009)
- An explicit commitment to expanding the health promotion workforce
- A key role for the IUHPE in providing global leadership and advice in relation to assuring standards and quality for those who work in health promotion

This chapter explores health promotion workforce capacity development, with a particular emphasis on addressing NCDs. Findings from the literature are discussed, including a scoping study on health promotion capacity in LMICs, and a review of two major initiatives on developing competency frameworks for health promotion, which could form the basis for implementing effective action on NCDs globally. The case is made for urgent investment in health promotion workforce development as a key element of the infrastructure for the implementation of strategic action on NCDs and population health improvement.

Capacity Development for Health Promotion Action on NCDs

NCDs affect people of all ages, nationalities and class and constitute the major burden of illness and disability in almost all countries of the world (Daar et al. 2007). However, the distribution and impact of NCDs and their risk factors is highly inequitable and imposes a disproportionately large burden on LMICs. The poor are more likely to die prematurely from NCDs (WHO 2010a) and this contributes to the widening health gaps both between and within countries (WHO 2008b). Without targeted and sustained interventions, these health inequities are likely to widen causing

even greater social and economic consequences (WHO 2010a).

One of the key gaps in taking action on NCDS is the lack of capacity of health systems (WHO 2010a). While 92 % of countries have developed at least one policy, plan or strategy to address NCDs, many are not implemented or are of insufficient quality (WHO 2010a). The delivery of effective NCD interventions is determined largely by the capacity of health systems and this particularly affects LMICs. This can be supported by building the knowledge and skills for the implementation of effective, affordable and feasible interventions in the context of local settings (IOM 2010).

In order to develop workforce capacity for health promotion action on NCDs it is necessary to explore the nature of the capacity that is required, together with what is known of existing capacity, and the factors which impact upon it, including, education and training needs and other resources required. Planning for workforce development needs to be informed by the most effective capacity development strategies. Models of workforce development are required that are congruent with the concepts and principles of health promotion and that build on the current knowledge, theory and evidence base.

Capacity development in relation to Health Promotion has been defined as:

> "the development of knowledge, skills, commitment, structures, systems and leadership to enable effective Health Promotion. It involves actions to improve health at three levels: the advancement of knowledge and skills among practitioners; the expansion of support and infrastructure for Health Promotion in organizations; and the development of cohesiveness and partnerships for health in communities. (Smith et al. 2006, p. 2)."

While much of the literature focuses on capacity development as a component of health promotion action, there is a growing awareness of the need to examine and take action on the first two levels as described above, i.e., health promotion practice and infrastructure development.

Catford (2005) indicates that while the concept of capacity varies for different types of organizations or levels, at a national level it commonly concerns infrastructure components including policies, sustainable funding, surveillance systems, leadership, research and evaluation capability, a skilled workforce, and mechanisms for program delivery. Thus, in health promotion capacity development there is a need to consider these common elements but also to ensure that each situation or context is specifically considered:

> "One of the complexities of health promotion is that there is no single 'one size fits all' in terms of intervention design. Responses have to be tailored to the issue, context and resources available. (Catford 2005, p. 2)."

This focus on context is also related to the shift noted in the literature away from the concept of "capacity building" focusing on individualized technical training, to a more developmental approach reflected in the increasing use of the term "capacity development," which fits well with the concepts of Health Promotion. Lin et al. (2009) propose a framework for health promotion capacity development, which is composed of multiple elements including; system governance (mandate for health promotion, strategic vision and leadership, institutional links and relationships), systems inputs (workforce, financing and funding, program delivery system, health information system), policy environment (healthy public policy and plans, health sector policy and plans) system outputs (programs and services designed to improve population health).

Models of workforce development have been developed which range from comprehensive systems-based models to more individual/team based approaches (New South Wales Health Department 2001; Council for Social Services in New South Wales (NCOSS) 2007; Scottish Executive Publications 2005; Skinner et al. 2003; Skinner et al. 2005; New Zealand Ministry of Health 2002; Roche 2002). The need to focus beyond the current workforce and look towards the future was highlighted in a World Health Organization (WHO 2010b) publication which emphasizes that it is critical that future plans for health promotion workforce development include mechanisms for adjustment to ongoing changing circumstances.

Another important feature of successful capacity development discussed in the literature

is that it should focus not only on needs but also identify, and build on, existing assets and strengths (Sparks 2007; Catford 2005; Roche 2002). All of these considerations are relevant for health promotion workforce capacity development with regard to tackling NCDs globally. Implementing effective health promotion action across diverse contexts, systems and settings which are undergoing rapid change, requires a flexible workforce with the required skills to anticipate and adapt to changing circumstances and respond to new challenges.

Capacity development to support the implementation of policy and evidence-based practice is key to strategic action on NCDs. It is important to consider the infrastructure required to support the sustainable implementation of effective health promotion practices at a scale and scope that will make a critical difference for population health. While recognizing that there have been significant developments in health promotion policy and research over the last 30 years, the situation regarding practice development is less clear. Investment in the human and technical resources required for the implementation of health promotion policies and programs is very variable globally with significant gaps in implementation and the translation of evidence into practice.

Closing the implementation gap requires aligning capacity to the delivery of effective population-based interventions for NCD prevention and control. This means developing capacity at both an organizational level and at the level of individual practitioners in order to bring about systemic level change. Translating from research into effective policy and practice requires not only good quality scientific research evidence but also the skills of effective implementation. There is an emerging implementation science which examines the adoption, implementation and scaling up of evidence-based interventions (Fixsen et al. 2005; Greenhalgh et al. 2005). This research emphasizes the importance of addressing not only the *content* of interventions but also the *context* and the *competencies* for effective implementation across a range of diverse settings. The scaling up and adoption of effective health promotion interventions in the community is dependent on the quality of implementation when interventions are disseminated across diverse cultural and economic settings outside of the research context. This calls for a closer focus on the process of implementing interventions in complex naturalistic settings and identifying the factors and conditions which can facilitate high quality implementation.

Implementation involves working creatively with local resources, engaging participation, mobilizing support, and successfully negotiating the process of collaboration and partnership-building with different stakeholders. Developing sustainable NCD health promotion initiatives requires the ability to foster collaboration across sectors that will bring about system transformation for endurable change. The resources and skills required for effective implementation tend to be underestimated and the leadership required for effective translation of plans into action needs to permeate all the way from the level of macro policy to local implementation. Dedicated resources and capacities are required for the effective implementation of policy and practice. A skilled and trained workforce with the necessary competencies to work at the level of population groups, communities, and individuals is recognized as being critical to effective health promotion implementation. Partnerships and cross-sectoral strategies that call for high-level expertise are needed in order to engage and facilitate the participation of diverse sectors (WHO 2005a). Building the capacity of the workforce in developing and implementing NCD prevention and health promotion interventions is fundamental to mainstreaming and sustaining action in this area.

Successive World Health Organization (WHO 2000, 2005a, b, 2009) and IUHPE world conferences on health promotion (for example, IUHPE 2010, 2007a, 2004) have focused on capacity development. The WHO seventh Global Conference on Health Promotion in Nairobi, Kenya, (WHO 2009), explored how efforts to build leadership, secure sustainable financing, develop knowledge and skills for intersectoral collaboration and effective delivery could be expanded to achieve a critical mass of capacity for health promotion globally. International developments in identifying core competencies for health promotion (Allegrante et al. 2009; Barry et al. 2009)

can usefully inform frameworks for workforce competency development and training in NCD prevention and health promotion.

A major IUHPE global initiative, the Galway Consensus Conference Statement (Allegrante et al. 2009; Barry et al. 2009), for example, refers to the need to develop a competent health promotion workforce globally in order to achieve population health improvement. The understanding that health promotion policies and interventions are only effective when they are made relevant to the context in which they are to be applied (De Castro Freire et al. 2007; IUHPE 1999, 2007b, c) is fundamental to the need for a skilled workforce capable of contextualizing policies and translating evidence into effective actions tailored to the realities of specific population groups, settings, and communities (IUHPE 2007a). Lin and Fawkes (2005) point out that even with infrastructure in place (e.g., staff), the implementation of policy innovations can still fail at the point of program delivery when there is not adequate capacity (e.g., skills, resources) to adapt to new approaches for health promotion. The development of the health promotion workforce capacity is, therefore, critical to the effective implementation of global and national policies on NCDs

Reports and declarations on addressing NCDs (e.g., UN 2011) clearly identify barriers to effective action as including insufficient human resources and inadequate or nonexistent training. The WHO Global Forum (WHO 2011a) also commented on what was described as:

> The largely untapped potential for health care workers to engage in health promotion and disease prevention (WHO 2011a, p. 8).

There is also reference to the need for multi-skill capacity and to have health workers able to integrate beyond a simple "one-skill approach" (Global Health Workforce Alliance 2011). Health promotion incorporates much of the skills and capacities required. A side event at the first Global Forum on Noncommunicable Diseases was titled; "Addressing Noncommunicable Disease - It takes a workforce" (Global Health Workforce Alliance 2011) which, it could be argued, could be expanded into the more specific slogan of "it takes a health promotion workforce."

Defining the Health Promotion Workforce

Globally the health promotion workforce is diverse, covering a wide range of functions, roles, and levels of activity. In many countries there is a lack of clarity as to who constitutes the core health promotion workforce. Dedicated health promotion posts have not been established in many countries and, therefore, the parameters of health promotion as a specialized field of practice are not well defined. Promoting the health of populations through the combined actions of the Ottawa Charter (WHO 1986) and subsequent WHO declarations requires a particular combination of knowledge and skills to ensure quality health promotion practice. It is becoming increasingly clear that both generic and specialist skills are needed in the development and implementation of evidence informed policy and practice. The strategic leadership and specialist skills required for the effective translation of research into effective and sustainable health promotion practice requires at least two different levels of the workforce: dedicated health promotion specialists who facilitate and support the development of policy and practice across a range of settings; and the wider health promotion workforce drawn from across different sectors such as health, education, employment, community, and nongovernmental organizations. Continuing professional development and training in health promotion is required at both levels to enhance the quality of practice and to update the skill set required to work within complex and changing social and political contexts.

A trained and competent health promotion workforce with the required knowledge, skills, and abilities in implementing policy and current knowledge into effective action tailored to local needs and contexts, is a vital component of the capacity needed by countries to address the NCD challenge. A sufficient, well-trained and organized health workforce is identified as being at the core of an effective response to NCDs (WHO 2008a, b, 2010a; IOM 2010; UN 2011). Workforce development is critical to building capacity for the effective delivery of health promotion NCD strategies. The level of development of health promotion practice varies across countries as health promotion covers a wide range of activities spanning specialist functions in leadership and technical roles, through to health and community workers, researchers, and individuals from different professions whose work is based on a "health promotion" perspective (Santa-María Morales and Barry 2007). Notwithstanding the diversity of the health promotion workforce, there is a specific body of knowledge, skills, values, and principles, which informs and underpins health promotion and makes it a distinctive area of practice. Many countries, however, lack the resources and support needed to build capacity and develop health promotion training and professional practice.

The IOM report (2010), commenting on the capacity for promoting cardiovascular health in developing countries, highlighted a lack of focused leadership and collaboration, uncertainty regarding the effectiveness and feasibility of interventions in LMIC contexts, and the lack of financial, technical, human, and institutional resources. This report outlines a number of essential functions that are required to address global cardiovascular health, all of which apply to NCDs more generally, including:

- Advocacy and leadership
- Developing policies
- Program implementation
- Capacity building
- Research focusing on evaluating approaches in developing countries that are context specific and culturally relevant
- Ongoing monitoring and evaluation
- Funding

Looking at each of these functions in turn, their relevance for the health promotion workforce is apparent. The development of a competency approach to workforce development assists in clarifying the specific knowledge, skill and values that are needed for effective practice. Ensuring that health promotion practice is informed by an agreed and defined body of knowledge, values, and skills is critical to building a competent and well-prepared workforce capable of addressing NCDs at the national and local levels.

Health Promotion Capacity Development in LMICs

Despite existing models of what constitutes health promotion capacity, and the emphasis on the need for workforce development, a lack of such capacity in health promotion, especially in LMICs, is widely recognized (IUHPE 2007b, c; Sparks 2007). Building a competent health promotion workforce is one of the priorities identified by the IUHPE in the report *Shaping the Future of Health Promotion*: *Priorities for Action* (International Union for Health Promotion and Education (IUHPE) and Canadian Consortium for Health Promotion Research 2007b). This report states that workforce capacity and capability for health promotion is well developed in only a few countries, and under resourced or entirely lacking in many.

Sparks (2007), in a report for the IUHPE, identified the major issues related to capacity for health promotion in low-income countries as being a lack of:

- Professionals trained in Health Promotion due to a lack of political priority given to Health Promotion and of structures to provide ongoing capacity building.
- Sustainable resources for capacity building in Health Promotion including funding and of education and training.
- Access to relevant information, evidence and training in an appropriate language/cultural context.
- Sharing of information, experiences and skills due to language, financial, or geographical barriers, costs associated with travel, etc.
- Linkages across health systems and with other sectors, which results in Health Promotion not being seen as relevant to multiple government departments.

The strengths and assets available to support health promotion capacity development in low-income countries were also identified in this report as being:

- Community knowledge, tradition and culture.
- Eagerness to learn and to build capacity.
- Low-cost infrastructure which can lead to more sustainable Health Promotion capacity building outcomes.

- Political commitment, particularly in countries which have a political and values-based commitment to working in participatory ways.
- Existing workforce including NGO leaders, academics and health professionals.
- Existing training and education.
- Internet and global communication/networks.
- Civil society partnerships including community organizations and partnerships at multiple levels with NGOs, the private sector, local foundations, and charitable organizations.

In addition to identified gaps and assets, there is reference to a lack of clarity in relation to capacity development for health promotion globally. Barry (2008), for example, notes that there is no clear picture globally of the extent of progress made in developing and strengthening health promotion capacity, particularly in LMICs. Mittelmark et al. (2006) reported that health promotion capacity is largely underdeveloped and that there is rarely reference to overcapacity in the literature. Lin and Fawkes (2005), in a mapping exercise undertaken for the WHO Regional Office for the Western Pacific Region, concluded that there is a need for investment in capacity related to all domains, but particularly professional development with appropriate and stable financing to build a skilled health promotion workforce.

These reports beg the question as to what are the current levels of capacity in the health promotion workforce globally, and specifically in LMICs, to address NCDs and what capacity development is required to support effective health promotion action.

Scoping Study on Health Promotion Capacity in LMICs

In Spring 2010, a scoping study was undertaken by the IUHPE, which aimed to explore current capacity for health promotion and the priority education and training needs for capacity development in LMICs (Battel-Kirk and Barry 2011). The sample for this scoping study comprised all countries defined by the World Bank (2010) as having low, lower middle or upper middle economic income levels, which were grouped into the global regions as defined by the IUHPE.

The final number of countries included in the study was 107 as contacts in some countries proved inaccessible. The sampling frame was developed using the IUHPE global network and an online questionnaire was designed to gather information on health promotion capacity. Following piloting, the questionnaire was made available to respondents via the Survey Monkey online research tool. Despite email reminders and an extension of the deadline for returning the questionnaires, the final responses numbered 37 from 34 countries, resulting in a response rate of 35 %.

The study, although limited by a low response rate, provides some insight into the levels of capacity for health promotion in LMICs and the education and training needs across the IUHPE global regions. The findings from this study complement those from the WHO report on NCDs (WHO 2010a) in providing an overview of the current health promotion capacity in LMIC contexts.

With regard to the infrastructure for health promotion, the scoping study found that health promotion formed part of overall health policies for the majority of those responding to the study but that a small number of countries reported having no health promotion policy of any type. While the term "Health Promotion" was reported as being used most frequently for health improvement activities, the study respondents reported a lack of clarity about what was meant by "Health Promotion" in their country and confusion about the differences between health promotion, public health and health education. These findings, which are also reflected in other studies (Lin and Fawkes 2005), highlight the difficulties of attempting to embed the complex concept of health promotion within multilingual and multicultural country contexts, and the need for the development of a shared understanding of health promotion, its core concepts and principles, as a basis for workforce capacity development.

In relation to the health promotion workforce, a majority of those responding to the study reported that there was an identifiable health promotion unit or section within the Ministries of Health in their countries, however, just over half indicated the existence of dedicated posts/job descriptions with the explicit title "Health Promotion". A large majority of respondents (94 %) in the scoping study endorsed the need for a dedicated health promotion workforce with specialized training in their country. Respondents reported that without such a dedicated workforce the "wrong approaches" are used and policies are developed which are not based on the local realities, but rather try to impose international models irrespective of local 'fit'. Examples given by respondents include:

> "Local thinking is not used to address local health problems'. Anthropological and/or sociological understanding of health issues is not an established culture."

> "The complexities of Health Promotion are often being reduced to a simplistic approach mainly based on media campaigns with a tendency to ignore or resist the parts of Health Promotion which focus on participation and empowerment."

In relation to existing assets and strengths, respondents to the scoping study viewed the "strong leadership provided by key individuals and organizations," followed by "commitment of the existing workforce" as the most important existing strength or asset for capacity building for health promotion in their country.

Dedicated funding for health promotion from governmental sources was reported by two thirds of those responding to the scoping study, with most referring to low levels of sustained funding from this source. A significant majority (89 %) reported that funding for health promotion activities was also available from other sources, mainly major international donors. Few details were provided of the amount of funding available from donors, which was reported as being "variable or depended on specific projects," "small and non-sustained" and that "Health Promotion is not an explicit priority within this type of funding." Overall, funding for health promotion, irrespective of source, was described as small or limited, project specific and not sustained.

While the majority of respondents reported the existence of some form of health promotion education training in their countries, most (56 %) considered that what was available was not adequate to build and maintain capacity for health promotion. The health promotion education and training currently available, however, was considered to be relevant and culturally appropriate to their country context by 74 % of those responding to the scoping study. The strong support for a dedicated workforce must be considered in the context of the barriers to capacity development identified by respondents, including a lack of shared understanding regarding health promotion and clear job descriptions for health promotion practitioners. "Basic foundation courses in health promotion" and "Continuing Professional Development" were identified as the types of training and education most required, with health promotion practitioners as the key target group. Respondents also identified "developing competencies and professional standards" as being among the priorities for action by global organizations taking the lead on capacity development in health promotion.

A lack of academic leadership and qualified teachers was reported by respondents together with a general lack of funding for training and education. Future capacity development strategies will need to explore the most effective way to address the education and training needs in LMICs in order to develop and strengthen a skilled cadre of health promotion practitioners. "Supporting the establishment of regional and national level training and education networks/forums" was identified as a priority activity, which should be undertaken by the lead organizations in relation to health promotion capacity development at global level.

Implications for Health Promotion Capacity to Address NCDs in LMICs

The findings of the IUHPE scoping study, while clearly limited, do provide a "snap shot" of the current capacity for health promotion and the training and education needed for effective health promotion action on NCDs. There is, for example, clear indication of support for a dedicated workforce with specialized training, but also of limited and unsustained funding and the existence of few dedicated practitioners with health promotion in their job title or job description across many of the

LMICs surveyed. The importance of developing and disseminating agreed definitions and understandings of health promotion is indicated in order to ensure that all involved in workforce capacity development have a shared terminology, and understanding of the core concepts, values, principles and knowledge base that underpins a health promotion approach to NCDs.

These findings can be compared to those in the WHO report (2010a) where 80 % of countries were reported as having funding for NCD prevention and health promotion. However, one third of low-income countries reported having no funding whatsoever for NCD prevention and control in the WHO report (2010a), which would appear to concur with the findings from the scoping study. In the WHO report 2010a, government sources of funding were the most commonly reported (85 %) but again proportionately fewer low-income countries receive funding from government sources. Approximately 65 % of low-income countries reported receiving government revenues for NCDs, which is very similar to the 68 % identified in the scoping study as receiving funding for health promotion. International donors were also identified as important sources of NCD funding in the WHO (2010a) report. However, it was also noted that this was despite the generally limited funding provided to this area of work by international development agencies, a finding which reflects the comments of respondents to the scoping study.

The lack of sustained funding emerges as a recognized barrier to workforce capacity development in LMICs. In developing a strategic approach to supporting capacity development globally, the issue of sustainability—both of funding and of action—must be a key consideration. In relation to funding, and particularly nongovernmental funding, raising the profile of health promotion as a valid capacity development approach with the major global development agencies, which is not currently the case, is indicated in both the scoping study and WHO report (2010a).

Balancing the prioritization of communicable diseases against the prevention of NCDs and longer-term health improvement is a difficult trade-off when funding and resources are scarce. However, it is recognized that the combined efforts of population-wide health promotion, prevention and effective treatment is needed to achieve the greatest health gains. To achieve the goals of tackling NCDs, it is clear that population-wide approaches are needed in order to address the causes rather than the consequences of chronic diseases and to address the health equity gap (WHO 2008a, b, 2010a, 2011a, b). Investment in chronic disease prevention and health promotion is essential for many LMICs struggling to reduce poverty and improve health (WHO 2005a, b, 2011a, b). International aid in the form of health development assistance could be channeled to build institutional capacity to promote health and respond to the challenges posed by NCDs in LIMICs. A greater focus is needed on funds for prevention and promotion and actions tackling the social determinants of NCDs. The case for sustainable investment in health promotion is supported by the fact that health promotion contributes to the global development agenda.

Strategies for capacity development in health promotion should include advocacy for sustainable funding and the adoption of health promotion as a priority within major global capacity development organizations and funding bodies, not limited to those with a remit for health. NCDs belong to the development agenda and, therefore, health promotion action on NCDs also belongs to the development agenda. A report from the Commonwealth Secretariat (2011) supports this argument suggesting that a major objective should be raising the priority accorded to NCDs in development work at global and national levels including; working with countries in building and disseminating information about the special relationship between NCDs, poverty and development, and calling on global development initiatives and related investment decisions to take into account the prevention and control of NCDs. This argument is further developed by the Young Professionals Chronic Disease Network who proposed to the UN High Level Meeting in September 2011 that governments, civil society organizations, development agencies, and the global public health community at large should reframe NCDs as a barrier to development by explicitly including NCDs as a target for "technical assistance, capacity building,

program implementation, impact assessment of development projects, funding, and other activities," as recommended by the Institute of Medicine. They also stressed the need to expand the next round of development targets beyond MDG-specific targets to a combination of human and economic development goals that explicitly address primordial, primary, secondary, and tertiary prevention and the treatment of NCDs.

Health promotion strategies fit well with the development approaches proposed by these diverse organizations and no doubt many others. This would appear to reinforce the development style approach of building on local and contexualized action with support for local leadership from global and regional organizations rather than the more traditional "top down interventions." The empowering and participative approaches espoused by a health promotion approach are well matched to localized development informed by global strategies and initiatives.

The inclusion of health promotion as a development activity is reinforced by the IUHPE scoping study finding that "strengthening community development" was reported as the Ottawa Charter action area most frequently employed to implement health promotion in LMICs by the majority of respondents. In contrast, among the main barriers to capacity development identified in this study, were references to a continuing emphasis on the biomedical approach and "traditional" approaches to health promotion. The emphasis on strengthening community action appears to mirror the WHO (2010a) report findings that 90 % of countries reported the existence of partnerships or collaborations for implementing key NCD prevention activities and control, including collaboration among health-care teams, patients, and families. The skills and competencies required to develop and sustain such partnerships, which are core to health promotion practice, are key to effective and efficient action on NCDs.

In light of the need for effective and efficient interventions, it is interesting to note that the focus of health promotion activities in the countries responding to the scoping study was considered as not being appropriate for best practice by a small majority of respondents (51 %).

Evidence of the effectiveness of health promotion is of particular relevance at this time of economic scarcity and future strategies must build on existing evidence of good practice and include reference to developing and disseminating more evidence of effectiveness. The development of evidence-informed practice requires investment in the training and continuing development of a cadre of health promotion practitioners with the specialized knowledge and skills to support effective implementation in complex settings.

The need for an informed and strategic approach to the development of the health promotion workforce in LMICs is apparent. There are frameworks available to support a competency based approach to workforce development for health promotion, which provide the foundations for shared understandings on the core concepts and principles of health promotion and the development of quality assurance mechanisms for health promotion practice, education and training. Employing a consensus building approach, such frameworks could provide a practical, action-oriented basis for health promotion workforce capacity building.

Competency Development in Health Promotion

Identifying and agreeing the core competencies for health promotion practice, education, and training offers a means of developing a shared vision of what constitutes the specific knowledge and skills required for effective health promotion practice (Allegrante et al. 2009; Barry et al. 2009; Taub et al. 2009; Battel-Kirk et al. 2009; Shilton et al. 2008).

While definitions of competencies can vary, they generally describe a set of knowledge, skills, abilities and values, often referred to as "know how" and "show how" in the international literature. Based on international definitions and particularly the work of Shilton et al. (2001), health promotion competencies may be defined as: "a combination of the essential knowledge, skills and values necessary for the practice of health promotion" (Barry et al. 2012). Core competencies are

described as: "the minimum set of competencies that constitute a common baseline for all health promotion roles. They are what all health promotion practitioners are expected to be capable of doing to work efficiently, effectively and appropriately in the field" (Australian Health Promotion Association 2009).

Competencies that are specific to health promotion are based on the core concepts, principles and actions of health promotion as defined in the Ottawa Charter for Health Promotion (WHO 1986) and subsequent World Health Organization declarations (WHO 1988, 1991, 1997, 2000, 2005a, 2009). Health promotion competency development can play an important role in:

- Underpinning future developments in health promotion training and course development
- Informing continuing professional development
- Developing professional standards and accreditation systems to assure quality
- Consolidating health promotion as a specialized field of practice
- Ensuring accountability to the public for the standards of health promotion practice.

Health promotion core competencies provide a basis for ensuring that there are clearly agreed guidelines for the knowledge, skills, and values required to plan, implement, and evaluate health promotion actions efficiently, effectively, and appropriately. They provide a common language and foster shared understandings of health promotion core concepts and practices and thereby advance greater recognition of the value of adopting a health promotion approach to population health improvement.

Development of Global Health Promotion Competencies

There is an emerging international literature on the competencies required for health promotion practice (Dempsey et al. 2010). A number of countries have made significant progress in delineating competencies for health promotion (Battel-Kirk et al. 2009), including; Australia (AHPA 2009; James et al. 2007; Shilton et al. 2006, 2008; Howat et al. 2000), Canada

(Ghassemi 2009; Hyndman 2007; Moloughney 2006), New Zealand (New Zealand Health Promotion Forum 2000, 2004, 2011; McCracken and Rance 2000). Competencies have also been developed in a number of countries in Europe (Santa-María Morales and Barry 2007; De Castro Freire et al. 2007; Santa-María Morales et al. 2009), including the UK (PHRU 2008; Health Scotland 2003, 2005; Skills for Health 2004), the Netherlands and Estonia (Santa-María Morales et al. 2009). Significant developments have also taken place in the USA, which focus on health education (Gilmore et al. 2004, 2005), including the development of accreditation systems (AAHE, NCHEC and SOPHE 1999; NCHEC, SOPHE and AAHE 2006). In Europe, accreditation systems for health promotion have been developed in the UK, Estonia, and the Netherlands (Santa-María Morales et al. 2009) and at a pan-European level by the CompHP Project (Barry et al. 2012).

Building on these international developments, the 2008 Galway Consensus Conference (Barry et al. 2009; Allegrante et al. 2009), sought to promote international collaboration on the development of core competencies in health promotion and the strengthening of common approaches to capacity building and workforce development. Organized by the IUHPE in collaboration with the Society for Public Health (SOPHE), the US Centers for Disease Prevention and Control (CDC), and global experts, the Galway Conference (Allegrante et al. 2009) participants reached agreement on core values and principles and identified eight domains of core competency required for effective health promotion practice. The Galway Consensus Statement (GCS), which focused on the broad domains of core competency, was seminal in providing an overall framework for global developments. The eight core domains of competency included *catalyzing change*, *leadership*, *assessment*, *planning*, *implementation*, *evaluation*, *advocacy* and *partnerships* (Allegrante et al. 2009).

In 2009, the GSC together with eight commissioned background papers and five sets of commentaries from the field, was published in tandem issues of the IUHPE journal, Global Health Promotion (Vol. 16, No. 2, June 2009) and SOPHE's journal Health Education and Behavior (Vol. 36, No.3, June 2009). The commentaries incorporated international perspectives from Africa, Australia, Canada and Latin America. Following these publications a global consultation was undertaken in collaboration with the IUHPE Regional Vice Presidents and the WHO Regional Offices on the likely impact of the GCS on health promotion practice, education and workforce development in their regions. Responses were received from over 116 individuals and organizations from around the world. In general, the initiative was welcomed and was viewed as being supportive of national and regional developments. The feedback commented on the need for a greater focus on cultural appropriateness of the competency domains, and the inclusion of core values and ethical elements, communication, knowledge base, addressing health inequities, and making competency development part of a continuous development process rather than the imposition of rigid standards. The domains of core competency identified in the Galway Consensus Statement, combined with the feedback received to date, provides a useful framework to guide further developments in specific regions and countries.

The CompHP Project: Developing a Core Competency Framework for Health Promotion in Europe

Building on the Galway Consensus Statement, a pan-European initiative—the CompHP Project (Barry et al. 2012)—was established in 2009 for a three year period with funding from the Health Programme of the European Union. The Project aimed to develop competency-based standards and an accreditation system for health promotion practice, education and training in Europe. The CompHP Project adopted a consensus building approach and aimed to work in collaboration with practitioners, policymakers and education providers from across the geographical spread in Europe. Based on an extensive process of collaboration and consultation, the CompHP Project produced three Handbooks, which present the

Fig. 28.1 Core Competencies
Framework for Health Promotion

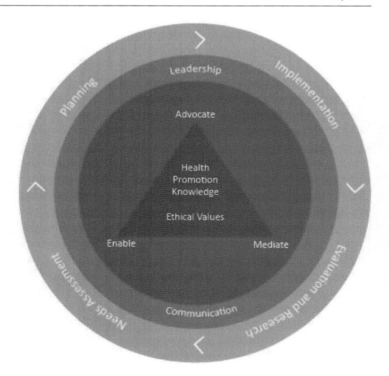

core competencies and professional standards required for ethical and effective health promotion practice and a competency-based accreditation framework to assure the quality of such practice (Barry et al. 2012).

The rationale for the CompHP Project lay in the fact that health promotion is an evolving field in Europe with a diverse and growing workforce drawn from a broad range of disciplines. Despite this diversity, however, it is recognized that there is a need to agree at a pan-European level on the specific body of skills, knowledge, and expertise that represents, and is distinctive to, health promotion practice (Barry 2008; Battel-Kirk et al. 2009). Operating across a variety of settings and a wide range of political, economic, and social contexts, the CompHP Project sought to unify and strengthen health promotion workforce capacity across Europe.

While job titles and academic course titles in different countries may not always include the term "health promotion," the CompHP Core Competencies are designed to be relevant to all practitioners whose main role reflects the definition and principles of health promotion as defined in the Ottawa Charter (WHO 1986). Whatever

their formal designation, the CompHP Core Competencies Framework emphasizes that health promotion practitioners require specific education and training together with ongoing professional development to maintain the particular combination of knowledge and skills required to ensure quality health promotion practice.

The CompHP Core Competencies Framework for Health Promotion (Dempsey et al. 2011) comprises 11 domains of core competency (Fig. 28.1). Ethical Values and the Health Promotion Knowledge base underpin all health promotion action detailed in the nine other domains. Ethical Values are integral to the practice of health promotion and inform the context within which all the other competencies are practiced. The Health Promotion Knowledge domain describes the core concepts and principles that make health promotion practice distinctive. The remaining nine domains are: Enable Change, Advocate for Health, Mediate through Partnership, Communication, Leadership, Assessment, Planning, Implementation, Evaluation and Research.

Each of these domains deals with a specific area of health promotion practice and their associated competency statements specifies the skills required for competent practice. It is the combined application of all the domains and the ethical values, which constitute the CompHP Core Competencies Framework for Health Promotion.

The CompHP Core Competencies Framework provides a common language and facilitates a shared understanding of what constitutes health promotion and its associated concepts and principles and provides clear guidelines for the knowledge, skills, and values necessary to practice effectively and ethically. While the CompHP Framework was designed as a pan-European framework, it could also provide a blueprint for global health promotion competency development.

Application of the Health Promotion Core Competencies to Action on NCDs

The CompHP Core Competencies Framework identifies a clear basis for developing the health promotion competencies required to address essential functions in tackling NCDs, through articulating the core knowledge, values, and skill base required for comprehensive and effective health promotion action.

Challenging the health inequities which contribute to and arise from the burden of NCDs calls for a rights and values-based approach to health promotion action, which is set out in the CompHP Core Competencies Framework. The Ethical Values domain articulates the health promotion principles of social justice and equity as being core to health promotion practice, and has as its foundation the understanding that "health is a human right which is central to human development." This domain outlines the individual competencies required by all practitioners to operate ethically in line with core health promotion principles, respecting the rights, worth and dignity of all, and all aspects of diversity. The competencies espouse a commitment to address health inequities and the prioritization of the needs of those experiencing poverty and social exclusion. The value base also emphasizes the need for health promotion action to address the political, economic, social, cultural, environmental, behavioral, and biological determinants of health and well-being. The Ethical Values domain provides a guide for all actions

which challenge health inequities and address the social determinants that underlie the burden of NCDs, especially in low-income countries.

CompHP Core Competencies Domain: Ethical Values Underpinning Health Promotion Core Competencies
Ethical values and principles for health promotion include a belief in equity and social justice, respect for the autonomy and choice of both individuals and groups, and collaborative and consultative ways of working.

Ethical health promotion practice is based on a commitment to:

- Health as a human right, which is central to human development
- Respect for the rights, dignity, confidentiality, and worth of individuals and groups
- Respect for all aspects of diversity including gender, sexual orientation, age, religion, disability, ethnicity, race, and cultural beliefs
- Addressing health inequities, social injustice, and prioritizing the needs of those experiencing poverty and social marginalization
- Addressing the political, economic, social, cultural, environmental, behavioral, and biological determinants of health and well-being
- Ensuring that health promotion action is beneficial and causes no harm
- Being honest about what health promotion is, and what it can and cannot achieve
- Seeking the best available information and evidence needed to implement effective policies and programs that influence health
- Collaboration and partnership as the basis for health promotion action
- The empowerment of individuals and groups to build autonomy and self respect as the basis for health promotion action
- Sustainable development and sustainable health promotion action
- Being accountable for the quality of one's own practice and taking responsibility for maintaining and improving knowledge and skills

In order to deliver effective health promotion interventions the workforce must be equipped with the necessary multidisciplinary knowledge base of health promotion core concepts, theory and research and their applications in practice. In the Knowledge domain, practitioners are called on to demonstrate an understanding of the broad determinants of health, and the current theories, models and evidence which underpin effective practice. The impact of social and cultural diversity on health and the implications for health promotion action is emphasized. The Knowledge domain requires practitioners to not only know what works in health promotion, but also to have an understanding of why and how to add to the existing knowledge base. In order to practice effectively, practitioners are expected to understand the systems, policies and legislation that impact on health. NCDs can be prevented and controlled using available knowledge (WHO 2005b) and the Knowledge domain provides practitioners with a sound theoretical foundation for health promotion action to tackle NCDs. In addition, the dissemination of this knowledge can be a critical component of capacity building (IOM 2010).

The three domains of Enable Change, Advocate for Health, and Mediate through Partnership reflect the

CompHP Core Competencies Domain: Knowledge Base Underpinning Health Promotion Core Competencies

The core competencies require that a health promotion practitioner draws on a multidisciplinary knowledge base of the core concepts, principles, theory and research of health promotion and its application in practice.

A health promotion practitioner is able to demonstrate knowledge of:

- The concepts, principles and ethical values of health promotion as defined by the Ottawa Charter for Health Promotion (WHO 1986) and subsequent charters and declarations

- The concepts of health equity, social justice, and health as a human right as the basis for health promotion action
- The determinants of health and their implications for health promotion action
- The impact of social and cultural diversity on health and health inequities and the implications for health promotion action
- Health promotion models and approaches which support empowerment, participation, partnership and equity as the basis for health promotion action
- The current theories and evidence which underpin effective leadership, advocacy and partnership building and their implication for health promotion action
- The current models and approaches of effective project and program management (including needs assessment, planning, implementation and evaluation) and their application to health promotion action
- The evidence base and research methods, including qualitative and quantitative methods, required to inform and evaluate health promotion action
- The communication processes and current information technology required for effective health promotion action
- The systems, policies and legislation which impact on health and their relevance for health promotion

three strategies of Advocate, Enable, and Mediate which are at the core of the Ottawa Charter (WHO 1986). Health promotion practitioners are encouraged to act as *advocates* ensuring that the conditions favorable to health are in place, as *enablers* to facilitate individuals, communities, and population groups to achieve their fullest health potential and overcome health inequities and as *mediators* to arbitrate between competing interests in society for the pursuit of health. These domains constitute the core health promotion strategies in addressing the political and economic challenges posed by NCDs globally. These domains outline the competencies that equip practitioners to: implement the actions needed to enable individuals, groups, communities, and organizations to build capacity to improve health and reduce health inequities; to advocate with, and on behalf of these individuals, groups, communities, and organizations to improve health and well-being; and to work collaboratively across disciplines, sectors, and partners to enhance the impact and sustainability of health promotion action. Taken together these domains support the development of effective action on NCDs, through enabling individuals, communities, and societies to be active participants in health promotion action.

CompHP Core Competencies Domain: Enable Change
Enable individuals, groups, communities, and organizations to build capacity for health promotion action to improve health and reduce health inequities.

A health promotion practitioner is able to:

1. Work collaboratively across sectors to influence the development of public policies which impact positively on health and reduce health inequities
2. Use health promotion approaches which support empowerment, participation, partnership and equity to create environments and settings which promote health
3. Use community development approaches to strengthen community participation and ownership and build capacity for health promotion action
4. Facilitate the development of personal skills that will maintain and improve health
5. Work in collaboration with key stakeholders to reorient health and other services to promote health and reduce health inequities

While there have been increasing international advocacy efforts to raise awareness of NCDs, including in LMICs (WHO 2008a, b, 2011a, b; IMO 2010), the challenge remains that of convincing

CompHP Core Competencies Domain: Advocate for Health
Advocate with, and on behalf, of individuals, communities, and organizations to improve health and well-being and build capacity for health promotion action.

A health promotion practitioner is able to:

1. Use advocacy strategies and techniques which reflect health promotion principles
2. Engage with and influence key stakeholders to develop and sustain health promotion action
3. Raise awareness of and influence public opinion on health issues
4. Advocate across sectors for the development of policies, guidelines and procedures across all sectors which impact positively on health and reduce health inequities
5. Facilitate communities and groups to articulate their needs and advocate for the resources and capacities required for health promotion action

CompHP Core Competencies Domain: Mediate Through Partnership
Work collaboratively across disciplines, sectors, and partners to enhance the impact and sustainability of health promotion action.

A health promotion practitioner is able to:

1. Engage partners from different sectors to actively contribute to health promotion action
2. Facilitate effective partnership working which reflects health promotion values and principles
3. Build successful partnership through collaborative working, mediating between different sectoral interests
4. Facilitate the development and sustainability of coalitions and networks for health promotion action

national governments and development assistance and donor agencies that investment in prevention and promotion strategies is critical to the effective implementation of a comprehensive approach to NCD control. Skills in using effective advocacy strategies to engage with, and influence, key stakeholders, including policy-makers, communities, individuals, and the non-health sector, is crucial in developing and sustaining health promotion action on NCDs. Health promotion advocacy efforts will need to be more targeted in order to ensure that effective health promotion strategies are integrated into existing health policies and programs and effectively communicated to the wider community of stakeholders and the general public.

Because the determinants of NCDs extend beyond the health sector, coordinated intersectoral policy approaches are required. The need for health promotion practitioners to have the required competencies to engage in effective partnerships through working collaboratively and mediating across sectors to influence the development of healthy public policies has been underscored in a number of NCD global reports and action plans. Likewise, the use of integrated health promotion approaches which create supportive environments for change, strengthening community action and facilitating the development of health lifestyles, personal skills, and the reorientation of health services are core to the health promotion essential function in addressing NCDs. All of these competencies and skills, underpinned by a core set of ethical values and multidisciplinary knowledge base, as outlined in the CompHP Core Competencies Framework, are needed to implement effective health promotion action (Barry et al. 2012).

Effective communication is essential to health promotion action on NCDs. The exchange of information can be used to inform, but also to influence, individual and community decisions that enhance health. The competenices outlined in the CompHP Communication domain provide a guide to the communication skills required by all health promotion practitioners. At the population level, health communication and education strategies are essential to effecting NCD-related behavior change. Public communication interventions that are coordinated with policy changes can enhance the effectiveness of both approaches.

The IOM report (2010) recommends maximizing communication and coordination among countries with similar resources and cultural conditions in order to help determine locally appropriate best practices, encourage innovation, and promote dissemination of knowledge in the battle against NCDs. Greater communication among stakeholders can avoid unnecessary duplication of efforts and facilitate the sharing of effective practice.

CompHP Core Competencies Domain: Communication

Communicate health promotion action effectively, using appropriate techniques and technologies for diverse audiences.

A health promotion practitioner is able to:

1. Use effective communication skills including written, verbal, nonverbal, and listening skills
2. Use information technology and other media to receive and disseminate health promotion information
3. Use culturally appropriate communication methods and techniques for specific groups and settings
4. Use interpersonal communication and groupwork skills to facilitate individuals, groups, communities, and organizations to improve health and reduce health inequities

CompHP Core Competencies Domain: Leadership

Contribute to the development of a shared vision and strategic direction for health promotion action.

A health promotion practitioner is able to:

1. Work with stakeholders to agree a shared vision and strategic direction for health promotion action
2. Use leadership skills which facilitate empowerment and participation (including team work, negotiation, motivation, conflict resolution, decision-making, facilitation and problem-solving)

3. Network with and motivate stakeholders in leading change to improve health and reduce inequities
4. Incorporate new knowledge to improve practice and respond to emerging challenges in health promotion
5. Contribute to mobilizing and managing resources for health promotion action
6. Contribute to team and organizational learning to advance health promotion action

Leadership at global and national level is recognized as being essential in addressing the NCD challenge (WHO 2008a, b; IMO 2010). Effective leadership involves working with others in creating an environment in which effective policies and practices can be developed and implemented (WHO 2010a). The CompHP Leadership domain outlines the skills and abilities needed to influence, motivate, and enable others to contribute towards leading change and mobilizing resources for effective health promotion action. This involves inspiring people to develop and achieve a shared vision and strategic direction for health promotion action. Building and supporting national level leadership is a vital part of strengthening country level capacity to respond to NCDs.

Engaging the local workforce to implement health promotion interventions and deliver health promotion services is fundamental to progressing action on population-wide interventions for NCDs. Progress is dependent on building the skills and competencies of local health promotion practitioners to plan, develop, manage, and maintain evidence-informed interventions in partnership with key stakeholders.

The CompHP Core Competencies domains of Needs Assessment, Planning, Implementation, Evaluation and Research support the need to improve the knowledge and skills for effective implementation. The Needs Assessment domain outlines for practitioners the competencies required to carry out a systematic assessment to determine the nature and extent of health needs and assets in a population, the underlying causes and factors influencing those needs, and the resources which are required to respond to them (Nutbeam 1998). The Planning domain outlines the development of measurable goals and objectives based on the needs assessment, while the Implementation domain guides the translation of plans into the delivery of effective actions that are culturally appropriate, empowering, and participatory. The Evaluation and Research domain addresses the competencies needed to measure the process, impact, and outcomes of interventions and demonstrate their effectiveness.

CompHP Core Competencies Domain: Assessment
Conduct assessment of needs and assets in partnership with stakeholders, in the context of the political, economic, social, cultural, environmental, behavioral, and biological determinants that promote or compromise health.

A health promotion practitioner is able to:
1. Use participatory methods to engage stakeholders in the assessment process
2. Use a variety of assessment methods including quantitative and qualitative research methods
3. Collect, review and appraise relevant data, information and literature to inform health promotion action
4. Identify the determinants of health which impact on health promotion action
5. Identify the health needs, existing assets and resources relevant to health promotion action
6. Use culturally and ethically appropriate assessment approaches
7. Identify priorities for health promotion action in partnership with stakeholders, based on best available evidence and ethical values

There is an urgent need for investment in the development and dissemination of health promotion evaluation and research processes in LMICs.

CompHP Core Competencies Domain: Planning

Develop measurable health promotion goals and objectives based on assessment of needs and assets in partnership with stakeholders.

A health promotion practitioner is able to:

1. Mobilize, support, and engage the participation of stakeholders in planning health promotion action
2. Use current models and systematic approaches for planning health promotion action
3. Develop a feasible action plan within resource constraints and with reference to existing needs and assets
4. Develop and communicate appropriate, realistic and measurable goals and objectives for health promotion action
5. Identify appropriate health promotion strategies to achieve agreed goals and objectives

CompHP Core Competencies Domain: Implementation

Implement effective and efficient, culturally sensitive, and ethical health promotion action in partnership with stakeholders.

A health promotion practitioner is able to:

1. Use ethical, empowering, culturally appropriate and participatory processes to implement health promotion action
2. Develop, pilot and use appropriate resources and materials
3. Manage the resources needed for effective implementation of planned action
4. Facilitate program sustainability and stakeholder ownership of health promotion action through ongoing consultation and collaboration
5. Monitor the quality of the implementation process in relation to agreed goals and objectives for health promotion action

CompHP Core Competencies Domain: Evaluation and Research

Use appropriate evaluation and research methods, in partnership with stakeholders, to determine the reach, impact and effectiveness of health promotion action.

A health promotion practitioner is able to:

1. Identify and use appropriate health promotion evaluation tools and research methods
2. Integrate evaluation into the planning and implementation of all health promotion action
3. Use evaluation findings to refine and improve health promotion action
4. Use research and evidence-based strategies to inform practice
5. Contribute to the development and dissemination of health promotion evaluation and research processes

Research capacity is essential to monitor NCDs and their determinants, in order to provide the foundation for advocacy, policy development and effective action. Further research is needed on what NCD intervention approaches are both feasible and effective within the low resource settings of LMICs. This includes developing research on adapting and translating what works to the realities of implementation in LMIC settings, and the development of innovative research approaches that are context specific and culturally relevant. While the strength of evidence on the effectiveness of interventions in low-income settings is variable, and absent in some cases, the adaptation of current knowledge, together with the development of the country-specific knowledge base, are crucial elements for effective capacity development. Many countries lack sufficient local data and research to inform local decision-making and the prioritization of action. The development of health promotion evaluation and research capacity, using methods adapted to the realities of LMIC settings, are critical to this process. In addition, integrating evaluation into the planning and implementation of all health promotion action means that the findings can be used to improve local knowledge and strengthen the practice base. Research should underpin all actions and is a critical element of the overall package of global NCD efforts. A systematic approach is needed to ensure that the development and dissemination of the knowledge and evidence base, which includes robust program evaluations and population surveillance at country level, is a core component of national health policy (IUHPE 2011).

Conclusions

Comprehensive and integrated action is needed to prevent and control noncommunicable diseases (WHO 2008a, b, 2011a, b). Building partnerships and successful collaborations with the key stakeholders across all sectors, including international agencies, NGOs, and academia is an essential part of the prevention and control of NCDs (WHO 2008a, b; IOM 2010). Improving country capacity has been identified as essential to tackling the global crisis presented by the rise in NCDs. Capacity needs to be developed and strengthened by improving the competencies of the local health promotion workforce and thereby increasing the capacity of countries to monitor, plan, and implement health promotion policies and programs to tackle NCDs.

A skilled health promotion workforce is vital to ensure that the recommendations and goals of global action strategies on NCDs are addressed. An adequate and appropriately trained workforce to implement and sustain innovative and effective health promotion intervention efforts is critical in reducing the burden of NCDs. The strengthening of the overall health promotion workforce, especially in LMICs, is needed to build capacity in the areas of NCD health promotion action, prevention, and related research. A workforce that is well equipped to address NCDs needs to include education and training in the broader systemic and social determinants of health together with the necessary knowledge, skills, and abilities to participate in the policy making process, implement effective interventions and develop and sustain partnerships across

sectors. Developing and strengthening the capacity for researching and implementing health promotion policies and practices in the field of global NCDs is a strategic investment to achieve global health and development.

The NCD policy agenda and advocacy efforts need to take urgent action on building workforce capacity and training health promotion practitioners and researchers in the field of NCDs, both in high and low-income countries. Having qualified human resources is essential to deliver quality health promotion actions, and this includes workforce education and training in the development and implementation of evidence-informed policy and practice. A competent and skilled workforce is a crucial element of building capacity for addressing NCDs in LMICs and closing the gap on the growing health inequities within and between countries. Strengthening workforce capacity involves addressing the provision of dedicated health promotion training, including basic courses, degree programs, and continuing professional development, together with the inclusion of health promotion in the curricula of health and other professionals. Gaps in the current curricula of health professional training with regard to NCDs need to be identified and closed. This action can then inform systematic plans to develop future health promotion leaders and a workforce that is better prepared with the competencies for effective action at a population level on NCDs (IOM 2010). The implementation of core competency frameworks for health promotion practice and education provide a useful tool for workforce capacity development in this field.

As explored in this chapter, health promotion capacity is underdeveloped in many countries around the world and there is an urgent need to invest in building, strengthening, and maintaining the health promotion workforce if population health goals in the area of NCDs are to be achieved. The negative impact of the economic downturn on the funding of public health policies, infrastructure and workforce development makes the case all the more urgent. This applies in relation to both high-income countries and in LMICs where investment in health promotion and prevention work has contracted severely due to health budget cuts. Further advocacy efforts are needed with governmental and nongovernmental agencies in order to underscore the importance of investing in the health promotion and public health workforce and strengthening their capacity for innovation and program implementation if progress is to be made in addressing NCDs and achieving population health improvement.

References

Allegrante, J. P., Barry, M. M., Airhihenbuwa, C. O., Auld, E., Collins, J. L., Lamarre, M. C., Magnusson, M., McQueen, D., & Mittlemark, M. (2009). Domains of core competency, standards, and quality assurance for building global capacity in health promotion: The Galway consensus conference statement. *Health Education and Behavior, 36*(3), 476–482. Retrieved April 2012, from http://heb.sagepub.com/content/36/3/476.full.pdf+html

American Association for Health Education, National Commission for Health Education Credentialing, Inc., & Society for Public Health Education (AAHE, NCHEC, and SOPHE). (1999). *A competency-based framework for graduate-level health educators.* Allentown PA: National Commission for Health Education Credentialing, Inc.

Australian Health Promotion Association. (2009). *Core competencies for health promotion practitioners.* Queensland, Australia: Australian Health Promotion Association. Retrieved April 2012, from http://www. healthpromotion.org.au/images/stories/pdf/core%20 competencies%20for%20hp%20practitioners.pdf

Barry, M. M. (2008). Capacity building for the future of health promotion. *Promotion and Education, 15*(4), 56–58.

Barry, M. M., Allegrante, J. P., Lamarre, M. C., Auld, M. E., & Taub, A. (2009). The Galway consensus conference: International collaboration on the development of core competencies for health promotion and health education. *Global Health Promotion, 16*(2), 05–11.

Barry, M.M., Battel-Kirk, B., Davison, H., Dempsey, C., Parish, R., Schipperen, M., Speller, V., Zanden, van der, G., Zilnyk, A., and the CompHP Project Partners (2012). *The CompHP Project Handbooks.* Paris: International Union for Health Promotion and Education (IUHPE). Retrieved May 2013, from http:// www.iuhpe.org/uploaded/CompHP/CompHP_ Project_Handbooks.pdf

Battel-Kirk, B., & Barry, M. M. (2011). *Health promotion workforce capacity and education and training needs in low and middle income countries,* Paris: International Union for Health Promotion and Education (IUHPE). Retrieved April 2012, from http://www.iuhpe.org/uploaded/Publications/Books_ Reports/RRS/RSS_1-2011.pdf

Battel-Kirk, B., Barry, M. M., Taub, A., & Lysoby, L. (2009). A review of the international literature on health promotion competencies: Identifying frameworks and core competencies. *Global Health Promotion, 16*(2), 12–20. Retrieved April 2012, from http://ped.sagepub.com/content/16/2/12.full.pdf+html

Catford, J. (2005). The Bangkok conference: Steering countries to build national capacity for health promotion. *Health Promotion International, 20*(1), 1–6. Retrieved April 2012, from http://www.bvsde.paho.org/bvsacd/cd41/bangkok.pdf

Commonwealth Secretariat. (2011). *Progress report: Commonwealth secretariat road map on non-communicable diseases.* London: Commonwealth Secretariat. Retrieved April 2012, from http://www.thecommonwealth.org/files/236498/FileName/HMM(G)(11)4Update_on_Commonwealth_Road_Map.pdf

Council for Social Services in New South Wales. (NCOSS). (2007). *Models of workforce development,* Australia: NCOSS. Retrieved April 2012, from http://www.ncoss.org.au/projects/workforce/workforce-development-models.pdf

Daar, A. S., Singer, P. A., Persad, D. L., Pramming, S. K., Matthews, D. R., Beaglehole, R., et al. (2007). Grand challenges in chronic non-communicable diseases. *Nature, 450*(22), 494–496.

De Castro Freire, S. B., Costongs, C., & Hagard, S. (2007). *Building the capacity for public health and health promotion in central and Eastern Europe.* Brussels: EuroHealthNet.

Dempsey, C., Barry, M. M., Battel-Kirk, B., & the CompHP Project Partners. (2010). *Developing competencies for health promotion – A literature review.* Paris: International Union for Health Promotion and Education (IUHPE). Retrieved April 2011, from http://www.iuhpe.org/uploaded/Activities/Cap_building/CompHP/CompHP_LiteratureReviewPart1.pdf, http://www.iuhpe.org/uploaded/CompHP/CompHPLiteratureReviewPartIIAppendices.pdf

Dempsey, C., Barry, M. M., Battel-Kirk, B., & the CompHP Project Partners. (2011). *Developing a European consensus on core competencies for health promotion.* Paris: International Union for Health Promotion and Education (IUHPE). Retrieved April 2012, from http://www.iuhpe.org/uploaded/European_Consensus_on_Core_Competencies_for_HP.pdf

Fixsen, D. L., Naoom, S. F., Blasé, K. A., Friedman, R. M., & Wallace, F. (2005). *Implementation research: A synthesis of the literature.* Tampa, FL: Louis de la Parte Florida Mental Health Institute, University of South Florida, The National Implementation Research Network.

Ghassemi, M. (2009). *Development of Pan-Canadian discipline-specific competencies for health promoters – Summary report consultation results,* Canada: Health

Promotion Ontario. Retrieved April 2012, from https:// www.cancercare.on.ca/escoop/includes/HPO competenciespaper_Apr07_finalg_pdf.pdf

Gilmore, G. D., Olsen, L. K., & Taub, A. (2004). *National health educator competencies update project, 1998–2004: Technical report*. Allentown, PA: American Association for Health Education (AAHE).

Gilmore, G. D., Olsen, L. K., Taub, A., & Connell, D. (2005). Overview of the national health educator competencies update project. 1998–2004. *Health Education & Behavior, 32*(6), 725–737.

Global Health Workforce Alliance. (2011). *Addressing noncommunicable diseases - It takes a workforce*! Summary of discussions at the side event at the first global forum on noncommunicable diseases, UN, New York, 19 September 2011. Retrieved April 2012, from http://www.who.int/workforcealliance/knowl-edge/resources/NCDevent_Sep2011_report.pdf

Greenhalgh, T., Robert, G., Bate, P., Kyrakidou, O., Macfarlane, F., & Peacock, R. (2005). *Diffusion of innovations in health service organisations: A systematic literature review*. Oxford: Blackwell.

Health Scotland (2003). *Competencies for the health promotion practitioners: Interim report*. Edinburgh: Health Scotland.

Health Scotland (2005). *Competencies for health promotion practitioners*. Edinburgh: Health Scotland. Retrieved May 2013, from http://www.healthscotland.com/uploads/documents/5128-CompHPP130206.pdf

Howat, P., Maycock, B., Jackson, L., Lower, T., Cross, D, Collins, J., et al. (2000). Development of competency based university health promotion courses. *Promotion and Education, 7*(1), 7–33.

Hyndman, B. (2007). *Towards the development of competencies for health promoters in Canada: A discussion paper*, Canada: Health Promotion Ontario. Retrieved April 2012, from http://hpo.squarespace.com/storage/HP%20competenciespaper%20Apr%2007.pdf

Hyndman, B. (2009). Toward the development of skills-based health promotion competencies: The Canadian experience. *Global Health Promotion, 16*(2), 51–55.

International Union for Health Promotion and Education. (2011). *Advocating for health promotion approaches to non-communicable diseases - Key messages from the international union for health promotion and education in the lead up to the united nations high level meeting on NCDs, New York, September 2011*. Paris: International Union for Health Promotion and Education (IUHPE). Retrieved April 2012, from http://www.iuhpe.org/uploaded/Activities/Advocacy/IUHPE%20Key%20Messages%20_LONG_WEB.pdf

International Union for Health Promotion and Education (IUHPE). (2010). *20th conference on health promotion and health education (2010). Health, equity and sustainable development*, 11–15 July 2010, Geneva, Switzerland.

International Union for Health Promotion and Education (IUHPE). (2007a). *19th world conference on health promotion and health education: Health promotion comes of age: Research, policy & practice for the 21st century*, 10–15 June 2007, Vancouver, Canada.

International Union Health Promotion and Education and Canadian Consortium for Health Promotion Research. (2007b). *Shaping the future of health promotion: Priorities for action*. Paris: International Union for Health Promotion and Education (IUHPE). Retrieved April 2012, from http://www.iuhpe.org/uploaded/About%20us/ Statements/SFHP_ENG.pdf

International Union for Health Promotion and Education (IUHPE). (2007c). *Strategic directions 2007–2013*. Paris: IUHPE (www.iuhpe.org).

International Union for Health Promotion and Education (IUHPE). (1999). *The evidence of health promotion effectiveness: Shaping public health in a New Europe*. A report for the European Commission, Paris: International Union for Health Promotion and Education (IUHPE). Retrieved April 2012, from http://www.iuhpe.org/uploaded/Publications/Books_Reports/EHP_part1.pdf

International Union for Health Promotion and Education (IUHPE). (2004). *18th world conference on health promotion and health education: Health 2004*. 26–30 April 2004, Melbourne, Australia.

Institute of Medicine (IOM). (2010). *Promoting cardiovascular health in the developing world: A critical challenge to achieve global health*, Washington, DC: The National Academies Press. Retrieved April 2012, from http://www.nap.edu/catalog.php?record_id=12815#toc

James, R., Howat, P., Shilton, T., Hutchins, C., Burke, L., & Woodman, R. (2007). *Core health promotion competencies for Australia*. Perth, Australia: The Centre for Behavioural Research in Cancer Control, Curtin University. Retrieved April 2012, from http://www.phaa.net.au/documents/healthpromo_core_hp_com-petencies_2007.pdf

Lin, V., Falkes, S., Lee, T., Engelhardt, K., & Mercado, S. (2009). *Building capacity for health promotion conference - A working document*, 7th Global Conference on Health Promotion, Promoting Health and Development - Closing the Implementation Gap, Nairobi, Kenya, 26–30th October 2009. Retrieved April 2012, from http://www.who.int/healthpromotion/conferences/7gchp/Track5_Inner.pdf

Lin, V., & Fawkes, S. (2005). *National health promotion capacity mapping in the Western Pacific Region, final report*. Prepared for World Health Organization, Regional Office for the Western Pacific. Australia, La Trobe University School of Public Health. Retrieved April 2012, from http://hpe4.anamai. moph.go.th/hpe/data/mission/WHOHealthPromotionCapacityMap-pingReportfinalAug05.pdf

McCracken, H., & Rance, H. (2000). Developing competencies for health promotion training in Aotearoa-New Zealand. *Promotion and Education, 7*(1), 40–43.

Mittelmark, M. B., Wise, M., Nam, E. W., Santos-Burgoa, C., Fosse, E., Saan, H., Hagard, S., & Tang, K. C. (2006) Mapping national capacity to engage in health promotion: Overview of issues and approaches.

Health Promotion International, 21(suppl. 1), 91–92. Retrieved April 2012, from http://heapro.oxfordjournals.org/content/21/suppl_1/91.short

Moloughney, B. (2006). *Development of a discipline-specific competency set for health promoters: Findings from a review of the literature.* Canada: Health Promotion Ontario. Retrieved April 2012, from http://hpo.squarespace.com/storage/lit%20review%20-%20health%20promoter%20competencies%20pdf%20-%20april%202006.pdf

National Commission for Health Education Credentialing, Inc., (NCHEC), Society for Public Health Education (SOPHE) & American Association for Health Education (AAHE). (2006). *A competency-based framework for health educators- 2006.* Whitehall, PA: National Commission for Health Education Credentialing, Inc.

New South Wales Health Department. (2001). A framework for building capacity to promote health. Sydney and New South Wales, Australia: Health Department. http://www0.health.nsw.gov.au/pubs/2001/pdf/framework_improve.pdf

New Zealand Health Promotion Forum. (2000). *Health promotion competencies for Aotearoa-New Zealand.* New Zealand: Health Promotion Forum. Retrieved April 2012, from http://www.hpforum.org.nz/resources/HPCompetenciesforAotearoaNZ.pdf

New Zealand Health Promotion Forum. (2004). *A review of the use and future of health promotion competencies for Aotearoa-New Zealand.* New Zealand: Health Promotion Forum. Retrieved April 2012, from http://www.hpforum.org.nz/resources/competenciesreportJan04.pdf

New Zealand Health Promotion Forum. (2011). *Health promotion competencies for Aotearoa-New Zealand.* Retrieved April 2012, from http://www.hpforum.org.nz/assets/files/Health%20Promotion%20Competencies%20%20Final.pdf

New Zealand Ministry of Health. (2002). Auckland, New Zealand: Mental health (alcohol and other drugs) workforce development. Retrieved August, 2010, from http://www.countiesmanukau.health.nz/funded-services/mental-health/Workforce-Development/Publications/MentalHealthWorkforceDevelopmentFramework2002.pdf\

Nutbeam, D. (1998). *Health Promotion Glossary.* Geneva: World Health Organization.

Public Health Research Unit (PHRU). (2008). *A career framework for public health.* London: PHRU. Retrieved April 2012, from http://www.sph.nhs.uk/sph-files/PHSkills-CareerFramework_Launchdoc_April08.pdf

Roche, A. M. (2002). Workforce development: Our national dilemma. In A. M. Roche, & J. McDonald (Eds.), *Catching clouds: Exploring diversity in workforce development for the alcohol and other drug field* (pp. 7–16). Adelaide, Australia: National Centre for Education and Training on Addiction (NCETA). Retrieved April 2012, from http://nceta.flinders.edu.au/files/9412/5548/1891/EN93.pdf

Santa-María Morales, A., & Barry, M. M. (2007). *A scoping study on training, accreditation and professional*

standards in health promotion. IUHPE/EURO Sub-Committee on Training and Accreditation in Europe. Paris: International for Health Promotion and Education (IUHPE). Research report series (Vol. II, p. 1). Retrieved April 2012, from http://www.iuhpe.org/upload/File/RRS_1_07.pdf

Santa-María Morales, A., Battel-Kirk, B., Barry, M. M., Bosker, L., Kasmel, A., & Griffiths, J. (2009). Perspectives on health promotion competencies and accreditation in Europe. *Global Health Promotion, 16*(2), 21–31. Retrieved April 2012, from http://ped.sagepub.com/content/16/2/21.full.pdf+html

Scottish Executive Publications. (2005). *The national strategy for the development of the social service workforce in Scotland: A plan for action 2005–2010.* Edinburgh, Scotland. Retrieved April 2012, from http://www.scotland.gov.uk/Resource/Doc/76169/0019065.pdf

Shilton, T., Howat, P., James, R., Burke, L., Hutchins, C., & Woodman, R. (2006). *Revision of health promotion competencies for Australia. Final report.* Perth, Australia: Western Australian Centre for Health Promotion Research, Curtin University.

Shilton, T., Howat, P., James, R., Hutchins, C., & Burke, L. (2008). Potential uses of health promotion competencies. *Health Promotion Journal of Australia, 19*(3), 184–188.

Shilton, T., Howat, P., James, R., & Lower, T. (2001). Health promotion development and health promotion workforce competency in Australia: An historical overview. *Health Promotion Journal of Australia, 12*(2), 117–123.

Skills for Health. (2004). *National occupational standards for public health guide.* Bristol: Skills for Health. http://www.wales.nhs.uk/sitesplus/documents/888/EnglishNOS.pdf

Skinner, N., Freeman, T., Shoobridge, J., & Roche, A. (2003). *Development issues for the alcohol and other drugs non-government sector: A literature review.* Australia: The National Research Centre on AOD Workforce Development (NCETA).

Skinner, N., Roche, A., O'Connor, J., Pollard, Y., & Todds, C. (2005). *Workforce development 'TIPS' (Theory Into Practice Strategies): A resource kit for the alcohol and other drugs field.* Australia: National Research Centre of Alcohol and Other Drugs (NCETA).

Smith, B.J., Kwok, C., & Nutbeam, D. (2006). WHO health promotion glossary: New terms. *Health Promotion International, 21*(4), 340–345. Retrieved April 2012, from http://heapro.oxfordjournals.org/content/21/4/340.full.pdf+html

Sparks, M. (2007). *Brief report of gaps and assets for capacity building in low-income countries.* Paris: International Union for Health Promotion and Education (IUHPE).

Taub, A., Allegrante, J. P., Barry, M. M., & Sakagami, K. (2009). Perspectives on terminology and conceptual and professional issues in health education and health promotion credentialing. *Health Education & Behavior, 36*(3), 439–450.

United Nations. (2011). *Political declaration of the high level meeting of the general assembly on the presevation and control of non communicable diseases*. New York, NY: United Nations. Retrieved April 2012, from http://www.un.org/ga/search/view_doc.asp?symbol=A/66/L.1

World Bank. (2010). *Classification of economic income*. Retrieved June 2010, from http://data.worldbank.org/about/country-classifications

World Health Organization. (1986). *The Ottawa charter for Health Promotion*. Geneva: World Health Organization. Retrieved April 2012, from http://www.who.int/healthpromotion/conferences/previous/ottawa/en/index.html

World Health Organization. (1988). *Adelaide Recommendations on Health Public Policy*. Geneva: World Health Organization. Retrieved April 2012, from http://www.who.int/healthpromotion/conferences/previous/adelaide/en/index.html

World Health Organization. (1991). *Sundsvall statement on supportive environments for health*. Geneva: World Health Organization. Retrieved April 2012, from http://www.who.int/healthpromotion/conferences/previous/sundsvall/en/

World Health Organization. (1997). *Jakarta declaration on leading health promotion into the 21st century*. Geneva: World Health Organization. Retrieved April 2012, from http://www.who.int/healthpromotion/conferences/previous/jakarta/en/index.html

World Health Organization. (2000). *Mexico statement on bridging the equity gap*. Geneva: World Health Organization. Retrieved April 2012, from http://www.who.int/healthpromotion/conferences/previous/mexico/en/index.html

World Health Organization. (2005a). *Sixth global conference on health promotion*: *Policy and partnership for action*: *Addressing the determinants of health*, Bangkok, Thailand, 7–11 August 2005. Retrieved June 2011, from http://www.who.int/healthpromotion/conferences/6gchp/en/index.html

World Health Organization. (2005b). *Preventing chronic diseases*: *A vital investment*. Geneva: World Health Organization. Retrieved March 2012, from http://www.who.int/chp/chronic_disease_report/en/

World Health Organization. (2008a). *Prevention and control of noncommunicable diseases*: *implementation of the global strategy*. *Report by the secretariat*. Geneva: World Health Organization. Retrieved February 2012, from http://www.who.int/nmh/media/Prevention_and_control_of_noncommunicable_diseases.pdf

World Health Organization. (2008b). *2008–2013 Action plan for the global strategy for the prevention and control of noncommunicable diseases*. Geneva: World Health Organization.

World Health Organization. (2009). *Seventh global conference on health promotion*: *Promoting health and development*: *Closing the implementation gap*, Nairobi, Kenya. 26–30th October 2009. Retrieved April 2012, from http://www.who.int/healthpromotion/conferences/7gchp/en/index.html

World Health Organization. (2010a). *Global status report on noncommunicable diseases*. Geneva: World Health Organization. Retrieved April 2012, from http://whqlibdoc.who.int/publications/2011/9789240686458_eng.pdf

World Health Organization. (2010b). *Models and tools for health workforce planning and projections. Human resources for health observer. Issue no 3*. Geneva: World Health Organization.

World Health Organization. (2011a). Addressing the challenge of noncommunicable diseases. WHO Global Forum 27th April 2011, Moscow, Russian Federation. Retrieved April 2012, from http://www.who.int/nmh/events/global_forum_ncd/forum_report.pdf

World Health Organization. (2011b). Rio political declaration on social determinants of health. World conference on social determinants of health, Rio de Janeiro, Brazil, 19–21 October, 2011. Retrieved July 2012, from http://www.who.int/sdhconference/declaration/en/

Young Professionals' Chronic Disease Network. (2011). *The YP—CDN manifesto on non communicable diseases*: *The social injustice issue of our generation*. YP-CDN. Retrieved April 2012, from http://ypchronic.org/sites/default/files/Youth_Manifesto_on_NCDs.pdf

Jürgen M. Pelikan, Christina Dietscher, and Hermann Schmied

Introduction: What Will This Contribution Focus on?

This chapter focuses on the role of health promotion in and by hospitals in addressing non-communicable diseases (NCDs). Today, the four main NCDs account for 36 million deaths worldwide, and according to WHO (2008), the majority of these deaths could be prevented by eliminating shared risk factors, mainly tobacco use, unhealthy diet, physical inactivity, and the harmful use of alcohol. In this respect, comprehensive strategies to tackle NCDs have been developed that include a combination of primary prevention interventions targeting whole populations (such as health campaigns, food and tobacco labeling, sodium reduction in food), improvements of early detection, and access to essential healthcare interventions for NCD patients (compare WHO 2000). The traditional role of hospitals in these strategies is the treatment of acute events or stages of diseases, but if applying concepts of health promotion, hospitals can, in addition, apply specific interventions to contribute to a better quality of life and improved prognosis of their patients (secondary prevention), and they

can contribute to primary prevention as well. Against this background, and in line with our specific expertise, we will focus on the contribution of hospitals in tackling NCDs by health promotion, and for this reason, we will concentrate on countries with a developed hospital sector, such as members of the OECD. For low- and middle-income countries it is unfeasible to invest in the development of an expensive tertiary care sector, although high-technology interventions would also be required for the treatment of acute events or advanced stages of NCDs. But there is consensus that "best buy" interventions within the healthcare system, for these countries, are programs for the early detection of NCDs, screening interventions, access to primary healthcare, and a better availability of essential drugs, such as aspirin, for the treatment of cardiovascular diseases (Samb et al. 2010, World Economic Forum and the Harvard School of Public Health 2011).

By addressing the intersecting sets or overlapping content areas which exist between NCDs, health promotion, and hospitals, we will (as illustrated in Fig. 29.1) argue that NCDs are, at least in the more developed countries which are marked by well-developed differentiated healthcare systems, and whose populations have a good life expectancy, the main cause for hospital treatment. We will demonstrate that approaches to addressing NCDs—especially with regard to primary and secondary prevention—greatly overlap with health promotion approaches and show that (health promoting) hospitals can have an important role in applying these health promotion

J.M. Pelikan (✉) • C. Dietscher • H. Schmied
Ludwig Boltzmann Institute Health Promotion Research, Health Promoting Hospitals, Untere Donaustraße 47/3, 1020 Vienna, Austria
e-mail: juergen.pelikan@lbihpr.lbg.ac.at;
christina.dietscher@lbihpr.lbg.ac.at;
hermann.schmied@lbihpr.lbg.ac.at

D.V. McQueen (ed.), *Global Handbook on Noncommunicable Diseases and Health Promotion*,
DOI 10.1007/978-1-4614-7594-1_29, © Springer Science+Business Media, LLC 2013

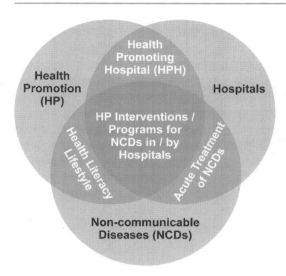

Fig. 29.1 Overlapping content areas of non-communicable diseases, health promotion, and hospitals

interventions to address NCDs in a systematic and comprehensive way. The application of such strategies can, not least, contribute also to better quality of care and better clinical outcomes.

An Introduction to NCDs

The traditional, historically developed definition of "NCDs" is that they are not caused by infection, and can therefore not be treated by antibiotic or antiviral medication. As this chapter is about the contribution of (hospital-based) health promotion in tackling NCDs, some comments need to be made to this definition from a health promotion perspective:

First of all, the term NCDs is often used as a synonym to chronic (curable as well as non-curable) diseases with a risk for lifelong progression and the need for repeated treatment over continued periods of time: "Chronic diseases include heart disease, stroke, cancer, chronic respiratory diseases and diabetes. There are many other chronic conditions and diseases that contribute significantly to the burden of disease on individuals, families, societies and countries. Examples include mental disorders, vision and hearing impairment, oral diseases, bone and joint disorders, and genetic

disorders" (WHO 2005). But infectious diseases too can become chronic in the sense of developing lifelong conditions with a risk for progression. Such diseases include, for example, HIV/AIDS and some cancers (one in five cancers is estimated to be due to infection, such as cervical cancer which is related to the human papilloma virus, or gastric cancer which is related to *Helicobacter pylori*). Non-communicable and infection-caused chronic diseases have in common that their prevention, cure, or the mitigation of progression strongly rely on the combination of the availability and quality of professional prevention and treatment strategies and on citizens' and patients' health literacy and ability for effective self-management (while the infectious ones require additional efforts to avoid transmission). Thus, the health promotion strategies we will introduce in this chapter are not limited to NCDs in the strict sense of the word, but more generally to chronic diseases.

The current discussion on NCDs has a strong focus on lifestyles, genetic predispositions, and external environmental factors, but hardly refers to the role of psychological factors in the etiology of some NCDs (e.g., via stress-induced changes in the hormonal status and a reduced capability of the immune system) which is however well researched and commonly accepted (e.g., Lugini and Pagani 2012). Furthermore, the role psychological concepts (such as Bandura's self-efficacy, Ajzen's theory of planned behavior, Prochaska and DiClemente's transtheoretical model) may have in the prevention and treatment-of NCDs, is also underrepresented in the discussion. From a health promotion perspective, we will therefore argue to follow a comprehensive, somato-psycho-social concept of health in addressing, preventing, and treating NCDs.

Compared to other types of diseases, NCDs are today considered as one of the most pressing challenges for public health and healthcare around the globe because of their high and rising prevalence, their life- and quality of life-threatening potential, and the economic loss they cause.

While NCDs, over the last decade, used to be discussed as mainly a problem of the high-income countries (labeled as "diseases of civilization"), current data clearly show that—not least because of the global trend towards urbanization and the globalization of Western lifestyles—the majority of NCDs, in age-standardized figures, occurs now in low- and middle-income countries (756 deaths in 100,000 males, and 565 in 100,000 females, which is 65 % higher for men and 85 % higher for women than in high-income countries) (WHO 2011). This amount has doubled since 1990 (compare Murray and Lopez 1997).

In comparison to other causes of death, NCDs account for 90 % of all deaths in high-income regions such as Australia, the European Union, or North America (not least due to the high life expectancy and the high degree of urbanization), while the relative risk of an NCD-related death is considerably lower in low-income and middle-income countries, as other common causes such as communicable diseases or childbed mortality are still considerably widespread. Furthermore, the risk to die from an NCD under the age of 60, which is only 13 % in high-income countries, rises to 41 % in low-income countries (WHO 2010).

Worldwide, NCD-related risk factors account for 48 % of healthy life years lost (DALYs). However, there are huge differences between regions of the world. While in low-income countries only 10 % of DALYS are related to these factors, the proportion rises to 30.6 % in middle-income countries and to even 42.4 % in high-income countries (WHO 2005).

By that, NCDs cause poverty for individuals and families and increase economic and social inequality. A loss of income due to NCDs can be a tragedy for a family, especially in low- and middle-income countries, but also often in vulnerable population groups in high-income countries. And NCDs cause enormous financial burdens for countries by high healthcare costs and absenteeism or decreased productivity in the workplace (Bloom et al. 2011).

While all parts of the globe are increasingly affected by NCDs, the priorities for action, and the available means to implement healthcare, public health and health promotion strategies differ with regard to regions of the world: High-income countries dispose of the well-developed healthcare systems needed for prevention, early detection, and high-quality continuous treatment of NCDs, including the application of health promotion strategies; lower- and low-income countries, however, still need to build up the healthcare infrastructure that is needed for the early detection and basic treatment of the population, for immunization, dealing with accidents and emergency situations, and safe pregnancy and birth. Thus, although NCDs are a problem of already high and still rising importance also in low-income countries too, our contribution on the role of health promotion in hospitals (and healthcare) in fighting NCDs will focus on high-income countries because these are the regions of the world where these strategies can be effectively applied, and add to the effectiveness of healthcare.

The etiology and treatment of NCDs share (in addition to individual factors like genetic predispositions) a few common aspects (which however also apply to some chronic communicable diseases) that make them (also) addressable by health promotion.

1. *Behavioral and lifestyle factors* are commonly understood as important risk factors for the development of many types of NCDs, including most cardiovascular diseases, some chronic lung diseases, some cancers, and type 2 diabetes. There is broad consensus that nutritional habits, physical inactivity, smoking, and alcohol consumption are the most important lifestyle factors with regard to their effects on the metabolic and physiological processes of relevance for NCDs, including effects on blood pressure (responsible for 12.8 % of deaths globally), blood glucose (5.8 % of deaths), overweight and obesity (4.8 % of deaths), and high cholesterol (4.5 % of deaths). Altogether, lifestyle-related effects account for 45.9 % of deaths worldwide, and even for 65.2 % of deaths in high-income countries (WHO 2009). Overall, lifestyle-related risk factors are highest in upper-middle-income countries which have the highest prevalence in smoking, overweight, and obesity, while their alcohol consumption comes second after high-income countries.

2. *Living environments* represent a second important risk factor for NCDs for at least two reasons: First of all, the risky lifestyles related to NCDs (especially fast-food consumption

and sedentary lifestyles) are most prevalent in high- and upper-middle-income urban areas, so the global trend towards urbanization will almost automatically lead to an increase in NCDs. Second, some NCDs, such as some lung diseases or cancers, are related to exposures to specific environmental pollutants which, too, are partly related to urbanization (such as fine particles caused by the continuous increase in traffic, industry, and domestic fuel) (WHO 2009).

3. The fact that lifestyles and living environments play such a big role in the etiology of NCDs naturally draws the discussion to the *socioeconomic determinants of health*, since socioeconomically disadvantaged groups of populations are usually less aware of and/or less empowered and able to live healthy lifestyles, and are also exposed to worse living and working environments, e.g., due to poor housing and more hazardous work conditions. In addition, risky lifestyles like smoking, alcohol, or unhealthy diets can, at least in part, be understood as problematic coping mechanisms of dealing with stress in the family, at work, or in societal settings.

4. While the three aspects outlined so far relate to the etiology of NCDs, the *availability and quality of healthcare* are of key importance for the adequate treatment and the quality of life of those already affected. While NCDs were, in the past, usually detected at relatively advanced stages, and were associated with almost unavoidable deterioration, with repeated severe crises and episodes that required frequent hospital treatment and often caused an early death, powerful drugs and treatment options (including preventive medicine and early detection), today, have transformed them into manageable conditions so that patients, if treated early and complying with or adhering to their treatment regimes, pursuing healthy lifestyles, and living in healthy environments, require less hospital care and can reach old age with a comparably good quality of life.

Thus, the healthcare sector and also hospitals, if committed to health promotion, can *effectively contribute not only to the curative* care of NCDs, but also to tackling behavioral and lifestyle factors, attitudes towards health and disease, living environments, and socioeconomic determinants of health, especially health literacy, relevant for NCDs.

What Is the Intersection or Overlapping Content Between NCDs and Health Promotion?

WHO's Ottawa Charter (1986) still provides a number of assumptions on health and health promotion that have proven to give sensible orientation for health policy and the development of healthcare settings over the last decades: "Health is created and lived by people within the settings of their everyday life" by "caring for oneself and others, by being able to take decisions and have control over one´s life circumstances." This, of course, holds true for healthy and less healthy, and even (chronically) ill, people, alike. "Health is a positive concept emphasizing social and personal resources, as well as physical capacities," and is, therefore, understood "as a resource for everyday life." Being defined as "complete physical, mental and social wellbeing" (WHO 1948), it represents a rather holistic—or comprehensive—concept. As such, health is determined by different social and environmental determinants; it can be endangered by many risk factors, but also strengthened by building up on, or developing, many kinds of personal or situational assets/resources. Therefore, "health promotion is the process of enabling people to increase control over, and to improve their health" (WHO 1986). This process is associated with seven guiding principles, i.e., it should be empowering, participatory, holistic, intersectoral, equitable, sustainable, and multi-strategical (Rootman et al. 2001:4). It can be related to three types of health promotion actions (advocate, enable, and mediate) in five action areas (WHO 1986). One of these action areas directly addresses people's personal health determinants (develop personal skills), aiming at improving what would, today, be called their health literacy. Four action areas relate to determinants in relevant environments of people. These are to "build healthy public policy," to "create supportive environments," to

Table 29.1 Four preconditions for general health behavior and disease-related self-care to be addressed by health promotion strategies

Impacting on general health behavior and disease-specific self-care by …		Addressing behavioral preconditions relating to …	
		Opportunity structures	Relevance structures
Addressing behavioral preconditions relating to …	Persons	*Enhancing knowledge* and *skills (health literacy) for …* • General health behavior • Patient behavior • Disease-specific self-care	*Addressing …* • Individual values, attitudes, and beliefs relating to personal selection of health-relevant options
	Situations	*Improving the availability of and access to relevant infrastructures*: • Patient information, education, and counseling • Health and social services to support self-care/self-management • Healthy goods (e.g., drugs, healthy nutrition) • Housing, sanitation	*Changing …* • Rules and regulations (e.g., smoking and food policies and legislation) and (financial) incentives/sanctions (e.g., by advocacy, lobbying) • Social values and norms (e.g., by campaigning)

Further developed from Pelikan and Halbmayer (1999), Pelikan (2007)

"strengthen community action," and, specifically for healthcare, to "reorient health services," although the Ottawa Charter is well aware that "health promotion goes beyond healthcare." The settings approach, which is understood as the most comprehensive health promotion approach, combines tackling the described personal and situational health determinants by "organizational change" as its preferred kind of intervention and by personnel development, teaching, and training interventions. The four resulting health promotion strategies are outlined in Table 29.1.

This scheme can be applied to different types of settings, including hospitals and health services, which are of specific importance for people suffering from chronic or non-communicable diseases. With regard to the prevention of NCDs (primary prevention), but also with regard to improving the self-care of those already affected (secondary prevention), hospitals can apply four different strategies:

• They can provide adequate patient information, education, and counseling that considers personal values and beliefs so as to enable informed, health-literate, and motivated citizens to adapt their health and disease behaviors for preventing, or living with, their NCD.
• They can aim at being easily accessible for diagnosis, treatment, and care, provide the necessary infrastructure to support the self-care of patients by education and training

(including also family members if needed), and support the health and well-being of their patients also via providing adequate settings (e.g., with regard to the nutrition offered and to tobacco-free environments).
• They can cooperate with communities with regard to the provision of healthy goods (drugs, nutrition) and environments (e.g., housing with adequate sanitation, clean drinking water).
• They can advocate for supportive legal regulations (such as smoking bans, food policies), societal values, and norms that support individual health behaviors and need to be addressed by lobbying and campaigning.

What Is the Intersection Between NCDs and Hospitals?

In this section, we address two questions—first of all, why hospitals should be considered as important partners in dealing with NCDs, and second, why NCDs are of high relevance to hospitals.

Why Are Hospitals Relevant for Dealing with NCDs?

Hospitals, today, can be understood as the *core organization of modern healthcare* systems in developed countries.

While their specific responsibilities for *patients'* *cure and care* may differ between countries with different healthcare systems (especially with regard to community outreach) or by type of owner, they usually deal with tertiary care which is often related to highly specialized and high-tech interventions (in contrast to basic or primary care, and partly also to specialized/secondary care). Thus, especially in cases of severe illness, such as severe NCD episodes, they can be life-saving for their patients, but depending on their understanding of the comprehensiveness of treatment, they can also contribute to primary and secondary prevention and strongly impact on their patients' quality of life.

Being the core organization of health systems, hospitals also have an important role in the *vocational training and further education of healthcare professionals*. Thus, they are highly relevant for shaping medical doctors', nurses', and therapists' perceptions of illness and health, diagnosis, treatment, and care. In light of NCDs, WHO-Euro (2012) explicitly calls for an inclusion of aspects of health promotion and disease prevention in the curricula of health professionals so as to become agents of change in "advertising" NCD risk reduction strategies.

Hospitals also engage in *clinical research*. By the research questions they pose, and by the research methodology they apply, they have a strong impact on the kind of knowledge and evidence that is produced as the basis for professional decisions by healthcare professionals around the globe. Although there is already a wealth of evidence on health promotion interventions in healthcare (compare, e.g., Tønnesen et al. 2005), further studies resulting in specific recommendations for specific clinical disciplines would be desirable to enable further change in clinical practice.

But hospitals are not only responsible for treating their patients. They also employ *a high number of staff*. Especially large hospitals usually have several thousand employees, and work in hospital settings is related with a number of occupational health hazards, such as night and shift work, continued high levels of stress, and exposure to biological, chemical, and nuclear substances, that are known risk factors for NCDs.

In addition to standard occupational health and safety measures, there are many examples from the international HPH network that demonstrate the feasibility of comprehensive health promotion and primary prevention strategies for hospital staff, including screening for early detection and tackling lifestyles—the latter being important also because hospital staff has to be considered as important role models for their patients.

The dealing with harmful substances makes hospitals an *environmental risk factor* also for the communities they serve if waste, wastewater, and emissions are not well managed (Weisz et al. 2011). Thus, by environmental management, and considering principles of sustainability, they can contribute to the primary prevention of NCDs in their communities.

And, last but not least, healthcare professionals, especially medical doctors, are often part of decision-making bodies—they can use their expert status for *advocacy*, e.g., for supportive legislation and for environmental changes. For example, the WHO European NCD strategy 2012–2016 refers to hospitals as strong partners in population-wide NCD strategies (World Health Organization—Regional Office for Europe 2012).

The aspects outlined above make hospitals highly relevant settings not only for the treatment and early detection of NCDs but also for the primary prevention of these.

Why Are NCDs Highly Relevant for Hospital Care?

As outlined, NCD patients, today, account for the majority of hospital patients in high-income countries. Demographic trends and prognoses with regard to lifestyle developments and environmental risk factors (including health impacts of climate change) make a further increase of NCD patients in the next decades most likely.

This situation represents a problem to modern high-tech medicine. In light of NCDs, the main merits of medical treatment for individual patients and population health alike do not lie in the application of high-tech interventions but widely in contributions to primary, secondary, and tertiary prevention, early detection, and the continuous support of patients with the aim to reduce the number and gravity of severe episodes, and to stabilize or even increase patients' quality of life for many years by improving their ability for self-care and for leading healthy lifestyles. This is why health promotion strategies are so relevant for NCDs.

In part, healthcare has already reacted to these demands, e.g., by the introduction of new medical specialties (such as allergology, pain management), specialized nurses (e.g., diabetes nurse, cancer nurse), the continuous expansion of rehabilitative care, and the implementation of case managers who support the continuity and effectiveness of treatment. Furthermore, disease-specific patient information, education, and training interventions can, in some cases (e.g., for diabetes, for chronic obstructive pulmonary disease (COPD)), already be considered as part of the routine treatment process. All these efforts add to the better support of patients and to better and more sustainable clinical outcomes and quality of life of patients.

However, hospitals see their NCD patients usually only during comparably short and severe episodes during which the available manpower and resources need to be concentrated on the necessary clinical interventions. Therefore, there is only limited time available for giving relevant information, education, and counseling, which is also very costly if provided by highly specialized clinical staff (so hospitals rather tend to prescribing related interventions offered by other providers). Still, as self-management and integrated and continuous care play such important roles in mitigating the progression of NCDs, best-quality medical and nursing care provided during acute or severe episodes, which are a necessary crisis intervention, are not sufficient to stop the progression of the disease or to enhance the quality of life of the patient. Further efforts in this respect are needed in light of epidemiological developments.

For this reason, with regard to effectively addressing NCDs, hospitals either need to further expand their services towards health promotion by including patient empowerment and contributing to better continuity of care or need to strengthen their cooperation with other providers following the same purpose.

We show in the next sections that health promotion can not only contribute to the (primary) prevention of NCDs but also to improving clinical outcomes and the quality of life of patients suffering from NCDs. For this reason, hospitals can and should take up health promotion not only in their daily business but also in their teaching/training and research.

How Has Health Promotion Been Integrated into the Hospital Setting by the HPH Movement?

When WHO, in 1986, launched its Ottawa Charter with the subtitle "Towards a new public health," health services were the only setting dedicated an own action area in the document because their role in improving public health was seen crucial. In the explanation of this action area, i.e., the "reorientation of health services," the Charter demands that the role of the health sector must move "beyond its responsibility for providing clinical and curative services. … This mandate should support the needs of individuals and communities for a healthier life, and open channels between the health sector and broader social, political, economic and physical environmental components."

In the late 1980s WHO-Euro initiated, based on this political statement, *concept* developments which soon focused on hospitals as the core organization of healthcare systems (Milz and Vang 1989, World Health Organization 1991). A first model hospital project in Vienna, Austria (Nowak et al. 1998), and a European pilot hospital project with 20 participating hospitals from 11 countries followed (Pelikan et al. 1998). The *projects* proved the feasibility of the HPH concept in different health systems and types of hospitals and led to the Vienna Recommendations (1997) as a framework orienting HPH networks and hospitals.

After establishing an international *network* of HPH already in 1990, WHO-Euro, in 1995, launched the policy of implementing national and regional networks of health promoting hospitals to further spread the concept (Pelikan et al. 2001).

Since 2005, the movement is being established also in other continents than Europe, and since 2007, it is open to other health services than hospitals. Since 2008, HPH is an international association according to Swiss law, linked to WHO by a memorandum of understanding (2011) and annual work plans. Today, the international network consists of approximately 1000 hospitals organized in 39 networks, including some individual members in areas without an established national/regional network, in five continents.

The conceptual basis of HPH has been formulated in 18 *HPH core strategies* (Pelikan et al. 2005, 2006) and 5 *standards for health promotion* (Groene 2006). The concept addresses health promotion for patients, staff, and inhabitants in the communities served by hospitals. For *patients*, it aims at improving the quality of routine care by taking patients' quality of life seriously and by making them good coproducers of their health, and by supplementary services which include information and education for disease management and lifestyle development, as well as interventions to improve the disease-specific living conditions in the community after discharge (e.g., the support of self-help groups, the availability of medical devices). For *staff*, the concept focuses on improving the working conditions and, again, on supplementary services in form of interventions to prevent, or cope with (occupational) disease, and to improve the living conditions for staff (e.g., by having a hospital kindergarten which is open around the clock). For *citizens* in the community, the concept is about adequate access to the hospital, and continuity and cooperation within the healthcare network (so as to allow integrated and continuous care), about expanding information and education offers to inhabitants, about making the hospital a healthy environment for its community (e.g., by minimizing waste and emissions, and energy consumption), and about contributions to health promoting community development (e.g., in the form of advocacy work).

For implementing the comprehensive concept, strategies and standards of HPH respectively for capacity building in hospitals (compare Pelikan et al. 2012; Dietscher 2012) seven additional implementation strategies (Pelikan et al. 2005)

and standard 1 (Groene 2006) were proposed. These connect HPH to organizational development and *quality management*. Following Donabedian's quality concept (Donabedian 1966), the desired health promotion outcomes— better health of patients and staff (and citizens)— are to be achieved by health promotion structures and processes which have to be defined, measured, and intervened following a quality cycle. A more complex model has been developed for purposes of *evaluation* and been used in the "Project on a Retrospective Internationally Comparative Evaluation Study of HPH" (PRICES-HPH) (Dietscher et al. 2011; Pelikan et al. 2011).

The *applicability* of health promotion strategies in a given hospital differs according to its type, its mission and role according to the function of hospitals in different healthcare systems (e.g., community strategies are more widespread in NHS systems), and the intentions of its owner. But, according to their scope, all hospitals do have some potential for applying at least parts of the concept. And, for strategies they cannot perform themselves, they can make referrals and build alliances or coalitions with other providers.

Dealing adequately with NCDs is not just part of the HPH concept, but member organizations of HPH are already widely active in addressing NCDs, as data from PRICES-HPH clearly demonstrate. The four major groups of NCDs—diabetes, chronic heart disease, cancer, and asthma—are also on top of the diseases addressed by 180 HPH member hospitals from 27 national/regional HPH networks that answered the questionnaire for the study (compare Fig. 29.2).

Data from PRICES-HPH also show that hospitals address numerous risk factors for NCDs by information, education, counseling, and training (compare Fig. 29.3). Of those lifestyles considered most relevant for NCDs, overweight/ obesity (85 %), tobacco (81 %), and nutrition (78 %) are most widely addressed, while physical inactivity (68 %) and alcohol (62 %) seem to be somewhat less on the agenda (compare Fig. 29.3).

PRICES-HPH also produced results showing that certain health promotion capacities of hospitals make a difference in successfully implementing

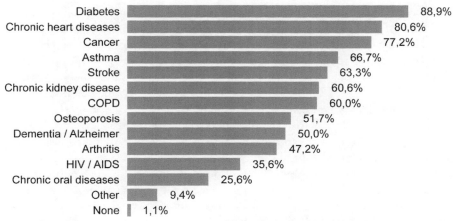

Source: "PRICES-HPH" study, n = 180 hospitals

Fig. 29.2 For which groups of chronic patients (and their relatives) does the hospital provide information, education, counseling, or training to improve patients' self-management of their condition?

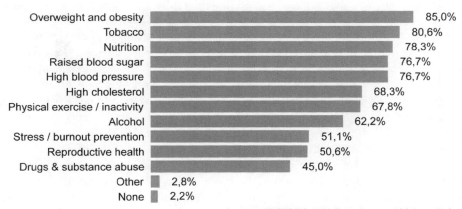

Source: "PRICES-HPH" study, n = 180 hospitals

Fig. 29.3 For which lifestyle issues or risk factors does the hospital provide information, education, counseling, or training offers for patients (and relatives)?

health promotion interventions. These hospital capacities can be effectively supported by HPH regional/national network strategies (Pelikan et al. 2012, Dietscher 2012).

Summing up, the HPH network has proven that hospitals can successfully move towards a more health promoting orientation and practice, including a better and more health promoting care and prevention of NCDs. Therefore, orientation at and capacity building for health promotion in hospitals is an important precondition for an improved, more systematic, comprehensive, and sustainable integration of single health promotion interventions for NCDs into the clinical routine of hospitals. Concrete examples are provided below.

Selected Examples for Addressing NCDs in Hospitals/Healthcare According to Health Promotion Principles

In this section, we provide concepts and selected examples for the two main approaches how hospitals can address NCDs in their patients, i.e., by expanding the scope of treatment and care by including secondary prevention of patients diagnosed with NCDs, and by supporting the primary prevention of these.

Addressing Specific NCDs by Health Promoting Secondary Prevention

From a health promotion perspective, a first expansion of "standard" treatment and care requires the provision of optimum living conditions for patients in the hospital (HPH core strategy 1—empowerment for health promoting living in the hospital, and a better integration of patients in treatment decisions and treatment by empowering them for coproduction in healthcare (HPH core strategy 2—empowerment for coproduction). These strategies can be strengthened by a supportive physical hospital setting, including the availability of adequate (privacy-ensuring) rooms for doctor–patient or nurse–patient communication (HPH core strategy 3—creating a health promoting hospital setting).

Furthermore, specific medical conditions will require specific healthcare and patient responses so as to mitigate progression, or even improve patients' the health and quality of life. In this respect, specific recommendations are available for all main groups of NCDs, i.e., heart diseases, metabolic syndrome and diabetes, respiratory disease, and cancer. We refer to some of these below.

In order to improve mid- and longer term clinical outcomes and quality of life, such strategies need, from a health promotion perspective, to also include the improvement of patients' health literacy and the empowerment of patients for adequate self-care; or, in more clinical terminology, patients need to be

supported in complying or adhering to their treatment and self-care regimes. Within the HPH concept, corresponding interventions relate to strategy PAT-4—empowerment for coping with specific diseases (also after discharge)—and to standards 2 and 3, "patient assessment" and "patient information and intervention" (compare Groene 2006).

In relation to NCDs, self-care, which can be defined as a naturalistic decision-making process that patients use (in real-world settings) in the choice of behaviors that maintain their physiological stability (symptom monitoring and treatment adherence), and the response to symptoms when they occur (Riegel et al. 2004). Selfcare includes different aspects of the patients' attitude and behavior, such as following the advice of providers to take medications, eat a specific diet, exercise, engage in preventive behaviors, actively monitor themselves for signs and symptoms, evaluate observed changes, decide to take action, implement a treatment strategy, and evaluate the response to the treatment implemented. Self-care is not synonymous with treatment adherence or compliance. Instead, treatment adherence is subsumed as one component of self-care (Riegel and Dickson 2008). Related interventions can, today, be widely regarded as elements of standard care for many chronic illness and NCDs.

However, the patients' ability for self-care may be challenged by a multitude of factors relating to the individual patients such as comorbid conditions that complicate medication taking, lifestyle adherence including diet, symptom monitoring, and decision making (Riegel and Carlson 2002), but also depression, anxiety, age-related issues, impaired cognition, sleep disturbance, or poor health literacy (Riegel & Carlson). In this respect, programs to support self-care need to consider the individual backgrounds and needs of the patients in order to be effective (e.g., by supporting the mental health of NCD patients, by using interpreting services for nonnative speakers, or by supporting the organization of social services or financial support for socioeconomically disadvantaged groups of patients). According to Bodenheimer et al. (2002), self-management education not only includes traditional patient education but also involves helping patients to set achievable goals and learn techniques of problem-solving that will improve their outcomes and quality of life. Furthermore, based on a literature review, Coulter and Ellins (2007) conclude that health literacy is central to better involving patients in their care so that they recommend that all strategies to strengthen patient engagement should aim to improve health literacy.

Hindering factors for effective self-care include also funding schemes (such as Medicare) that do not reimburse for patient education and counseling or for the coordination of care, inappropriate discharge management (e.g., lacking information on activity level, diet, discharge medications, follow-up appointment, weight monitoring, and what to do if symptoms worsen), and lacking time in clinical practice (Beasley et al. 2004). Therefore, it makes sense that HPH also takes an advocacy role for making health system conditions conducive to supporting the empowerment of patients for better self-care.

Furthermore, self-care after discharge may be hindered by the patients' living conditions in so far as these are of relevance to their health condition (e.g., quality of housing—compare HPH core strategy 6—creating health promoting living conditions in the community). The public health literature suggests numerous strategies for the improvement of housing conditions, e.g., in relation to asthma, and other respiratory diseases, injuries, and mental health that make it worthwhile for hospitals to engage in advocacy work for adequate housing conditions in the populations they serve (compare Krieger and Higgins 2002).

Addressing General Health and Primary Prevention of NCDs by Health Information, Education, and Counseling

As outlined, there is rich and strong evidence for the contributions of lifestyles to the genesis of many NCDs. For this reason, hospitals can become strong partners in the primary prevention of NCDs if they routinely screen for their patients' lifestyle habits and related risk factors, and provide adequate follow-up intervention, as is for example intended by the UK initiative "Making every contact count" (Ion 2011). In the HPH concept, this type of intervention corresponds to principle HPH strategy 5 (empowering for lifestyle improvements; compare Pelikan et al. 2005, 2006) and to standards 2 and 3, "patient assessment" and "patient information and intervention" (compare Groene 2006). One example for the feasibility of this approach is the "Data model" that was developed in a multicenter study involving 11 clinical specialists from HPH member hospitals in different countries (Tønnesen et al. 2008). Based on a simple assessment tool, medical records were screened for lifestyle-related risk factors of patients. The conclusions from the study are that the basic registration of lifestyle factors for adult patients is possible and clinically relevant, and according to a study by Oppedal et al. (2010) that built up on the Data model, nearly all patients assessed in a Norwegian hospital had one or more health risk factors with the potential to aggravate clinical outcomes, so the authors identified a significant need, and potential, for health promoting interventions.

Another study, also from within the HPH network, shows that not only such interventions are desirable from a clinical perspective, but also patients would accept to be screened that way, and to receive targeted health education (specifically with regard to alcohol use, diet, physical activity, and weight), corresponding to their screening results (Haynes 2008). According to the study by Haynes, the majority of patients participating in the survey agreed that the hospital is a good place for patients to receive health education (87 %) and also that the hospital should provide patients with details of community organizations that provide health education (83 %), but only one-third of respondents reported actually having received health education while being in the hospital. So, for many patients, a teachable moment has been missed (compare McBride et al. 2003 for the concept of "teachable moment").

Selected examples for the feasibility and effectiveness of targeted primary prevention of NCDs by health information, education, and counseling include not least UNICEF's and WHO's well-established and well-researched baby-friendly hospital initiative that takes into account the strong evidence for the positive effects of breastfeeding on the health of mothers (reduced risks for ovarian and breast cancer) and children (e.g., reduced risk of childhood infections; reduced risks of becoming obese or of acquiring diabetes in later life) (UNICEF & WHO 2009). The initiative builds up on the hospital's important role in the initiation and maintenance of breastfeeding: Women who are informed about breastfeeding already during pregnancy (in outpatient clinics) and who receive specific support during and immediately after birth are much more likely to take up and maintain breastfeeding than those without this support (Merten et al. 2005; Renfrew et al. 2009). On the basis of the evidence, the provision of effective breastfeeding support to mothers should routinely be included in the quality criteria for maternity services.

Examples for other lifestyle interventions along the "SNAPW" (smoking, nutrition, alcohol, physical activity, and weight) spectrum range from brief interventions to specific targeted interventions in which the hospital cooperates with other healthcare providers in a concerted approach. Tønnesen et al. (2005) summarized specific recommendations for the hospital-based support of lifestyle changes that basically include six steps for each lifestyle. These are the identification of patients with problems in specific lifestyle areas, the documentation in patient records, the provision of oral and written information, specific targeted advice and recommendation, specific interventions, and an ensured follow-up (compare Table 29.2).

Research on the evidence usually covers only part of the range of possible interventions. For example, with regard to brief interventions, a review by the Cochrane drugs and alcohol group concludes that there are benefits of delivering brief interventions to heavy alcohol users admitted to general hospital wards in terms of reduction in alcohol consumption and death rates (McQueen et al. 2011). However, the literature suggests that in general moderate to high intensive interventions, involving group sessions over a prolonged period of time, are more likely to bring about desired lifestyle changes than

brief interventions alone. Therefore, a review on SNAPW interventions (which however had its main focus on primary healthcare) concludes that, since the necessary intensity of interventions usually cannot be provided in clinical practice, referral mechanisms to more intensive services need to be in place (Dennis et al. 2012). In this respect, health promotion in hospitals has been described as an interface to diverse actors in the healthcare field that need to systematically cooperate in bringing about desired lifestyle changes (Meyer et al. 2011). With regard to such targeted cooperation, collaboration between specialized (outpatient) hospital wards and community nurses has, e.g., proven effective in tackling obesity in children (compare Kolsgaard et al. 2011).

Although clinicians see the need for (Johansson et al. 2010), patients are in favor of and examples show the feasibility and effectiveness of addressing lifestyle changes in the hospital, the necessary services are currently often not provided because they are not covered by financing systems in healthcare, especially by DRG models. However, research shows that an inclusion of health promotion services in DRG models is feasible at least in principle. The DRG study by Tønnesen et al. (2007) suggested codes for health promotion services that proved to be applicable for international use.

Another hindering factor for routinely screening patients for lifestyle risks, and offering corresponding health promotion interventions, is the lacking qualification of staff. The initiative "Making every contact count" in Yorkshire and the Humber in the United Kingdom which aims at improving the public health impact of health services, therefore, starts off with a systematic training of healthcare staff in lifestyle monitoring and interventions, based on a prevention and lifestyle behavior change competence framework (NHS Yorkshire and the Humber 2011), as a first large-scale intervention.

Wider Health Promotion Strategies in the Primary Prevention of NCDs

Health behavior—as one important risk factor for acquiring NCDs—can, not least, be supported by healthcare staff acting as role models for

Table 29.2 Six steps to address lifestyles with health promotion (based on Tønnesen et al. 2005)

	Tobacco	Alcohol	Nutrition and weight	Physical activity
Identifying patients with …	… tobacco consumption	… harmful and dependent alcohol consumption according to ICD-10 criteria	• … undernutrition or a risk to become undernourished • Overweight	… a need for counseling on physical activity
Documenting …	… thorough tobacco history			
Providing oral and written information to patients on …	• Damaging effects • Health benefits of reduced consumption or cessation • Possibilities of assistance to stop or reduce consumption			
Giving advice and recommendations …	… with regard to cessation	… to stop or reduce consumption	… on diet and physical training	… on exercise in accordance with international guidelines
Offering specific interventions	• Establishing smoking cessation services • Integration of smoking cessation counseling as part of treatment	• For consumers with harmful intake: brief interventions • For consumers with dependent intake: referral so specific services	• Initiation of relevant nutrition treatment and continued observation of body weight and food intake throughout the patient's stay in hospital • Screening for diabetes and other complications • Systematic training programs for relevant patients	Systematic training programs for relevant patients (heart and lung patients, diabetes, surgery, psychiatry, overweight, and underweight)
Ensuring follow-up/ continuity of care		Secure follow-up in primary care	Communication of information on discharge (to own doctor, home care, general practitioner)	Follow-up and counseling in connection with subsequent contacts with the department

their patients. Thus, from a health promotion perspective, lifestyles need to be addressed not only in patients but also in staff.

Another main risk factor for NCDs is the exposure to environmental risks which play a role in hospital settings, too, as patients (and to some extent also inhabitants in the surrounding communities) may be exposed to threats like secondhand smoke, and unhealthy food or beverages in hospital canteens and vending machines. Hospitals should therefore eliminate or reduce these exposures on their own grounds (HPH core strategy 3—creating a health promoting hospital setting for patients). And they can further expand their positive health impact by the professional management of their hazardous (nuclear, chemical, and biological) wastes, wastewater, and emissions that can also be considered as risk factors for the development of some NCDs. In addition, health services can use their expert voice to advocate for health promoting community development or for changes in legislation (HPH core strategy 6—contributing to a healthy community) (e.g., with regard to vending regulations for tobacco and alcohol products, or food labeling).

Selected Studies on Effective Approaches to Tackle Specific NCDs

In the following, we summarize selected studies on effective approaches to tackle specific NCDs that are relevant for the different discussed HPH strategies and standards.

Health Promotion for Heart Patients

Ischemic heart disease is one of the biggest disease groups in the hospital sector and is the source of large, and ever-increasing, pressure of demand on the healthcare sector (Tønnesen et al. 2005). There is broad consensus that the risk to acquire a heart disease is related to four individual—and modifiable—factors. These include tobacco consumption, physical inactivity, an unhealthy diet, and psychosocial factors (Meyer et al. 2011).

According to European Action on Secondary and Primary Prevention by Intervention to Reduce Events (EUROASPIRE), a longitudinal study by the European Society of Cardiology with three surveys so far (1995/1996; 1999/2000; and 2006/2007) that monitored selected clinical indicators of heart patients, as well as selected lifestyles and their blood pressure management, there is a high prevalence of numerous modifiable cardiovascular risk factors in patients with manifest coronary heart disease, including high smoking and obesity rates, and poor self-management of blood pressure. The authors of the study conclude that there is a compelling need for more effective lifestyle management of patients with coronary heart disease, and demand more investments in prevention, since, according to the study, blood pressure management remained unchanged, and almost half of all patients remained above the recommended lipid targets, despite a substantial increase in antihypertensive and lipid-lowering drugs in the survey period (Kotseva et al. 2009).

There are several patient education models that might be promising in this respect. One such model is "heart schools" that teach patients the knowledge and skills they need for effective lifestyle changes. Such schools are, for example, widely offered by Swedish hospitals (Meyer et al. 2011). There is evidence that patients attending these schools are more likely to stop smoking than those that do not (Bellman et al. 2009). However, the heart schools have, so far, proven to be ineffective with regard to optimizing blood pressure, exercise behavior, cardiac symptoms, the quality of life of patients, or a reduction of readmission rates (ibid.). In contrast, a model described by Muñiz et al. (2010) that builds on the personal relation between the patient, his/her doctor, and next of kin showed effects also with regard to the reduction of the body mass index, and of waist circumference and cholesterol, as well as to an increase in physical activity: The intervention included a personalized interview at discharge with the patient and his/her next of kin, which resulted in a signed agreement regarding prevention procedures and therapeutic aims, and a follow-up interview with the patient 2 months after discharge in order to review the agreement, adapt treatment if needed, and reinforce the intervention. It seems that this kind of "witnessed commitment," as a result of coaching (and not educating) patients, increases chances to keep up the motivation for actual lifestyle changes. Amongst HPH member hospitals, heart conditions were, according to PRICES-HPH data, among the top NCDs addressed by patient education strategies, with 81 % of answering hospitals being active in that field.

Health Promotion for Patients with Diabetes

Studies estimate that there will be a 69 % increase in the number of adults with diabetes in developing countries and a 20 % increase in developed countries between 2010 and 2030 (Shaw et al. 2010). Effective strategies for primary and secondary prevention are therefore strongly needed.

Since the quality of life of patients with diabetes depends so strongly on their blood sugar level, which in turn is strongly dependent on the patients' self-management of their condition, diabetes is probably the one disease with the longest experiences, and best developed and best researched models in empowering patients for self-care: patient education with the aim to maintain near-normoglycemia and to avoid hypoglycemia, as well as complications such as ulcers, intraocular bleeding, or renal failure can today be considered as the norm in diabetes care. Therefore, there is a multitude of guidelines and recommendations available, including the guidelines by the International Diabetes Federation which is an umbrella organization of more than 200 national diabetes associations (International Diabetes Federation 2005). However, the effectiveness of such interventions is based on some preconditions: A systematic review by Loveman et al. (2008) concludes that education is most effective if delivered by a team of educators, with some degree of reinforcement of that education made at additional points of contact. They also state that there are some prerequisites to effective education, such as sufficient time and resources for the educators to fulfil the needs of any structured educational program, or a clear program at the outset. Because of the specialists and know-how available, hospitals are, in principle, well equipped to provide such diabetes education teams and structured educational programs, and as data from the PRICES-HPH study show, almost 90 % of the answering hospitals do provide such services.

Health Promotion for Patients with Respiratory Diseases

The two main respiratory diseases in the NCD group are asthma and COPD. Of the four main groups of NCDs, according to PRICES-HPH data, these two were, with 66.7 % for asthma and 60 % for COPD, least often, but still by a majority of HPH hospitals, addressed with patient education strategies.

With regard to *asthma*, data suggest that at least in the developed countries a peak has been reached with regard to mortality. However, asthma remains a major public health concern (American Lung Association 2011a). Health education interventions to tackling asthma are well researched, and there is evidence that they are effective with regard to reducing hospital

admissions, night attacks, and emergency ward visits, as well as the quality of life, the functional capacity, and workability of patients (compare Tønnesen et al. 2005).

The *COPD*-related mortality, on the other hand, is still increasing. For the USA, data suggest that COPD has moved from the fourth leading cause of death to the third (American Lung Association 2011b). As COPD is an age-related disease, Mannino and Buist (2007) conclude that, as a result of global demographic trends, a rise in COPD can be expected even if every smoker on the planet were to stop today.

Against this background, a multitude of strategies and guidelines for the prevention, treatment, and mitigation of COPD have been developed by medical societies (e.g., Qaseem et al. 2011 in cooperation with the American College of Physicians, the American College of Chest Physicians, the American Thoracic Society, the European Respiratory Society), public health and health planning institutes (e.g., NICE Clinical Guidelines, 2011), and international initiatives (e.g., Global Initiative for Chronic Obstructive Lung Disease— GOLD 2011).

From a health promotion perspective, the Western Australian *model of care for COPD* is an example of specific interest. It represents a fundamental shift away from an acute focus to an integrated approach across the continuum of care. The aim is to develop optimal pathways of care and the management of long-term conditions through self-management, disease management, and case management. It comprises five standards that include COPD prevention, early diagnosis, management of stable COPD, treatment and support during acute exacerbations, and care and support at the end of life. In this model, patient education and peer-led interventions play an important role especially with regard to managing stable COPD. They were found to reduce bed demand and the frequency of hospitalization for COPD patients, and there is also evidence from other studies that patient education and increased self-care in COPD have positive effects with regard to reductions in the utilization of healthcare services and improved health status (compare, e.g., Bourbeau et al. 2003, Moullec et al. 2012).

The Western Australian strategy also considers that many people with COPD also have other conditions (co-morbidities), and therefore demands the implementation of *integrated programs to meet the complex needs of these people*.

Since environmental factors (such as exposure to fine dust, secondhand smoking, and other environmental pollutants) have a strong role in the etiology of both asthma and COPD, hospitals should, from a health promotion perspective, in addition to diagnosis, treatment, and care, and the provision or the prescription of professional patient education, also engage in advocacy work for creating healthy environments, and in reducing their own admissions as one strategy towards more sustainable health services.

Health Promotion for Patients with Cancer

Cancers occur in many different forms and require many different treatment strategies. However, they have in common that patients diagnosed with cancer are usually confronted with the probability to die, and with the need for fundamental changes of their lives, which is related to a high level of mental strain. Therefore, in consideration of the somato-psycho-social concept of health on which health promotion is based, strategies to support cancer patients should include psychosocial support and counseling. Furthermore, since the survival of cancer patients depends not least on adequate and sufficient nutrition, there should be support and clinical standards in that direction too. And there is increasing evidence that physical activity supports the mental well-being and overall quality of life of cancer patients (compare Tønnesen et al. 2005). (Health promoting) Hospitals, therefore, should include psychological services for cancer patients, and they can initiate or support rehabilitation groups for patients recovering from cancer. According to PRICES-HPH data, 77.2 % of the HPH hospitals do provide support for cancer patients to improve self-care.

Discussion and Conclusions

Hospitals in OECD countries who deal with great number of NCD patients in acute episodes of their patient career can make relevant contributions to tackling NCDs by integrating health promotion measures into their everyday routines. Thereby, they can not only improve the clinical outcomes, health literacy, self-care resources, and quality of life for their NCD patients but also contribute to the primary prevention of NCDs. Most of the possible health promotion measures make sense from a clinical quality perspective, but have effects which are of interest also from the perspective of population and public health.

Hospitals can integrate health promotion measures for NCDs much better and more systematically and sustainably if they follow a general and comprehensive HPH approach by reorienting their services and settings in line with health promotion principles and by building specific health promotion capacities to support the implementation and application of specific health promotion measures in their everyday work. And, in line with the Ottawa Charter, clinical experts and hospital organizations can use their standing for advocacy work to support the change of health systems in more educative, preventive, and promotive directions, which are relevant preconditions for better treating NCD patients.

But since NCDs create longer lasting patient careers with different needs for services in and outside the hospital, more complex approaches are needed. There is broad consensus that NCD strategies require concerted approaches, involving all sorts of actors within and partly also outside the healthcare system. Quite a number of more or less related and overlapping innovative models for improving care of chronic diseases have been suggested, discussed, and partly implemented in different countries (compare Singh and Ham 2006). The most widespread model is the "Chronic Care Model" (CCM). The aim of the CCM is to transform the daily care for patients with chronic illnesses from acute and reactive to proactive, planned, and population based (Wagner et al. 2001,

Coleman et al 2009). A meta-analysis of 112 CCM studies (Tsai et al. 2005) concludes that interventions based on the elements of the CCM are associated with improved outcomes and care processes for people with asthma, diabetes, heart failure, and depression. In 2002 WHO adapted this model to focus more on community and policy aspects of improving chronic care. The Innovative Care for Chronic Conditions Model (WHO 2002) focuses on improving care at three different levels: micro level (individual and family), meso level (healthcare organization and community), and macro level (policy) (Epping-Jordan et al. 2004).

Care and delivery models for chronic diseases use different labels, including managed care, integrated care, disease management, coordinated care, and case management, but determining which models are most successful is difficult because they are not based on agreed-upon definitions and because of their partly overlapping components (Battersby and The SA HealthPlus Team 2005).

There is quite some overlap between the components included in these models, but there are also differences with regard to the way health promotion is included, to the specific role of hospitals, and to the available practical experiences with actual implementation and evidence on outcomes. In any case, because of their health system embeddedness, the potential contributions of hospitals to tackling NCDs by health promotion measures depend only in part on how their owners, management, and professionals use the leeway they usually have for strategic decisions on the services they provide. To a large degree, their opportunities are determined by the local and national healthcare schemes they are a part of. Thus, the Ottawa Charter's principle of reorienting health services is still relevant and in need for implementation.

References

American Lung Association. (Ed.). (2011). *Trends in asthma morbidity and mortality. Chronic bronchitis and emphysema*. Retrieved September 12, 2012, from http://www.lung.org/finding-cures/our-research/trend-reports/asthma-trend-report.pdf

American Lung Association. (Ed.). (2011) *Trends in COPD (Chronic bronchitis and emphysema):*

Morbidity and mortality. Retrieved September 12, 2012, from http://www.lung.org/finding-cures/our-research/trend-reports/copd-trend-report.pdf

Battersby, M. W., & The SA HealthPlus Team. (2005). Health reform through coordinated care: SA HealthPlus. *BMJ, 330*, 662–666.

Beasley, J. W., Hankey, T. H., Erickson, R., Stange, K. C., Mundt, M., Elliott, M., et al. (2004). How many problems do family physicians manage at each encounter? A WReN study. *Annals of Family Medicine, 2*, 405–410.

Bellman, C., Hambraeus, K., Lindback, J., & Lindahl, B. (2009). Achievement of secondary preventive goals after acute myocardial infarction: A comparison between participants and nonparticipants in a routine patient education program in Sweden. *The Journal of Cardiovascular Nursing, 24*, 362–368.

Bloom, D. E., Cafiero, E. T., Jané-Llopis, E., Abrahams-Gessel, S., Bloom, L. R., Fathima, S., et al. (2011). *The global economic burden of noncommunicable diseases*. Geneva: World Economic Forum.

Bodenheimer, T., Lorig, K., Holman, H., & Grumbach, K. (2002). Patient self-management of chronic disease in primary care. *JAMA: The Journal of the American Medical Association, 288*(19), 2469–2475.

Bourbeau, J., Julien, M., Maltais, F., Rouleau, M., Beaupre, A., Begin, R., et al. (2003). Reduction of hospital utilization in patients with chronic obstructive pulmonary disease. A disease-specific self-management intervention. *Archives of Internal Medicine, 163*, 585–591.

Coleman, K., Austin, B. T., Brach, C., & Wagner, E. H. (2009). Evidence On The Chronic Care Model In The New Millennium. *Health Affairs, 28*(1), 75–85. doi:10.1377/hlthaff.28.1.75.

Coulter, A., & Ellins, J. (2007). Effectiveness of strategies for informing, educating, and involving patients. *BMJ, 335*, 24–27.

Dennis, S. M., Williams, A., Taggart, J., Newall, A., Wilson, E. D., Zwar, N., et al. (2012). Which providers can bridge the health literacy gap in lifestyle risk factor modification education: A systematic review and narrative synthesis. *BMC Family Practice, 13*, 44. doi:10.1186/1471-2296-13-44.

Dietscher, C. (2012). *Interorganizational networks in the settings approach of health promotion – The case of the International Network of Health Promoting Hospitals and Health Services (HPH)*. Dissertation, University of Vienna.

Dietscher, C., Schmied, H., Röthlin, F., & Pelikan, J. M. (2011). *Project on a retrospective, internationally comparative evaluation study of HPH (PRICES – HPH): Characteristics of national/regional networks of the International Network of Health Promoting Hospitals (HPH)*. The PRICES – HPH network survey. Report 1. LBIHPR Working Paper Series #11. Vienna: Ludwig Boltzmann Institute Health Promotion Research.

Donabedian, A. (1966). Evaluating the quality of medical care. *The Milbank Memorial Fund Quarterly, XLIV*(3), 166–206.

Epping-Jordan, J. E., Pruitt, S. D., Bengoa, R., & Wagner, E. H. (2004). Improving the quality of health care for chronic conditions. *Quality & Safety in Health Care, 13*(4), 299–305.

Global Initiative for Chronic Obstructive Lung Disease (GOLD). (2011). *From the global strategy for the diagnosis, management and prevention of COPD.* Retrieved September 12, 2012, from http://www.goldcopd.org/

Groene, O. (2006). *Implementing health promotion in hospitals: Manual and self assessment forms.* Copenhagen: World Health Organization – Regional Office for Europe.

Haynes, C. L. (2008). Health promotion services for lifestyle development within a UK hospital – Patients' experiences and views. *BMC Public Health, 8*, 284. doi:10.1186/1471-2458-8-284.

International Diabetes Federation. (2005). *Global guideline for type 2.* Brussels: International Diabetes Federation.

Ion, V. (2011). Making every contact count: A simple yet effective idea. *Perspectives in Public Health, 131*(2), 69–70.

Johansson, H., Weinehall, L., & Emmelin, M. (2010). If we only got a chance. Barriers to and possibilities for a more health-promoting health service. *Journal of Multidisciplinary Healthcare, 3*, 1–9.

Kolsgaard, M. L., Joner, G., Brunborg, C., Anderssen, S. A., Tonstad, S., & Andersen, L. F. (2011). Reduction in BMI z-score and improvement in cardiometabolic risk factors in obese children and adolescents. The Oslo adiposity intervention study - a hospital/public health nurse combined treatment. *BMC Pediatrics, 11*, 47. doi:10.1186/1471-2431-11-47.

Kotseva, K., Wood, D., De Backer, G., De Bacquer, D., Pyörälä, K., Keil, U., et al. (2009). Cardiovascular prevention guidelines in daily practice: A comparison of EUROASPIRE I, II, and III surveys in eight European countries. *Lancet, 373*, 929–940.

Krieger, J., & Higgins, D. L. (2002). Housing and health: Time again for public health action. *American Journal of Public Health, 92*(5), 758–768.

Loveman, E., Frampton, G. K., & Clegg, A. J. (2008). The clinical effectiveness of diabetes education models for Type 2 diabetes: A systematic review. *Health Technology Assessment, 12*(9), 1–116. iii.

Lugini, D., & Pagani, M. (2012). From stress to functional syndromes: An internist's point of view. *European Journal of Internal Medicine, 23*, 295–301.

Mannino, D. M., & Buist, A. S. (2007). Global burden of COPD: risk factors, prevalence, and future trends. *Lancet, 370*(9589), 765–773.

McBride, C. M., Emmons, K. M., & Lipkus, I. M. (2003). Understanding the potential of teachable moments: The case of smoking cessation. *Health Education Research, 18*(2), 156–170.

McQueen, J., Howe, T. E., Allan, A., Mains, D., & Hardy, V. (2011). Brief interventions for heavy alcohol users admitted to general hospital wards. *Cochrane Database Systematic Reviews (Online)* (8), CD005191.

Merten, S., Dratva, J., & Ackermann-Liebrich, U. (2005). Do baby-friendly hospitals influence breastfeeding duration on a national level? *Pediatrics, 116*(5), e702–e708. doi:10.1542/peds.2005-0537.

Meyer, C., Göpel, E., Siegrist, J., Heiss, C., Kelm, M., & Rassaf, T. (2011). Lifestyle modification programs protecting cardiovascular health in Germany and SwedenA qualitative interview study. *Bundesgesundheitsblatt, Gesundheitsforschung, Gesundheitsschutz, 54*(2), 213–220.

Milz, H., & Vang, J. (1989). Consultation on the role of health promotion in hospitals. *Health Promotion International, 3*(4), 425–427.

Moullec, G., Lavoie, K. L., Rabhi, K., Julien, M., Favreau, H., & Labrecque, M. (2012). Effect of an integrated care programme on re-hospitalization of patients with chronic obstructive pulmonary disease. *Respirology, 17*, 707–714. doi:10.1111/j.1440-1843.2012.02168.x.

Muñiz, J., Gómez-Doblas, J. J., Santiago-Pérez, M. I., Lekuona-Goya, I., Murga-Eizagaetxebarría, N., de Teresa-Galván, S. S. E., et al. (2010). The effect of post-discharge educational intervention on patients in achieving objectives in modifiable risk factors six months after discharge following an episode of acute coronary syndrome, (CAM-2 Project): A randomized controlled trial. *Health and Quality of Life Outcomes, 8*, 137.

Murray, C. J., & Lopez, A. D. (1997). Global mortality, disability, and the contribution of risk factors: Global burden of disease study. *Lancet, 349*(9063), 1436–1442.

NHS Yorkshire and Humber. (2011). *Prevention and lifestyle behaviour change. A competence framework.* Retrieved June 29, 2012, from http://www.yorksandhumber.nhs.uk/document.php?o=6994

NICE Clinical Guidelines. (2011). *Chronic obstructive pulmonary disease: Management of chronic obstructive pulmonary disease in adults in primary and secondary care.* Retrieved May 17, 2012, from http://publications.nice.org.uk/chronic-obstructive-pulmonary-disease-cg101

Nowak, P., Lobnig, H., Krajic, K., & Pelikan, J. M. (1998). Case study Rudolfstiftung Hospital, Vienna, Austria – WHO-model project "Health and Hospital". In J. M. Pelikan, M. Garcia-Barbero, H. Lobnig, & K. Krajic (Eds.), *Pathways to a health promoting hospital. Experiences from the European pilot hospital project 1993–1997* (pp. 47–66). Werbach-Gamburg: G. Conrad Health Promotion Publications.

Oppedal, K., Nesvåg, S., Pedersen, B., Skjøtskift, S., Kari, A., Aarstad, H., et al. (2010). Health and the need for health promotion in hospital patients. *European Journal of Public Health, 21*, 744–749. doi:10.1093/eurpub/ckq148.

Pelikan, J. M. (2007). Health promoting hospitals – Assessing developments in the network. *Italian Journal of Public Health, 5*(4), 261–270.

Pelikan, J. M., Dietscher, C., Krajic, K., & Nowak, P. (2005). Eighteen core strategies for health promoting hospitals. In O. Groene & M. Garcia-Barbero (Eds.), *Health promotion in hospitals. Evidence and quality management* (pp. 48–67). Copenhagen: World Health Organization – Regional Office for Europe.

Pelikan, J. M., Dietscher, C., Schmied, H., & Röthlin, F. (2011). A model and selected results from an evaluation study on the International HPH Network (PRICES-HPH). *Clinical Health Promotion, 1*(1), 9–15.

Pelikan, J. M., Garcia-Barbero, M., Lobnig, H., & Krajic, K. (Eds.). (1998). *Pathways to a health promoting hospital. Experiences from the European pilot hospital project 1993–1997.* Werbach-Gamburg: G. Conrad Health Promotion Publications.

Pelikan, J. M., & Halbmayer, E. (1999). Gesundheitswissenschaftliche grundlagen zur strategie des gesundheitsfördernden krankenhauses. In J. M. Pelikan & S. Wolff (Eds.), *Das gesundheitsfördernde krankenhaus. Konzepte und beispiele zur entwicklung einer lernenden organization* (pp. 13–36). Weinheim: Juventa.

Pelikan, J. M., Krajic, K., & Dietscher, C. (2001). The health promoting hospital (HPH): Concept and development. *Patient Education and Counseling, 45,* 239–243.

Pelikan, J. M., Krajic, K., Dietscher, C., & Nowak, P. (2006). *Putting HPH policy into action. Working paper of the WHO Collaborating Centre on Health Promotion in Hospitals and Health Care.* Vienna: WHO Collaborating Centre for Health Promotion in Hospitals and Health Care.

Pelikan, J. M., Schmied, H., & Dietscher, C. (2012). Improving organizational health: The case of health promoting hospitals. In G. F. Bauer & O. Hämmig (Eds.), *Bridging occupational, organizational and public health.* New York, NY: Springer.

Qaseem, A., Wilt, T. J., Weinberger, S. E., Hanania, N. A., Criner, G., van der Molen, T., et al. (2011). Diagnosis and management of stable chronic obstructive pulmonary disease: A clinical practice guideline update from the American College of Physicians, American College of Chest Physicians, American Thoracic Society, and European Respiratory Society. *Annals of International Medicine, 155*(3), 179–191.

Renfrew, M. J., Dyson, L., McCormick, F., Misso, K., Stenhouse, E., King, S. E., et al. (2009). Breastfeeding promotion for infants in neonatal units: A systematic review. *Health Technology Assessment, 13*(40), 1–146. iii–iv.

Riegel, B., & Carlson, B. (2002). Facilitators and barriers to heart failure self-care. *Patient Education and Counseling, 46,* 287–295.

Riegel, B., Carlson, B., Moser, D. K., Sebern, M., Hicks, F. D., & Roland, V. (2004). Psychometric testing of the self-care of heart failure index. *Journal of Cardiac Failure, 10,* 350–360.

Riegel, B., & Dickson, V. V. (2008). A situation-specific theory of heart failure self-care. *The Journal of Cardiovascular Nursing, 23,* 190–196.

Rootman, I., Goodstadt, M., Hyndman, B., McQueen, D. V., Potvin, L., Springett, J., et al. (2001). *Evaluation in health promotion. Principles and perspectives* (European Series, Vol. 92). Copenhagen: WHO Regional Publications.

Samb, B., Desai, N., Nishtar, S., Mendis, S., Bekedam, H., Wright, A., et al. (2010). Prevention and management of chronic disease: A litmus test for health-systems strengthening in low-income and middle-income countries. *Lancet, 376*(9754), 1785–1797.

Shaw, J. E., Sicree, R. A., & Zimmet, P. Z. (2010). Global estimates of the prevalence of diabetes for 2010 and 2030. *Diabetes Research and Clinical Practice, 87,* 4–14.

Singh, D., & Ham, C. (2006). *Improving care for people with long-term conditions. A review of UK and international frameworks.* University of Birmingham Health Services Management Centre/NHS Institute for Innovation and Improvement. Retrieved September 16, 2012, from http://www.birmingham.ac.uk/Documents/college-social-sciences/social-policy/HSMC/research/long-term-conditions.pdf

Tønnesen, H., Christensen, M. E., Groene, O., O'Riordan, A., Simonelli, F., Suurorg, L., et al. (2007). An evaluation of a model for the systematic documentation of hospital based health promotion activities: Results from a multi-centre study. *BMC Health Services Research, 7,* 145. doi:10.1186/1472-6963-7-145.

Tønnesen, H., Fugleholm, A. M., & Jørgensen, S. J. (2005). Evidence for health promotion in hospitals. In O. Gröne & M. Garcia-Barbero (Eds.), *Health promotion in hospitals: Evidence and quality management* (pp. 21–45). Copenhagen: WHO-Regional Office for Europe.

Tønnesen, H., Roswall, N., Odgaard, M. D., Pedersen, K. M., Larsen, K. L., Mathiassen, B., et al. (2008). Basic registration of risk factors in medical records. Malnutrition, overweight, physical inactivity, smoking and alcohol. *Ugeskrift for Laeger, 170*(20), 1747–1752.

Tsai, A. C., Morton, S. C., Mangione, C. M., & Keeler, E. B. (2005). A Meta-Analysis of Interventions to Improve Care for Chronic Illnesses. *Am J Manag Care, 11*(8), 478–488.

Wagner, E. H., Austin, B. T., Davis, C., Hindmarsh, M., Schaefer, J., & Bonomi, A. (2001). Improving Chronic Illness Care: Translating Evidence Into Action. *Health Affairs, 20*(6), 64–78. doi:10.1377/hlthaff.20.6.64.

Weisz, U., Haas, W., Pelikan, J. M., & Schmied, H. (2011). Sustainable hospitals: A socio-ecological approach. *Gaia, 20*(3), 191–198.

WHO (1946). Preamble to the constitution of the World Health Organization as adopted by the International Health Conference, New York, 19–22 June, 1946, signed on 22 July 1946 by the representatives of 61 States (Official Records of the World Health Organization, no. 2, p. 100) and entered into force on 7 April 1948.

World Economic Forum and the Harvard School of Public Health. (2001). *From burden to "Best Buys": Reducing the economic impact of non-communicable diseases in low- and middle-income countries.* Geneva: World Economic Forum.

World Health Organization. (2002). *Innovative care for chronic conditions: Building blocks for action.* Geneva: World Health Organization.

World Health Organization (Ed.). (1986). *Ottawa charter on health promotion. Towards a new public health.* Geneva: World Health Organization.

World Health Organization (Ed.). (1991). *The Budapest declaration on health promoting hospitals.* Copenhagen: WHO-Regional Office for Europe.

World Health Organization (Ed.). (1997). *Vienna recommendations on health promoting hospitals.* Copenhagen: WHO-Regional Office.

World Health Organization (2000). *Prevention and control of noncommunicable diseases.* 51st World Health Assembly, Eighth plenary meeting, 20 May 2000. Geneva: World Health Organization

World Health Organization. (2005). *Preventing chronic diseases: A vital investment.* Geneva: World Health Organization.

World Health Organization. (2008). *2008–2013 Action plan for the global strategy for the prevention and control of noncommunicable diseases.* Copenhagen: World Health Organization – Regional Office for Europe.

World Health Organization. (2009). *Global health risks. Mortality and burden of disease attributable to selected major risks.* Geneva: World Health Organization.

World Health Organization. (2010). *Global status report on non-communicable diseases.* Geneva: World Health Organization.

World Health Organization. (2011). *Noncommunicable diseases country profiles 2011.* Geneva: World Health Organization.

World Health Organization – Regional Office for Europe. (2012). *Action plan for implementation of the European strategy for the prevention and control of noncommunicable diseases 2012 – 2016.* Copenhagen: World Health Organization – Regional Office for Europe.

World Health Organization & United Nations 'Children's Fund. (2009). *Baby-friendly hospital initiative. Revised, updated and expanded for integrated care. Section 1: Background and implementation.* Geneva: World Health Organization.

Author Biographies

Thomas Abel is a Medical Sociologist and Professor for Health Research at the Institute of Social and Preventive Medicine of the University of Bern, Switzerland, and chair of the division of Social and Behavioural Health Research. Prior to his appointment in Bern he was Professor for Public Health and Epidemiology at the Ludwig-Maximilians-University in Munich (1993–1995), and Lecturer and Research Assistant in Medical Sociology at the Philipps-University, Marburg, Germany (1986–1993). His academic degrees include a Habilitation at the Philipps-University (Department of Medicine, 1993), a Ph.D. from the University of Illinois in 1989, and a Master's (1980) and a Dr.phil. (1984) degree from the Justus Liebig-University. Thomas Abel has published widely on theoretical and empirical challenges in social science applied in public health. As the editor in chief he has led the International Journal of Public Health from 2000 to 2011. He has also served as reviewer and consultant for major national and international research institutions and funding agencies.

Dr. Karim Abu-Omar works as a researcher at the Institute of Sport Science and Sport of the Friedrich-Alexander-University, Erlangen-Nürnberg. He has an M.A. degree in Sociology and did his Ph.D. in Medical Sociology at the University of Alabama at Birmingham (UAB), USA. His research interests include health promotion policy development and implementation, and physical activity surveillance.

Laurie M. Anderson, Ph.D., M.P.H., currently serves as Affiliate Associate Professor in the Department of Epidemiology, School of Public Health and Community Medicine, University of Washington, Seattle, USA. Dr. Anderson was a senior researcher at the Washington State Institute for Public Policy where she worked in the areas of public health and health care policy under the direction of the state legislature. Prior to joining the Institute, she worked for the US Centers for Disease Control and Prevention where she supported the work of the US Task Force on Community Preventive Services by conducting reviews on program effectiveness in the areas of public health nutrition, obesity prevention and control, and early childhood development.

Dr. Anderson is a member of the US Department of Health and Human Services Healthy People 2020 Workgroup on Social Determinants of Health, a member of the Society for Research Synthesis Methods, an Associate Editor of the Journal of Research Synthesis Methods, and an Editor with the Cochrane Collaboration Public Health Review Group. She received her doctorate in public health from University of California, Los Angeles, and master's degree in epidemiology from Emory University in Atlanta.

Rebecca Armstrong (Ph.D., M.P.H.) is an Associate Director of the Jack Brockhoff Child Health and Wellbeing program and manages the public health evidence and knowledge translation research group (which incorporates the Cochrane Public Health Group (CPHG)). Rebecca helps to coordinate the activities of the CPHG, is a systematic review author, develops and facilitates training courses on evidence-informed decision making, and manages a research program exploring the effectiveness of knowledge translation strategies. Her research interests are the development of methods for synthesis of complex public health interventions and the effectiveness of knowledge translation and exchange in public health settings.

Margaret M. Barry, Ph.D., is Professor of Health Promotion and Public Health and Head of the WHO Collaborating Centre for Health Promotion Research at the National University of Ireland. She has published widely in health promotion and works closely with policymakers and practitioners on the development, implementation, and evaluation of mental health promotion interventions and policies at national and international levels. As Global Vice President for Capacity Building, Education and Training of the IUHPE from 2007 to 2010, and continuing, she is coordinating international collaborative work on the development of core competencies for health promotion, including a major European Commission-funded initiative in the European region. Professor Barry has served as board member of a number of international and European steering groups, research councils, and scientific committees and has acted as expert adviser on mental health promotion policy development in Ireland, Northern Ireland, Scotland, the UK, New Zealand, and Canada. She is coauthor of *Implementing Mental Health Promotion* (Barry and Jenkins, 2007). She completed her primary degree and doctoral studies in Psychology at Trinity College, Dublin; she has held previous posts as Lecturer in Psychology at the University of Birmingham, UK; Trinity College, Dublin, and as Deputy Director of the Health Services Research Unit at University College, North Wales.

Barbara Battel-Kirk (B.Sc., M.Sc., Health Promotion) is an independent consultant on health promotion and multidisciplinary public health with a particular interest in competency-based approaches to capacity building. Battel-Kirk has worked in the academic, voluntary, and statutory sectors in Ireland, the UK, and Canada as a health promotion practitioner in a variety of settings, as lecturer in health promotion at graduate and postgraduate levels and as a researcher and project manager. Battel-Kirk has worked on a number of projects and initiatives focusing on capacity-based approaches to health promotion and multidisciplinary public health in the UK and at European and global level and is currently the project coordinator of a major EU-funded initiative entitled "Developing competencies and professional standards for health promotion capacity building in Europe (CompHP)." Publications include a comprehensive literature review on health promotion competencies (2009), a global scoping study on health promotion capacity (2011), and a report on the development of a Pan European Accreditation Framework (in press).

Adrian Bauman is the Sesquicentenary Professor of Public Health, University of Sydney, Australia. He is Director of the Prevention Research Collaboration (PRC), part of the School of Public Health. His research interests are in primary prevention, and in particular in physical activity and health, and in the new area of the health consequences of sitting time. Recent work focuses on research translation, and the dissemination of evidence-based prevention.

Professor Fiona Bull is Director of the Centre for Built Environment and Health at The University of Western Australia and Visiting Professor at Loughborough University working with the National Centre for Physical Activity and Health and Visiting Professor at the UKCRC Centre for Diet and Activity Research (CEDAR), Institute of Public Health, Cambridge, UK. She has over 25 years of experience in public health with a focus on prevention of chronic disease and specifically lifestyle-related risk factors including physical inactivity. Her research and public health work extends across both developed and developing countries. Professor Bull has received over US$15 million in research funding and authored over 150 peer-reviewed publications, book chapters, and scientific reports. Outputs of her research have informed local, state, and national policy and practice. In addition, Professor Bull has long-standing involvement in civil society activities as member of Heart Foundation committees, WA State Physical Activity Task Force, Founding Chair of Global Advocacy for Physical Activity (GAPA), and President Elect of the International Society for Physical Activity and Health.

Belinda Burford (Ph.D., B.Sc. (Hons)) is a Research Fellow with the CPHG, where she is a methodological advisor for Cochrane Reviews with the CPHG and provides guidance for review authors. Belinda is also involved in a number of methodological projects across the Cochrane Collaboration that seek to address issues facing authors of complex systematic reviews. She also contributes to teaching in evidence-informed decision making in public health. Belinda has a multidisciplinary background, with a Ph.D. in Medicine and training in molecular biology, medicinal chemistry, and electrophysiology. She has also worked in international clinical study design and publication development within the private sector.

Bronwyn Carter is a Research Assistant in the School of Public Health at La Trobe University. She has qualifications and experience in nursing, rehabilitation, management and teaching. She completed her MPH with La Trobe University and is pursuing her interests in public health policy and research.

Stefano Campostrini is full professor of Social Statistics and Dean of the Graduate School at the University of Ca' Foscari of Venice (Italy), formerly professor at Pavia, associate professor at Padua, and research fellow at Edinburgh (Scotland). His main research interests are in the application of statistics as support to decision-making processes in health and social policies

and intervention. He has been principal investigator in many research projects concerning evaluation, needs analysis, information systems, and quality of life. His international experience has focused particularly on the study of behavioral risk factors for health, and the evaluation of health promotion. In this regard he has collaborated with several international institutions. He has helped build the Italian surveillance system "PASSI," serving in the National Coordinating group at the National Institute for Health. He has published over a hundred scientific works and has been on the scientific committees of several international and national congresses. He has promoted a global network on the behavioral risk factor surveillance, now a Global Working Group of the International Union for Health Promotion and Education. Stefano Campostrini is the Chair of this group, named "World Alliance for Risk Factor Surveillance" (WARFS).

Evelyne de Leeuw, M.Sc., M.P.H., Ph.D., is professor and chair of Community Health Systems and Policy at Deakin University, Victoria, Australia. She also acts as senior evaluation advisor to the Healthy Cities programme in WHO/Europe, and implementation expert consultant for Healthy Cities in WHO/Western Pacific. She teaches community health promotion in the Deakin Medical School for which she has developed novel reflective cloud-based learning technologies. Previously she was based in Denmark, France, and the Netherlands. Other recent books cover Healthy Cities (with Jean Simos) and health political science (with Carole Clavier).

Ligia de Salazar is currently the director of the Public Health Development Foundation—FUNDESALUD; in Colombia, until 2012 she was senior professor and researcher of the School of Public Health, Universidad del Valle, Cali-Colombia, and director of the Center for Evaluation of Public Health Policy and Technologies, CEDETES, at the same University. She has been Leader and Regional Coordinator of the Latin American Regional Project of Health Promotion Effectiveness, promoted by the International

Union for Health Promotion, IUHPE, 2002–2008. She has been coordinator of national and international projects as well as consultant for several institutions, invited as temporary professor in Latin American Universities. Dr. Salazar has been member of different committees and scientific associations such as PAHO Health Scientific Advisory Committee, CAIS; Healthy Lifestyles, Healthy People, HLHP, PAHO-CDC (2005); and Latin American Surveillance Network for nontransmissible Chronic Diseases (2005). She has been associate editor of the International Journal of Public Health, 2012–2014. She received two grants from the International Development Research Centre in Canada to obtain the Master degree in Community Health at Liverpool University, England, and the Ph.D. in Evaluation Research at McGill University, Canada. Her research and academic interest has been evaluation research and public health surveillance, as well as strategies to articulate science, politics, and society.

Colette Dempsey, B.A. (Hons), M.A., Health Promotion, works as a researcher at the Health Promotion Research Centre (HPRC) at the National University of Ireland, Galway. She graduated with a B.A. in Economics and Health Promotion (1997) and an M.A. in Health Promotion (1999) from NUI, Galway. She worked as a researcher in the HPRC from 2000 to 2002 and rejoined the HPRC in 2008. Colette was the lead researcher on the workpackage "Developing Core Competencies for Health Promotion Practice in Europe" on the CompHP Project, where she worked closely with Professor Margaret Barry and Ms Barbara Battel-Kirk. She contributes to the teaching of Health Promotion across a number of courses at NUI, Galway, and also has significant experience in the voluntary sector. Colette is involved in workforce development at a national level in Ireland through the Association for Health Promotion Ireland. In addition to her work on workforce development and health promotion competencies, she has a particular research interest in mental health promotion and promoting health in the early years and has a number of publications in these areas.

Christina Dietscher, Ph.D., Sociologist, is a senior researcher at the Ludwig Boltzmann Institute Health Promotion Research in Vienna, Austria. Her areas of expertise are health promotion in settings, especially hospitals and schools, and evaluation of health promotion in these settings. Her present research interests include the effectiveness of health promotion networks in the settings approach, especially of networks of health-promoting hospitals, the implementation of health promotion programs, such as baby-friendly hospitals, into hospitals, and concepts of health-promoting and health-literate organizations.

Jodie Doyle (M.P.H., Grad. Dip. Health. Prom.) is Managing Editor of the CPHG. She manages the editorial process of reviews from registration with the CPHG through to publication on The Cochrane Library. Jodie is also a systematic review author, and participates in the facilitation of workshops on systematic review development. Jodie enjoys the challenges associated with coordinating teams of international authors, ensuring contextual richness, and the provision of useful information to end users of systematic reviews, locally and globally.

Dr. Michael Eriksen is the founding Dean of the Institute of Public Health at Georgia State University. He is also director of Georgia State University's Partnership for Urban Health Research and Center of Excellence in Health Disparities Research. Prior to his current position, Dr. Eriksen served as a senior adviser to WHO in Geneva and director of the CDC's Office on Smoking and Health (1992–2000). Previously, he was director of behavioral research at the M.D. Anderson Cancer Center. He has served as an advisor to the Bill & Melinda Gates Foundation, the Robert Wood Johnson Foundation, the American Legacy Foundation, and the CDC Foundation. He has published extensively on tobacco prevention and control and is lead author on the fourth edition of The Tobacco Atlas. He has served as an expert witness of behalf of the US Department of Justice and the Federal Trade Commission in litigation against the tobacco industry. He is editor in chief of Health Education

Research. He is a recipient of the WHO Commemorative Medal on Tobacco or Health and a Presidential Citation for Meritorious Service, awarded by President Clinton. He is a past president and Distinguished Fellow of the Society for Public Health Education.

Annika Frahsa works as a research assistant and lecturer at the Institute of Sport Science and Sport of the Friedrich-Alexander-University, Erlangen-Nürnberg. She has studied political science in Erlangen and is currently a Ph.D. candidate at the Friedrich-Alexander University, Erlangen-Nürnberg. Her research interests include health promotion and empowerment among socially disadvantaged population groups.

Professor John Frank is trained in Medicine and Community Medicine at the University of Toronto, in Family Medicine at McMaster University, and in Epidemiology at the London School of Hygiene and Tropical Medicine. He was Professor (now Emeritus) at the University of Toronto since 1983 and founding Director of Research at the Institute for Work and Health in Toronto from 1991 to 1997. In 2000, he was appointed inaugural Scientific Director of the Canadian Institutes of Health Research—Institute of Population and Public Health. In July 2008, he became Director of a new Edinburgh-based research unit: the Scottish Collaboration for Public Health Research and Policy. The Collaboration seeks to develop and robustly test novel public health policies and programs to equitably improve health status in Scotland. He holds a Chair at the University of Edinburgh in Public Health Research and Policy. His broad research and professional interests concern the determinants of population and individual health status, and especially the causes, remediation, and prevention of socioeconomic gradients in health. Publications include 25 books, monographs, and book chapters; over 150 peer-reviewed journal articles; and 65 other scientific publications.

Katherine L. Frohlich is Associate Professor at the Département de médecine sociale et préventive and Research Associate with the Institut de Recherche en Santé Publique, Université de Montréal (IRSPUM). She currently holds a CIHR New Investigator award for her work on social inequities in smoking. Her current research interests include social inequities in health-related practices, social theory in social epidemiology and health promotion, and the sociology of smoking. Her latest publications focus most specifically on conceptual and theoretical issues with relation to neighborhood and health research, population-level research, and social inequities in smoking.

Dr. Peter Gelius works as a research assistant and lecturer at the Institute of Sport Science and Sport. He has studied political science in Erlangen, Germany, and at Duke University (Durham, NC/USA) and has a Ph.D. from Friedrich-Alexander University, Erlangen-Nürnberg. His research interests include comparative political science and theories of the policy process as they relate to health promotion policy development/implementation and physical activity promotion for older people and disadvantaged populations.

Dr. Ruth Jepson is currently the Senior Scientific Advisor at the Scottish Collaboration for Public Health Research. She also has an academic position at the University of Stirling where she is Codirector of Centre for Public Health and Population Health (CPHPH). The CPHPH was established in June 2010. It has two Codirectors (Dr. Ruth Jepson and Professor Andrew Watterson) and four program leads. In the past 12 months, members of the Centre have successfully secured funding for 24 projects worth around £700,000. Within the Centre she is also lead for the Physical Activity, Diet and Health Programme. Her current research interest and activities are focused on helping people to become more physically active, particularly in the outdoor environment and as part of their everyday lives. She also has an interest in roust evaluation of policy interventions, such as alcohol brief interventions.

Since joining the University of Stirling as a Senior Research Fellow in 2006, she has been involved in grants totaling over 1.4 million pounds. Her scientific publications include around 40 peer-reviewed publications and a further 30 scientific publications.

Darwin R. Labarthe is Professor of Preventive Medicine, Department of Preventive Medicine, Northwestern University Feinberg School of Medicine. He is a graduate of Princeton University (1961), the College of Physicians and Surgeons, Columbia University (1965), and the School of Public Health, University of California, Berkeley (M.P.H., 1967; Ph.D., 1974). His principal appointments have been the following: Faculty in Epidemiology, University of Texas School of Public Health, Houston (1970–1974, 1977–1990); and successive positions at the CDC Atlanta (2000–2011). At CDC he led the development of the strategic plan, A *Public Health Action Plan to Prevent Heart Disease and Stroke*, and was founding Director of the Division for Heart Disease and Stroke Prevention (2006–2011). His professional activities focus on epidemiology and prevention of cardiovascular diseases. He has published more than 200 research articles and book chapters and the textbook, *Epidemiology and Prevention of Cardiovascular Diseases: A Global Challenge* (Jones and Bartlett Publishers, 2011).

Ronald Labonté holds a Canada Research Chair in Globalization and Health Equity at the Institute of Population Health, Professor in the Faculty of Medicine, at the University of Ottawa. His work over the past 15 years has focused on the health equity impacts of contemporary globalization. He chaired the Globalization Knowledge Network for the WHO Commission on the Social Determinants of Health (2004–2007) and the Working Group on global influences of the European-WHO review of social determinants of health (2011–2012). He has published extensively. Recent books as an editor and author include *Major Works in Global Health* (Sage, 2011); *Globalization and Health: Pathways, Evidence and Policy* (Routledge, 2009); *Health Promotion in Action: From Local to Global Empowerment* (Macmillan, 2008); *Critical Perspective in Public Health* (Routledge, 2007);

and *Fatal Indifference: The G8, Africa and Global Health* (University of Cape Town Press/ IDRC Books, 2004). Before joining academia full-time in 1999, he enjoyed a 25-year career in health education, health promotion, and community development. His present areas of research interest are in global primary health care reform, medical tourism, health worker migration, global health diplomacy, the political economy of neoliberalism and health, and social determinants of health equity.

Marie-Claude Lamarre is the Executive Director of the International Union for Health Promotion and Education (IUHPE), based in Paris. In this capacity she contributes to the advocacy efforts and knowledge and best practice dissemination needed to support NCD prevention and control from a health promotion perspective, and to mobilize the technical expertise of the IUHPE Global network and partners to support the implementation of health promotion strategies and actions to reduce NCDs and health inequalities at the global, regional, and local levels.

Dr. Becky H. Lankenau is the retired Director of the World Health Organization (WHO) Collaborating Center for Physical Activity and Health at the Centers for Disease Control and Prevention (CDC), in Atlanta, Georgia, USA. She also served as Senior Health Scientist and External Relations Coordinator in the Physical Activity and Health Branch at CDC. Dr. Lankenau has worked for over 40 years in a broad spectrum of public health activities across multiple sectors including industry, academia, government, and voluntary organizations. Examples of her past efforts include the planning and execution of a World Congress on Productivity, consultation on prevention and management of multiple risk factors for chronic diseases, and development of an evaluation system for comprehensive health care services for indigent children. She has either given presentations or participated in projects in 23 countries, and has additionally visited 30 other countries. At earlier stages of life, Dr. Lankenau also worked in public relations, fashion modeling, and radio and fashion merchandising. She is now serving as a senior consultant in the areas of physical activity promotion, chronic disease prevention, and health promotion.

Raphael Lencucha is an Assistant Professor of Public Health and a Research Affiliate at the Prentice Institute on Global Population and Economy at the University of Lethbridge, Alberta, Canada. Dr. Lencucha has conducted research on the negotiation of the Framework Convention on Tobacco Control and the relationship between global trade and tobacco control. He is currently conducting research on the relationship between trade and tobacco control in four African countries, Brazil, and the Philippines. He will be joining the Faculty of Medicine at McGill University, Quebec, Canada, in August 2013.

Vivian Lin is Chair of Public Health at La Trobe University in Melbourne and former head of the School of Public Health from 2000 to 2005. She was previously the Executive Officer for the Australian National Public Health Partnership. She has held senior positions within the NSW, Victorian, and federal governments in Australia, where she has had responsibility for policy, planning, and program development across a wide range of issues. She is Vice President for Scientific Affairs for the IUHPE, deputy chair of the Chinese Medicine Board of Australia, and member of the Global Agenda Council for Healthcare for the WEF. She consults for the World Bank, WHO, and the UK Dept. for International Development, particularly in China and the Asia Pacific region, on health systems and health promotion. She is senior editor for health policy for *Social Science and Medicine*. Her education was at Yale (B.A.) and UC Berkeley (M.P.H. and Dr.P.H.). Her research interests are in political economy and social determinants of health, health system development, and public health policy. She has published widely.

Dr. Erma Manoncourt is the current Vice President for Communications in IUHPE (2010–2013) and Cochair of the IUHPE Global Working Group on Social Determinants of Health. Currently the President of Management and Development Consulting, Incorporated, she has worked over 30 years in international development providing technical assistance in management/leadership, strategic planning, training and facilitation skills, communication for development, and research, monitoring, and evaluation for behavior and social change interventions. As a specialist in behavior and social change, she worked more than 15 years in Sub-Saharan Africa, and the Caribbean in community-based development, nutrition, and health programming, evaluating family planning and women's health programs. At UNICEF, she served as the Country Representative in the Arab Republic of Egypt, Deputy Representative in India, and Chief, Program Communication/Social Mobilization in New York. Prior to joining the United Nations, she was an Assistant Professor at Tulane University School of Public Health and served as the Director of the Southeast Regional Support Centre, which provided training/technical assistance to mental health and substance abuse programs in the southeastern United States and the Caribbean. She holds a Ph.D. in Public Health from the University of North Carolina—Chapel Hill, with a specialization in Health Behavior.

David V. McQueen is a global consultant in health promotion, based in Atlanta, GA, USA, and retired from 20 years at the CDC in Atlanta where he served government as Chief of the behavioral risk factor surveillance system (BRFSS), Director of the Division of Adult and Community Health (DACH), and Associate Director for Global Health Promotion. He has held Professorships on the faculties of the University of Edinburgh, where he directed the Research Unit in Health and Behavioral Change, 1983–1992, and The Johns Hopkins University, SHPH, 1972–1983. He also brings rich NGO experience as a globally elected Board Member of the International Union of Health Promotion and Education as well as serving for 8 years as the Vice President for Science and 4 years as President; he is currently the Immediate Past President of IUHPE. He has served on numerous consultancies and committees with the World

Bank, WHO, the Canadian Government, as well as other public and private agencies. He brings editorial experience as a member, present and past, of several editorial boards. He is widely published in academic journals and the author/ editor of several books. He is currently an Adjunct Professor in the Department of Behavioral Sciences and Health Education at Emory University in Atlanta.

K.S. Mohindra is a global health researcher and consultant. She holds a Ph.D. in public health (Université de Montréal) and has worked on collaborative research projects in Asia, Africa, and Latin America. Her research is transdisciplinary and involves investigating global and local factors that influence the health of poor women and marginalized populations in low- and middle-income countries. She is the author of Women's Health and Poverty Alleviation in India.

Dr. Sania Nishtar, Founder and President of Heartfile and Pakistan's first female cardiologist, is a global health expert and a proponent of health reform. She is founder of the NGO think tank Heartfile, Pakistan's Health Policy Forum and Heartfile Health Financing. Internationally, she is a member of many Expert Working Groups and Task Forces of WHO; a member of the board of IUHPE, the Alliance for Health Policy and Systems Research, the WEF's Global Agenda Council, the Ministerial Leadership Initiative for Global Health, and the Clinton Global Initiative; and is Chair of GAVI's Evaluation Advisory Committee. She is a regular plenary speaker at global health meetings and is a key health policy voice in Pakistan, the author of Pakistan's first health reform plan, and the country's first national public health plan for NCDs. She has authored 6 books, and more than 100 peer-reviewed articles. She is the recipient of Pakistan's Sitara e-Imtiaz, a presidential award, Global Innovation award, the European Societies Population Science Award, and many accolades of the International Biographical Centre, Cambridge, and the American Biographical Centre. Sania Nishtar is a Fellow of the Royal College of Physicians and has a Ph.D. from Kings College, London.

Jürgen M. Pelikan, Ph.D., is emeritus professor at the Institute of Sociology at the University of Vienna/Austria and adjunct professor at Centre for Environment and Public Health, Griffith University, Brisbane/Australia. He holds a position as key researcher at the Ludwig Boltzmann Institute Health Promotion Research, Vienna/ Austria, where he also is director of the WHO-CC for Health Promotion in Hospitals and Health care. Member Governance Board and chair Scientific Committee of International Conferences HPH; member Board of Trustees IUHPE; member editorial board Health Promotion International; Coeditor Clinical Health Promotion; former consultant to WHO HQ and EURO; former president of ESHMS. His research interests include theory of health and of health promotion, the settings approach in health promotion, health promoting and sustainable hospitals, quality and evaluation in health care, health literacy, and systems theory.

Tahna Pettman (Ph.D., B.HSc.) is a research fellow and capacity building coordinator in the public health evidence and knowledge translation research group (which incorporates the CPHG). Tahna has a background spanning health promotion policy, evaluation, and research across the public sector, academia, and primary health. Tahna develops and facilitates training courses in evidence-informed decision making, is involved in research that explores the effectiveness of knowledge translation strategies, and liaises with end users regarding use and usefulness of Cochrane public health reviews. Tahna is passionate about supporting evidence-informed public health decision making, generation of rigorous practice-based evidence (evaluation), and obesity prevention.

Louise Potvin is currently professor at the Department of Social and Preventive Medicine, Université de Montreal, and Scientific director of the Centre Léa-Roback sur les inégalités sociales de santé de Montréal. She holds the Canada research Chair in Community Approaches and Health Inequalities. This Chair aims at documenting how public health interventions in support to local social development contribute to the reduction of health inequalities in urban settings. Her main research interests are the evaluation of community health promotion programs and how local social environments are conducive to health. She was a member of the WHO-EURO Working Group on the Evaluation of Health Promotion. She is a globally elected member of the Board of Trustees of the International Union for Health Promotion and Education and a Fellow of the Canadian Academy of Health Sciences. In addition to having edited and coedited seven books, she has published more than 250 peer-reviewed papers, book chapters, editorials, and comments.

Johanna Ralston joined the World Heart Federation as Chief Executive Officer in February 2011. The World Heart Federation is headquartered in Geneva with 200 member cardiac societies and heart foundations in more than 100 countries and focuses on the global fight against heart disease and stroke, with a focus on low- and middle-income countries. Johanna also serves as senior strategic adviser and on the steering group of the NCD Alliance, of which the World Heart Federation is a founding member. Before joining the World Heart Federation Johanna was Vice President, Global Strategies at the American Cancer Society, where she was hired in 1999 to build the Society's global programs, eventually developing and overseeing cancer and tobacco control projects in more than 30 countries. Johanna's work in development and global health has also included positions at New York University and International Planned Parenthood Federation of Latin America, where she served as Program Development Adviser. She has presented at numerous conferences and has coauthored commentaries and other articles in journals including The Lancet and The Guardian. A citizen of the USA and Sweden, Johanna studied at Harvard Business School, and studied public health at Harvard and Johns Hopkins Bloomberg School of Public Health.

Dennis Raphael, Ph.D., is a Professor of Health Policy and Management at York University in Toronto. His research focuses on the health effects of social inequality and poverty, the quality of life of communities and individuals, and

the impact of government decisions on health and well-being. Dr. Raphael's recent research project The Social Determinants of the Incidence and Management of Type 2 Diabetes confirmed that living conditions account for much of the variation among Canadians in the incidence and prevalence of type 2 diabetes independent of the effects of weight and physical activity. He has also published two recent articles in Health Promotion International that explore how the political economy of nations shapes the availability of the prerequisites of health. He is editor of Social Determinants of Health: Canadian Perspectives, Tackling Health Inequalities in Canada: Lessons from International Experiences, and Health Promotion and Quality of Life in Canada, coeditor of Staying Alive: Critical Perspectives on Health, Illness, and Health Care, and author of Poverty in Canada: Implications for Health and Quality of Life and About Canada: Health and Illness. He is also coauthor of *Social Determinants of Health: The Canadian Facts*.

Irving Rootman is an Adjunct Professor in the School of Public Health and Social Policy at the University of Victoria and a Visiting Professor in Gerontology at Simon Fraser University. He was a Michael Smith Foundation for Health Research Distinguished Scholar and Professor from 2002 to 2007 at the University of Victoria. From 1990 to 2001, he was the Director of the Centre for Health Promotion at the University of Toronto. From 1973 to 1990, he was a researcher, research manager, and program manager for Health and Welfare Canada in health promotion and nonmedical use of drugs. He has been a Technical Advisor, Consultant, and Senior Scientist for the World Health Organization and a former member of the Health Promotion and Disease Prevention Advisory Board and the Health Literacy Committee of the US Institute of Medicine and Cochair of the Canadian Expert Panel on Health Literacy. He received his Ph.D. in sociology from Yale University in 1970. His areas of expertise are health promotion and literacy and health. He has published widely in both fields as well as in evaluation and nonmedical drug use. Most recently, he was the lead editor for the Third Edition of Health Promotion in Canada.

Prof. Dr. Alfred Rütten is the head of the Institute of Sport Science and Sport of the Friedrich-Alexander-University, Erlangen-Nürnberg. He was visiting research Professor at the Departments of Sociology and Medicine of the University of Alabama at Birmingham (USA), and visiting Professor of Public Health at the Department of Epidemiology and Public Health at Yale University, New Haven (USA). He has led several EU-funded projects dealing with issues of policy development in health promotion, among others the "Improving Infrastructures for Leisure-Time Physical Activity in the Local Arena—Good Practice in Europe (IMPALA)" and "Building Policy Capacities for Health Promotion through Physical Activity among Sedentary Older People (PASEO)" projects.

Hermann Schmied, M.P.H., is currently senior researcher at the Ludwig Boltzmann Institute Health Promotion Research in Vienna, Austria. His area of expertise is health promotion, and prevention and evaluation in health care, especially in the hospital sector. His present research interests are specific clinical health promotion topics, such as health promotion interventions in hospitals for heart disease patients or smoking cessation programs in the context of surgeries in hospitals, the sustainable or "green" hospital, as well as hindering and supporting factors for the implementation of health promotion programs in human service organizations/professional organizations.

Trevor Shilton is Director of Cardiovascular Health at the National Heart Foundation of Australia (WA). He is also Adjunct Associate Professor in the School of Population Health at the University of Western Australia. His principal research and health promotion interests are in advocacy, policy, and programs relating to physical activity and obesity, workforce development, Aboriginal health, and social marketing. Trevor has directed major community-wide initiatives, including social marketing campaigns in obesity, physical activity, and tobacco. He was the founding National President of the Australian Health Promotion Association (AHPA). He is Global

Vice President for Advocacy of IUHPE, and manages that organization's global advocacy. He is also Deputy Chair of GAPA, the Advocacy Council of ISPAH, and codirector of the Global Physical Activity Network GlobalPANet. Trevor has over 25 years experience in health promotion, and has published book chapters and over 35 papers in peer-reviewed journals. He has given many national and international conference presentations and workshops. He has participated in guideline and policy development in Australia, Canada, and the USA.

Michael Sparks is the current President of IUHPE, Assistant Editor of the journal *Health Promotion International*, and Postgraduate Coordinator of Health and Community Development at the University of Canberra in Australia. He is a past president of the Australian Health Promotion Association and is on the Editorial Board of the journals *Health Education Research* and *Osong Public Health and Research Perspectives*. Michael cochairs the Conference Organizing Committee for the IUHPE 21st World Conference on Health Promotion and Education to be held in Thailand in 2013 and is a member of the Organizing and Scientific Committees for the WHO Eighth Global Conference on Health Promotion in Finland in 2013.

Over the past 25 years Michael has been involved in public health as a health promotion practitioner, a policymaker, academic, and leader. He has undertaken consultancies with the WHO in the areas of health promotion, capacity building, healthy islands, and pandemic influenza. Michael has an ongoing interest in public health governance, social determinants of health, and the evolution of health promotion practice in the twenty-first century. He has published papers and editorials across a range of topics and seeks to maintain a broad awareness of the practice, research, and needs of the health promotion and health education communities.

Sylvie Stachenko is Professor at the University of Alberta School of Public Health and its inaugural dean from 2009 to 2012. Earlier she was Deputy Chief Public Health Officer of the Health

Promotion and Chronic Disease Prevention Branch at the Public Health Agency of Canada and Director of the WHO Collaborating Centre on Chronic Disease Policy. She also worked with the WHO Regional Office for Europe (EURO) as director of Health Policy and Services. She has led chronic disease policies at national level and internationally. She led policy efforts such as the joint WHO/Public Health Agency of Canada Policy observatory on chronic disease and participated in the development of a number of international policy documents. She is the recipient of many awards, including the Woman of Distinction Award for Science and Technology (YWCA), and is recognized as an Honorary Member of the Academy of Sciences (Moscow) and an Honorary Professor of the Society of Polish Internal Medicine (Poland). She earned a Doctorate in Medicine from McGill University in 1975 and was resident in family medicine at the Université de Montréal. She earned a Master's degree in Epidemiology and Health Services Administration from the Harvard School of Public Health in 1985.

Maria D. Stefan's capabilities and experience cut across the business, nonprofit, international, political, education, and sports/fitness/health arenas. Her involvement in the sports and fitness industry spans more than 25 years. As President of the CHASEAMERICA Group, she works with organizations to identify high-value strategic and global opportunities to expand reach, revenue, capacities, and leadership. Her firm has a specialist practice in the sports, fitness, nutrition, and health marketplace, helping organizations build stakeholder relationships and capabilities that drive public/private partnerships across the economic, environmental, and social dimensions of well-being and performance. She is also a Visiting Professor in the Masters of Sports Management at the IE Business School, in Madrid, Spain. Throughout her career, she has served on numerous boards and committees; she has published in the IUHPE Journal of Health Promotion and has spoken at the International Congress on Physical Activity and Health. She has a B.A., from Temple University, Philadelphia, PA, and holds a Graduate Certificate, from the Harvard Business School, Advanced Management Program for International Senior Executives.

Dr. Sandra Vamos is a former Associate Professor from the Faculty of Education at Simon Fraser University (SFU) in Vancouver, British Columbia, Canada. Her expertise developed through her experiences in Canada, Australia, and the USA, and includes health literacy, health education, healthy behaviors, health-promoting schools, curriculum development, and teacher preparation. A focus has been on guiding improvements in school health education to enhance health literacy through curricular innovations involving the coordinated school health program approach. Vamos previously served as a faculty member in the Department of Exercise Science, School Health Education Master of Science program at Southern Connecticut State University. In Connecticut, she participated in the National Health Education Assessment Project (HEAP) initiative designed to direct improvements in health education planning and delivery by aligning curriculum, instruction, and assessment. She also served as a faculty member and program coordinator at Canisius College in Buffalo, New York, where she developed both undergraduate and graduate health education programs.

Elizabeth Waters (D.Phil., M.P.H.) is the Jack Brockhoff Chair of Public Health and Director of the Brockhoff Child Health and Wellbeing Program at the University of Melbourne. Elizabeth also leads the Public Health Group of the Cochrane Collaboration, which seeks to summarize research evidence on "what works to make a difference to population health and health equity." The Jack Brockhoff Child Health and Wellbeing Program comprises over 40 transdisciplinary researchers involved with research and community partnerships on studies that are embedded with children and families, with a focus on solutions for child health issues that require understanding and commitment to addressing issues related to social and physical environments, cultural understandings, systems and services, policies and programs, health literacy, norms, and behaviors—across physical, mental, and social well-being. They focus on understanding not just what makes a difference, but how, why, for what cost, and for whom.

Lauren Weinberg grew up in New York and moved to the UK to study psychology and biology at the University of Edinburgh. She completed a Masters Degree at the University of Edinburgh in Global Health and Public Policy and a second one in Public Health, at the "Ecole des Hautes Etudes en Sante Publique" in Rennes, France. Her academic interests include public health promotion, policy, mental health, and non-communicable disease epidemiology.

Carrie Whitney is a Research Specialist for tobacco-control projects in the Institute of Public Health at Georgia State University. Carrie worked as the Lead Research Assistant for The Tobacco Atlas, Fourth Edition. The Atlas is a global tobacco-control resource, and Carrie assisted the lead author, Michael Eriksen, with researching, writing, and editing the publication that was launched at the World Conference on Tobacco OR Health in Singapore in March 2012. Carrie's other tobacco-related projects include coordinating surveys of smoke-free policies in restaurants and bars and use of alternate nicotine delivery systems, as well as coauthoring publications and textbook chapters. Carrie received her M.P.H. from Georgia State in 2010 with a focus on Health Promotion and Behavior, and in addition has worked on nonprofit fund-raising, and tobacco issues among various mental health populations.

Index

D.V. McQueen (ed.), *Global Handbook on Noncommunicable Diseases and Health Promotion*,
DOI 10.1007/978-1-4614-7594-1, © Springer Science+Business Media, LLC 2013